Pediatric Cardiology

Advanced Textbook Series

- *Pediatric Endocrinology*, Wellington Hung, M.D., Gilbert P. August, M.D., and Allen M. Glasgow, M.D.
- *Pediatric Gastroenterology*, edited by Mervin Silverberg, M.D.
- *Pediatric Cardiology*, Courtney L. Anthony, M.D. and Rica G. Arnon, M.D.

Textbook of

Pediatric Cardiology

Courtney L. Anthony, M.D.
Associate Professor of Pediatrics
Director, Section of Pediatric Cardiology
University of Tennessee Center for the Health Sciences
Memphis, Tennessee

Rica G. Arnon, M.D.
Associate Professor of Clinical Pediatrics
Mt. Sinai School of Medicine
New York, New York

MEDICAL EXAMINATION PUBLISHING CO., INC.
an Excerpta Medica company

Anthony, Courtney L.
Textbook of pediatric cardiology.

Rev. ed. of: Pediatric cardiology, 1979.
Bibliography: p.
Includes index.
1. Pediatric cardiology. I. Arnon, Rica G.
II. Title. [DNLM: 1. Cardiovascular diseases — In infancy and childhood. WS 290 A628r]
RJ421.A57 1983 618.92'12 83-8183
ISBN 0-87488-607-4

an Excerpta Medica company
3003 New Hyde Park Road
New Hyde Park, New York

Printed in the United States of America

Contents

Part IV Acquired Cardiovascular Problems

Part V Therapeutic Principles

Preface

In this new edition we have endeavored to follow the format begun in the first; specifically, to provide a basic core of information regarding the diagnostic evaluation and treatment of children with cardiovascular problems in a brief and lucid manner without unnecessary attention to some of the more sophisticated details. It is our hope that this type of presentation will make essential information readily accessible to the medical student, the house-officer, and all physicians providing primary pediatric care.

The basic format has been retained. There has been considerable expansion in keeping with increased knowledge, particularly in the areas of echocardiographic diagnosis and surgical treatment. A chapter on diseases of the pericardium has been added. Since surgical treatment is discussed under each of the individual lesions, we felt that a separate chapter on surgical aspects might be somewhat redundant and thus have eliminated it. This decision was in part influenced by the untimely death of our long-time friend and colleague, Dr. Robert G. Allen, who had been in charge of the cardiovascular and thoracic surgical program at Le Bonheur Children's Medical Center in Memphis, Tennessee, for over 25 years. His loss has been a great one to the many thousands of colleagues who worked with him and patients for whom he cared. We would like to dedicate this edition to his memory.

notice

The authors and the publisher of this book have made every effort to ensure that all therapeutic modalities that are recommended are in accordance with accepted standards at the time of publication.

The drugs specified within this book may not have specific approval from the Food and Drug Administration in regard to the indications and dosages that may be recommended by the authors. The manufacturer's package insert is the best source of current prescribing information.

Part I

DIAGNOSTIC TECHNIQUES

Chapter 1

MANIFESTATIONS OF CARDIOVASCULAR DISEASE IN INFANTS AND CHILDREN

The ultimate goal of treatment of cardiovascular disease at any age is the restoration of normal structure and function of the heart. This may not be a practical goal in selected instances, but the degree to which it is approached is significantly lessened by a delay in recognition of the problem. Myocardium which has been too long subjected to the effects of severe hemodynamic stress, abnormal rhythm, hypoxemia, or inflammation may be unable to recover even if the basic problem can be corrected. Accordingly, the theme underlying the remainder of this text is the preservation of normally functioning myocardium. It seems appropriate to begin with a discussion of the clues which serve as a warning that a cardiovascular problem may exist. These manifestations which may be signs of symptoms in the more traditional terminology ("subjective" or "objective" are the terms which our students now routinely utilize) vary in their presentations at different ages. It seems useful to discuss those manifestations common to the newborn and infant separately from those seen in the older child and adolescent (Table 1-1). Clearly, all of them overlap with the manifestations of noncardiovascular problems, and the alert physician will learn to think of circulatory disease even when the clues are subtle.

Newborns and Infants

Cyanosis

Whether due to central arterial hypoxemia or to inadequate tissue perfusion, cyanosis is a manifestation of the utmost magnitude, particularly in the newborn infant. Little experience is required to be able to differentiate this from acrocyanosis or the mottled, reticulated pattern of cutis marmorata routinely seen in normal newborns. It is essential to remember that fetal hemoglobin, with its higher affinity for oxygen, will show a greater degree of saturation at a given level of oxygen tension so that visible cyanosis in the newborn infant may be much less severe than in the older child with the same degree of hypoxemia. One should not be deluded that mild cyanosis in the newborn is of little concern. The mucous membranes and subungual regions are still the areas at which to look. The experienced observer learns to recognize cyanosis when all that can be detected is a minimal duskiness of the proximal nailbeds. Apparent improvement to the eye if the infant is allowed to breathe oxygen is deceptive and should not be an excuse to delay appropriate evaluation.

Table 1-1 Manifestations of Cardiovascular Disease in Pediatric Patients

Clue	Approach to Evaluation	Comments
Newborn and Infant		
Cyanosis	Obtain arterial blood gases in room air and while breathing 100% oxygen	May be mild in the newborn even in presence of severe hypoxemia
Respiratory distress	Evaluate when resting; careful auscultation of the lungs; chest x-ray	May occur in absence of overt congestive failure
Exercise tolerance	Careful feeding history	
Growth failure	Plot growth curve	Weight more affected than height
Congestive failure	Thorough physical exam; chest x-ray	Cardiomegaly always present in myocardial decompensation; look for excess sweating
Murmurs	Precise assessment of characteristics of murmur	Less diagnostic in newborn; often absent even with severe heart disease
Arrhythmias	Obtain EKG	Supraventricular tachyarrhythmia common in this age group
Older Children		
Cyanosis	As above	Noncardiac causes less common; less of an emergency than newborn but still calls for prompt evaluation
Congestive failure	As above	Clinical picture clearer than with infants; initial episode of failure after 1 year of age usually means acquired heart disease
Murmurs	As above	As child grows, murmur becomes more specific feature of the defect

Table 1-1 (continued)

Clue	Approach to Evaluation	Comments
Arrhythmias	As above	Sinus arrhythmia normal; premature beats common and may be insignificant
Syncope	Careful history re precipitating events; obtain EKG; exercise testing	Consider noncardiac causes
Exercise intolerance	Obtain detailed history about activity pattern with peer group	Many false positives exist; absence of this complaint does not exclude severe heart disease
Squatting	Evaluate presence of cyanosis; exercise intolerance, and activity pattern	Seen with lesions characterized by reduced pulmonary blood flow
Hypertension	Evaluate pulses and measure blood pressure in all extremities	Proper size cuff important; noncardiac causes more common
Chest pain	Careful history for nature of pain and pattern of occurrence; obtain EKG and chest x-ray	Cardiovascular chest pain rare in children except in pericarditis; benign chest wall pain common in adolescents

Any suggestion of cyanosis warrants determination of arterial blood gas tensions. These should be measured on an arterial sample since so-called arterialized capillary samples may be misleading. This is quick and easy, and necessary equipment is available in most hospitals today. If for any reason it is not possible to perform these measurements locally, the child should be promptly referred to an appropriate institution and not simply observed to see what will happen. It is not unusual to see an infant who appears only mildly cyanotic have an arterial pO_2 of less than 20 torr. Typically, in cyanosis of cardiac origin, the arterial pCO_2 is near normal although it may be somewhat reduced if severe hypoxemia has resulted in tachypnea. With milder degrees of hypoxemia the pH will be within normal limits; however, if the pO_2 is less than 25-30 torr, metabolic acidosis is to be expected and once started may progress rapidly. The child's decline would be precipitous at this point.

Even with assisted ventilation, relatively little improvement in the pO_2 is noted after breathing 100% oxygen in the child with a severe cyanotic heart defect, in contrast to the usual improvement in pulmonary hypoxemia (see Chap. 4). Confirmation of arterial hypoxemia warrants prompt referral to an institution having personnel and facilities for complete diagnostic evaluation and surgery. Watchful expectancy will lead only to disaster, especially in the newborn where the onset of acidosis may progress rapidly along an irreversible downhill course or where closure of the ductus arteriosus which may have been serving as the sole source of pulmonary blood flow will produce similar results. The newborn with arterial hypoxemia on a cardiac basis should be promptly evaluated by a cardiologist, even if this means transferring the infant to another hospital at 2 a.m., as the passage of only a few hours may prove fatal. Although the evaluation of the older infant with cyanosis is slightly less urgent, it should still be accomplished without undue delay as these children may suddenly and unexpectedly deteriorate.

Cyanosis in the Newborn is Always an Emergency

Respiratory Distress

Tachypnea and labored respiration may have many causes other than cardiac disease, and in the newborn infant disorders of respiration are more likely to be due to pulmonary or central nervous system causes. However, respiratory distress may be caused by the stiff lungs of infants with large left to right shunts and/or pulmonary edema; chronic tachypnea may also be seen in the hypoxemic infant. Cardiovascular disease should be diligently looked for even when respiratory distress is the sole presenting manifestation. The old wives' tale of the grandmother who insists that the young infant is breathing too rapidly has proven true time and time again, often to the embarrassment of the physician who could find nothing wrong. A slightly different type of respiratory disorder is apnea which, as a manifestation of cardiovascular disease, is limited to the premature infant. Commonly seen in prematures with large left to right shunts, usually through a patent ductus arteriosus, it is a manifestation the cause of which is poorly understood, but it is a uniform indication for more intensive management.

Like cyanosis, respiratory distress, particularly in the newborn, is a finding indicating an urgent need for thorough evaluation. A chest x-ray and measurement of arterial gas tension will in the vast majority of instances clarify the etiology of the distress. One would not expect to find respiratory distress on a cardiovascular basis if the chest x-ray reveals a cardiac silhouette of normal size and configuration with normal pulmonary vascular markings.

Exercise Intolerance

With or without arterial hypoxemia, the presence of a severe cardiac defect may limit the heart's ability to pump an adequate flow under conditions of increased demand. Although one cannot assess the infant's ability to run the 100-yard dash or climb stairs, his exercise capacity can still be evaluated by a careful history. Nursing or feeding from a bottle requires a great deal of caloric expenditure and consequently a significantly increased cardiac output. If the cardiac reserve is limited, the infant may appear hungry and begin to feed eagerly, only to tire out after a minute or two and have to stop and rest often with increased tachypnea. Evaluation of this manifestation requires detailed questioning as to the volume and frequency of feedings and time required to accomplish them. A 4-month-old infant who takes 2 oz of formula every 3 hr and requires 45-60 min to consume this amount tells us that he has a limited cardiopulmonary reserve and should be looked at critically. Gross motor milestones may be somewhat delayed in the older infant, but the normal variability in passing these milestones makes evaluation more difficult. In most severely ill infants, those with chronic congestive failure or severe hypoxemia, motor development may not seem to progress at all, whereas infants with milder abnormalities may show little apparent problem.

Growth Failure

Cardiac lesions associated with markedly increased pulmonary blood flow, chronic congestive failure, and/or severe arterial hypoxemia commonly result in an abnormal growth pattern. This pattern is characteristic, affecting weight far more significantly than height. The latter, although usually less than average, is generally still within normal limits, whereas the weight is usually well below the third percentile. Growth of the head generally progresses in keeping with the chronologic age and may give the false impression of hydrocephalus, unless these measurements are compared with a normal growth curve. Careful plotting and following the growth curve is an essential part of serial evaluation. The infant whose congestive failure is well controlled may remain small while growing along a curve which parallels the normal, whereas a weight curve which is falling further and further below the normal range indicates a need for intensive medical treatment or possible surgical intervention.

Congestive Heart Failure

Congestive heart failure will be discussed in more detail in a subsequent chapter. At this point we are concerned with the manifestations that result therefrom. It seems appropriate to mention that, as the term is used in this book, it will refer to alterations resulting from weakened pumping ability of the myocardium. Impaired myocardial contractility may result from a structural abnormality imposing excessive demands, from certain rhythm disorders, or from various metabolic or inflammatory conditions which render the myocardium unable to meet even normal resting requirements. The manifestations which result depend on the etiology of the congestive failure as well as on the age of the patient and duration that failure has been present. All of those discussed previously may be seen as a result of failure.

One should bear in mind that severe central hypoxemia is the result of the basic structural abnormality. Milder degrees of desaturation may result from the effects of pulmonary edema. Moderate-to-severe failure with poor tissue perfusion and increased oxygen extraction in the systemic capillary bed may also produce signs of cyanosis. In this instance, however, arterial oxygen tension is normal. Tachycardia at a rate inappropriate for the infant's state of activity is present in the absence of heart block, and hepatomegaly is common. Rales resulting from alveolar edema are heard not infrequently. However, edema limited to pulmonary interstitium is silent and better detected by x-ray. Peripheral edema may also occur but is less frequent than in older patients. When present, it is noted where subcutaneous tissue is more loosely attached (periorbital region, dorsum of hands and feet) or in areas of gravitational predilection (presacral region or abdominal wall). Peculiar to the infant is excess sweating resulting from increased sympathetic activity. This sweating is inappropriate to environmental temperature and most commonly involves the face and head. Frequently seen while the infant is feeding, it may occasionally be profuse during sleep. Pallor is common in more severe states of failure resulting from poor perfusion and peripheral vasoconstriction.

In teaching students and house officers about congestive failure, we have frequently noted a complete lack of awareness that a decompensated heart is a dilated heart. Although, as will be discussed later, some of the individual manifestations commonly associated with failure (e.g., pulmonary edema) may be seen in selected circumstances with normal cardiac size, true congestive failure (i.e., myocardial decompensation) implies the presence of cardiomegaly. One exception to this rule is the patient who is on positive-pressure ventilation where increased intrathoracic pressure may reduce cardiac filling and mask the dilatation, although some change in cardiac size is to be expected if serial films are reviewed.

Congestive Heart Failure Means Cardiomegaly

Heart Murmur

In the newborn period, particularly in the first week of life, the presence or absence of a heart murmur is one of the least useful indicators of cardiovascular abnormality. It is by no means rare to see a newborn with a potentially lethal cardiac defect with no murmurs. On the other hand, during this period of life physiologic (i.e., normal) murmurs are extremely common. These will be discussed in more detail in Chap. 2. If none of the other clues are present and if the cardiovascular examination is otherwise normal, the presence of a murmur per se is not necessarily a cause for urgent evaluation by a cardiologist. Almost all physiologic murmurs seen in the newborn will disappear within a few days to 3 or 4 months, and more specialized evaluation of the perfectly healthy infant can usually be deferred unless the murmur persists beyond this time or changes significantly in character. This is not to suggest that organic murmurs are not present within the first week of life. Murmurs resulting from any congenital heart disease may appear during the first few days; however, it is not infrequent for murmurs of some of the most common defects to be delayed for a week or more.

Differentiating between the organic and physiologic murmur requires some degree of experience. Presence of other clues is extremely helpful. As the infant passes out of the newborn period, organic murmurs characteristic of the individual congenital heart defects are more commmonly noted. Significant heart disease in the absence of a murmur is even more frequent when one is dealing with problems which primarily attack the myocardium such as endocardial fibroelastosis or myocarditis.

Arrhythmias

An occasional child is referred for cardiovascular evaluation because his heart is either beating too fast, too slow, or irregularly. EKG evaluation is essential to understanding the nature of the problem. In the healthy newborn the resting cardiac rate would generally range between 100-150 beats/min and only rarely exceed 200 beats/min even with vigorous crying. If these limits are exceeded on either low or high side, an EKG should be performed promptly. Individual rhythm disorders will be dealt with in a subsequent chapter. An excessively fast or slow heart rate should always be regarded as a potential emergency. Premature beats, both atrial and ventricular, are frequently encountered in the newborn period. If there is no evidence of underlying heart disease and no extracardiac causes such as hypoxemia or metabolic derangements, premature beats are generally benign, disappearing within 3-4 months and requiring no treatment. A thorough physical examination, EKG, and chest x-ray constitute the minimum data base required to make such a decision.

Children and Adolescents

In this age group the manifestations of cardiovascular disease are merging into a pattern more nearly like that seen in adults. A few specific comments, however, are in order.

Cyanosis

The general pattern and the recognition of cyanosis in the older child are essentially the same as in the infant although the degree of visible discoloration obviously bears a more direct relationship to the level of hypoxemia once fetal hemoglobin has been replaced. One should be aware of a peculiar plethoric appearance of the lips, cheeks, and distal phalanges which may indicate a degree of desaturation too mild to result in cyanosis. Children with cyanotic congenital heart disease who have survived infancy are, in general, in a more stable situation and less likely to undergo fulminant deterioration. For this reason, cardiovascular workup is not the emergency that it was in the newborn period. Cyanosis is nonetheless still a sign of severe cardiovascular disease, and a detailed evaluation of the situation should be undertaken without undue delay.

Congestive Heart Failure

As the initial manifestation of congenital heart disease, congestive heart failure is extremely unusual after the first yar of life. Recurrent episodes of failure due to incompletely treated or inoperable lesions may, of course, occur, but the first episode of failure occurring during childhood or adolescence is far more likely to be due to an acquired abnormality such as myocarditis, rheumatic fever, or some form of cardiomyopathy. Tachypnea or overt respiratory distress at rest in this age group are generally manifestations of congestive failure but may occasionally be seen in severely hypoxemic children. The same comments as were made regarding the findings in heart failure in infants could be made in the older child as well. Peripheral venous distension is now a readily recognizable manifestation of systemic venous overexpansion and may be a valuable clue in situations where the liver is difficult to palpate, such as in the child who guards his abdomen excessively.

Heart Murmurs

A murmur is the most frequent reason for cardiac evaluation during the childhood years. It should be stressed again that the absence of a murmur be no means indicates that the heart is normal. Detailed evaluation of murmurs will be discussed in Chap. 2 and specific murmurs discussed with the individual lesions. The physician seeing children should be aware that innocent murmurs are an extremely common and perfectly normal part of the cardiovascular examination in children and should not be construed to represent an abnormality. They fall into several specific types which can be easily recognized and will also be covered in Chap. 2.

Arrhythmias

Arrhythmias continue to be an occasional first, and sometimes the only, clue as they were in the infant group. One must understand that it is abnormal for the cardiac rhythm to be perfectly regular in children as neuroregulatory mechanisms are extremely active, particularly in relation to respiration (see sinus arrhythmia; Chap. 28). Tachycardia of any cause will override the normal rate variability. Clearly, anytime there is a question an electrocardiogram is mandatory. In this age group as in infancy, the presence of a pathologic rhythm disorder may or may not be associated with other cardiac abnormalities, and the latter should be carefully looked for. Premature beats are a frequent occurrence at any age and again, in the absence of underlying disease, are almost always benign. Of serious concern in the active child or teenager is the paroxysmal onset of an arrhythmia which may severely interfere with cardiac output and thus produce syncope and possible injury. Tachyarrhythmias are usually recognized by the child as palpatations, weakness, or a vague feeling of abdominal or thoracic discomfort. A sudden syncopal episode is rarely the result of a fast heart rate, being more commonly associated with abrupt slowing. Exercise testing may be invaluable in identifying benign irregularities of rhythm as well as provoking potentially serious pathologic ones.

Syncope

More commonly a manifestation of rhythm disturbance, syncope may also be the result of a severe valvular obstruction, particularly involving the semilunar valves. Children may have benign neurogenic syncope for the same reason that adults do, although less commonly. In general, syncope due to cardiovascular disease in children is related to exercise, and a careful history of precipitating events is crucial. This relation to exercise is characteristic of the obstructive valvular lesions and to a slightly lesser degree of the arrhythmias. So-called gray-out or presyncopal episodes consisting of lightheadedness, vertigo, or blurred vision without loss of consciousness are more difficult to evaluate but from a cardiovascular standpoint have the same significance as overt syncope.

Exercise Intolerance

The inability of the myocardium to meet increased tissue demands for oxygen is clearly part of the picture of congestive failure, but may be present even when the clinical examination indicates adequate compensation at rest. This may be seen in large left to right shunts, hypoxemia, valvular obstructive lesions, and certain rhythm disorders. As is true at any age, one must find out what the child's general lifestyle is before one can assess the true significance of apparent exercise intolerance. It is extremely common to hear a mother say that her child "tires more easily than other children" only to find a perfectly normal cardiac examination with an innocent murmur. Often what she is saying is that the child has gone at an extremely rapid pace throughout the day and by suppertime is exhausted, often falling asleep on the floor watching television. This is particularly common in the child who has recently begun school on a full-day schedule. The child who still requires a nap at 5 years of age or who spends more time in front of the television set than his playmates does not necessarily have a heart problem.

It is particularly difficult to evaluate exercise capability when the lifestyle is predominantly sedentary. The types of activities engaged in on a day-to-day basis must be carefully assessed, and it is of particular value to try and pin down performance levels and duration when engaged in peer group activity. In this light, another point is in order. The child who routinely fatigues rapidly when asked to perform calisthenics in physical education class, much to the consternation of teachers and parents alike, but who is able to play basketball or ride a bike without difficulty after school is more likely to be operating at the level of secondary gain rather than to be limited by his heart.

Squatting

Periods of squatting during play are occasionally the initial clue to a cardiovascular problem. They are generally associated with severe cyanotic congenital heart disease, and the other manifestations of the problem are usually clear. One must be careful to differentiate squatting as a symptom from squatting as a habit pattern common in the preschool-age child. The latter is of no importance, and if the examination does not show other evidence of heart disease, the squatting can be ignored. From a historic standpoint, evaluation of this complaint is closely tied in to evaluation of the child's exercise capacity as discussed previously.

Hypertension

With the obvious exception of coarctation of the aorta, hypertension is rarely the presenting finding or even an accompaniment of cardiovascular problems in children. A detailed discussion of the subject is outside the scope of this book. It is important to remind those caring for children that hypertension is a problem far more common than has been thought true in the past, and one which, in contrast to the adult, more often has a specific definable and treatable etiology such as a renal or endocrine disorder. However, within the last 10 years careful studies of large groups of adolescents revealed essential hypertension as the etiology in 40-50%.

Chest Pain

Chest pain is an extremely common complaint, particularly in the preadolescent and adolescent years, and rarely is due to cardiovascular disease in this age group. It is another symptom where careful history is critical. The discomfort associated with pericarditis is usually dull, aching, and substernal and often accentuated in the supine position, being relieved by sitting up and leaning forward. This should rarely be missed if a chest x-ray is combined with a careful physical examination. On rare occasions in children, chest pain may be associated with severe congenital aortic stenosis. This pain is usually classically anginal in character, being dull, crushing, substernal, and exercise-precipitated with relief upon resting. Depending upon the age of the patient, classic patterns of radiation may or may not be identified. The physical examination indicates the presence of the cardiovascular abnormality, thus there should be little confusion. Paroxysmal tachyarrhythmia should also be looked for. A far more commonly seen pattern, particularly in the adolescent female, is pain which is described as sharp or stabbing in nature and which may be located anywhere over the anterior thorax between the clavicles and the diaphragm. It is typically brief, lasting from a few seconds to minutes, rarely over an hour. It is often not exercise-precipitated, often occurring while the child is sitting quietly. Movement produces little change, and only occasionally is the discomfort affected by deep inspiration. It may occur daily and often repeats itself over a period of years, usually disappearing toward the end of adolescence. It is an aggravating symptom, primarily so because of the apprehension which it engenders. Although the etiology is not known, the pattern of discomfort is recognized as benign and self-limited. When this type of pain is combined with a normal examination, normal EKG, and normal chest x-ray, reassurance to the family is the only treatment required.

Chapter 2

TECHNIQUES OF EVALUATING THE CARDIOVASCULAR SYSTEM

When the clues suggest the cardiovascular system as a possible culprit, the physician, like a television detective, narrows his field of investigation and begins to look at the suspect in far more detail in an effort to learn its identity and the degree to which it is causing problems. Much like James Bond, he has a number of tools or techniques which he can call upon in his investigation to give him progressively sophisticated information about structure and function of the cardiovascular system. Beginning with the technique with which the physician has had the most experience, the physical examination, we will evaluate a number of these in the present chapter. Some are more widespread in their usage and, as such, would be expected to be present to some degree in the armamentarium of any physician caring for a child. These will be discussed in more detail. Those techniques which are more complicated and which generally would be utilized by the cardiologist will be covered briefly in order to provide the reader with a basic introduction to the subject upon which he can build if he so desires.

Physical Examination

Obviously all the principles which one has learned regarding the physican examination of a child would apply in this more limited area. Although examination of the cardiovascular system is probably the least uncomfortable of all portions of the general physical, some children are still apprehensive, and the examiner should approach in a friendly manner. It has been our practice with children in the age group of 1-3 years to examine them sitting in their mothers' laps if they appear at all frightened. This reassurance, combined with distracting play with keys, flashlights, and so forth, will calm the vast majority of frightened infants. The quality of the examination is only slightly compromised in this manner, and very commonly one is able to make friends with the child following which he or she can be induced to lie on the examination table without crying. The younger infant may be allowed to take his bottle; any noise produced by swallowing is far less distracting to the examiner than crying.

If one is to learn to do a thorough and accurate examination, he must initially learn to be consistent in his approach and to conduct his examination in the same sequence each time with active concentration on each step. In teaching our medical students about the cardiovascular examination, we try to impress them that the most important information which they will collect is gained from the Gestalt impression at the beginning. At this point the examiner gains much insight into whether or not the patient is experiencing real difficulties from a cardiovascular problem. This is best accomplished by observing the child sitting in the mother's lap or on the examination table while taking the history. One looks at the child's size and growth pattern as well as for any evidence of distress. The presence of cyanosis or sweating is usually noted. In a more specific sense, a closer inspection would include a search for the stigmata of the various birth defect syndromes, other congenital defects, or multisystemic disease which might involve the heart such as the Marfan or Down syndromes, and so forth.

Examination of the Heart

If the child is willing to lie quietly on the examination table, the precordium is generally inspected next. This is best done with the physicain standing at the foot of the table viewing the precordium somewhat tangentially. One primarily looks for asymmetry of the precordial region indicative of longstanding cardiac dilatation or for primary thoracic deformities which might alter the cardiac examination. A dilated hyperdynamic heart, present from early infancy, will deform the compliant anterior thorax in a pattern indicative of the ventricular stress. In other words, a dilated, chronically hyperfunctioning left ventricle will produce an asymmetrical deformity of the left precordium with the maximal protrusion near the midclavicular line. In contrast, right ventricular dilatation will usually bulge at the lower sternum and lower left sternal border. Obviously a diffuse bulge incorporating both areas can be seen when both ventricles are involved. At the same time, visible impulses produced by underlying cardiac activity are evaluated. Particularly with oblique lighting, abnormalities of the cardiac impulse against the chest wall may be detected. Thus, one might detect the presystolic impulse of a poorly compliant ventricle even when a fourth heart sound is not audible. Other thoracic deformities should be looked for such as pectus excavatum and the shallow depressions of the lower anterior ribs seen in patients with poorly compliant lungs as might occur in large right to left shunts (Harrison's groove).

Palpation

The next step should be a careful palpation of the entire precordial area to detect impulses due to the heart thrusting against the thorax, palpable heart sounds, or murmurs. The examiner should remember to make use of a peripheral arterial pulse to time palpated or auscultated events; it is far easier to confuse systole and diastole than one might think. Impulses due to anterior movement of the heart are best detected with the fingertips lightly placed in the intercostal spaces (Fig. 2-1A). A good approach for the right-handed examiner is to stand at the right side of the supine patient (with the patient's head to the examiner's left) and to place the fingers of his right hand in the left fourth, fifth, and sixth intercostal spaces at the anterior axillary line. One can then palpate in a progressively medialward direction until cardiac activity is detected. In this manner, the hand is advanced over to the lower left sternal border paying attention to all impulses and their configuration.

The traditionally used term PMI (point of maximal impulse) can be misleading as we have found that many students and house staff feel that it uniformly reflects the cardiac apex or left ventricle. It has a tendency to divert the examiner from further consideration of what the impulse actually represents, thereby losing much valuable information. We discourage students in our clinic from using this term and try instead to have them describe each palpable event in turn. In a normal child past early infancy the only event generally palpable over the lower precordium is the apex impulse which is usually located in either the fourth or fifth left intercostal spaces inside the midclavicular line. It may be somewhat diffuse, extending over an area as much as 3 or 4 cm in diameter, particularly if the child is apprehensive. This is a reflection of the smaller chest volume of the child, but it often comes as a surprise to the examiner more familiar with evaluating adults. The impulse should be monophasic, that is, each heartbeat should produce only one detectable impulse and should be of normal intensity based on a scale that can be gained only by experience.

The normal apical impulse is related to left ventricular activity; the right ventricle is not palpable other than in the first few months of life. The right ventricle impulse is felt best at the lower left sternal border, directly through the lower sternum, or in the subxiphoid region during held inspiration. This represents the right ventricular sinus or inflow portion and is the dominant impulse or PMI in the newborn period. It may occasionally be detected in a very thin-chested child who is apprehensive or for some other reason is in a high-output state. For the most part, detection of a right ventricular impulse past 6 months of age is an abnormal finding. However, it is not unusual to palpate a distensile systolic impulse in the second and third intercostal spaces at the left sternal border, representing the right ventricular outflow tract; in slender children this may be normal. In the pathologic situation it is of accentuated intensity and usually combined with an inflow tract impulse. In pulmonic stenosis, the maximum cephalad extent of the outflow tract impulse may give a valuable clue as to the level of the obstruction. The second heart sound is also frequently palpable in the same location following this outflow tract impulse, and its presence does not automatically denote pathology. Obviously it is accentuated in the presence of pulmonary hypertension.

Although impulses of the type under discussion are rare along the right sternal border in the normally positioned heart, this area should be carefully palpated. Occasionally abnormal impulses such as an unusually forceful atrial systole may be detected. Far more common in the pediatric patient is presence of a malpositioned heart, and recognizing this on palpation would be a valuable guide to the conduct of the auscultatory examination.

Abnormal ventricular impulses are variously described as lifts, taps, or heaves. The distinction between definition of these terms is not always clear. As mentioned previously, one should regard even a soft tapping impulse located over the right ventricular inflow tract with suspicion except in the first few months of life. The dilated hyperfunctioning ventricle will present a more diffuse, hyperdynamic, sustained impulse, probably best described as a heave. The typical left ventricular heave is maximal far lateral to the sternum, generally at or outside the midclavicular line, not uncommonly extending to the anterior or midaxillary line, and often displaced inferiorly to the sixth intercostal space or lower. In a medialward direction it may occasionally extend as far as the lower left sternal border. If the heave is pure left ventricle, then the impulse at the lower left sternal border will be significantly reduced in intensity, and there will be no detectable impulse beneath the sternum. The typical right ventricular heave would be maximal at the lower left sternal border or in the substernal region extending to the left with diminishing intensity and also palpable superiorly along the left sternal border. Significant dilatation of the right ventricle will produce posterior rotation of the interventricular septum, and the entire anterior surface of the heart may be made up of the right ventricle. The palpable impulse then extends so far laterally that the examiner may be confused into thinking that he is feeling a biventricular heave. This issue is best resolved by placing two hands on the precordium — one hand placed over the sternum or lower left sternal border and the other at the cardiac apex. If the heave is due solely to the right ventricle, it will lift the two hands synchronously, whereas a biventricular heave can be recognized by asynchronous impulses or by an area of reduced intensity between the two ventricles representing the interventricular septum. The latter does not seem to be a particularly useful finding in infants.

Other impulses can be palpated in the manner which we have described. Among these might be mentioned an aneurysm of either a ventricle or a pulmonary outflow tract (particularly after patch insertion in the surgical repair of tetralogy of Fallot) or impulses due to abnormally dilated great arteries. Palpation should be extended to include the lower edges of the middle posterior ribs on both sides where intercostal artery pulsations in coarctation of the aorta can often be detected. This evaluation is best carried out with the patient either prone or sitting and leaning slightly forward.

A thrill is a palpable murmur, and its detection serves merely to call the examiner's attention to the presence of a murmur and to give some indication as to its intensity. Prominent thrills can be detected regardless of the method of palpation, whereas faint ones are best recognized by placing the palm of the hand very lightly on the precordium (Fig. 2-1B). The precordium should be explored in a manner similar to that utilized in detecting cardiac impulses. One pays attention to the timing of the thrill in the cardiac cycle as well as to its location and radiation. In some thin-chested patients with markedly hyperdynamic cardiac impulses, it may be difficult to differentiate the impulse from a thrill. In most cases alternately palpating the area with the fingertips and the palm of the hand will clarify the issue. The examiner should not forget to palpate the suprasternal notch and carotid arteries for the presence of a thrill. In addition to the obvious radiation of the murmur of aortic stenosis to this region, thrills in the suprasternal notch may also be detected in pulmonic stenosis and patent ductus arteriosus. Palpation in these locations must of necessity be done with the fingertips, and one should remember not to exert undue pressure as partial compression of a vessel may produce a thrill leading to an erroneous interpretation.

Auscultation

Nowhere is it a truer statement than with auscultation of the heart that one must learn the technique well and practice it in a systematic manner with great concentration in order to be proficient. The examiner who places the stethoscope in the four traditional auscultatory areas and expects heart sounds and murmurs to jump out at him is going to miss the vast majority of information available. The entire precordium should be explored with the stephoscope in a manner similar to that described for palpation. The stephoscope is advanced from apex to lower left sternal border, to the base, along the right sternal border, and then to the secondary areas over the thorax and elsewhere. The examiner must be careful to concentrate on both phases of the cardiac cycle as well as the heart sounds at each location. He must also learn to consciously filter out unwanted noise in order to evaluate softer events. It comes as a great surprise to the student of cardiac examination that the aortic component of S_2 can be recognized while overlapped by the end of a murmur from a ventricular septal defect or pulmonic stenosis which is grade 4 or greater in intensity. This can be achieved only by mentally filtering out the murmur and consciously listening for the components of the second heart sound. It is relatively easy once one learns how.

Before discussing the individual auscultatory events, a few comments are in order regarding the selection of the stethoscope. The old joke about the most important part of the stethoscope being that which goes between the ear pieces is

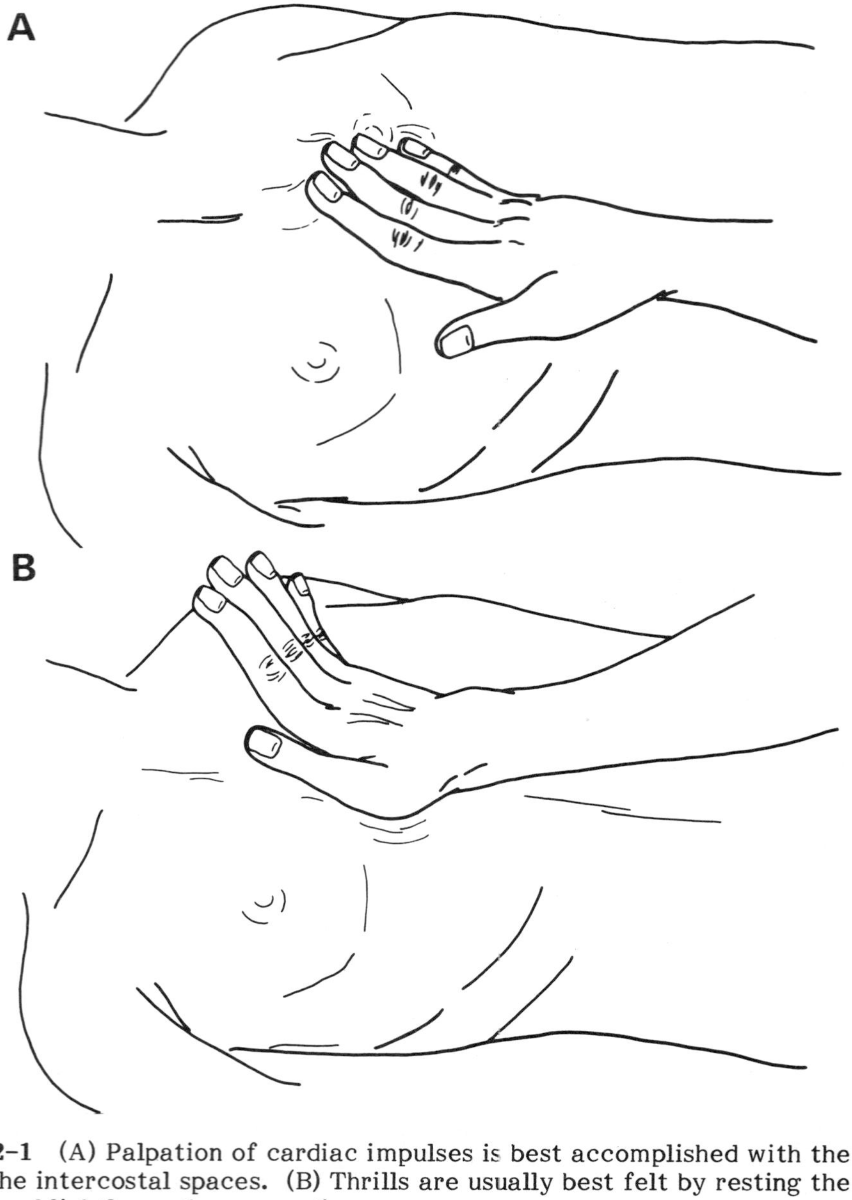

Figure 2–1 (A) Palpation of cardiac impulses is best accomplished with the fingertips in the intercostal spaces. (B) Thrills are usually best felt by resting the palm of the hand lightly on the precordium.

still a very true statement. Almost any stethoscope will be satisfactory as long as a few general principles are met. In examining children whose chest sizes vary over an extremely wide range, perhaps the most critical factor regarding the physical construction of the stethoscope is that the chest pieces be of an appropriate size. One must have available a bell and diaphragm which are sufficiently large to collect maximum of sound and small enough to make complete contact with the chest wall and not to overlap so large a portion of the precordium that accurate localization of events is not possible. A stephoscope designed for infants is not adequate for the larger child or adult. Thus, more than one size stethoscope should be available or one with multiple interchangeable chest pieces of various sizes. The tubing should be thick-walled to prevent kinking and of approximately one-eighth inch uniform internal diameter. If an instrument with two pieces of tubing is selected, the tubing must not rub together, although this is not a difficult problem to avoid. Ideal tubing length for convenience in examination without sacrificing information is approximately 10 inches. Ear pieces should be selected to fit the external auditory meatus comfortably and snugly enough to exclude ambient noise.

Most students are well aware that the bell-type chest piece is better suited for detecting low-frequency events, whereas the diaphragm selectively picks up the high frequencies. In practical application, most of the sounds and murmurs detectable in children fall within a frequency spectrum such as to be easily detected with the bell. This is true of such traditionally high-frequency events as second heart sounds and semilunar regurgitant murmurs. This is not to condemn auscultation with the diaphragm since some events are better heard with it. Both chest pieces should be utilized in auscultation, but the common practice of the inexperienced examiner of listening with just the diaphragm will result in his missing much.

Heart Sounds (Fig. 2-2)

First Heart Sound (S_1)

The first heart sound marks the onset of systole and is characteristically best heard at the apex or lower left sternal border. High-fidelity recordings have identified four components of which generally only the second and third are audible.

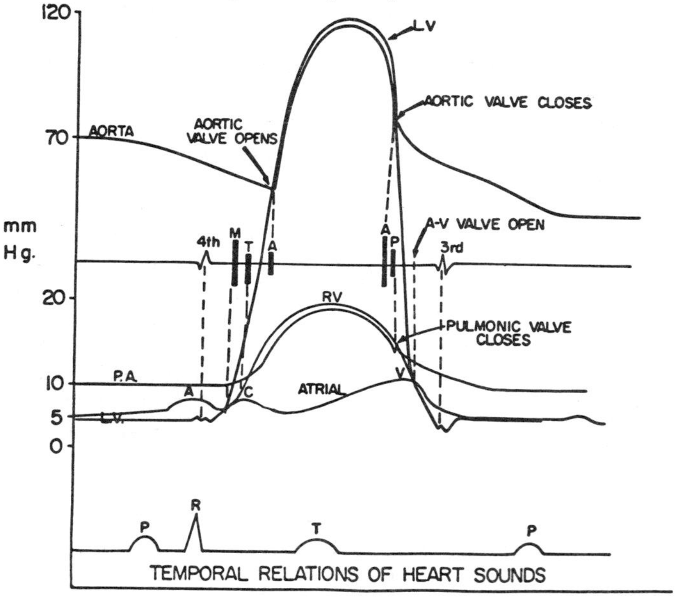

Figure 2-2 Diagrammatic representation of simultaneous EKG, phonocardiogram, and pressure tracings in the aorta, left ventricle, pulmonary artery, right ventricle, and atrium showing temporal relationships of pressure and sound events. M, T, and A are components of S_1; A and P are components of S_2. LV - left ventricle, RV - right ventricle.

Traditionally these components have been considered as representing mitral and tricuspid valve closure. Recent evidence suggests that this is not the case, rather that the entire first sound is related to vibration developing in myocardium, arterial wall, or the contained blood as tension is developed and blood is accelerated through the semilunar valves. The second and third components of S_1 may be separated by as much as 30-40 msec, thus it is not unusual to recognize two components of S_1. When such reduplication is due to splitting of S_1, the two components sound almost identical in intensity, pitch, and duration. Major points on which to concentrate when evaluating S_1 are the intensity (whether normal, increased, or decreased) and any reduplication. If the latter is present, the examiner must then decide whether this is due to two audible components of S_1 or whether it is related to a fourth heart sound preceding S_1 or an ejection click following it. This differentiation will be discussed later.

Second Heart Sound (S_2)

The second heart sound consists of two relatively high-frequency components which are best detected at the upper left sternal border. These components which are referred to as aortic (A_2) and pulmonic (P_2) appear to originate from vibrations in the rapidly decelerating column of blood rather than from any noise arising from physical contact of the closing semilunar valve cusps although this point is debated. A critically important point is that both components should always be audible in every normal child and adolescent. Absence of one component implies either severe obstruction to flow through one of the semilunar valves or marked malposition of the great arteries. Although best heard with a diaphragm, both components of S_2 are usually readily audible with the bell as well.

Splitting of S_2, that is, the audibility of both components, behaves in a characteristic manner. The width of this splitting increases in inspiration, generally to around 30-50 msec so that both components are easily heard, and then decreases during expiration to a point where they fuse and only one can be detected. Here again traditional concepts appear to be changing. It was originally thought that the reason for this so-called physiologic splitting was the increased filling of the right ventricle during inspiration with subsequent prolongation of ejection time. Recent highly sophisticated studies have indicated that right ventricular ejection time is not significantly prolonged during inspiration. Briefly stated, the column of blood flowing into the great arteries at the end of systole behaves primarily as an inertial system; thus, forward flow of this blood appears to exceed the duration of ventricular systole by a small interval known as the *hangout time*. The duration of this interval is dependent upon the impedance of the respective vascular bed. Pulmonary vascular impedance is significantly less than that in the systemic bed, hence the inertial flow from the right ventricle continues longer than that from the left and the pulmonic component characteristically follows the aortic. With inspiration there is a further decrease in pulmonary vascular impedance resulting in a greater right-sided hangout time and, therefore, a further delay in the pulmonic component. Increased right ventricular filling during inspiration would tend to increase the inertia of the ejected blood adding to the effect of decreased impedance. The decreased filling of the left heart during inspiration results in a slightly earlier aortic component, but this is a less significant factor in the inspiratory widening of S_2.

Although slight persistent splitting in expiration may be recognized in normal young adults, such persistence is generally abnormal in children. Occasionally the second sound may not fuse completely in the supine position, and in this case the child should be examined sitting and/or standing and persistent expiratory splitting not diagnosed unless it is present in the latter position. Another useful technique when splitting of S_2 is difficult to detect or expiratory closure uncertain is to tell the child to inspire when you raise your hand and expire when you lower it. The cycles should be regular and slightly deeper and slower than the child's normal breathing without pausing at end-inspiration or end-expiration. This will usually allow precise evaluation of S_2 in a child old enough to cooperate. As mentioned previously, the examiner must recognize the components of S_2, even when overlapped by a murmur, otherwise the erroneous impression of a single second heart sound may result.

Pathologically wide splitting may occur when right ventricular ejection is prolonged by pulmonic stenosis or when a combination of increased filling and decreased pulmonary impedance results in a longer hangout time as in atrial septal defect (Table 2-1). Delayed electrical activation of the right ventricle, as seen in severe right bundle branch block, pathologically widens the splitting, whereas left bundle branch block has the opposite effect. Decreased splitting may also be seen where pulmonary vascular impedance is significantly increased as in pulmonary hypertension.

Evaluation of S_2 involves not only the degree of splitting and its behavior during the respiratory cycle but also the intensity of both components. This is logically assessed only where both can be heard, that is, at the upper left sternal border, and in that location in children both components are of approximately the same intensity. Comparing the second heart sound in aortic and pulmonic areas has no value. The examiner must question whether or not both components are of the same intensity and if not then decide whether one is abnormally loud or abnormally soft. This requires some experience as one must build up a concept of normal intensity before he can make this decision. Diminution in intensity of one component may indicate obstruction to blood flow through the respective semilunar valve, whereas increased intensity may be associated with hypertension and impedance to flow in the vascular bed or to the aortic valve being abnormally close to the chest wall. As is true of all auscultatory events, S_2 is louder in children than adults and may lead the inexperienced to erroneously diagnose pulmonary hypertension.

Third Heart Sound (S_3)

The third heart sound is a low-frequency sound best heard at the apex or lower left sternal border and follows S_2 by an interval of 100-200 msec. It is often best heard in the semileft lateral decubitus position. The student can accurately simulate this sound for himself by moving his hand past his ear at a distance of 2 or 3 inches in a quiet room. The muffled sound which results is quite similar to S_3. Abrupt deceleration of blood entering the ventricles during the rapid filling phase is felt to be the origin of this sound. It is commonly heard in normal children and young adults, and its presence in this age group does not necessarily imply pathology. S_3 is accentuated when the filling rate exceeds ventricular distensibility, especially with dilated ventricles. Thus, it is frequently heard with significant volume overload of a ventricle or in the presence of congestive failure. In the latter situation the intensity of S_3 is generally thought to be increased; however, this may be related to alteration of the frequency spectrum toward the higher range.

The presence and intensity of S_3 are the major points for evaluation. It must also be differentiated from early diastolic murmurs such as those resulting from increased flow across an atrioventricular valve.

Table 2–1 Causes of Abnormal Splitting of S_2 in Children

I. Increased Width of Splitting

A. Delayed P_2

1. Delayed activation of right ventricle

Right bundle branch block
Ectopic beats of left ventricular origin
Left ventricular pacing

2. Prolonged right ventricular ejection time

Pulmonic stenosis
Right heart failure, severe
Atrial septal defect (controversial)

3. Increased capacitance or decreased impedance of pulmonary vascular bed

Idiopathic dilatation of pulmonary artery
Atrial septal defect
Partial anomalous pulmonary venous drainage

B. Early A_2

1. Decreased impedance to left ventricular ejection

Mitral regurgitation, acute
Ventricular septal defect (rare)

II. Decreased or Inaudible Splitting (Single S_2)

A. Early P_2

Pulmonary hypertension

B. Decreased intensity of A_2 or P_2

Pulmonic stenosis (severe)
Tetralogy of Fallot
Pulmonic atresia
Aortic atresia
Tricuspid atresia
Transposition of great arteries (inconstant finding)
Truncus arteriosus
Other cyanotic congenital heart lesions with severe pulmonary stenosis or atresia

III. Paradoxical Splitting of S_2 (A_2 Follows P_2, Split Decreases during Inspiration)

A. Delayed A_2

Left bundle branch block
Right ventricular pacing or ectopic beats
Preexcitation (WPW type B)
Aortic stenosis (rare)

Fourth Heart Sound (S_4)

The fourth heart sound is also a very low-frequency muffled event best audible at the apex and less commonly at the lower left sternal border. It occurs late in diastole preceding S_1, and if the heart sounds are recorded together with an electrocardiogram can be seen to begin 70 msec or more after the P wave of the EKG. It is also a ventricular filling sound resulting from the sudden deceleration of the blood entering the ventricle following atrial contraction. When audible with the stethoscope, it is uniformly pathologic and indicates loss of ventricular compliance as might result from severe hypertrophy, myocardial fibrosis, or chronic dilatation. It is rarely detected in children although we have seen it in some cases of severe longstanding semilunar valve stenosis.

Primarily one is interested in whether or not an S_4 is present. As mentioned previously it becomes important to differentiate from a split S_1. This is generally done very easily by increasing pressure with the bell of the stethoscope or by listening to the area in question with the diaphragm. Both maneuvers serve to filter out low-frequency sounds and will result in disappearance of S_4, whereas it will not affect audibility of a split S_1.

Gallop Rhythms

Whereas third and fourth sounds are often called gallop sounds, the typical galloping cadence results from the combination of an S_3 or the summation of S_3 and S_4 with tachycardia. As one might expect, this is most commonly the result of congestive heart failure. Use of the term *gallop rhythm* generally implies pathology, and since S_3 may be a normal event in children, we prefer to reserve this term for situations where tachycardia produces the typical cadence.

Ejection Sounds and Opening Snaps

Ejection sounds are relatively short, high-frequency events occurring early in systole at the onset of the ejection phase as blood is being accelerated into the aorta or pulmonary artery. They may follow the first sound by as much as 40 msec, although on occasion the interval is much shorter to the point where it is difficult to separate the click from S_1. Basically two types of ejection sounds can be identified: (1) Those originating from an arterial root probably representing an accentuated fourth component of S_1. Seen where there is significant dilatation of the main pulmonary artery or aortic root with poor compliance of the vessel wall, they are not uncommon in such lesions as tetralogy of Fallot, truncus arteriosus, idiopathic dilatation of the pulmonary artery, and severe pulmonary hypertension. Those originating from the pulmonary artery are best heard at the upper left sternal border, whereas aortic ejection sounds are more commonly recognized at the mid-left sternal border, upper right sternal border, and occasionally at the apex. There is no respiratory variation regardless of which artery is the origin of the sound. (2) The second type of ejection sounds is ejection clicks of semilunar valvular stenosis. These are really opening snaps and are the result of the sudden checking of the upward valve motion. They may be present in patients who have bicuspid aortic or pulmonic valves, even in the absence of any significant obstruction, but are more frequent when stenosis exists and then initiate a typical stenotic murmur. Their presence not only indicates a valvular abnormality but also indicates that the valve is relatively thin and mobile. Extremely dystrophic, rigid, calcified valves do not produce ejection clicks. The pulmonic valvular click is best heard at the mid-to-upper left sternal border and increases in intensity with expiration. This respiratory variation is due to increased diastolic filling of the right ventricle during inspiration producing a higher end-diastolic pressure with resultant partial elevation of the valve toward a domed position. With the onset of systole the remaining valvular excursion to its maximal limits is reduced and a softer click results. In expiration the valve remains in a full diastolic position until the onset of ejection. Its upward excursion is then greater and a louder click is heard. With increasing severity of stenosis the click moves closer to S_1. In contrast, aortic valvular clicks are best heard at the mid-left sternal border and apex, being less common in the aortic area at the upper right sternal border. In addition to the location, the other feature differentiating the aortic from the pulmonic valvular click is the absence of respiratory variation in the former.

One should also make mention of another type of systolic click which is not properly an ejection sound but is described here because it requires differentiation from those events already described. These are the mid-systolic clicks which may be single or multiple and are most commonly heard at the apex. They generally constitute part of the clinical picture of mitral valve prolapse and may or may not be accompanied by a late systolic crescendo murmur of mitral regurgitation. The significantly later timing in systole should cause little confusion in differentiation from ejection sounds.

The major point for evaluation in regard to ejection sounds is to recognize the origin and thus differentiate them from either a split S_1 or S_4-S_1 combination. The latter is generally not difficult as described previously. Whether arising from arterial root or semilunar valve, the ejection sound may appear similar to S_1 although it is of shorter duration and more snapping in character. Recognition of a dilated artery on chest x-ray may be of value. If due to semilunar stenosis, there is little confusion as the murmur accompanies the click.

The term *opening snap* has traditionally been reserved for the sound originating from a stenotic atrioventricular valve. Like the ejection click, it is of high frequency and snapping in quality. It is audible most frequently at the apex or lower left sternal border but may be detected at the base. As with the semilunar valvular clicks, the opening snap is due to sudden checking in the opening motion of the stenotic valve and occurs 30-150 msec after S_2. Opening snaps have been described in situations where there is excessive flow through a normal valve as in atrial or ventricular septal defects. The opening snap tends to occur somewhat earlier than S_3 and is accompanied by the murmur radiating from the stenotic valve. Confusion sometimes results in deciding whether an opening snap or a pathologically widely split S_2 is present. In the former circumstance, auscultation at the upper left sternal border will reveal a trilogy consisting of the two components of S_2 followed by the opening snap.

Murmurs

Murmurs are auscultatory manifestations of turbulent blood flow through abnormal pathways or areas of narrowing. The latter may be due to absolute narrowing from the normal or may be the result of relative stenosis, that is, to an excessive flow of blood across a normal area of narrowing. The entire precordium is examined using both bell and diaphragm as has been previously described. In each location both systole and diastole must be consciously listened to since very soft murmurs at the extremes of frequency range may be difficult to detect. This should be done in the supine position if feasible and then reexamined in the sitting and semileft lateral decubitus positions. Although almost all murmurs in children can be heard while the child is supine, an occasional one is inaudible unless the examination is also carried out in one of the two latter positions. The examiner should not forget to continue his auscultation over the back and both lateral aspects of the thorax or neglect to listen over peripheral arteries, especially the carotid vessels. As was true in discussing thrills, the stethoscope should be applied over a peripheral artery only with sufficient pressure to make adequate contact because audible murmurs may be produced by partial compression of an artery.

In addition to evaluating the presence or absence of murmurs a number of specific characteristics should be carefully defined for each murmur present.

1. Intensity: A scale of six grades is utilized and the basis of this grading system is outlined in Table 2-2.
2. Timing: The murmur should be identified as being systolic, diastolic, or continuous throughout the cardiac cycle. This often requires timing of the murmur with a peripheral or apical pulse. Occasionally, long murmurs may alter the usual cadence of heart sounds resulting in erroneous timing if the murmur is not correlated with some other event. The duration of the murmur should be described. It may be early, mid, or late in its phase of the cardiac cycle or may extend through the entire cycle. The murmur extending from S_1 all the way to S_2 is described as holosystolic (or pansystolic), whereas one occupying all of diastole is called holodiastolic (or pandiastolic) (Fig. 2-3). It is useful with other than the shortest murmurs to try and describe roughly the fraction of the cycle occupied by the murmur.
3. Maximal location: For almost all murmurs an area of maximal intensity can be identified.
4. Radiation: The murmur may transmit away from the area of maximal intensity in one of two ways. Of diagnostic importance is selective radiation occurring along lines of blood flow. As one maps the precordium with his stethoscope, he will identify that this type of transmission is much more prominent in one direction, whereas intensity falls off rapidly when the stethoscope is advanced from the maximal location in other directions. This selective radiation is of great value in assessing the etiology of the murmur. In contrast, loud murmurs will also radiate in a nonspecific circumferential manner much like the spread of ripples in a pond. This type of radiation drops off equally in intensity in all directions in contrast to the above. The distance over which the murmur transmits in this manner is related to the intensity of the murmur and the dimensions of the volume conductor through which it is being transmitted. A loud murmur in a very small child may be heard all over the thorax without the radiation imparting any diagnostic information. It is not too difficult to differentiate these two modes of spread.

Table 2-2 Gradation of Intensity of Murmurs

Grade 1:	Barely audible in quiet room by experienced examiner
Grade 2:	Soft but easily audible, limited radiation
Grade 3:	Moderately loud, moderate-to-wide radiation
Grade 4:	Loud, associated with palpable thrill
Grade 5:	Audible with stethoscope chest piece in incomplete contact with skin
Grade 6:	Audible with chest piece 1 cm away from skin

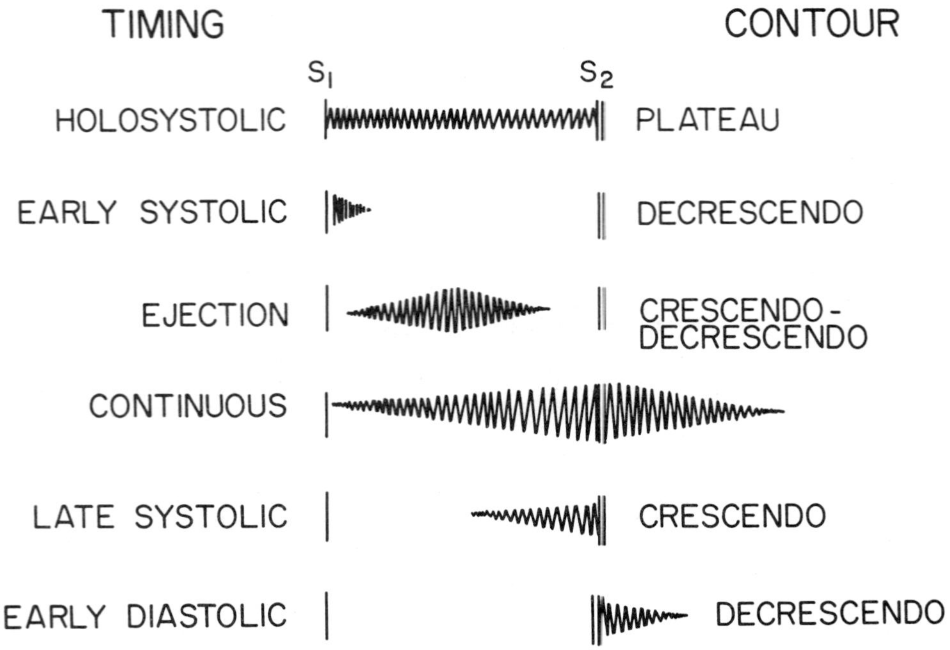

Figure 2–3 Phonocardiographic characteristics of several types of murmurs illustrating variations in timing, duration, and contour.

5. Pitch: Most murmurs in children consist of mixed frequencies in the middle range although some diagnostically important events are either very low or very high in pitch. Thus, this characterization is of importance.
6. Quality: The examiner should differentiate between the murmur which is blowing in character, being relatively free of vibrations, or that which is rough (harsh) in which the vibrations are a prominent feature. In the latter case the buzzing or vibratory components may occur close together, as is typical in murmurs of ventricular septal defects and aortic stenosis, or may be coarser and more widely spaced as is seen in innocent vibratory murmurs.
7. Contour: Murmurs which are due to the ejection of blood into an artery typically increase in intensity as the flow velocity across the semilunar valve increases; therefore, they are generally crescendo-descrescendo or diamond-shaped in contour (Fig. 2-3). In contrast, the regurgitant murmur due to either atrioventricular valvular regurgitation or a ventricular septal defect tends to be of a more even amplitude throughout systole (plateau type). A crescendo-decrescendo holosystolic murmur is not infrequently heard in patients with ventricular septal defects, particularly during infancy or early childhood years. The reasons for this are not clear. Other contour variations include the decrescendo murmur of semilunar valvular regurgitation or the tiny ventricular septal defect, the late systolic crescendo murmur of mitral valve prolapse, and the diastolic murmur of mitral stenosis which is generally of relatively even amplitude throughout most of diastole with presystolic accentuation following atrial contraction.
8. Change with altered position or other maneuvers: The examiner should note whether the murmur is louder in supine, sitting, or semidecubitus positions. It is characteristic of most innocent murmurs (v.i.) that they are audible at one position and disappear when that position is changed.

Frequently assessing the behavior of the murmur in response to various physiologic or pharmacologic maneuvers is of value in clarifying an uncertain finding. Isometric exercise or squatting increases the resistance to left ventricular ejection and will intensify the murmurs of mitral regurgitation or ventricular septal defect, whereas the murmur of left ventricular outflow tract obstruction, especially hypertrophic subaortic stenosis, will usually decrease in intensity. The Valsalva maneuver (forced expiration against a closed glottis) decreases cardiac filling and will diminish the intensity of many murmurs, especially those of obstructive lesions. The most marked decrease is seen in innocent murmurs; the ejection murmur of hypertrophic subaortic stenosis, on the other hand, becomes louder and is essentially the only one which so increases. This maneuver is easily performed in any child over the age of 3 or 4 years by either elevating his feet 6-10 inches above the table and asking him to hold them there (having him take a deep breath first) or by asking him to inspire deeply, hold his breath, and resist the downward pressure of the examiner's hand on his abdomen. Amyl nitrite produces a significant peripheral vasodilatation upon inhalation and increased cardiac output, increasing obstructive murmurs while diminishing those of valvular regurgitation or ventricular septal defect.

Although many different types of murmurs are recognized, they can all be generally divided into one of two groups: innocent or organic. Organic murmurs are those resutling from abnormalities in structure in the circulatory system and fall into many different patterns depending upon the nature of the abnormality. These will be discussed in more detail in the section dealing with specific lesion complexes. Innocent murmurs are normal events resulting from physiologic turbulence or vibrations within the heart or great vessels and are of no importance except for the confusion that they generate. They are present in at least 50-75% of normal children at one time or another under good conditions of examination. A closely related but perhaps not identical term is the so-called functional murmur. This generally refers to accentuations of normal murmurs under conditions of increased output such as with anemia, fever, anxiety, thyrotoxicosis, and so forth.

All of the innocent murmurs have certain features in common. With one exception they are all systolic in timing and are usually of short duration. They are usually soft, being of grade 3 or less in intensity, and are commonly altered in intensity with changes in body position. They will all decrease markedly in intensity or disappear with a good Valsalva maneuver. If the murmur is innocent, all the features of the examination as well as the EKG and chest x-ray are normal. However, the diagnosis of an innocent murmur is not a diagnosis of exclusion. In addition to the previously mentioned characteristics shared by all, there are at least six types of innocent murmurs which can easily be recognized by the experienced examiner (Table 2-3).

1. *Innocent ejection murmur:* These are short, early-to-mid systolic murmurs resulting from turbulence during ejection into an artery and have usually been regarded as pulmonic ejection murmurs. Recent high-fidelity recordings have demonstrated small gradients across both right and left ventricular outflow tracts in early systole (so-called impulse gradients) in normal individuals. It may be that many of the innocent ejection murmurs originate from the left heart. They are

Table 2-3 Innocent Murmurs

Murmur	Type	Location	Special Characteristics	Resembles
Basal ejection	Ejection	Upper left sternal border	Little radiation	Pulmonic stenosis; atrial septal defect
Physiologic pulmonary flow murmur of newborn	Ejection	Upper sternal border bilateral	Radiates to back and axillae	Peripheral pulmonic stenosis
Vibratory (Still's)	Early systolic	Lower left sternal border	Radiates to upper sternal border and apex; coarsely vibratory, twanging	Tiny ventricular septal defect
Venous hum	Continuous	Neck and upper sternal border, bilateral	Two intensity peaks; louder in inspiration; not audible when supine; varies with head position	Patent ductus arteriosus Arteriovenous malformation
Supra-clavicular bruit	Ejection	Neck	Decreases with hyperextension of shoulders	Aortic stenosis
Cardio-respiratory	Systolic	Left sternal border	Actually a respiratory sound; disappears with held respiration	Ventricular septal defect; mitral regurgitation

They are heard best at the upper left sternal border giving rise to the previous concept of pulmonic murmur. They are blowing in quality and are of crescendo-decrescendo contour with relatively little radiation. On occasion very faint transmission to the back may be present. This murmur is accentuated in high-output states. Differentiation from semilunar valvular stenosis or atrial septal defect is required. These pathologic conditions are generally identified by associated features to be described later. This type of murmur seems to have a bimodal age distribution being common in infancy and early childhood years and again during adolescence.

2. *Physiologic pulmonary flow murmur of the newborn:* This is also a short early-to-mid systolic crescendo-decrescendo blowing murmur which is heard maximally at the base on either side of the sternum but differs from the previous murmur in that it radiates widely over the entire thorax including the axillae. Radiation is prominent even though the murmur may be only of grade-2 intensity at the base. This murmur has its origin in the normal development of the pulmonary arteries. At birth and for a variable period thereafter, the first-order right and left pulmonary arteries are somewhat small relative to the main pulmonary artery due to the fact that in the fetus the majority of the blood ejected into the main pulmonary artery crosses the ductus arteriosus to the descending aorta and blood flow to the lungs is small. There is a physiologic hypoplasia of the right and left pulmonary arteries, and small gradients across these vessels have been demonstrated. The murmur, because of its wide radiation, resembles peripheral pulmonic stenosis, and differentiation between the physiologic and pathologic murmur in the newborn is almost impossible except in the rare incidence where pathologic peripheral pulmonic stenosis might be sufficiently severe as to produce detectable right ventricular overload. It is recognized most often in prematures but is not uncommon in a full-term infant. Over a period of a few months the pulmonary arteries enlarge relative to the main pulmonary artery, and the physiologic murmur disappears.

3. *Innocent vibratory murmur (Still's murmur):* Still's murmur is an early systolic, coarsely vibratory murmur of short duration audible maximally at the mid-to-lower left sternal border. Occasionally, some high-frequency overtones are present, giving the murmur a peculiar twanging quality. It may remain localized or may radiate to the upper left sternal border and/or apex. Its origin is debated although recent evidence suggests that it originates from the acceleration of blood into the left ventricular outflow tract. The inexperienced examiner may confuse it with a ventricular septal defect, but the short duration of the Still's murmur and the fact the it begins after S_1 are differentiating features. This murmur is most frequently recognized in the late preschool and early school-age child.

4. *Venous hum:* Resulting from turbulence in venous return through the jugular and superior vena caval system, this is a low-frequency, continuous systolic and diastolic murmur audible maximally in the neck but in children usually recognized

at the upper right or left sternal border or both. Two peaks of intensity, one in systole and one in diastole, are recognized, giving the characteristic double-diamond contour. The diastolic component is generally louder, and there is accentuation during inspiration. Because of its continuous nature and maximal intensity at the base of the heart, it is often confused with the murmur of patent ductus arteriosus. The venous hum is heard only in the upright position and disappears when supine. It can be obliterated by occlusion of the jugular system on the ipsilateral side. Flexion of the head reduces the intensity markedly, whereas the extension of the head or rotation to the contralateral side accentuates the murmur by increasing tension on the vein. If a venous hum is audible in the supine position, one should consider an abnormal increase in blood flow through this portion of the venous bed or some area of localized obstruction. Although not common in young infants, it may be heard at any age.

5. *Supraclavicular or carotid bruits:* Up to 50% of normal children will show a short, early systolic crescendo-decrescendo murmur in the supraclavicular fossa or over the carotid vessels. Although generally soft, they can occasionally be as loud as grade 3 and show a somewhat harsh quality. These bruits are thought to originate from turbulent flow into the brachiocephalic vessels. In contrast to aortic stenosis, from which they must be differentiated, there is relatively little murmur heard below the clavicles. Hyperextension of the shoulders in the sitting position with the elbows flexed to 90° will commonly cause the murmur to decrease in intensity or disappear entirely. It will also decrease with a Valsalva maneuver, although this may be hard to recognize because of the contraction of the neck muscles that is produced. There does not seem to be any age predilection for this murmur. More recently, analysis of turbulent flow utilizing pulsed Doppler echocardiography has shown that some brachiocephalic bruits, originally thought to be innocent, actually originated from minor abnormalities of the aortic valve. Standard echocardiography, utilizing M-mode or two-dimensional techniques, may also help in the differentiation. If there is any question, the child should probably be followed at infrequent intervals.

6. *Cardiorespiratory murmur:* These are soft, blowing systolic murmurs heard best at the apex or lower left sternal border with varying intensity. Careful auscultation reveals that the murmur is present only during inspiration and disappears with held respiration, differenting it from murmurs of atrioventricular valvular regurgitation or ventricular septal defect. They are not murmurs at all, but are breath sounds in a segment of lung which is being intermittently compressed by the heart. There is no age specificity.

As one learns to recognize characteristic innocent murmurs, there is usually little confusion with murmurs originating from organic heart disease. Reassurance to the family is the only treatment required for innocent murmurs. The fact that they are normal events should be stressed. Also, it is a good idea to mention that, although innocent murmurs generally eventually disappear, they may remain audible for years and that this persistence is of no importance. It is a bad idea to tell the family that the child will outgrow the murmur as this implies some definable change that is expected to take place. The parents are often disturbed when the murmur remains audible several years later, the implication being that some type of normal developmental alteration has failed to occur.

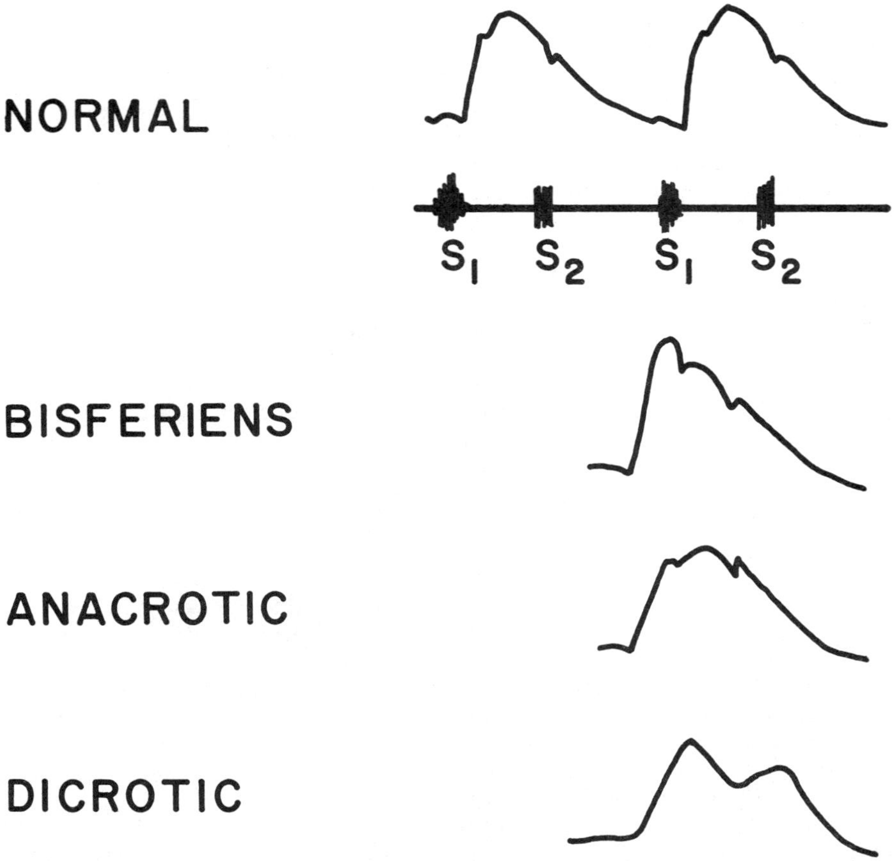

Figure 2-4 Normal and abnormal carotid arterial pulse waveforms. See text for discussion.

Examination of Peripheral Pulses

Arterial Pulsations

Peripheral arterial pulses are palpated best with the child lying quietly in a supine position with the fingertips applied over the artery with sufficient pressure to feel the pulse well but not to compress the artery since this may not only produce thrills but also may obliterate the pulse. The examiner should be concerned with the pulse amplitude, that is, how strong the pulse is, as well as the contour of the waveform. Under the later characteristic, we would consider rate of rise and fall-off of the pulse wave as well as the number of impulses per cardiac cycle. The normal arterial pulse is monophasic with only one impulse per cycle (Fig. 2-4). This occurs shortly after S_1 or the apex impulse. A biphasic or twice-beating pulse may fall into several patterns, all of which are abnormal (Fig. 2-4). A rapidly rising pulse with two palpable waves during systole is described as bisferious and may be seen in aortic regurgitation, particularly when there is a mild degree of associated stenosis, or in idiopathic hypertrophic subaortic stenosis. Less commonly a prominent anacrotic notch on the upstroke of the pulse wave may be palpable in patients with severe stenosis. More frequently this lesion produces a pulse which is of low amplitude and slow rising (so-called pulsus parvus et tardus). This will be discussed in more detail in the section on aortic stenosis, but it is well to mention at this point that the typical pulses associated with this abnormality are more characteristically seen in the adult. Children with severe aortic valve obstruction not uncommonly have normal arterial pulse waves. The final type of double pulse may be seen when peripheral resistance and arterial diastolic pressure are low as in high-output states or aortic regurgitation. This type of pulse is characterized by a single systolic impulse followed by a diastolic wave and is described as a dicrotic pulse.

The type of pulse-wave evaluation just mentioned is best carried out by examination of the carotid arteries. The pulse wave in these vessels more accurately reflects events occurring near the aortic valve. The obvious exception is the infant in whom the short, fat neck and lack of cooperation make it almost impossible to palpate the carotids. In the older child the pulses are examined with the head very slightly extended, palpating between the sternocleidomastoid muscle and the angle of the mandible. In the infant the examination is generally limited to the extremity pulses; these should be evaluated in older children as well. It is preferable to evaluate the brachial and femoral pulses, palpating first both brachial arteries simultaneously and then the right brachial and femoral artery together. The brachial pulses are best felt either in the medial aspect of the antecubital fossa or in the groove between biceps and triceps muscles on the medial aspect of the upper arm. The axillary pulse can also be easily evaluated. Femoral pulses are easily detected in the fossa ovalis beneath the inguinal ligament, particularly if the leg is slightly externally rotated.

In addition to the waveform characteristics, the examiner is also concerned with determining relative amplitude and timing in all extremities. All four extremity pulses should be of equal intensity and nearly synchronous. Although in the adult the radial and femoral pulses occur closer together in time with the brachial pulse somewhat earlier, this is probably not true in the infant and young child where body proportions are different. For this reason we feel that the brachial pulses are preferable to the radial pulse in this type of examination. In addition, the smaller diameter of the radial artery results in loss of information about waveform and amplitude, particularly in infants. A significant decrease in femoral pulse intensity or delay in the femoral pulse as compared to the upper extremities is indicative of coarctation of the aorta. Asymmetry of the upper extremity pulses may be seen in some types of coarctation as well as in supravalvular aortic stenosis or in localized obstruction to the brachiocephalic vessels. Every so often a particularly chubby or restless infant will be encountered in whom the femoral pulses are difficult to palpate. The presence of a normal dorsalis pedis or posterior tibial pulse is good evidence against a significant aortic coarctation.

Venous Pulses

Venous pulses are often neglected in children because they are more difficult to evaluate, particularly in the infant. Important information can be gained from careful inspection of the pulsations which originate in the jugular veins. This is best carried out with the head and thorax elevated between 15-30°; greater elevation may be necessary if the venous pressure is increased. If a beam of light is shined obliquely across the anterolateral aspect of the neck, the venous wave can be identified. The normal waveform is illustrated in Fig. 2-5. The A wave which precedes the first heart sound is due to atrial contraction. As the atrium relaxes, pressure decreases, but there may be a secondary hump following S_1 referred to as the C wave. In the jugular veins, this may be due to two factors: (1) transmission of the carotid arterial pulse to the veins and (2) retrograde transmission of a positive wave produced in the right atrium by upward displacement of the tricuspid valve at the onset of systole. The further decline of venous pressure following the C wave is referred to as the X descent and results from further atrial relaxation as well as inferior displacement of the ventricles in systole. As the right atrium becomes filled with blood, there is a third positive-pressure wave called the V wave. At the onset of diastole and emptying of the atrium a second rapid decrease in pressure called the Y descent occurs.

Many conditions will alter the venous wave configuration. Obstructions to atrial emptying will increase the height of the A wave. Large A waves are seen intermittently in complete atrioventricular block when the atrium attempts to contract during ventricular systole. A large A wave may also accompany an S_4 in the presence of a poorly compliant right ventricle. Tricuspid regurgitation will produce a large systolic wave which obliterates the normal V wave and encroaches upon the X descent.

Another useful point in the evaluation of jugular venous pulses is the ability to obtain a rough estimate of the central venous pressure. With the patient elevated as previously described the vein is emptied by compression and then released. The level to which the vein is distended can be measured in reference to the right atrium. The latter is usually estimated as located at the fourth or fifth intercostal spaces at the mid-thoracic level.

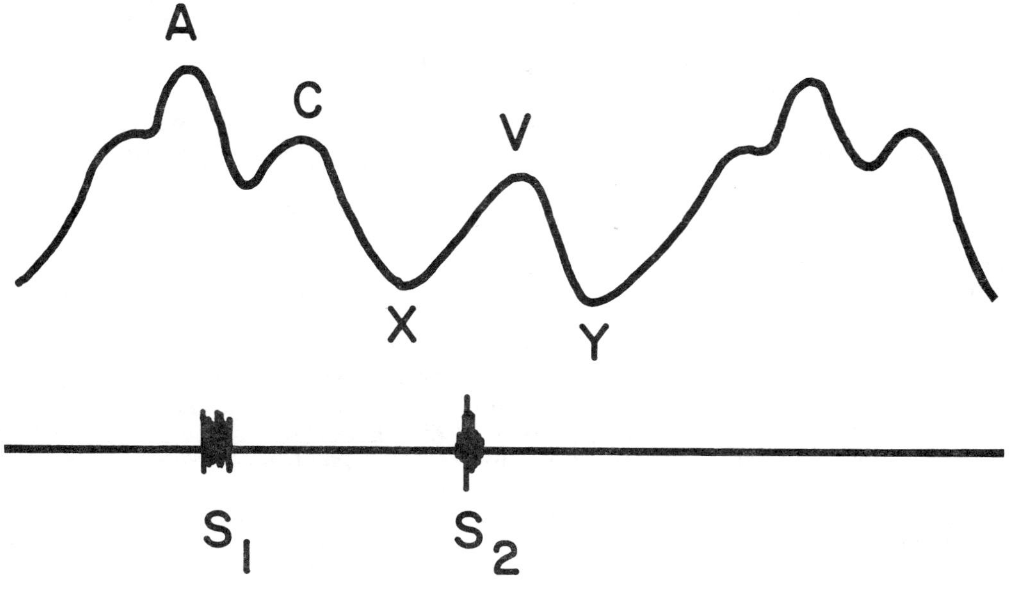

Figure 2-5 Normal jugular venous waveform. Significance of the individual deflections is discussed in the text.

Measurement of Blood Pressure

As was true of the palpation of peripheral pulses, blood pressure should also be measured in both arms and one leg. Since the most common cause of high or low blood pressure in children is iatrogenic due to improper cuff size, the examiner should be sure the cuff fits properly. An adequately fitting blood pressure cuff has an air bladder whose width extends two-thirds to three-fourths of the length of the upper arm or thigh. In addition, the length of the air bladder should be sufficient to extend at least halfway around the circumference of the extremity and preferably completely encircle it. Thus, many of the so-called newborn blood pressure cuffs available commercially are inadequate because the air bladder is too short to cover a sufficient portion of the circumference. The cuff should be applied snugly around the extremity, without tension, prior to inflating. A wide assortment of cuff sizes is currently available so that folding should not be necessary. The cuff should be inflated to a level of approximately 20-30 mmHg (torr) above systolic and smoothly deflated at a rate of 2-3 mm/sec. Undue delay in deflating the cuff should be avoided since this will produce discomfort and may render the child uncooperative. The chest piece of the stethoscope should be of a proper size to make adequate contact without undue pressure on the extremity. Normal values are shown in Fig. 2-6.

The five phases of Korotkoff sounds are described in Table 2-4. Ideally, one uses phases 1 and 4 in the assessment of systolic and diastolic blood pressure, but in children phase 4 may be difficult to detect so that complete disappearance may have to be used as the end point. The leg pressure is best measured with the child prone and the knee slightly flexed, with the foot resting on a small pillow or sand-bag since resting the toes on the table may produce tension of the muscles around the popliteal fossa. The examiner listens over the popliteal fossa and takes the blood pressure in the same manner as in the upper extremities.

If an infant is actively struggling and moving about, no method of blood pressure recording will be accurate, and attempts should be deferred until the child is quiet or has been sedated. There are a number of devices which use the Döppler ultrasonic principle for detection of flow, and these can be used to recognize a systolic blood pressure. Some of these utilize external speakers with sufficient amplification to overcome most ambient noise which may interfere with the use of a conventional stethoscope. These devices are of particular value in a small infant, especially the premature.

When auscultatory blood pressure cannot be obtained, other methods may have to be utilized. Palpation of the pulse as the cuff is deflated provides a fairly accurate estimation of systolic blood pressure, but the diastolic pressure cannot be evaluated in this manner. Another common practice in infants is to obtain a flush blood pressure. In this technique the cuff is placed about the extremity in the usual manner, the distal extremity snugly wrapped with an elastic bandage to the level of the knee or elbow, and the cuff is inflated above the anticipated systolic levels. The elastic bandage is then removed, and if the cuff has been adequately inflated, the extremity will appear pale. The cuff is deflated stepwise rather than in a continuous manner as described previously. It is most useful to reduce the pressure in 5-mm increments, allowing at least 2-3 sec and not more than 5 sec between each step. The end point is a prominent reactive hyperemia which usually appears within 1 or 2 sec. This technique roughly approximates mean blood pressure rather than systolic or diastolic. Regardless of the method utilized, it is important to take the blood pressure in all extremities in the same way. It is of little value to obtain auscultatory blood pressure in the upper extremities and then measure flush pressure in the legs since the values will not be comparable.

A

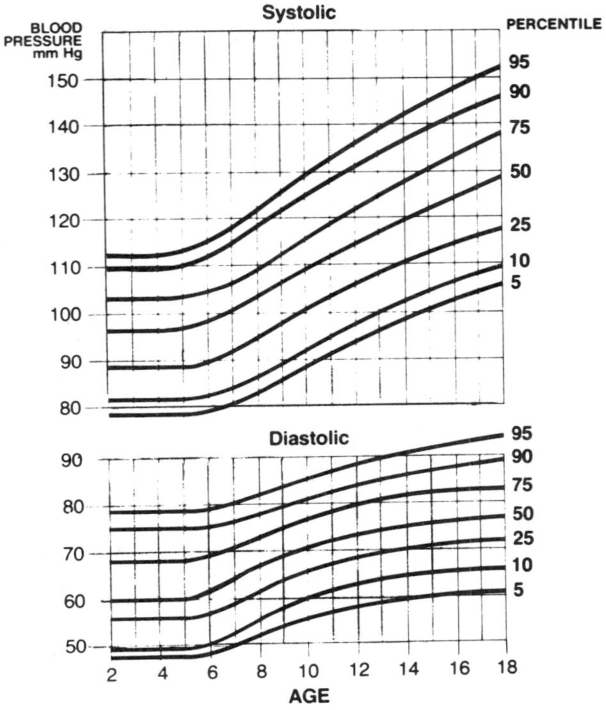

B

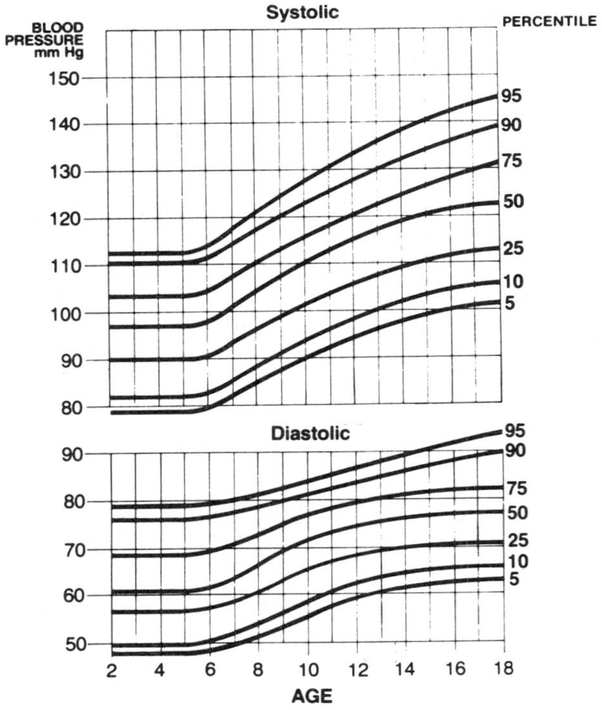

Figure 2-6 (A) Percentiles of blood pressure in boys (right arm, seated). (B) Percentiles of blood pressure measurement in girls (right arm, seated). (Reproduced with permission from Pediatrics 59:108, 1977 [Suppl.]).

Table 2-4 Korotkoff Sounds

Phase	Characteristics	Hemodynamic Significance
1	Clear, tapping sound	Cuff pressure lowered to arterial peak systolic
2	Phase 1 + swishing sound	
3	Accentuation of phase 2	Flow through partially compressed artery
4	Abrupt muffling of sounds	Loss of phase-1 sound as diastolic pressure approached; decrease in phase-3 sounds as flow period increases and velocity decreases
5	Disappearance of sounds	Artery no longer compressed

Additional Areas of Evaluation

Lungs

As the examiner listens over the lung fields for radiation of murmurs, he should evaluate the presence of adventitious sounds, particularly rales which might denote congestive heart failure. These may be missed unless the patient takes a deep inspiration. The presence of respiratory infection may provide some confusion in estimating the significance of a cardiovascular defect. Careful assessment of the presence of the former is, therefore, important. Inspiratory stridor may be due not only to respiratory infection but also to mediastinal vascular anomalies, and expiratory wheezing may be due to heart failure.

Abdomen

Of primary importance in abdominal evaluation is the estimation of liver size and position. Abnormalities in the position of the liver may suggest not only cardiac malposition but should also call to mind the possibility of serious congenital heart malformations. Palpation of the liver is best achieved by gentle pressure utilizing a rolling motion across the inferior edge. In normal infants, the edge can be felt as much as 2-3 cm below the right costal margin, although in older children the liver is not usually palpable except on deep inspiration. The examiner should be careful to estimate the total height of the liver by percussion since hyperinflation of the lungs will push the liver further into the abdomen and give a false impression of hepatomegaly. Tenderness, which may occur with acute distention or abnormal hepatic pulsation, should also be evaluated. The spleen is generally not enlarged in congestive failure or congenital heart defects. Splenomegaly may occur in bacterial endocarditis and should be carefully looked for. Palpation of the kidneys, although not directly related, may suggest the presence of associated congenital abnormalities. Bruits in the abdominal aorta or liver should be listened for. In slender children the abdominal aortic pulse may be palpated and evaluated; this should be done gently as this maneuver usually produces some discomfort. Palpation of the abdominal aorta is of particular importance when coarctation of the aorta is suspected because the uncommon occurrence of abdominal coarctation may be detected in this manner.

Extremities

As previously described, all four extremities should be evaluated for cyanosis. In some unusual circumstances this may involve only one, two, or three extremities. The presence of clubbing of the distal phalanges should also be looked for. In its early stages, this presents as a shininess of the skin at the base of the nail, followed by loss of the nailbed angle and, subsequently, overt enlargement of the distal phalanges and prominent convexity of the nail as shown in Fig. 2-7. Other extremity anomalies which may relate to the cardiovascular system as part of a syndrome (e.g., the Holt-Oram syndrome) may be detected. Nodules of acute rheumatic fever may be identified over extensor surface of the extremities and vertebral processes and in the postoccipital region.

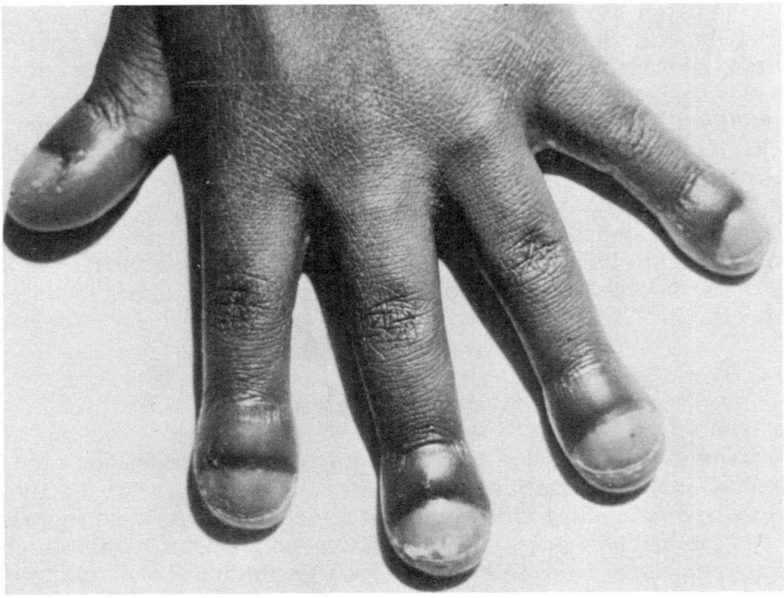

Figure 2-7 Marked clubbing of the fingers in a child with cyanotic congenital heart disease.

Skin

In addition to comments previously made, the examiner should not forget to look the skin over carefully for other less common manifestations such as the lesions of bacterial endocarditis (petechiae, splinter hemorrhages, Osler nodes, and Janeway lesions). Skin rashes may be noted occasionally, such as the typical erythema marginatum of acute rheumatic fever. Less common skin manifestations may point toward a multisystemic disorder with cardiac involvement (e.g., the adenoma sebaceum of tuberous sclerosis).

Eyes

Ocular abnormalities may be part of many somatic syndromes. In addition, congenital anomalies of the eye such as colobomata may not uncommonly accompany heart disease. The dislocated lens of Marfan syndrome and cataracts as seen in the congenital rubella syndrome are important manifestations that should not be missed. Conjunctivae are a good place to look for petechiae in bacterial endocarditis. Examination of the fundus may disclose vessel anomalies of importance as well as the Roth spots of bacterial endocarditis.

Head

Some final comments are in order regarding the evaluation of the head in general. Obviously, many types of cranial anomalies may be seen, either as part of a general syndrome involving the heart or as associated but not related findings. In either event, evaluation of the impact of the cardiovascular lesion on a child's overall health may be rendered more difficult by the presence of a severe central nervous system anomaly which usually accompanies marked alteration in head structure. One often overlooked examination is auscultation of the head. This should be carried out over the occiput, the area over the anterior fontanelle, and both parietal regions. In children, auscultation of the eyeballs is somewhat difficult and generally is not necessary. If one makes a habit of listening to the head in all patients, soft systolic bruits will frequently be noted and may not be of any significance. A continuous bruit suggests the possibility of an intercranial atriovenous malformation. Large arteriovenous malformations, generally draining into the vein of Galen, are a not infrequent cause of congestive heart failure in the newborn period or may produce cardiomegaly, basal ejection murmurs, and signs of a high-output state in older patients. The physician may be tricked into believing that a cardiac defect is responsible unless he remembers to listen for intracranial bruits.

Electrocardiography

The recording of electrical activity generated by the heart has been one of the major contributions to the field of cardiology in this century. From the early studies of Einthoven, surface electrophysiological recording has progressed to the point where there are now extremely sophisticated methods available utilizing simultaneous recordings from 150 or more points which are then computer processed to obtain the maximum information content. These methods are complicated and for the most part suitable only for research purposes. The basic scalar electrocardiogram (EKG) remains the mainstay of clinical cardiology, and it is the purpose of this section to provide the basics of interpretation of the electrocardiogram in children. Many excellent and detailed discussions of the subject are available, and some of these are referenced at the end of the chapter for the reader who wishes to explore in more depth.

In the resting state the myocardial cell is in a polarized state as shown in Fig. 2-8. Excitation of this cell results in the initiation and propagation of a wave of depolarization due to ion flux across the cell membrane. This depolarization wave is propagated along the length of the myocardial cell. The resulting difference in potential between the two ends of the cell can be viewed as a dipole as illustrated in Fig. 2-9. This dipole will have not only magnitude but also direction, depending upon the orientation of the cell in space, and can be represented as a vector. At each instant of time, the total cardiac electrical activity is the result of a tremendous number of simultaneous dipole vectors, the vast majority of which cancel each other out. The electrical activity recorded at the body surface is, therefore, the result of the algebraic summation of thousands of these vectors at an infinite number of points throughout the cardiac cycle. At any one given instant, this net magnitude and direction of cardiac electrical activity can be thought of as represented by a single vector.

The body surface electrocardiogram can be visualized as looking at this resultant activity from a number of different sites. Electrical activity recorded by the individual electrodes is considered as being directed along a theoretical line connecting the electrode with the center of cardiac electrical activity. This line is referred to as the lead axis. These lead axes are assumed to bear a certain mathematical relationship to each other which does not correspond to an anatomic line between the electrode position and the cardiac center. Since at any given instant the resultant vector of electrical activity may be directed along a line which is not parallel to the given lead axis, the electrical activity seen by that lead will be the result of projection of the resultant vector on the lead axis. Properly, the scalar electrocardiogram as implied by its name records only potential magnitude. The recording of multiple leads allows the interpreter to construct the concept of direction.

Lead Systems

Many different electrode positions have been utilized, but the following are the standard for clinical scalar electrocardiography. In most institutions when recording pediatric electrocardiograms, tracings are obtained along 13 lead axes. From a historic standpoint, electrodes were initially placed on the four extremities, and the potential difference between three different pairs of electrodes was recorded

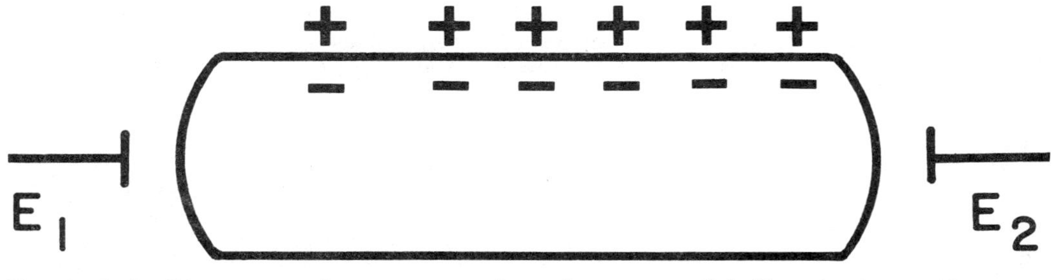

Figure 2-8 Diagrammatic representation of a myocardial fiber in the resting state. The surface of the cell is positive with respect to the interior. There is no difference in potential between electrodes E_1 and E_2.

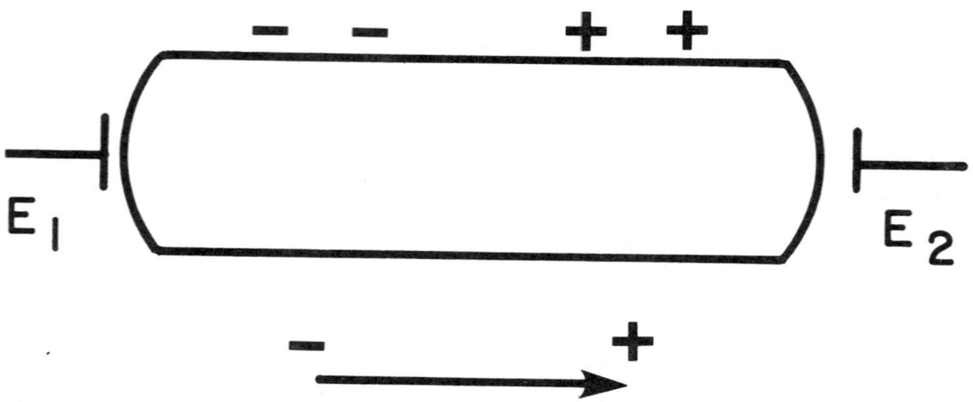

Figure 2-9 Depolarization of myocardial fiber following excitation of the end adjacent to electrode E_1. The direction of spread of the depolarization wave is from right to left. At this point in time, electrode E_2 has a positive potential with respect to E_1. This potential difference can be represented as a dipole vector having direction and polarity as shown at the bottom of the figure.

(with the right leg electrode being a ground). These were referred to as the bipolar limb leads and are still utilized; they are obtained as follows.

Lead I: Left arm potential minus right arm potential
Lead II: Left leg potential minus right arm potential
Lead III: Left leg potential minus left arm potential

Subsequently, the unipolar limb leads were developed. These record the potential difference between an exploring electrode placed either on the right arm, left arm, or left leg and the remaining limb electrodes connected so as to form a central terminal with 0 potential. They are referred to as leads aVR, aVL, and aVF, respectively. The a refers to electrical technique of augmentation of the recorded potentials. Thus, utilizing four limb electrodes, electrical activity is recorded along six lead axes, each of which is considered as passing through the center of cardiac electrical activity and bearing a relationship to the other as illustrated by the hexaxial system in Fig. 2-10. The lead axes divide a 360° circle into 30° segments. There are three pairs of mutually perpendicular leads. The convention of expressing the lead axis direction in terms of degrees around the circle is illustrated as is the positive end of each lead axis. This hexaxial system is considered as describing the electrical activity in the frontal plane, incorporating the left-right and the superior-inferior directions as shown. Work performed subsequent to the original description of this axis system has indicated that the lead relationship is more complicated than Fig. 2-10 illustrates. However, the simple hexaxial system is commonly accepted as being sufficiently accurate for ordinary clinical work at the present time.

In addition to the limb leads, the electrocardiogram is commonly recorded from seven positions over the anterior thorax in children. Other lead positions have been utilized in both children and adults, but for the most part only seven are necessary. An exploring electrode is placed over the precordium, and the potential difference recorded between this electrode and the limb electrodes constructed into a common ground terminal. Standard lead positions are referred to as leads V_1 through V_6 illustrated in Fig. 2-11. Placing the electrode in mirror-image

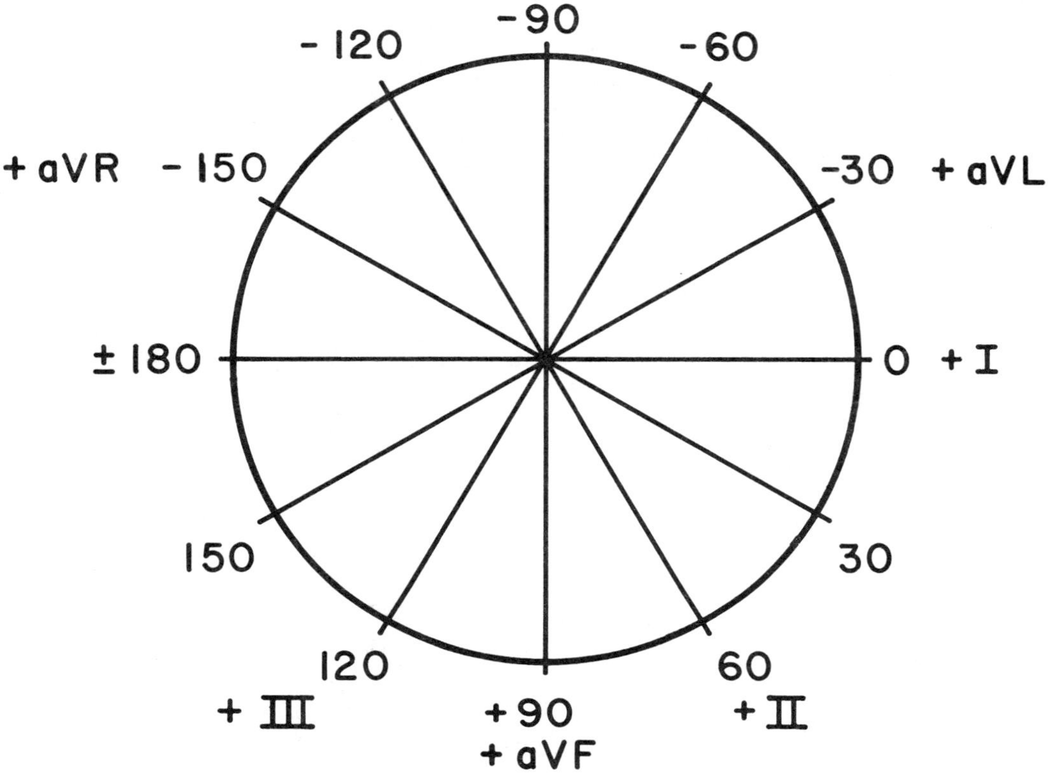

Figure 2–10 Orientation of limb lead axes.

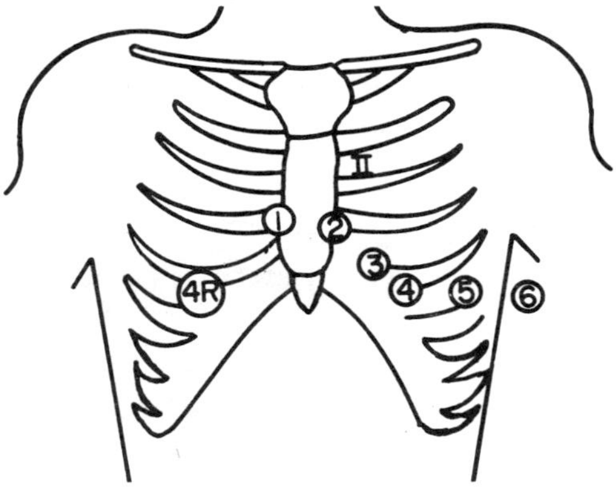

Figure 2–11 Precordial electrode positions. Leads V_1 and V_2 are recorded in the fourth intercostal space at the right and left sternal borders, respectively. V_4 is in the left fifth intercostal space at the midclavicular line; V_3 is located at the midpoint of a line connecting V_2 and V_4. V_5 and V_6 are at the same level as V_4 in the anterior and midaxillary lines, respectively. V_4R is in the same position as V_4 over the right hemithorax.

positions over the right anterior thorax allows the recording of leads V_3R through V_6R (V_1 and V_2 become V_2R and V_1R, respectively). Lead V_4R is commonly recorded together with the left chest leads in pediatric practice. Remaining right chest leads may be utilized if there is dextrocardia. As illustrated in Fig. 2-12, the theoretical relationship between chest lead axes is less straightforward than has been postulated for the limb leads. This axis system describes cardiac activity in the horizontal (or transverse) plane, incorporating left-right and anterior-posterior directions.

Generation of the Cardiographic Waveform

At the start of each cardiac cycle all myocardial cells are in the polarized state. The wave of depolarization which will eventually spread to all cells is initiated in the sinoatrial node (SA node) in the right atrium, near the orifice of the superior vena cava. The spread of this excitation wave throughout the heart is controlled by means of specialized tissue referred to as the conduction system (Fig. 2-13). Depolarization waves spread through the atria in a manner not yet completely understood but felt to be primarily along the internodal tracts. The resultant direction of this atrial depolarization wave is leftward, inferior, and anterior, directed toward the atrioventricular node (AV node). As atrial cells are depolarized, the surface electrodes record a low-voltage deflection known as the P wave (Fig. 2-14). As the depolarization wave reaches the AV node, the atria have completed their depolarization. The wave then passes along the conduction system from the AV node through the His bundle and the bundle branches to the Purkinje network and subsequently to the ventricular myocardial cells. Electrical potentials generated by depolarization along the His-bundle-branch-Purkinje system are too small to be recorded by surface techniques. They can be detected by intracardiac recording as described later. Ventricular myocardial cells are depolarized from the endocardial surface outward to the epicardium.

A larger amplitude deflection known as the QRS complex is recorded. The initial portion of the QRS complex is due to the depolarization of the interventricular septum from left ventricular to right ventricular side and is directed rightward, anteriorly, and superiorly. Subsequently, excitation of the ventricular walls occurs nearly simultaneously. Since the left ventricle possesses greater mass in the older child or adult, the resultant electrical forces are directed toward the left and posteriorly. Figure 2-15 shows this sequence of ventricular depolarization in the generation of the QRS complex. The process of repolarization is less well

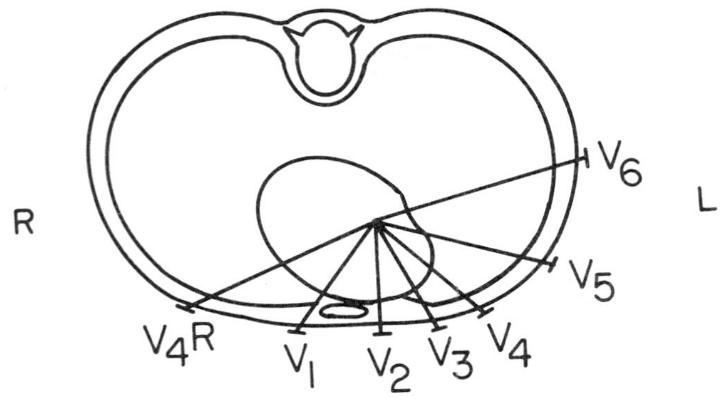

Figure 2-12 Theoretical orientation of the precordial lead axes to the heart.

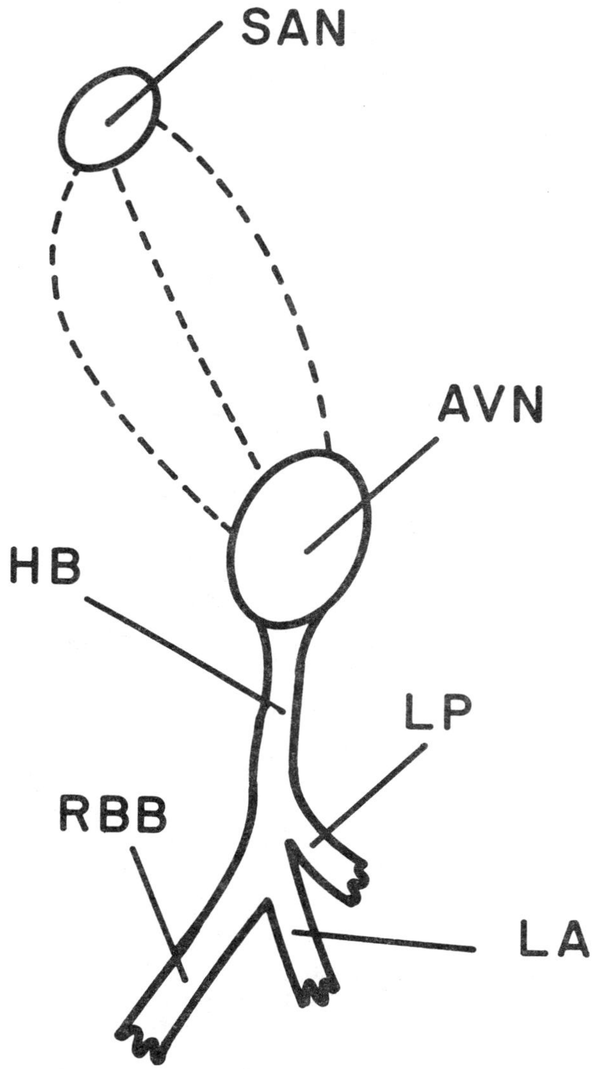

Figure 2–13 Diagrammatic representation of the conduction system, SAN - sinoatrial node, AVN - atrioventricular node, HB - His bundle, LA - anterior fascicles of left bundle branch, LP - posterior fascicles of the left bundle branch, RBB - right bundle branch. Dashed lines indicate internodal tracts.

understood. Although the dipole is oppositely directed, depolarization proceeds from epicardium to endocardium, producing a deflection known as the T wave which is generally directed toward the major portion of the QRS complex.

A concept of considerable practical value in the evaluation of congenital heart disease is determination of the average direction of electrical forces known as the mean electrical axis (MEA). This is most often determined for the QRS forces, but P and T wave axes may be calculated as well. Maximal precision in determining the axis requires careful measurement of the amplitude of the deflections and plotting on a coordinate system. This time-consuming and complicated if conduction defects are present. For clinical purposes, this degree of precision is not

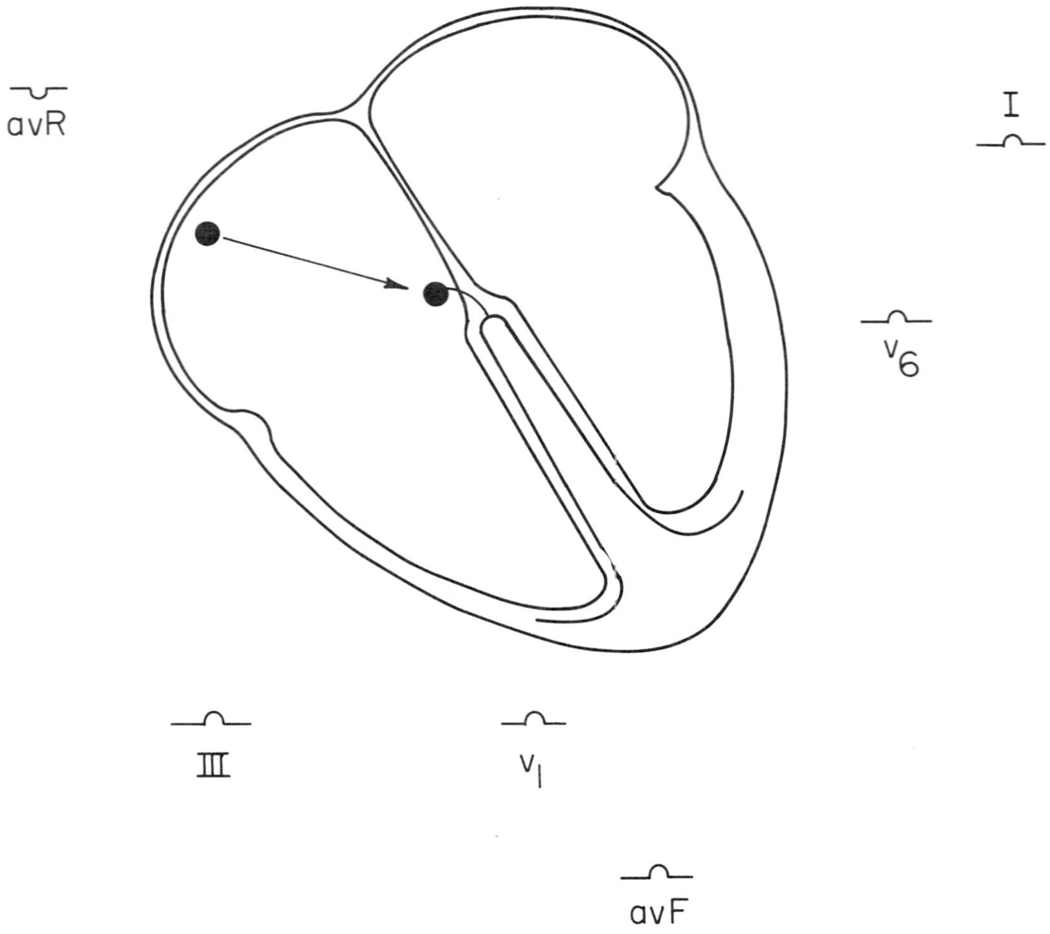

Figure 2-14 Generation of the normal P wave. Solid circles represent sinoatrial and atrioventricular nodes. Overall leftward, inferior, and anterior direction of spread of the atrial excitation wave results in P-wave configuration as shown in selected leads.

required, and the approximate axis can be determined by simple inspection. The hexaxial lead system in the frontal plane lends itself readily to this determination. Because of irregular spacing of the lead axes in the horizontal plane, mean axis determination is far less precise and not generally reported.

Certain basic concepts must be kept in mind. A depolarization dipole moving along a line perpendicular to a given lead axis and equidistant from the two ends of the axis will produce a 0 voltage deflection in that lead (Fig. 2-16). If the dipole is moving toward the positive electrode and is closer to it than to the negative end, the EKG records a positive (upward) deflection. If closer to and moving toward the negative end, a negative (downward) deflection is recorded. A dipole moving away from the positive end but closer to it is shown as a positive voltage on the EKG but progressively returning toward the 0 or isoelectric baseline, and the opposite is true for a dipole close to but moving away from the negative end. The frontal plane QRS axis is usually determined by following these steps:

1. The QRS complex in the perpendicularly oriented lead pair, I and aVF, is initially inspected. This will allow the interpreter to locate the axis within one of the 90° quadrants of the frontal plane.
2. Those leads whose perpendiculars run through the quadrant determined in step 1 are inspected and the algebraic sum of the deflections in the QRS complex determined. If the deflections in a given lead show an algebraic sum of 0, the QRS axis lies along the perpendicular to that lead. Otherwise, it lies between two lead axes, and in this manner can be narrowed down to a 30° segment which more than suffices for clinical purposes. In the presence of conduction defects, the individual deflection of the QRS complex may not be of equal duration. If the difference in width of the deflections is significant (more than 20 msec) estimation of MEA based on deflection amplitude done may not be accurate. Under such circumstances, one must visually estimate the algebraic sum of the areas enclosed by the individual deflections. This is a complicated

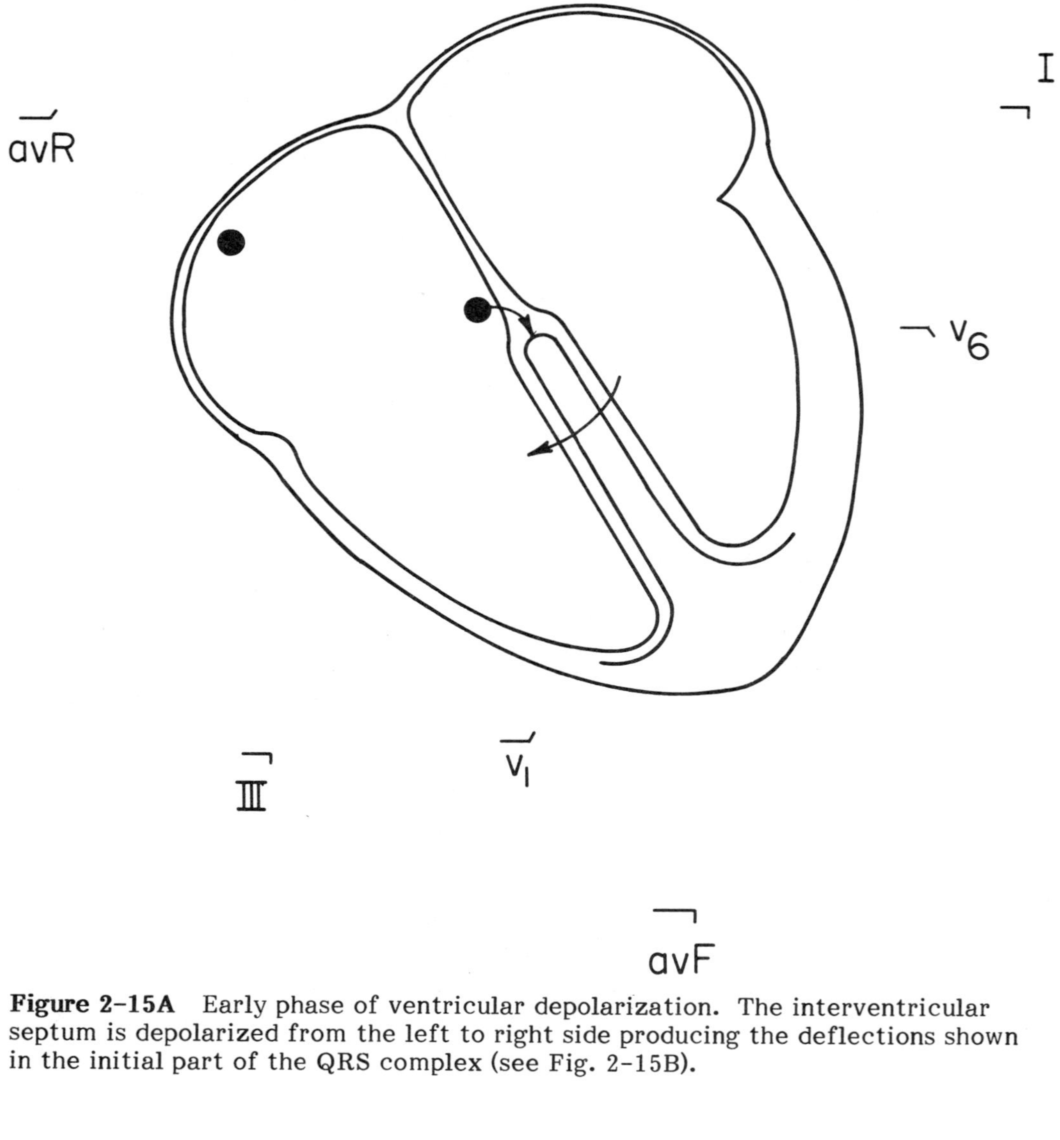

Figure 2–15A Early phase of ventricular depolarization. The interventricular septum is depolarized from the left to right side producing the deflections shown in the initial part of the QRS complex (see Fig. 2-15B).

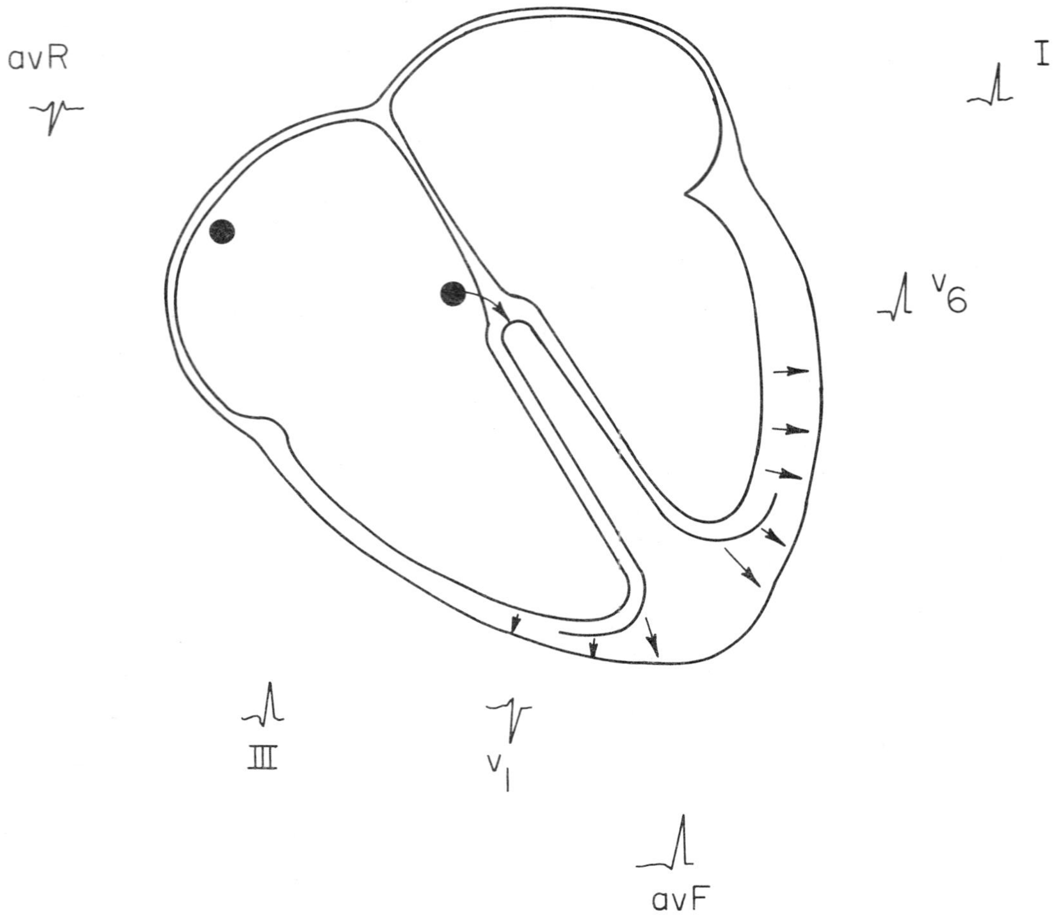

Figure 2-15B Completion of ventricular depolarization. As a result of greater myocardial mass of the left ventricle, the net forces are directed leftward, posteriorly, and inferiorly.

business which results in only a gross estimate of MEA. When the conduction defect affects only a portion of the QRS complex (e.g., RBBB), estimation of the overall MEA may be less informative than analyzing the direction of the vectors representing each deflection.

Two examples should serve to illustrate the methods involved. Inspection of Fig. 2-17 shows totally upright (i.e., positive) QRS complexes in leads I and aVF. Recording of a totally positive QRS complex in lead I means that the electrical forces lie in a semicircle extending from +90° - -90° closer to the positive end of lead I. In the same manner, lead aVF indicates that the same forces must lie between 0° - +180° toward the positive end of aVF. Since leads I and aVF are mutually perpendicular, they overlap in the left inferior quadrant which extends from 0° - +90° as illustrated. The lead axes of leads III and aVL have perpendiculars (leads AVR and II, respectively) which pass through the left inferior quadrant. Since the complex in lead III is positive, this limits the QRS axis to the arc between +30° and +90°. One does not need to look at lead III, however, since the algebraic

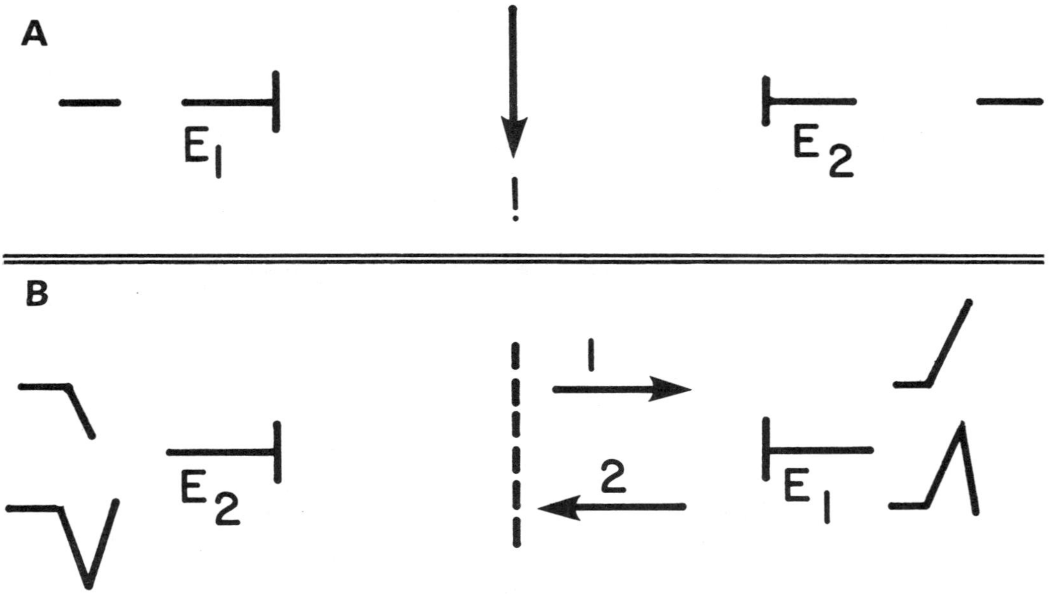

Figure 2–16 Effect of the position and movement of a dipole on the EKG complex. In each portion of the figure, a depolarization dipole is depicted as moving along the path indicated by the arrows with the positive end of the dipole toward the head of the arrow. The dashed lines are equidistant from the recording electrodes E_1 and E_2. (A) The dipole is moving along a line perpendicular to and equidistant from E_1 and E_2. No change in potential is detected by either electrode and thus no deflection is recorded. (B) Arrow 1 indicates a dipole moving toward E_1 and located closer to it. E_1 detects an increase in potential and a positive (upright) deflection is recorded, whereas E_2 records a negative (downward) deflection. If the dipole subsequently moves in the opposite direction as indicated by arrow 2, the recorded deflections return toward the baseline.

sum of positive and negative deflection in aVL is approximately 0. The average direction of the QRS forces is perpendicular to lead AVL (i.e., along the lead axis of II), and since it is directed in the left inferior quadrant, it must be located at approximately +60°.

In contrast, look at the complexes recorded in Fig. 2-18. Perusal of lead I and aVF shows the former to be predominantly negative and the latter to be positive in direction. These conditions can be met only if the mean electrical axis is in the right inferior quadrant (i.e., between +90° and +180°). Lead aVR is also positive, further narrowing the range to between +120° and +180°. The negative complex in lead II restricts the possibilities of the mean electrical axis to between +150° and 180°. Simple inspection reveals that the electrical forces project nearly equally on both leads II and aVF, and the MEA must be approximately halfway between. This method would place the mean axis at approximately +165° and is probably accurate within ±5°. Further precision is not necessary for clinical purposes.

As mentioned previously, because of the inconstant relationship between the chest lead axes, determination of an MEA for the horizontal plane is quite difficult. From a clinically useful standpoint, one calculates the frontal plane axis

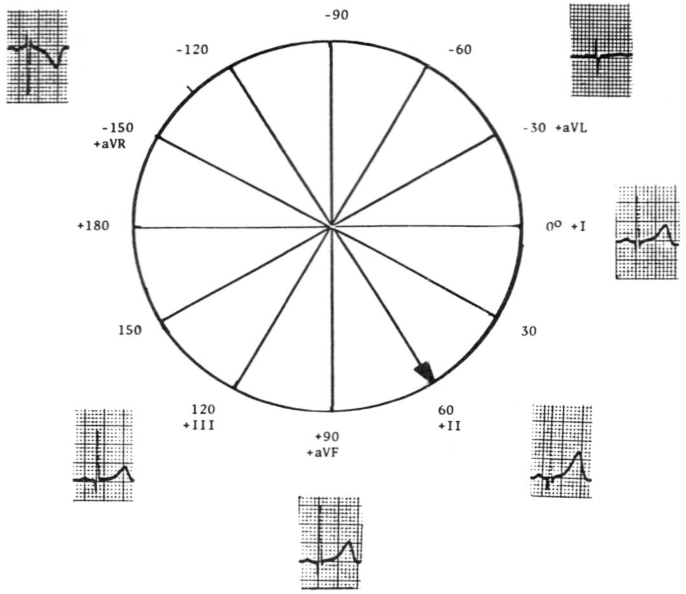

Figure 2–17 Mean electrical axis of +60°. Determination of the axis position from the leads illustrated as discussed in the text.

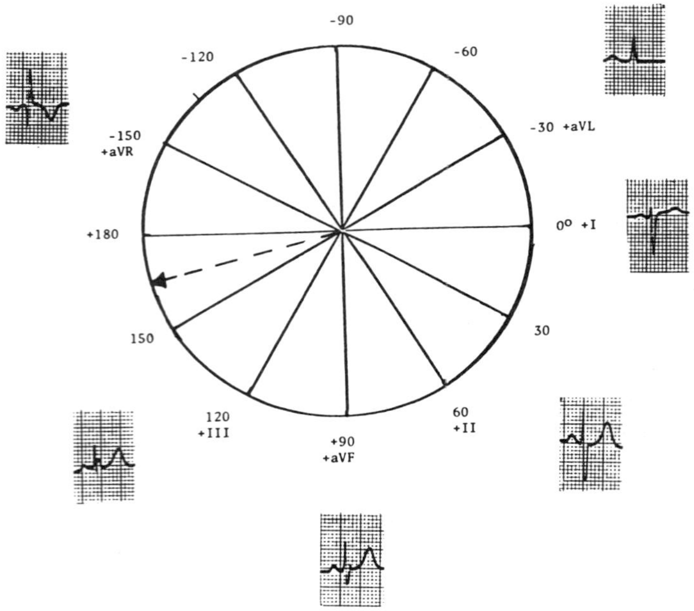

Figure 2–18 Mean electrical axis of +165°. See text for details.

as described previously and then looks at lead V_2 for an indication as to whether this vector is directed anterior or posteriorly.

Normal Electrocardiogram

The primary feature of the pediatric electrocardiogram is the wide range of normality which is noted and the way in which this range shifts with increasing age. Thus, what is a normal EKG for a newborn would be grossly abnormal for an adult. The interpreter must have a good grasp of the change in normal patterns if he is to accurately evaluate pediatric tracings. This subject is beautifully covered in the text by Park and Guntheroth to which the reader is referred for more detailed analysis than is possible here. Another noteworthy characteristic of the pediatric EKG is the voltages recorded in children, particularly in the chest leads, which are generally larger than in adults.

As previously mentioned, the P wave is normally directed leftward, inferiorly, and anteriorly, being upright in leads I, II, III, and aVF. Although usually upright in aVL, biphasic complexes may occasionally be seen, and a negative P wave is normally recorded in lead aVR. This deflection is also usually upright in the chest leads, although leads V_1 and V_4R may not infrequently record a small biphasic or inverted deflection. Generally accepted standards indicate a maximum height of 2.5-3 mm at full standardization (0.25-0.3 mv), with average duration of 0.06 ± 0.02 sec, thus the upper limit of normal for P-wave duration would be 0.1 sec or 2.5 small squares at the usual paper speed of 25 mm/sec. There does not seem to be any significant change in direction, magnitude, or duration of the P wave with increasing age, although these details are not fully worked out.

There is a general increase in the AV nodal delay throughout childhood. Various intracardiac studies have suggested this to be at both the level of the AV node and the His bundle. The standard scalar electrocardiogram, therefore, records tendency toward a longer PR interval with advancing age. Normal values are shown in Table 2-5.

The QRS complex reflects the physiologic changes in the ventricular myocardium which take place throughout childhood. As a result of the high impedance to right ventricular output in the fetus, right ventricular myocardial mass exceeds that of the left, and the EKG reflects right ventricular dominance in the full-term newborn. As illustrated in Fig. 2-19, the right chest leads show a prominent initial R wave which usually exceeds the S wave in magnitude (R/S ratio greater than 1). Relatively prominent S waves are seen in the left chest. The mean QRS vector is directed anteriorly and inferiorly and somewhat rightward, producing a normal right axis deviation in this age group.

The transition toward the typical adult pattern is a gradual one throughout most of the first two decades of life. Electrical dominance of the left ventricle is generally recognized by the end of the first year, and the average child at this age shows R and S waves of equal magnitude in lead V_1, in contrast to the uniformly dominant R waves earlier in infancy. This transition is illustrated in Figs. 2-20 - 2-22. Recent studies in the normal premature infant demonstrated less physiological right ventricular dominance than is seen in the full-term infant.

The ST segment should show an isoelectric J point (junction between the QRS complex and ST segment). This is best determined by comparison with the baseline following termination of the T wave since the PR segment may be distorted by atrial repolarization events. In leads where the T wave is upright, the ST segment has a slightly upward slope. The T waves show an orientation similar to the direction of major ventricular depolarization forces and are upright in the inferior and leftward limb leads. Major age-related differences are noted in the precordial

Table 2-5 Normal Values for EKG Intervals and Q-Wave Magnitude

Cycle Length, Heart Rate, and Q-T Interval Average (and Upper Limits)
(Ashman and Hull, 1941)

CYCLE LENGTH (SEC.)	HEART RATE PER MIN.	AVERAGE Q-T (SEC.)	CYCLE LENGTH (SEC.)	HEART RATE PER MIN.	AVERAGE Q-T (SEC.)
1.50	40	0.45(0.49)	0.85	70	0.36(0.38)
1.40	43	0.44(0.48)	0.80	75	0.35(0.38)
1.30	46	0.43(0.47)	0.75	80	0.34(0.37)
1.25	48	0.42(0.46)	0.70	86	0.33(0.36)
1.20	50	0.41(0.45)	0.65	92	0.32(0.35)
1.15	52	0.41(0.45)	0.60	100	0.31(0.34)
1.10	55	0.40(0.44)	0.55	109	0.30(0.33)
1.05	57	0.39(0.43)	0.50	120	0.28(0.31)
1.00	60	0.39(0.42)	0.45	133	0.27(0.29)
0.95	63	0.38(0.41)	0.40	150	0.25(0.28)
0.90	67	0.37(0.40)	0.35	172	0.23(0.26)

P-Q (P-R) Interval, with Rate and Age: Average (and Upper Limits of Normal)
(Ziegler, 1951; Alimurung and Massell, 1956; Ashman and Hull, 1941)

RATE	0-1/12 YEAR	1/12-6/12 YEAR	6/12-1 YEAR	1-3 YEARS	3-8 YEARS	8-12 YEARS	12-16 YEARS	ADULT
<60						0.16 (0.18)	0.16(0.19)	0.17(0.21)
60- 80					0.15 (0.17)	0.15 (0.17)	0.15(0.18)	0.16(0.21)
80-100	0.10(0.12)				0.14 (0.16)	0.145(0.16)	0.15(0.17)	0.15(0.20)
100-120	0.10(0.115)			(0.15)	0.13 (0.155)	0.145(0.15)	0.15(0.16)	0.15(0.19)
120-140	0.10(0.11)	0.105(0.14)	0.11 (0.14)	0.12(0.14)	0.125(0.15)	0.14 (0.15)		0.15(0.18)
140-160	0.09(0.11)	0.10 (0.13)	0.105(0.13)	0.11(0.14)	0.12 (0.14)			(0.17)
160-180	0.10(0.11)	0.10 (0.12)	0.10 (0.12)	0.10(0.12)				
>180	0.09	0.09 (0.11)	0.10 (0.11)					

QRS Duration: Average (and Upper Limts) for Age
(Ziegler, 1951)

Years:	0-1/12	1/12-6/12	6/12-1	1-3	3-8	8-12	12-16	ADULT
Seconds:	0.05(0.065)	0.05(0.07)	0.05(0.06)	0.06(0.07)	0.07(0.08)	0.07(0.09)	0.07(0.10)	0.08(0.10)

"Ventricular Activation Time" in Seconds: Average
(and Upper Limits of Normal)
(Ziegler, 1951)

LEAD	0-1/12 YEAR	1/12-6/12 YEAR	6/12-1 YEAR	1-3 YEARS	3-8 YEARS	8-12 YEARS	12-16 YEARS	ADULT
V_1	0.015(0.03)	0.02 (0.03)	0.02 (0.03)	0.015(0.03)	0.015(0.025)	0.015(0.03)	0.015(0.03)	0.02(0.03)
V_{5-6}	0.02 (0.03)	0.025(0.035)	0.025(0.04)	0.03 (0.04)	0.03 (0.04)	0.035(0.045)	0.035(0.045)	0.04(0.05)

Q Voltages According to Lead and Age: Mean (and Upper Limits)
(Ziegler, 1951; N.Y. Heart Assoc., 1953)
(Measured in Millimeters, When 1 mv. = 10 mm. Paper)

LEAD	0-1/12 YEAR	1/12-6/12 YEAR	6/12-1 YEAR	1-3 YEARS	3-8 YEARS	8-12 YEARS	12-16 YEARS	ADULT
III	2 (5)	3 (8)	3(8)	3 (8)	1.5(6)	1 (5)	1(4)	0.5(4)
aVF	2 (4)	2 (5)	2(6)	1.5(5)	1 (5)	1 (3)	1(3)	0.5(2)
V_5	1.5(5)	1.5(4)	2(5)	2 (6)	2 (6)	2 (4.5)	1(4)	0.5(3.5)
V_6	1.5(4)	1.5(4)	2(5)	2 (4.5)	1.5(4.5)	1.5(4)	1(2.5)	0.5(3)

Reproduced with permission from Guntheroth WG, Pediatric Electrocardiography, 1965, W.B. Saunders Co., Philadelphia.

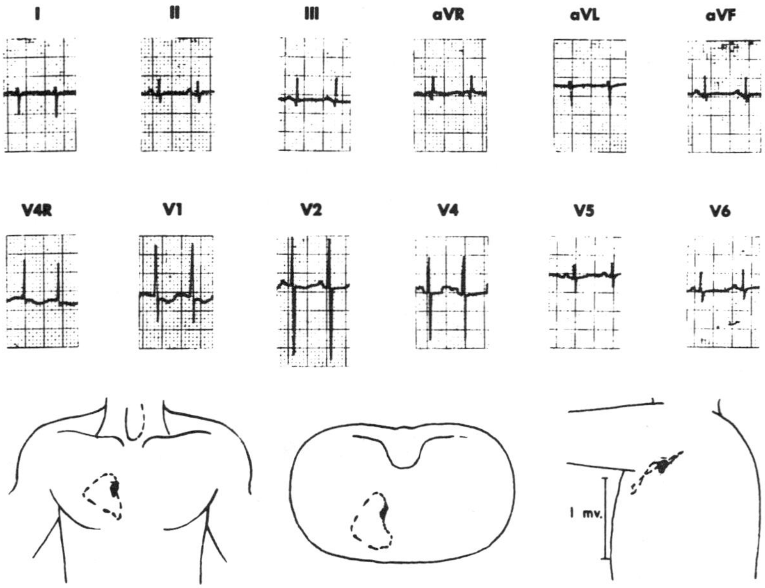

Figure 2-19 Electrocardiogram and vectorcardiogram from a normal 2-day-old infant. (Reproduced with permission from Guntheroth WG, Pediatric Electrocardiography, 1965, W. B. Saunders Co., Philadelphia.)

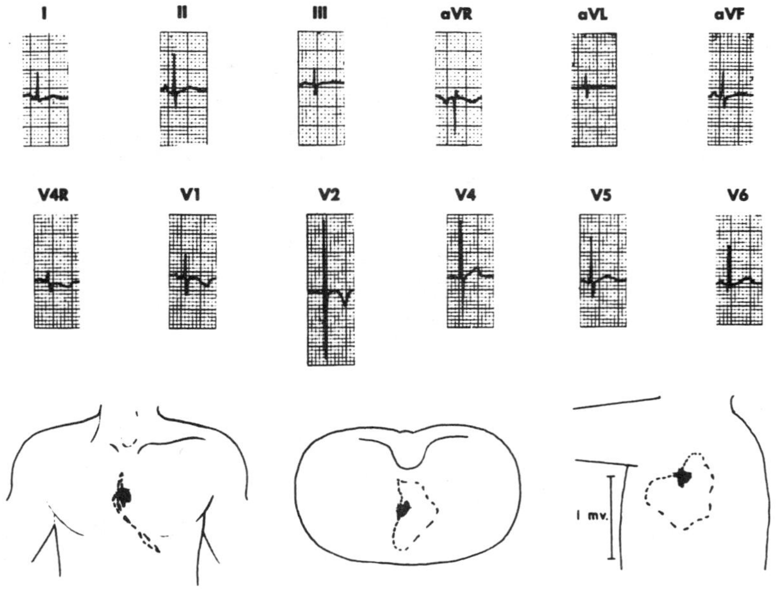

Figure 2-20 Normal 14-month-old infant. (Reproduced with permission from Guntheroth WG, Pediatric Electrocardiography, 1965, W. B. Saunders Co., Philadelphia.)

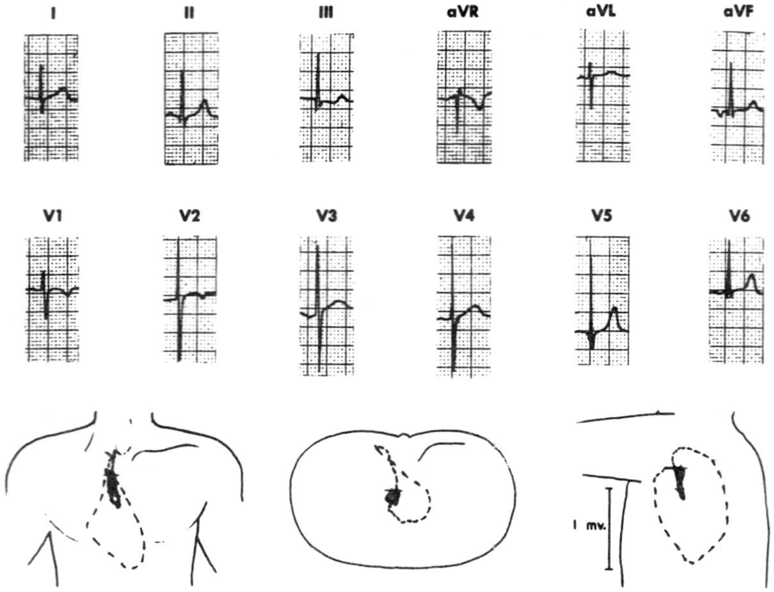

Figure 2–21 Normal 5-year-old child. (Reproduced with permission from Guntheroth WG, Pediatric Electrocardiography, 1965, W.B. Saunders Co., Philadelphia.)

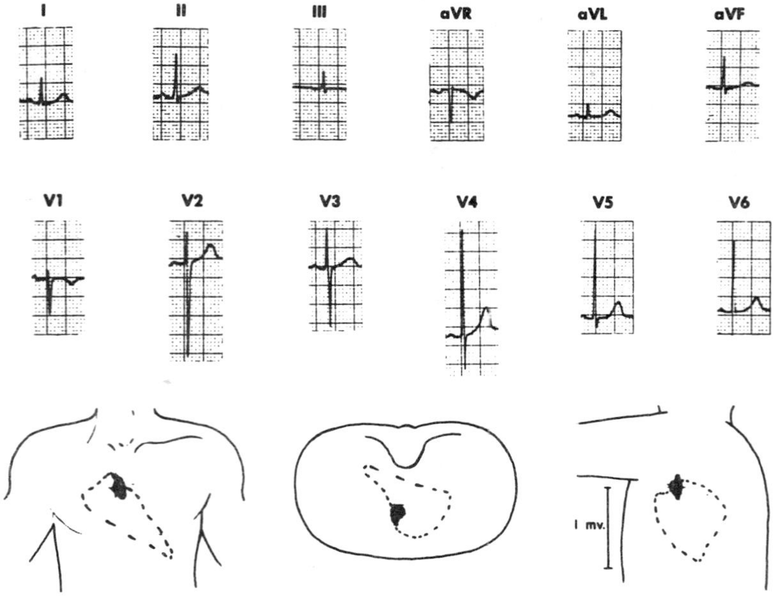

Figure 2–22 Normal 10-year-old child. (Reproduced with permission from Guntheroth WG, Pediatric Electrocardiography, 1965, W.B. Saunders Co., Philadelphia.)

leads. Full-term newborns characteristically show a T wave which is directed leftward and anterior, being upright in all chest leads. Generally, by 4 days of age the direction of the T wave has shifted more posteriorly and leftward so that inversion in right precordial leads is the rule. This may extend as far to the left as leads V_2 or V_3 without being abnormal. Persistence of an upright T wave in lead V_1 past the end of the first week of life is abnormal and will be discussed further subsequently. Toward the end of the first decade T-wave orientation is more variable, and upright deflections may be occasionally seen in the right chest leads in normal individuals.

It has been known for many years that black children tend to have T waves which are more posteriorly directed, being inverted further to the left than in Caucasian children. This persistent juvenile pattern is often seen as late as the third decade of life. More recently, studies of racial variation have indicated larger leftward QRS forces in black children, with the depth of the S waves in right chest leads achieving statistical significance.

Myocardial Hypertrophy

It is in the recognition of hypertrophy that the electrocardiogram achieves its greatest usefulness in pediatrics. Traditionally, recognized alterations have been based on the concept that an increased muscle mass produces larger electrical forces directed toward that region of the myocardium. Some highly sophisticated studies have revealed that the volume of blood contained within a chamber may also affect the magnitude of electrical forces. The electrocardiogram can no longer be looked upon as recognizing only hypertrophy rather than dilatation. Nonetheless, hypertrophy of the free wall of a chamber results in increased electrical forces directed toward it with greater cancellation of forces arising from the opposite side of the heart. Depending on the chamber involved, hypertrophy may result in increased voltage, a change in the orientation of forces, or both.

Atrial Hypertrophy

Right Atrial Hypertrophy

Right atrial hypertrophy results in a P wave which is tall and pointed but of normal duration (Fig. 2-23) and is best recognized in leads II and V_1. The P wave is excessively tall if it exceeds 2.5 mm at full standardization. Duration should not exceed 0.1 sec.

Left Atrial Hypertrophy

The left atrium is normally depolarized following the right, and hypertrophy of this chamber produces prolongation of the P wave (greater than 0.1 sec) with the appearance of two distinct peaks (Fig. 2-24). In lead V_1 there is usually a biphasic wave with the terminal negative peak (the so-called P-terminal force) of significantly greater magnitude and duration than the initial positive deflection. The abnormal P-terminal force will usually incorporate an area of at least 1 mm^2 at normal standardization and paper speed.

Biatrial Hypertrophy

A combination of the features already mentioned is noted with P waves appearing broad and notched. Generally, the initial peak representing the right atrium is taller and pointed.

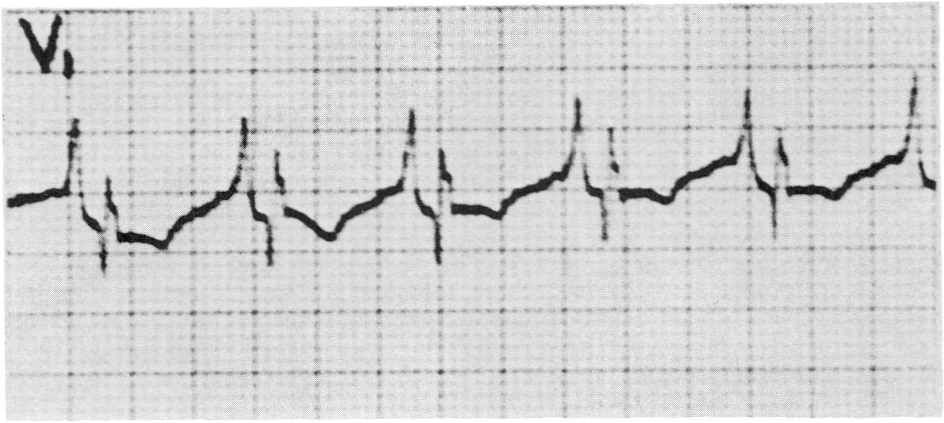

Figure 2-23 Lead V_1 in a 12-year-old boy with massive left ventricle to right atrial shunt. Tall pointed P waves indicate marked right atrial hypertrophy.

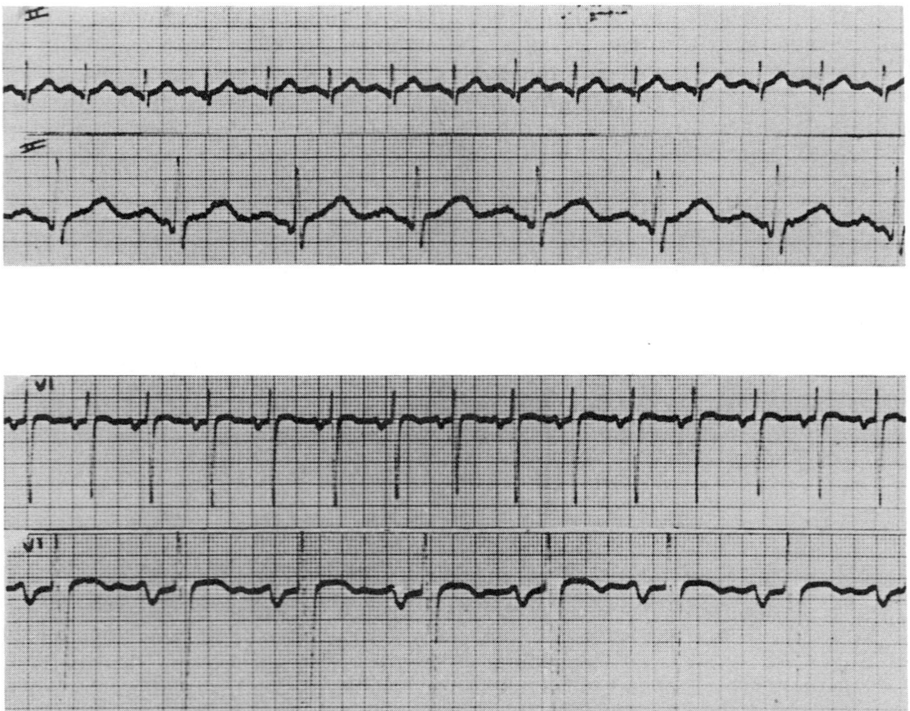

Figure 2-24 Leads II (top) and V_1 (bottom) from a patient with mitral stenosis. The bottom strip of each lead pair is taken at twice the usual standardization and at a paper speed of 50 mm/sec. Lead II reveals a P wave of slightly prolonged duration with notching. The prominent negative P-terminal force is clearly evident in lead V_1, indicative of left atrial hypertrophy.

Ventricular Hypertrophy

Right Ventricular Hypertrophy (RVH)

In the newborn and young infant, RVH presents primarily as an accentuation of the normal pattern. As such, it may be somewhat difficult to recognize unless rightward-anterior QRS forces definitely exceed the upper limits of normal (see Table 2-6 and Fig. 2-25). Right axis deviation generally accompanies right ventricular hypertrophy but is usually not outside the normal range in this age group. Even in the newborn, a pure R wave (i.e., a totally positive deflection) exceeding 1 mv (10 mm) in leads V_4R or V_1 is highly suggestive of right ventricular hypertrophy. These abnormal rightward forces are generally reflected in the left chest leads by deep S waves. Although this subject is not totally settled, there is a general concensus that upright T waves in the right chest leads after 1 week of age reflect right ventricular hypertrophy, at least during the first decade of life. In general, these T waves point leftward and anterior and are upright in all chest leads, in contrast to the situation in severe left ventricular hypertrophy. This abnormal T-wave direction may be seen in the absence of overt abnormalities in the QRS complex; however, rightward QRS forces are usually relatively prominent. Q waves in the right chest leads reflecting abnormal direction of septal depolarization may be of several different etiologies (Table 2-7), one of which is severe right ventricular hypertrophy. These Q waves are accompanied by excessive free-wall forces producing tall R waves in the right and deep S waves in the left chest leads.

In the older child abnormalities of QRS voltage still constitute the most overt criteria for right ventricular hypertrophy. Milder degrees may be recognized by relative shifting of the direction of forces toward the right and anterior. Even in the face of voltages which do not exceed normal values, one may see an R/S ratio in V_1 greater than upper limits of normal with a relative decrease in the same ratio in left chest (Fig. 2-26). In the limb leads, right axis deviation generally occurs. To oversimplify, voltage changes are more important in the diagnosis of right ventricular hypertrophy in the young infant, whereas orientation changes may become prominent in the older child. An occasional patient is seen with excessive forces directed to the right and posteriorly. This pattern of so-called indeterminant ventricular hypertrophy most often reflects right ventricular hypertrophy. In severe degrees of hypertrophy, ST segment depression and deeply inverted T waves in the right chest leads resulting in a wide QRS-T angle (so-called right ventricular strain) may be seen.

In the past, there have been attempts to divide right ventricular hypertrophy into patterns of systolic overload and diastolic overload. The former was thought to be manifested by tall positive complexes in the right chest leads with both initial and terminal forces so directed (i.e., a tall, pure R wave) and deep S waves in the left chest leads (Fig. 2-27). These are usually accompanied by repolarization abnormalities or right ventricular strain. On the other hand, dilatation of the right ventricle due to diastolic overload was represented by prominent rightward terminal QRS forces with the initial portion of the QRS normally directed. In other words, leads V_4R and V_1 would usually show a rSR' complex. The left chest leads showed only a prominent S wave but not to the degree usually seen in systolic overloading (Fig. 2-26). There are many exceptions to these concepts, and the degree of separation cannot be regarded as absolute. More accurately the systolic overload patterns are due to more severe degrees of right ventricular hypertrophy which, in the pediatric age group, are usually due to increased right ventricular pressure, whereas diastolic overload is seen in milder right ventricular hypertrophy usually associated with lesions producing primarily dilatation of the

Table 2–6 Normal Values for Magnitude of R and S Waves and R/S Ratio

R Voltages According to Lead and Age: Mean (and Upper Limits)
(Ziegler, 1951; Manning and Smiley, 1964; N.Y. Heart Assoc., 1953)
(Measured in Millimeters, When 1 mv = 10 mm. Paper)

LEAD	0-1/12 YEAR	1/12-6/12 YEAR	6/12-1 YEAR	1-3 YEARS	3-8 YEARS	8-12 YEARS	12-16 YEARS	YOUNG ADULTS
I	4 (8)	7 (13)	8 (16)	8 (16)	7 (15)	7 (15)	6 (13)	5.5(13)
II	6 (14)	13 (24)	13 (27)	12.5(23)	12.5(22)	13.5(24)	13.5(24)	9 (25)
III	8 (16)	9 (20)	9 (20)	9 (20)	9 (20)	9 (24)	9 (24)	5.5(22)
aVR	3 (7)	3 (6)	2.5(6)	2 (6)	1.5(5)	1.5(4)	1.5(4)	1 (4)
aVL	2 (7)	4 (8)	4.5(10)	4.5(10)	3 (10)	2.5(10)	2.5(12)	2.5(9)
aVF	6.5(14)	9.5(20)	9.5(16)	8 (20)	10 (19)	10 (20)	11 (21)	5 (23)
V_1	15 (25)	11 (20)	10 (20)	9 (18)	7 (18)	6 (16)	5 (16)	3 (14)
V_2	21 (30)	21 (30)	19 (28)	16 (25)	13 (28)	10 (22)	9 (19)	6 (21)
V_5	12 (30)	17 (30)	18 (30)	19 (36)	21 (36)	22 (36)	18 (33)	12 (33)
V_6	6 (21)	9.5(20)	13 (20)	12 (24)	13.5(24)	14 (24)	13.5(22)	10 (21)

S Voltages According to Lead and Age: Mean (and Upper Limits)

LEAD	0-1/12 YEAR	1/12-6/12 YEAR	6/12-1 YEAR	1-3 YEARS	3-8 YEARS	8-12 YEARS	12-16 YEARS	ADULT
I	4.5(10)	3.5(9)	3.5(9)	3 (8)	2 (8)	1.5(8)	1.5(8)	1 (6)
V_1	10 (20)	7 (18)	8 (16)	13 (27)	13.5(30)	16 (26)	15 (24)	9.5(23)
V_2	20 (35)	16 (30)	17 (30)	21 (34)	23 (38)	23 (38)	23 (48)	14 (36)
V_6	3.5(12)	2 (6)	2 (4)	1.5(4)	1 (4)	1 (4)	1 (5)	1 (13)

R/S Ratio According to Age: Mean, Lower and Upper Limits of Normal
(Ziegler, 1951; Sokolow and Lyon, 1949)

LEAD		0-1/12 YEAR	1/12-6/12 YEAR	6/12-1 YEAR	1-3 YEARS	3-8 YEARS	8-12 YEARS	12-16 YEARS	ADULT
	LLN*	0.5	0.3	0.3	0.5	0.1	0.15	0.1	0.0
V_1	Mean	1.5	1.5	1.2	0.8	0.65	0.5	0.3	0.3
	ULN†	19	S=0	6	2	2	1	1	1
	LLN	0.3	0.3	0.3	0.3	0.05	0.1	0.1	0.1
V_2	Mean	1	1.2	1	0.8	0.5	0.5	0.5	0.2
	ULN	3	4	4	1.5	1.5	1.2	1.2	2.5
	LLN	0.1	1.5	2	3	2.5	4	2.5	2.5
V_6	Mean	2	4	6	20	20	20	10	9
	ULN	S=0	S=0	S=0	S=0	S=0	S=0	S=0	S=0

* Lower limits of normal.
† Upper limits of normal.

Reproduced with permission from Guntheroth WG, Pediatric Electrocardiography. W. B. Saunders Co., Philadelphia.

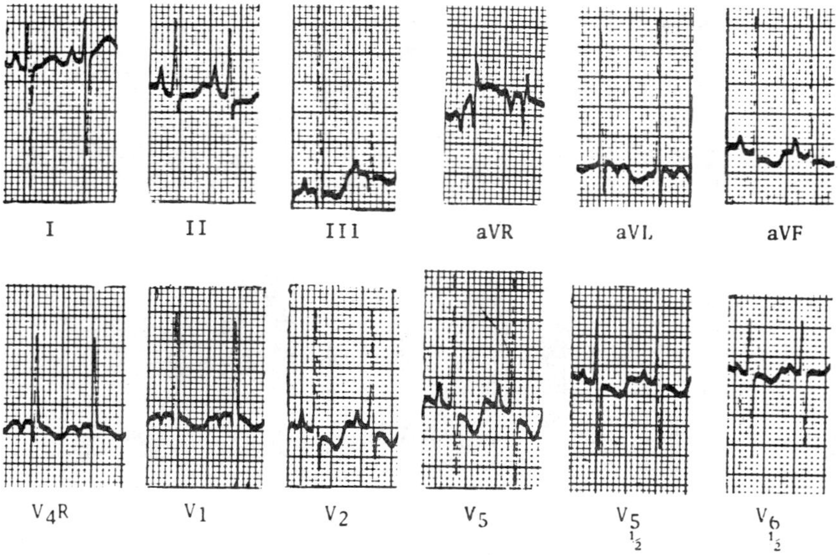

Figure 2–25 Electrocardiogram from a newborn infant with severe pulmonary hypertension. Tracing shows marked right ventricular hypertrophy. Q waves in leads V_4R and V_1 are due to hypertrophy. Tall pointed P waves indicate right atrial hypertrophy as well. In this and all subsequent tracings in this text, 1/2 indicates that the lead was recorded at 1/2 the usual gain.

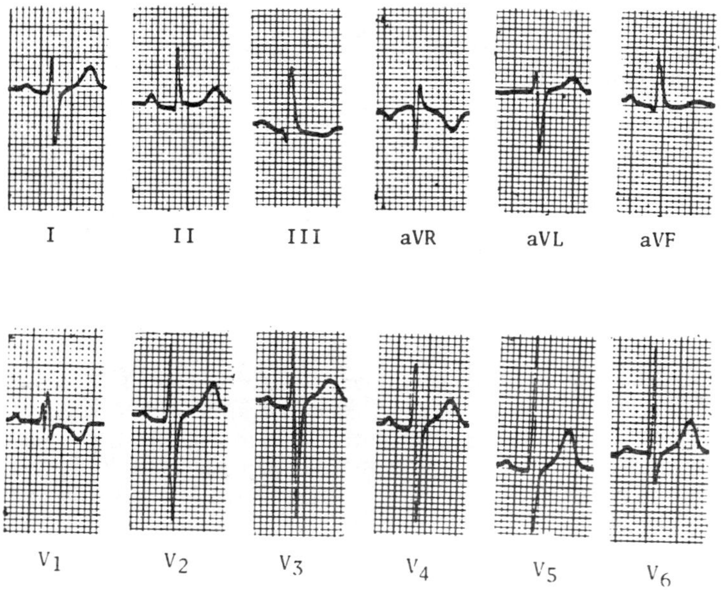

Figure 2–26 The presence of right axis deviation and a relative prominence of rightward-anterior forces as manifested by an increased R/S ratio in V_1 and prominent S in V_6 are indicative of mild right ventricular hypertrophy in a child with an atrial septal defect. Duration of the QRS complexes is normal so no conduction defect is involved.

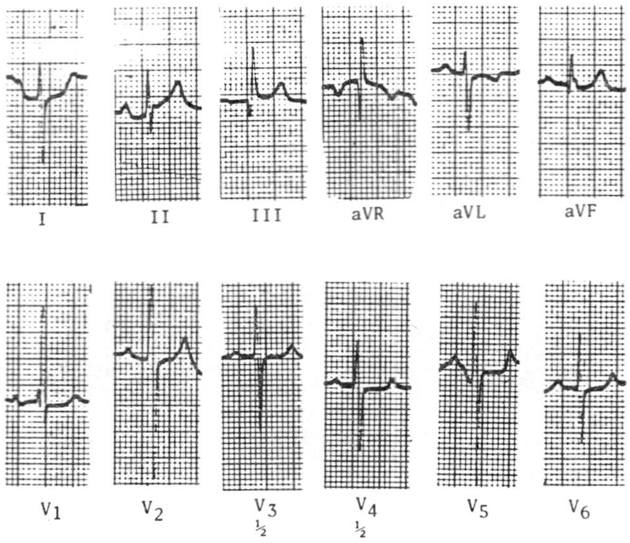

Figure 2-27 Severe right ventricular hypertrophy in an older child is indicated by right axis deviation, tall R wave in V_1, and deep S in V_6.

right ventricle such as atrial septal defects. However, this may also be seen with mild forms of pulmonic stenosis. The diastolic overload pattern closely resembles that seen in right bundle branch block (v.i.), but in the former the duration of the QRS complex never exceeds the limits of normal. It has been shown that the velocity of spread of the excitation wave is normal in contrast to right bundle branch block, and the slightly delayed depolarization of the right ventricle results from a longer pathway.

Left Ventricular Hypertrophy (LVH)

In the newborn and young infant ventricular hypertrophy is usually represented by a simple change in orientation of QRS forces resulting in a tracing which appears more mature than expected for age. Rightward and anterior forces are less prominent than normal. R-wave voltages in the left chest leads (and conversely S waves in the right chest) may exceed the upper limits of normal but frequently do not, and one simply sees decreased R/S ratios in lead V_1 (Fig. 2-28). In older children, left ventricular hypertrophy is recognized primarily by excessive leftward-posterior voltage (Fig. 2-29). This must be approached with caution since children, as mentioned previously, characteristically show prominent forces, and the interpreter should be careful about diagnosing left ventricular hypertrophy on voltage alone, particularly if it is only slightly excessive. The upper limits of normal used in Tables 2-5 and 2-6 represent two standard deviations from the mean. Thus, 2.5% of the normal population would be expected to be outside the limits. The common practice in adult cardiology of summing right-sided S waves and left-sided R waves and regarding a sum of more than 35 mm (3.5 mv) as being abnormal has little validity in childhood. Most children would have left ventricular hypertrophy by this criterion. In contrast to the situation with right ventricular hypertrophy, left ventricular hypertrophy does not normally produce left axis deviation. The direction of electrical forces in left ventricular hypertrophy shifts more posteriorly but only slightly more superiorly if at all. Left axis deviation in

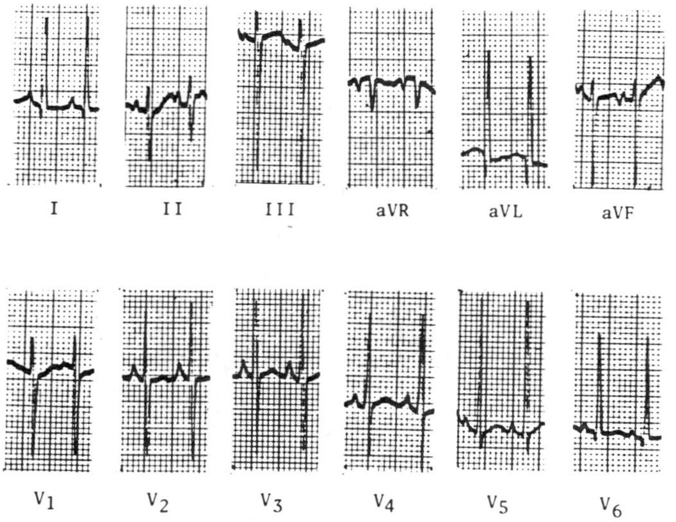

Figure 2–28 Electrocardiogram from a 4-day-old infant. QRS forces are directed leftward and posteriorly, indicative of left ventricular hypertrophy in this age group. Left axis deviation and somewhat prominent P waves are consistent with the known diagnosis of tricuspid atresia.

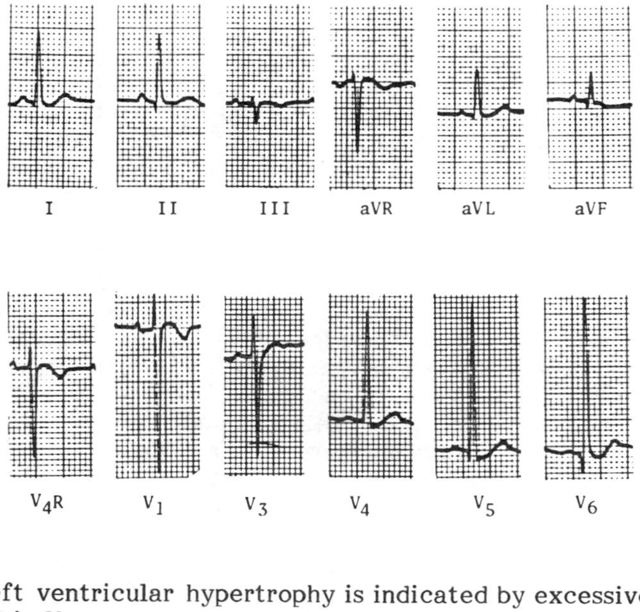

Figure 2–29 Left ventricular hypertrophy is indicated by excessively tall R wave in V_6 and deep S in V_1.

Table 2-7 Causes of Q Waves in V_1

Anteroseptal myocardial infarction
Malposition of interventricular septum
Ventricular inversion
Single ventricle
Conduction abnormalities
Left bundle branch block
Wolff-Parkinson-White syndrome type B
Severe right ventricular hypertrophy

the pediatric patient is the result of an abnormality of the sequence of spread of the excitation wave and not due to the increased muscle mass itself.

In lesions producing significant diastolic overloading of the left ventricle, there is a tendency toward prominent Q waves in leads V_5-V_6 due to septal hypertrophy, whereas repolarization changes (left ventricular strain) are uncommon in these conditions. However, there are far too many exceptions to this classification for it to have any value. It is best to state that congenital heart lesions producing volume overloading of the left ventricle such as a ventricular septal defect usually show normal ST segments and upright T waves in the left chest leads, and the presence of ST segment depression with inverted T waves should be viewed with suspicion as a possible indicator of an unrecognized associated abnormality.

Combined Ventricular Hypertrophy (CVH)

In many cases combined ventricular hypertrophy is sufficiently obvious as to be easily diagnosed, but at times the EKG manifestations may be very subtle even though hypertrophy of both ventricles is clearly demonstrated by other techniques. There is little difficulty if overt voltage criteria for both right ventricular and left ventricular hypertrophy are present. When difficulties exist, they occur because the forces due to hypertrophy of both ventricular walls cancel each other to an unusual degree. Frequently, one may recognize obvious hypertrophy of one ventricle with involvement of the other chamber indicated only by a relative prominence of forces in the opposite direction. Tall R waves in leads V_4R and V_1 diagnostic of right ventricular hypertrophy would normally be associated with deep S waves and a low R/S ratio in the left chest leads. If the latter are not seen, but rather left-sided QRS complexes appear relatively normal (particularly if the R-wave voltage exceeds 75% of the upper limits of normal), one should be suspicious that combined ventricular hypertrophy may be present. Frequently, extremely wide equiphasic QRS complexes are seen in the mid-precordial leads. The presence of such complexes with the total height of R + S waves exceeding 60 mm (6.0 mv) is highly suggestive of combined ventricular hypertrophy (Fig. 2-30). Such a wide complex may occasionally be seen in just one chest lead, and this by itself is not sufficient for a diagnosis of combined ventricular hypertrophy. One word of caution is in order. Occasionally a patient is encountered who demonstrates tall, pure R waves in all chest leads. This is more often the manifestation

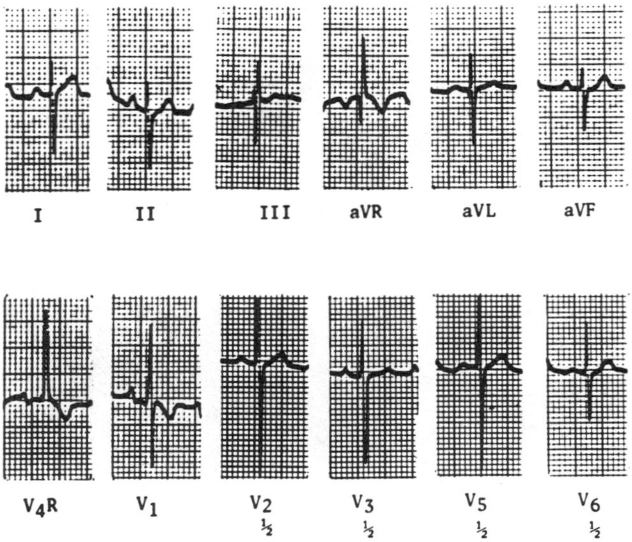

Figure 2–30 Combined ventricular hypertrophy. Right ventricular hypertrophy is clearly indicated by the tall right-sided R waves, together with a deep S in V_6. In addition, the tall R in V_6 suggests associated left ventricular hypertrophy, and confirmatory evidence is found in the wide equiphasic QRS complexes in V_2 - V_5.

of severely dilated and hypertrophied right ventricle than it is due to combined ventricular hypertrophy (Fig. 2–31).

Abnormalities in the Sequence of Ventricular Depolarization

This section will deal with alteration in the spread of the excitation wave through the conduction system distal to the bifurcation of the His bundle (i.e., through the bundle branches and Purkinje network) and with abnormal pathways by which the excitation wave reaches the ventricular myocardium. Abnormalities of conduction through the atrioventricular junction will be discussed in the chapter on arrhythmias.

Right Bundle Branch Block (RBBB)

Lesions producing a block in conduction through the right bundle branch result in a significant delay in depolarization of the right ventricular free wall. Depolarization of the interventricular septum and left ventricular wall is not altered so the initial and major forces are normal, but prominent terminal rightward and usually anterior forces are seen. The terminal forces are prolonged, and the duration of the QRS complex exceeds the upper limits of normal. In the right chest leads rsR' or rSR' complexes are recorded with wide S waves in V_6 (Fig. 2–32). In the limb leads, these terminal rightward forces may be directed superiorly, horizontally, or inferiorly. The T wave is usually directed opposite to the terminal vector. With the exception of a slurred S wave in lead I, abnormalities noted in the limb leads are variable in right bundle branch block.

It has been traditional to divide the EKG pattern of right bundle branch block into complete and incomplete forms. The latter was diagnosed on the basis of

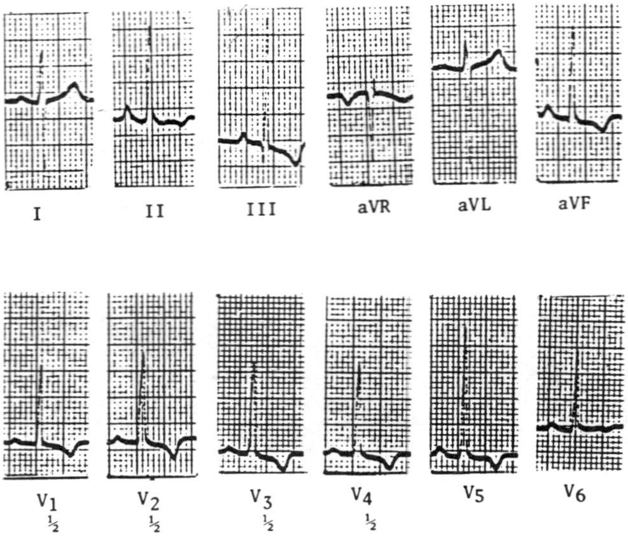

Figure 2–31 Electrocardiogram from a 26-year-old female with severe pulmonic stenosis. Right ventricular hypertrophy is clearly indicated by the tall right-sided R waves. The left chest leads might lead one to think that combined ventricular hypertrophy is present, but the absence of negative forces in any of the leads indicates that this unusual precordial lead pattern is due to a severely dilated and hypertrophied right ventricle rather than combined ventricular hypertrophy.

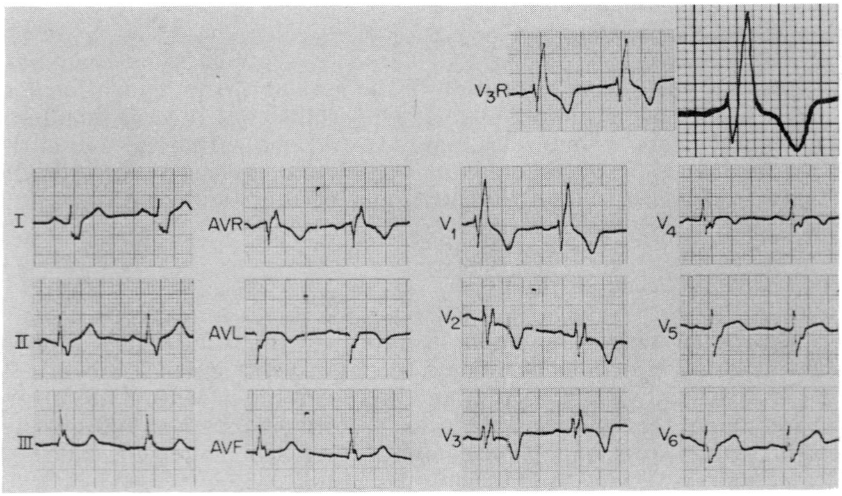

Figure 2–32 Right bundle branch block. The terminal rightward conduction delay is indicated by the wide, slurred R' deflections in V_3R and V_1 and the wide S waves in leads I and V_6. (Reproduced with permission from Moss AJ, Emmanouilides GC, Practical Pediatric Electrocardiography, 1973, J.B.Lippincott Co., Philadelphia.)

delayed rightward terminal forces where the total duration of the QRS complex did not exceed the upper limits of normal. We think that this is a confusing concept which may be inaccurate in implying the presence of a lesion of the right bundle branch when in reality the EKG pattern is due to other factors. For this reason we prefer to consider the presence of terminal rightward QRS forces (rsR' in V_1) as indicative of right ventricular conduction delay (RVCD), which is a broad category encompassing several different mechanisms (Table 2-8). A small terminal rightward deflection in V_1 may be seen in normal infants and children due to depolarization of the posterobasal left ventricle and superior interventricular septum; the r' does not usually exceed the initial rightward forces. Increased terminal rightward forces in the absence of minimal QRS duration are usually a manifestation of RVH (v.s.); prolonged QRS duration related to widened terminal forces is seen with RBBB and also following ventricle right ventriculotomy, with resultant delay in depolarization of the lateral RV free wall. The distinction between the various causes of RVCD on the surface electrogram is not always easy, and intracardiac electrocardiography (v.i.) may be required.

Left Bundle Branch Block (LBBB)

Complete left bundle branch block involving all fascicles of the left bundle branch system is extremely uncommon in children. It is probably noted most commonly following surgery for relief of subvalvular aortic stenosis. The entire QRS complex is affected, and in general there is a wide, slurred complex directed to the left and posteriorly (Fig. 2-33). Since primary innervation of the interventricular septum is derived from the left bundle branch distribution, septal activation is affected and usually progresses from right to left in left bundle branch block. Normal septal Q waves in the left chest leads are usually absent, and Q waves may be seen in the right chest leads. T waves are usually directed opposite to the major QRS forces and thus are inverted on the left.

Far more commonly seen are conduction delays involving only one fascicle of the left bundle branch system (Fig. 2-34). These are referred to as hemiblocks or fascicular blocks. The anterior fascicle is distributed primarily toward the base of the anterolateral papillary muscle of the left ventricle and from that point to the lateral free wall. If there is a delay in conduction through this division, the excitation wave first passes down the posterior fascicle to the diaphragmatic surface, and initial forces are directed rightward and inferiorly giving Q waves in leads I and aVL. The excitation wave then spreads over the free wall of the left ventricle, and the major QRS forces are directed leftward and superiorly with overall left axis deviation in the frontal plane of around -60°. QRS duration may vary from normal to slightly increased. The chest leads are not significantly altered.

Table 2-8 Etiology of Right Ventricular Conduction Delay

Normal variant
Right ventricular hypertrophy
Right bundle branch block
Ventriculotomy

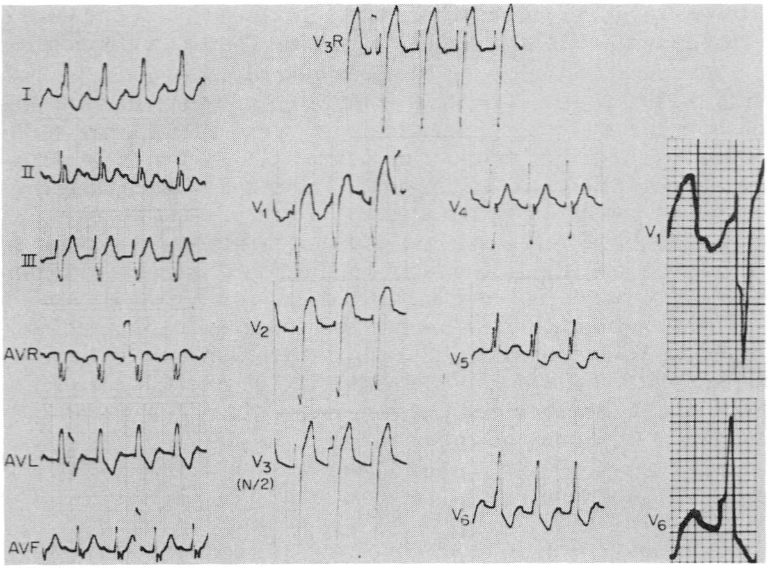

Figure 2–33 Left bundle branch block. QRS duration is prolonged with slurring of the entire complex and orientation in a leftward-posterior direction. (Reproduced with permission from Moss AJ, Emmanouilides GC, Practical Pediatric Electrocardiography, 1973, J.B. Lippincott Co., Philadelphia.)

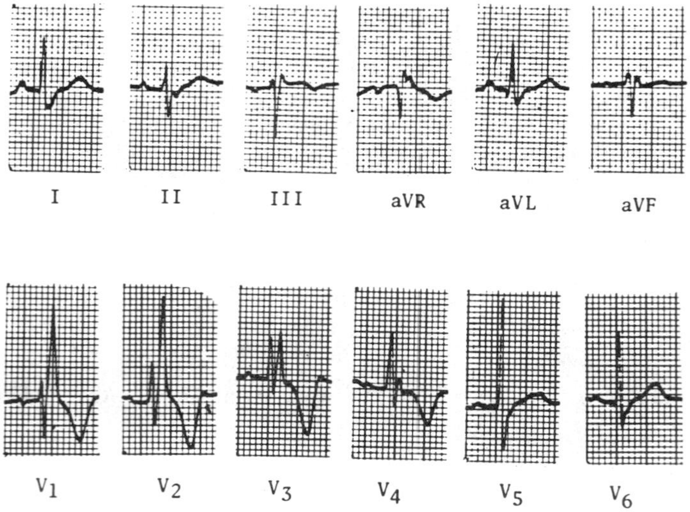

Figure 2–34 Bifascicular block. The presence of left axis deviation with initial forces directed rightward and inferiorly (small Q waves in leads I and aVL) indicate left anterior fascicular block. In addition, a typical pattern of right bundle branch block is noted.

Conduction delay involving the anterior fascicle may occur following surgery, especially closure of a ventricular septal defect. The identical EKG pattern is associated with several congenital heart defects, including endocardial cushion defects and tricuspid atresia. Available evidence suggests that the cause is an abnormal course of the conduction system rather than slowing of conduction velocity.

Left posterior fascicular block is less commonly noted. The excitation wave initially activates the free wall producing initial forces (up to 20 msec in duration in the adult) directed leftward and superiorly, generally in the vicinity of -45° with the major portion of the QRS complex directed rightward and inferiorly. An overall right axis deviation usually around $+120^{\circ}$ is noted.

Combined Bundle Branch Blocks

In general combined bundle branch blocks are uncommon in children. Depending upon the degree of involvement, blocks in both the right and left bundle branch system could produce so-called complete or 3° atrioventricular block which will be discussed in the chapter on arrhythmias. In the pediatric age group, complete AV block is usually the result of disease of the AV node rather than the bundle branch system. One combination is worthy of comment as it is occasionally seen in the postoperative patient. After extensive intracardiac surgery, particularly for repair of tetralogy of Fallot, a pattern of right bundle branch block and left anterior fascicular block may be seen (Fig. 2-34). This association is not difficult to recognize since the former affects the chest leads and the latter the limb leads. If this pattern is truly due to damage to both the proximal right bundle branch and the anterior fascicle of the left bundle branch, it is of some concern as there is an increased incidence of progressing to complete AV block or sudden death. It is important in this case to differentiate proximal right bundle branch block from that resulting from more peripheral interruption as with extensive ventriculotomy since the latter has far less serious implications. Intracardiac studies of the conduction system may be necessary to make this differentiation. The same pattern is also commonly encountered in association with endocardial cushion defects where again it appears to be related to the cause of the conduction system.

Bundle Branch Block and Ventricular Hypertrophy

In general, the diagnosis of ventricular hypertrophy is rendered more difficult in the presence of bundle branch block as the criteria for the diagnosis of hypertrophy are based on a normal sequence of excitation of the ventricles. Since left bundle branch produces a delay involving the entire QRS complex, ventricular hypertrophy is not generally recognized in the presence of left bundle branch block. Some workers have reported detecting greater rightward direction in the major QRS forces when right ventricular hypertrophy coexists with left bundle branch block. This was described utilizing vectorcardiography (v.i.) and really cannot be recognized on the scalar electrocardiogram.

With some reservation and caution certain comments may be made regarding ventricular hypertrophy in the presence of right bundle branch block since the latter does not alter the initial portion of the QRS complex. Such evaluation is better made with vectorcardiography, but changes may be recognized on a scalar electrocardiogram as well. The presence of associated right ventricular hypertrophy cannot be reliably diagnosed on the basis of the magnitude of the terminal rightward forces since the delay in right ventricular depolarization results in unmasking these forces. In other words, forces due to right ventricular depolarization are not opposed by simultaneous left ventricular depolarization, and in some instances of pure right bundle branch block the terminal rightward forces may be very prominent. However, right ventricular hypertrophy may alter the initial forces, directing them abnormally to the right and anterior for age. This would produce a pattern of wide, slurred pure R wave (rR' pattern) in lead V_1 with the slurred S wave in the left chest leads showing more depth than in pure right bundle branch block (Fig. 2-35).

There are a number of exceptions to this statement, and totally upright complexes in the right chest leads in pure right bundle branch block may be seen. That the concept has some validity is borne out by patients with tetralogy of Fallot who undergo open heart surgery. These patients demonstrate right ventricular hypertrophy preoperatively and usually develop a right bundle branch block pattern at surgery. In the immediate postoperative period a wide rR' complex is seen in lead V_1. As right ventricular hypertrophy recedes following surgery, there is gradual development of an S wave which increases in depth until a typical rSR' configuration of pure right bundle branch block is seen. Left ventricular hypertrophy in the

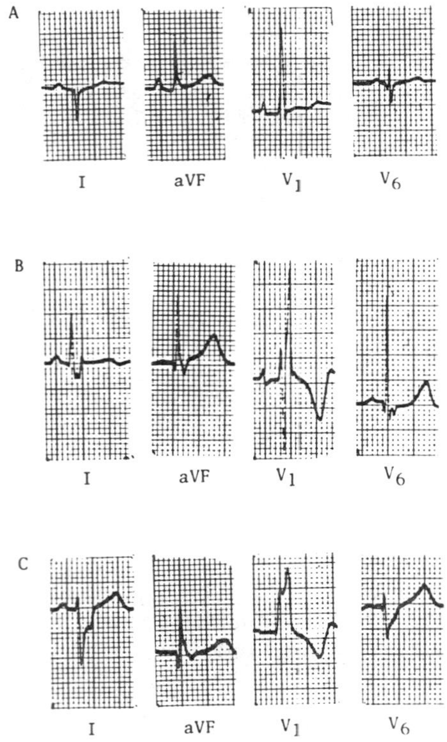

Figure 2–35 (A) Right axis deviation and right ventricular hypertrophy in a child with tetralogy of Fallot. (B) Postoperative tracing from the same child reveals the presence of right bundle branch block and a movement of the frontal plane axis to within normal limits. There is no longer any evidence of right ventricular hypertrophy. (C) In contrast, this postoperative tracing from a 4-year-old child with tetralogy shows that in addition to right bundle branch block, the initial QRS forces remain deviated strongly rightward and anteriorly, a finding suggestive but not diagnostic of right ventricular hypertrophy.

presence of right bundle branch block may be recognized on the basis of excessive leftward and posterior forces as previously described. Here again caution is indicated since these forces may be prominent due to the unmasking effect of delayed right ventricular depolarization. Minimal increases in leftward-posterior forces should not be taken as clearly abnormal.

Preexcitation

As the name inplies, the various forms of preexcitation are the result of premature activation of ventricular myocardium via an aberrant pathway. These pathways may enter or leave the normal conduction system at one of several points (Fig. 2-36) or may be totally separate, connecting atrial and ventricular myocardium directly. In either event, there is partial or complete bypass of the AV node. The most commonly seen form of preexcitation is the Wolff-Parkinson-White (WPW) pattern which results from an excitation wave passing from atrium directly to ventricular myocardium by way of a bypass tract known as bundle of Kent. This bridge of specialized tissue is more frequently located on the posterior aspect of the heart on either the left or right side. The major EKG manifestations are a short PR interval and slurring of the upstroke of the QRS complex known as the delta wave, which usually takes off at or very shortly after the end of the P waves so that the shortening of the PR interval is due to encroachment on the PR segment by the delta wave. The QRS complex is widened by the presence of the delta wave, but the total interval from onset of the P wave to the end of QRS complex (the PJ interval) is normal. The T wave is usually opposite in direction to the major portion of the QRS complex.

Although exceptions exist, WPW patterns are generally divided into two groups, depending upon the direction of the delta wave. If the delta wave is directed strongly anteriorly and is upright in all chest leads, the pattern is referred as type A (Fig. 2-37). In general the major QRS forces are also directed strongly anteriorly, giving a false picture of right ventricular hypertrophy. In contrast, type-B WPW (Fig. 2-38) is characterized by a delta wave directed leftward and somewhat posteriorly, generally manifesting itself as an initial negative deflection in the right chest leads, but positive in the left. Again the QRS forces are usually directed in a manner similar to the delta wave, and a pattern of pseudo-left ventricular hypertrophy may be produced. It should be noted, however, that because of the anomalous pathway of entry into the myocardium, the diagnosis of ventricular hypertrophy in the presence of WPW is unreliable.

Frequently, patients may demonstrate this type of preexcitation only intermittently and in some cases may show a bigeminy pattern with a normal beat followed by an aberrantly conducted one. The generally held concept is that the excitation wave enters the ventricle by two pathways: the anomalous bundle and the normal conduction system. Depolarization of the ventricle may be achieved by two different routes in the same beat producing a fusion beat. The abnormal contour of the QRS complex will vary, depending on how much of the ventricle is depolarized by the wave front which enters through the anomalous bundle.

The preexcitation pattern would be of academic interest only were it not for the fact that at least 40% of these patients have paroxysmal tachyarrhythmias, usually supraventricular. The characteristic EKG pattern associated with tachyarrhythmias is known as the Wolff-Parkinson-White syndrome. Another type of preexcitation pattern is manifested soley by an extremely short PR interval. The P wave and QRS complex are normal. When associated with paroxysmal tachyarrhythmias, it is known as a Lown-Ganong-Levine syndrome. This is thought to be due to the presence of fibers which bypass the AV node and permit early entry into the His-Purkinje system.

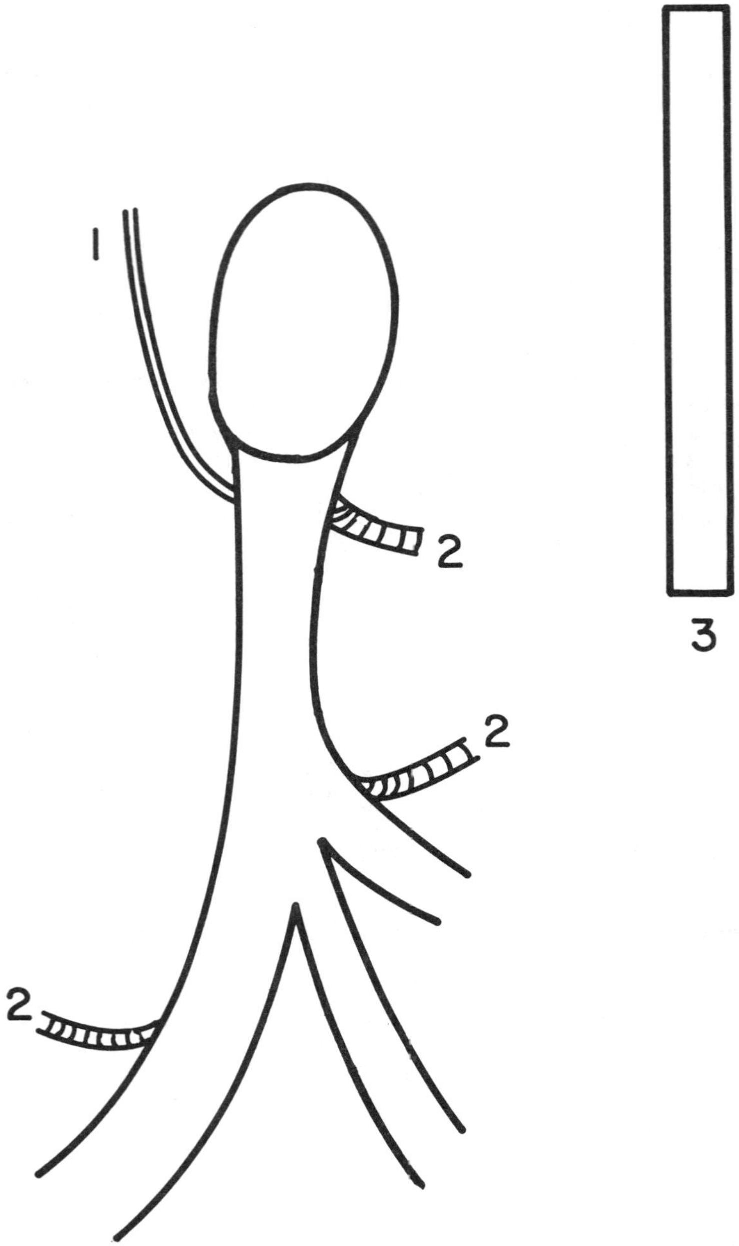

Figure 2-36 Bypass tracts in preexcitation. 1 - fibers from the atrium entering the bundle of His directly, bypassing the AV node (James fibers). 2 - Maheim fibers which are postulated to exit prematurely from the conduction system at any one of several locations providing a path for premature ventricular excitation. 3 - Bundle of Kent connecting arterial and ventricular myocardium directly. These may be located on either the left or right side.

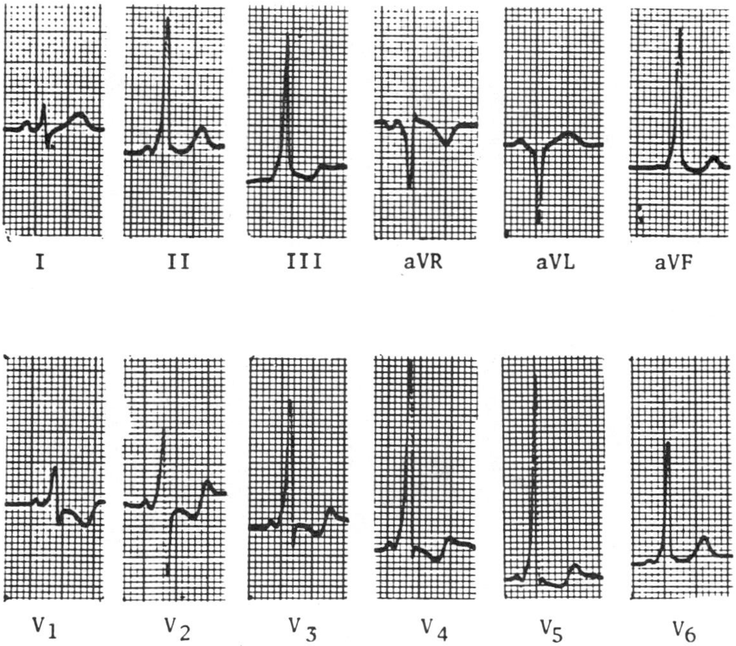

Figure 2-37 Preexcitation of the Wolff-Parkinson-White type. Note the extremely short PR interval with widening of the QRS complex due to a slurring of the initial portion (delta wave). The delta wave is directed anteriorly (upright in all chest leads) consistent with type A - WPW.

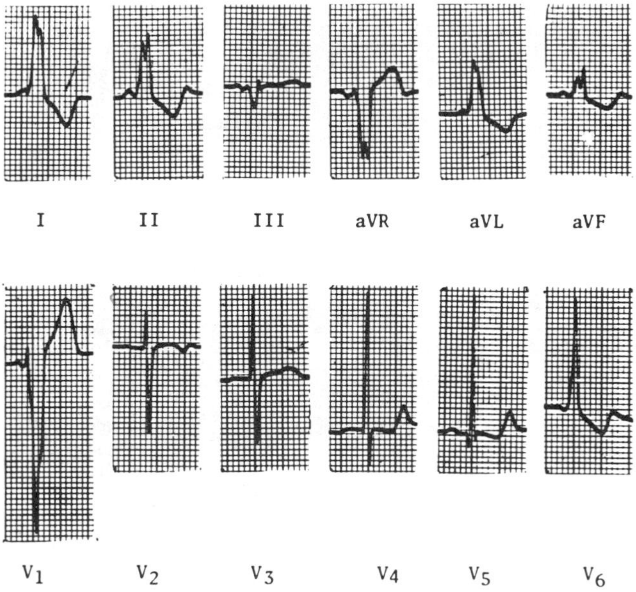

Figure 2-38 Wolff-Parkinson-White, type B. The delta wave is directed further leftwards than in the preceding figure and is at least partially negative in lead V_1. Note the sudden resumption of normal conduction in leads V_2-V_5 with a return to preexcitation in lead V_6.

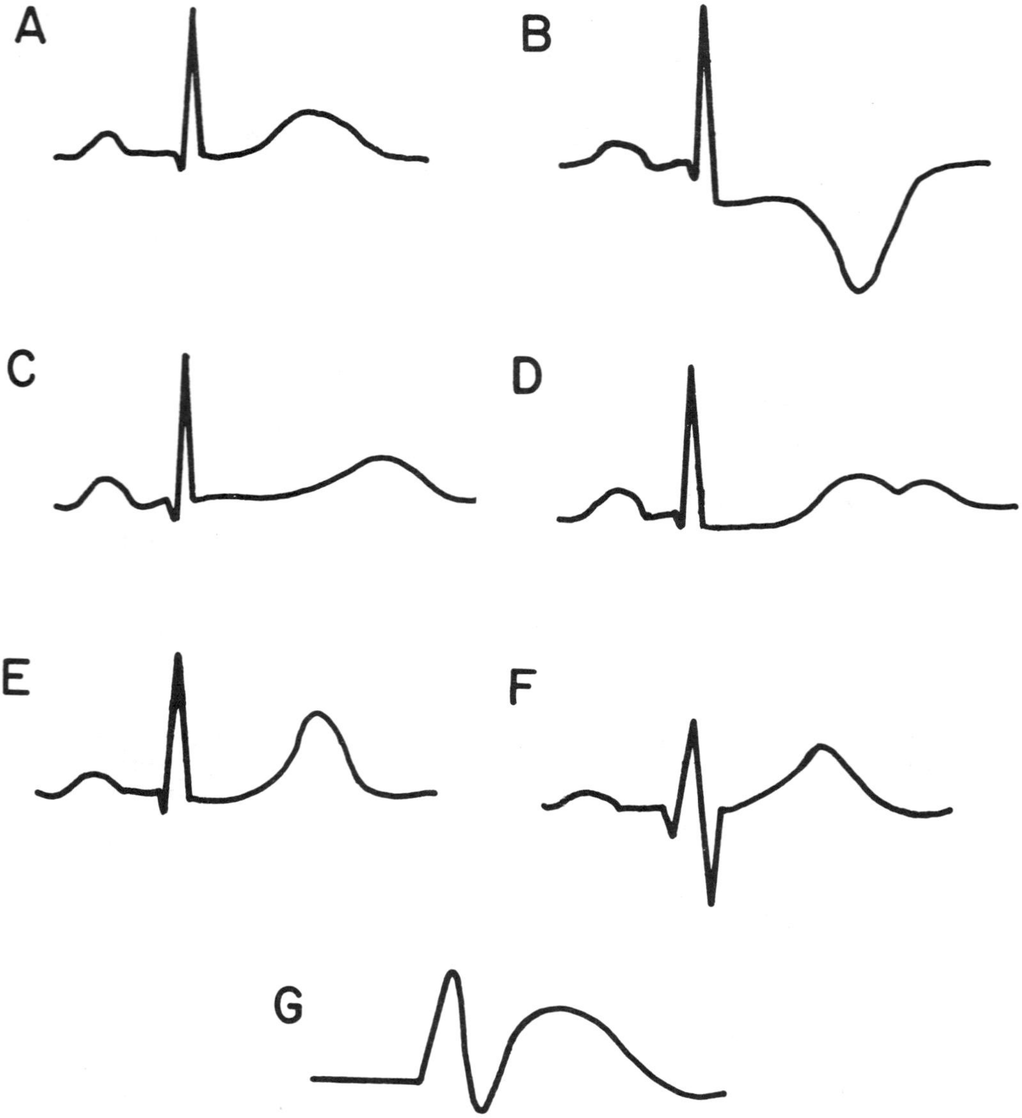

Figure 2-39 (A) Normal electrocardiogram cycle. (B) Myocardial ischemia. There is horizontal depression of the ST segment and a prominently inverted T wave. (C) Hypocalcemia. The QT interval is prolonged due to an increase in the ST segment. (D) Hypokalemia. The ST segment is slightly depressed, and a U wave is seen as a secondary positive hump on the down slope of the T wave. (E-G) Progressive degrees of hyperkalemia. Tall symmetrical T waves are seen with mild elevation of serum potassium. When the level exceeds 7 mEq/L, there is flattening of the P waves and prolongation of both the PR and QRS duration. Above 9 mEq/L, P waves are not seen and the QRS-T complex resembles a sinusoidal waveform.

Primary Repolarization Changes (Fig. 2-39)

In addition to abnormalities of ST segment or T waves associated with ventricular hypertrophy or disorders in the sequence of excitation of the ventricles, abnormalities of repolarization may be seen in a number of other conditions which may or may not affect the rest of the EKG complex. Basically these conditions can be divided into four main groups: ischemia, drug effects, metabolic effects, and inflammation.

Ischemia

In the presence of acute myocardial ischemia, the ST segment is typically depressed 1 mm or more below the baseline and is either horizontal or downward slanting. The T wave is generally inverted in these leads. These changes are noted in the leads reflecting the area of ischemic myocardium, and reciprocal elevation of the ST segment may be seen in leads on the opposite side. The EKG abnormalities reflect an imbalance between coronary arterial perfusion and myocardial demand and may be seen not only in primary abnormalities of the coronary arterial tree but also in severe tachyarrhythmias where coronary flow may be compromised or during exercise in the presence of significant hypertrophy when myocardial wall tension interferes with adequate perfusion.

Drug Effects

Digitalis

The typical EKG pattern seen in patients on various forms of digitalis consists of a shortening of the QT interval, together with sagging of the ST segment, often pulling down the initial portion of the T wave. There may be slight depression of the J point, but this is minimal. These EKG changes reflect the presence of digitalis in the myocardium and are neither indicative of toxicity nor adequate digitalization. Some prolongation of the atrioventricular conduction time manifested as an increase in the PR interval may be seen, primarily due to the increased vagal effect of this group of drugs. The problem of digitalis toxicity will be considered in a later chapter.

Quinidine

When present in excessive amounts, quinidine may produce widening of the QRS complex and T wave with increased QT interval. The amplitude of the T wave may be depressed.

Procainamide

EKG effects are similar to those described under quinidine.

Propranolol

There are no specific EKG changes due to propranolol. Because of the beta-adrenergic blockade which it produces, there may be a slowing of the cardiac rate and some prolongation of the atrioventricular conduction.

Metabolic Effects

Hyperkalemia

Earliest demonstrated changes are an increase in amplitude of T wave with peaking. As serum levels of potassium increase, the PR interval is lengthened, and the QRS complex widened. At severe levels of hyperkalemia, the P wave disappears, and the widened QRS complex and T wave resemble a sinusoidal waveform.

Hypokalemia

In contrast to hyperkalemia, low serum potassium levels produce a broad T wave of low amplitude with prominent U waves. These are low-amplitude deflections which follow the T wave. The QT interval may be lengthened and QRS amplitude decreased. At the extremes of hypokalemia, the ST segment may be depressed and the T wave inverted.

Hypercalcemia

In hypercalcemia the QT interval is decreased, and there is a tendency toward premature beats and occasional runs of ventricular tachycardia.

Hypocalcemia

In hypocalcemia the QT interval is prolonged due to lengthening of the ST segment. The T wave is unaffected.

Inflammatory Diseases

EKG abnormalities in pericarditis and myocarditis are frequently nonspecific and may consist of diffuse T-wave flattening with little else. Occasionally patients with acute myocarditis will show some generalized diminution in QRS amplitude. Approximately 25% of patients with acute pericarditis will evolve a typical sequence of EKG changes showing initially diffuse ST segment elevation noted primarily in the precordial and leftward limb leads. T waves are usually not affected at this point, and the pattern must be differentiated from a normal variant known as early repolarization in which the J point is somewhat elevated but the ST segment generally sags back close to the baseline before rising at the onset of a T wave. The entire ST segment is significantly elevated in patients with pericarditis. Around the end of the first week of illness, the ST segments have generally again become isoelectric, and T waves have inverted. T-wave inversion progresses over the next 3-4 weeks with the inverted waves achieving greater amplitude. The pattern then remains stable over the next 1-2 months, following which there is a gradual return to normal.

Vectorcardiography

Although traditional methods of displaying the vectorcardiogram (VCG) suggest a totally new technique of studying cardiac electrical activity, this is basically a simple extension of the principles just discussed. As previously mentioned, the EKG is a scalar record depicting only the magnitude of electrical forces as projected on a given lead axis. The horizontal dimension on the EKG record is time. A sense of direction is inferred from the presumed orientation of the various lead axes. If the deflections of the standard EKG were sliced up into a given number of points, the forces at each point of time could be represented as a vector in both the frontal and horizontal planes by placing a dot on either lead axis coordinate system in such a location that the projection on the lead axes reflected the magnitude of forces at that time. If an arrow is then drawn from the center of the coordinate system to that point, the same information is depicted as a vector with a given magnitude and defined direction (Fig. 2-40).

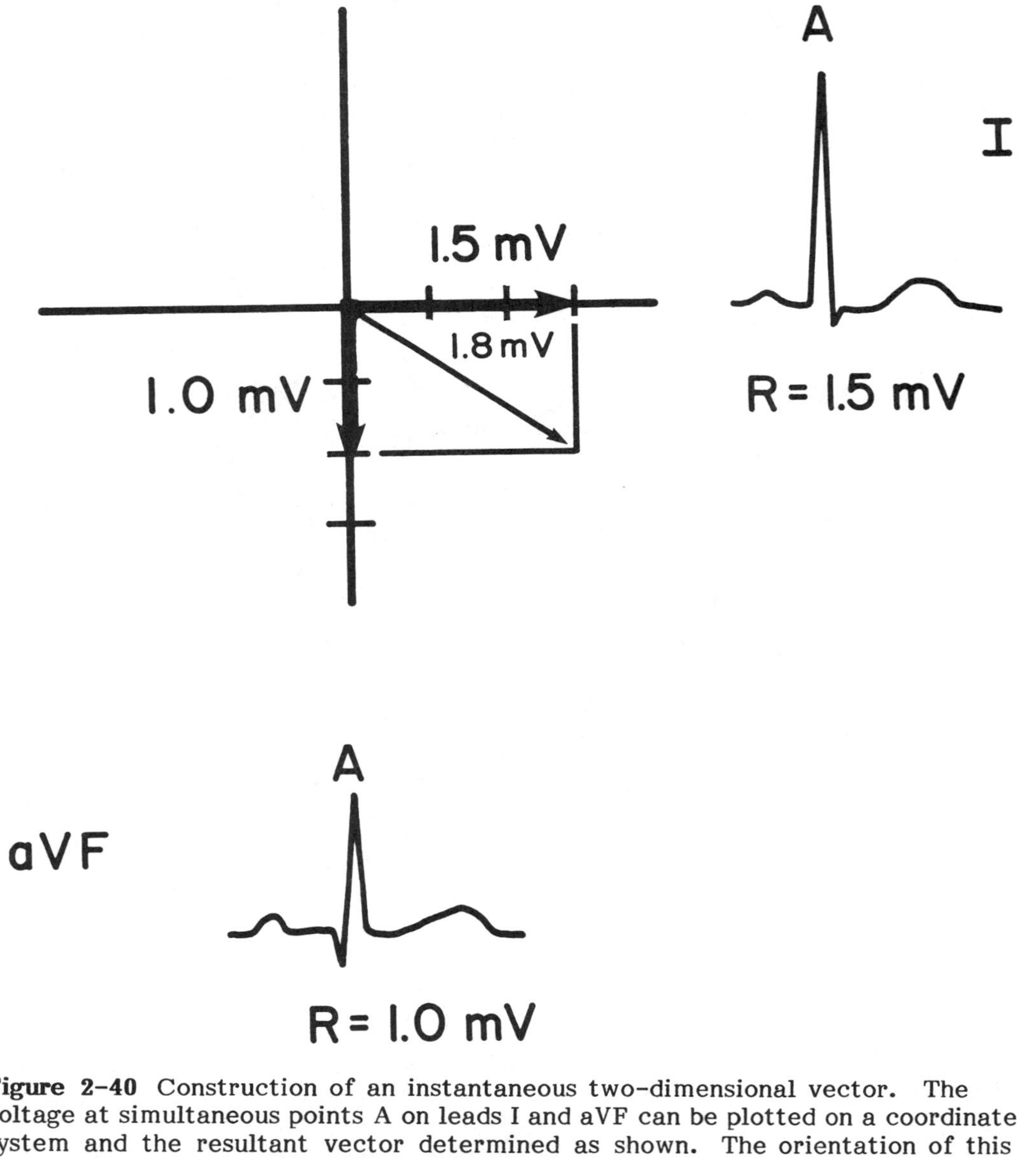

Figure 2-40 Construction of an instantaneous two-dimensional vector. The voltage at simultaneous points A on leads I and aVF can be plotted on a coordinate system and the resultant vector determined as shown. The orientation of this vector could be indicated by the angle between it and either lead axis and its magnitude = $\sqrt{X^2 + Y^2}$ where X equals the voltage in lead I and Y equals the voltage in aVF.

Three scalar electrocardiographic leads are recorded. Since the simplest type of coordinate system on which to construct any type of graphic representation is one in which the coordinates are perpendicular, various types of lead systems have been devised in an effort to achieve recordings along three axes which are orthogonal (i.e., mutually perpendicular). Theoretical considerations of these lead systems are beyond the scope of this book, and the interested reader is referred to the references at the end of the chapter. In our institution, we use the Frank lead system which has the advantage of simplicity and ease of application with only eight electrodes being required (Fig. 2-41). The three leads recorded are referred to as x, y, and z, and their orientation and polarity are shown in Fig. 2-42. Combination of any two leads allows the information to be depicted in one of three planes (Fig. 2-43). For example, Fig. 2-44 shows the magnitude of electrical forces recorded simultaneously in leads x and y. A vector can be drawn from the center of the lead axes to a point on the frontal plane, such that the projections of this vector on the two leads are of the correct magnitude.

This is the process by which the recording device constructs the standard loop presentation. At a number of equal intervals of time, which are dependent upon recording device utilized, the magnitude of deflection in each of a pair of leads is

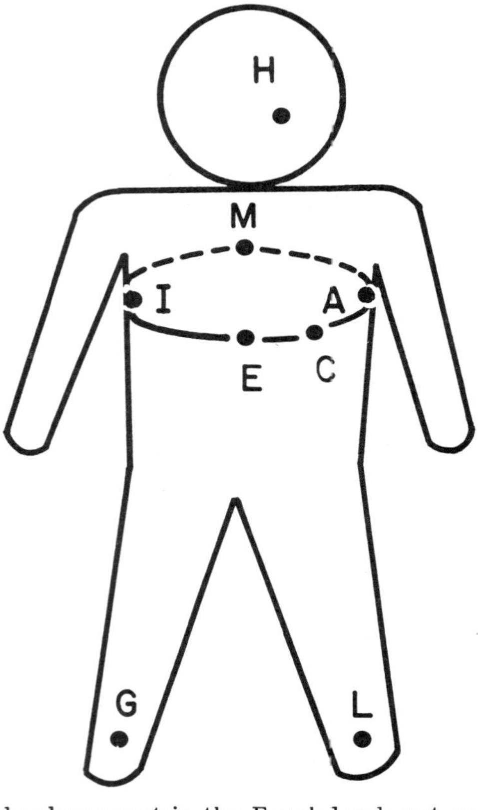

Figure 2–41 Electrode placement in the Frank lead system. The E electrode is placed directly over the sternum at the level of the anterior fifth intercostal space. Electrodes A, M, and I are located at the same transverse thoracic level in the left midaxillary, midspinal, and right midaxillary lines, respectively. Electrode C is also at the same level halfway between E and A. The H electrode is placed on the head or neck.

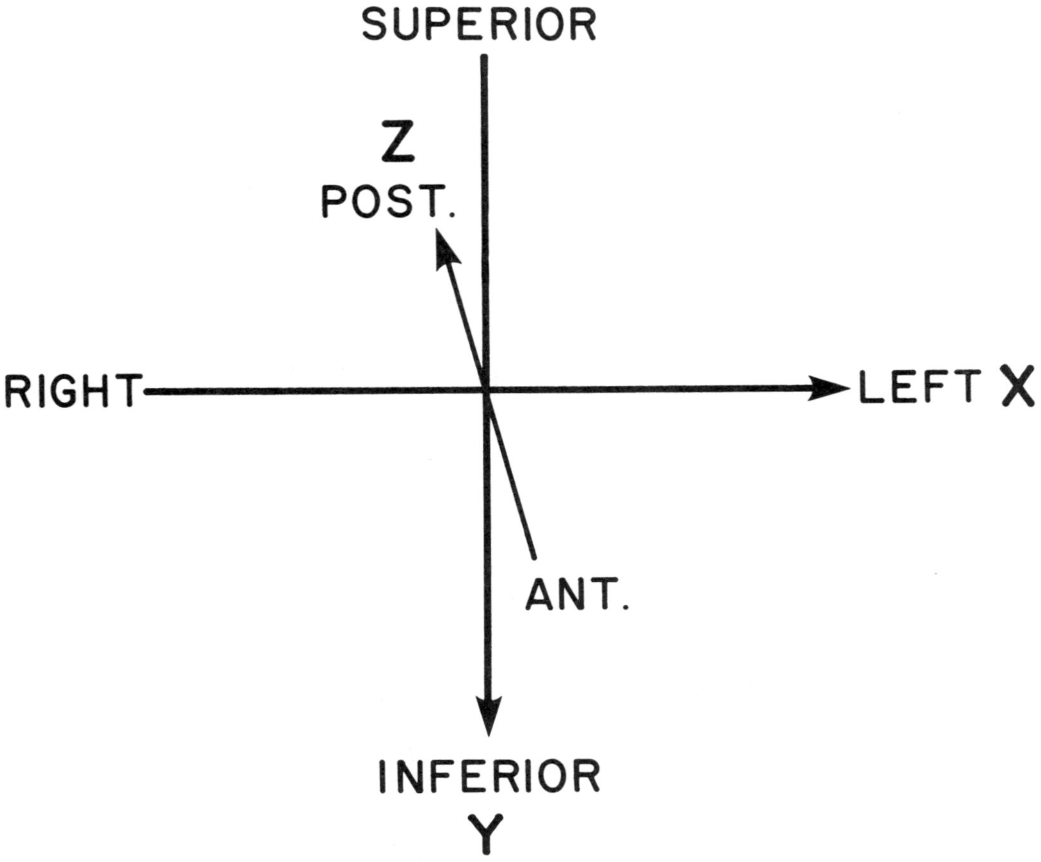

Figure 2–42 Spatial orientation of Frank leads X, Y, and Z.

put together to yield the appropriate resultant vector in the plane under consideration. With planar recording techniques this vector is usually characterized utilizing polar coordinates, that is, as magnitude (length) and direction, with the latter described by the angle of deviation from the horizontal axis of that plane. This is done for a number of sequential time points. Multiple instantaneous vectors are produced radiating out from the center from the lead axes as in Fig. 2-45.

If a loop is drawn starting at the center and the axes (E point) connecting the tip of each of these vectors and returning back to the E point, we then have the usual loop presentation seen in vectorcardiography. Most recording devices interrupt this loop at a number of given time points which are controlled by the device. There are a number of conventions for altering the shape of the instantaneous marks so that a directional sequence of change can be ascertained. This is referred to as the direction of loop rotation. With appropriate calibrations, the magnitude of the vector at each time point is measured as the distance along the line connecting the E point with a point on the loop, and the direction of forces at that point are determined by measuring the angle between that line and the positive portion of the horizontal axis (i.e., the x axis in the frontal and horizontal planes and the z axis in the sagittal plane). The major (i.e., largest) vector in a given

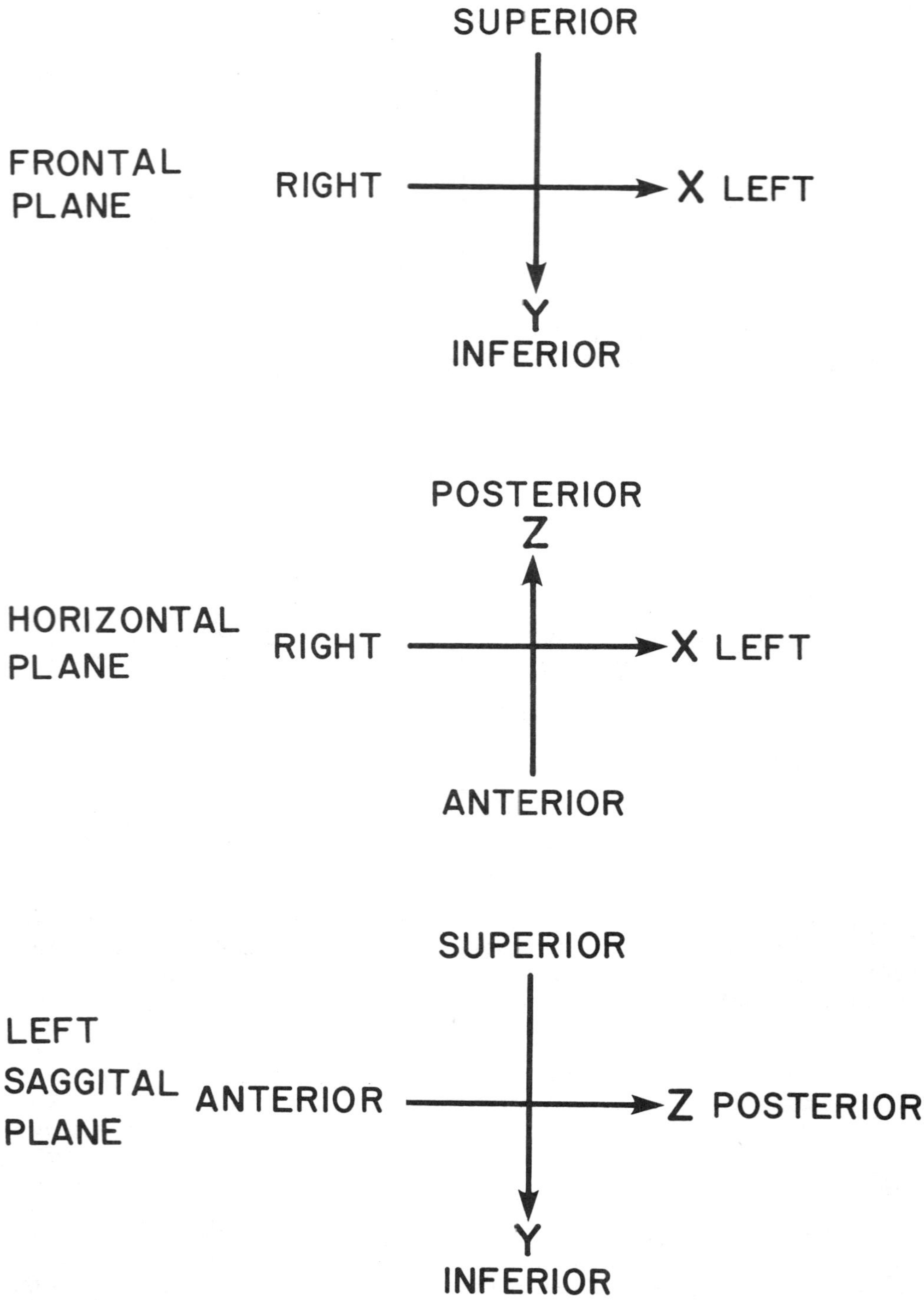

Figure 2-43 Two-dimensional (planar) recording is achieved by combining two of the three scalar leads in the manner shown. Spatial orientation of the three planes is as indicated.

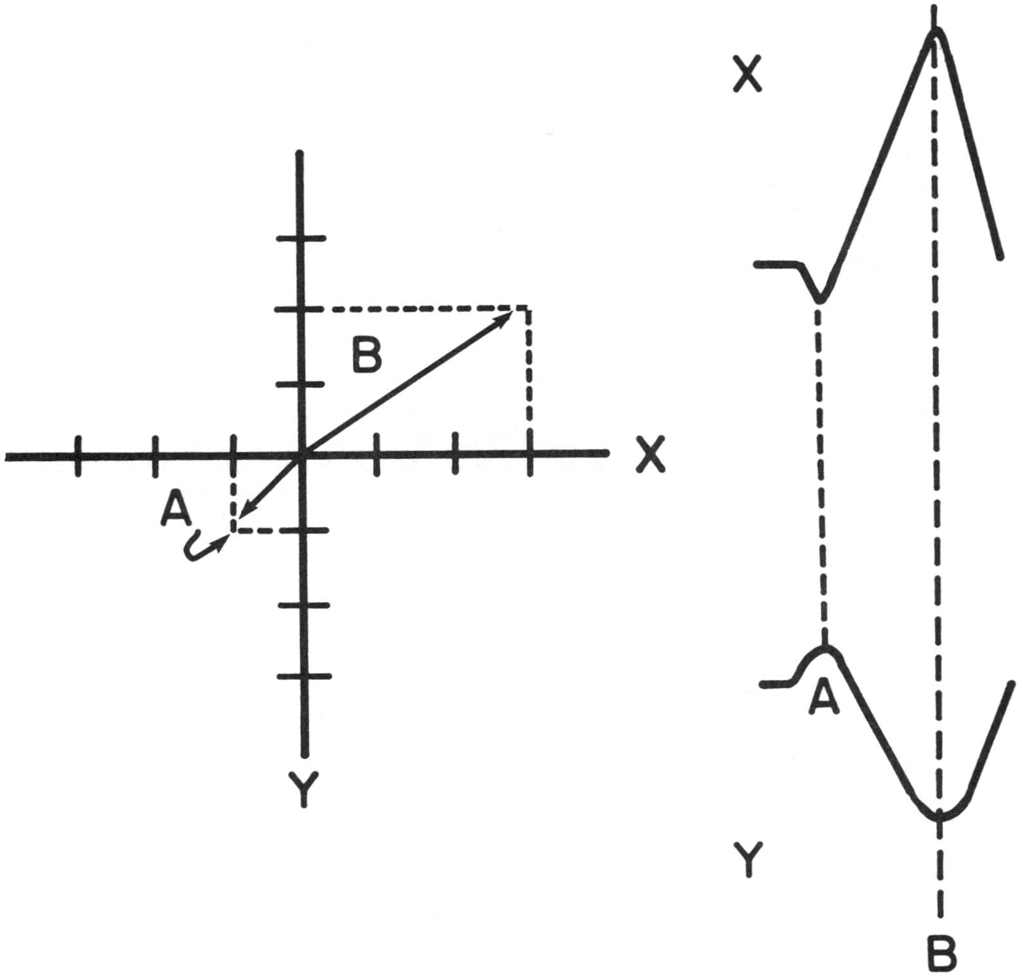

Figure 2-44 Vectors A and B display the magnitude and direction of electrical forces at two sequential time points in simultaneously recorded leads X and Y. This frontal plane display indicates that the initial QRS forces are directed to the right and inferiorly, whereas the major forces are oriented leftwards and superiorly.

plane usually reflects the largest deflection on the scalar leads, as illustrated in Fig. 2-46.

The magnitude and direction of this vector are of great importance in the diagnosis of ventricular hypertrophy. The average direction of electrical forces (the mean electrical axis) is represented by the vector which divides the area enclosed within the loop in half. This may or may not correspond to the major vector, depending upon the particular loop configuration. In addition to more precisely detecting the direction of cardiac electrical forces, the VCG offers the following advantages over scalar techniques:

1. The magnitude of forces at far shorter time intervals can be evaluated.
2. The sequence of change of direction of forces is clearly shown.

3. Rate of the directional change can be evaluated as an approximation to the velocity of the spread of the excitation wave through the myocardium.

Since with most recording systems only one cardiac cycle is recorded at a time, vectorcardiography is of relatively little value in the evaluation of arrhythmias.

Ideally, of course, one would like to study electrical forces generated by the heart in three dimensions, but appropriate devices for this representation do not exist. With computer assistance it is easy to calculate the magnitude and orientation of each of the instantaneous vectors in three-dimensional space (v.i.).

The Normal Vectorcardiogram

Although the magnitude of forces is of great importance, much information can be gained by simple inspection of the three loops. As the information obtained increases with more sophisticated techniques, so does the complexity of tables of normal values. For children, these tables now occupy many pages and are far too extensive to be included in a book of this type. The interested reader is referred to the work by Liebman cited in the bibliography. In our discussion we will concern ourselves primarily with alteration in loop configuration.

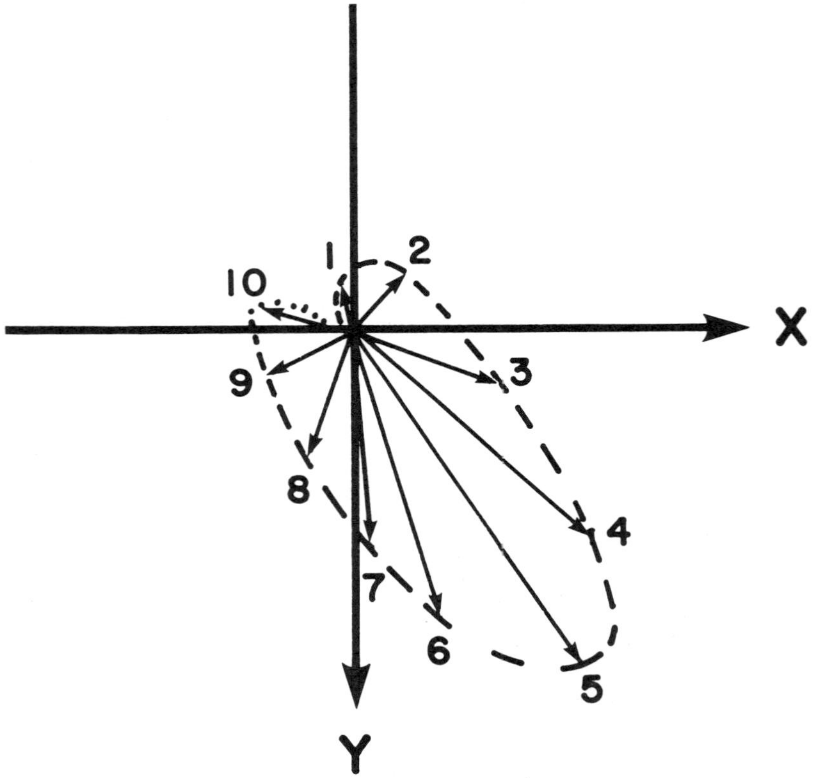

Figure 2–45 Sequential vectors for multiple time points throughout the QRS complex can be constructed as illustrated in the preceding figure. Connecting the tips of these vectors in the manner shown produces the typical vectorcardiogram loop display.

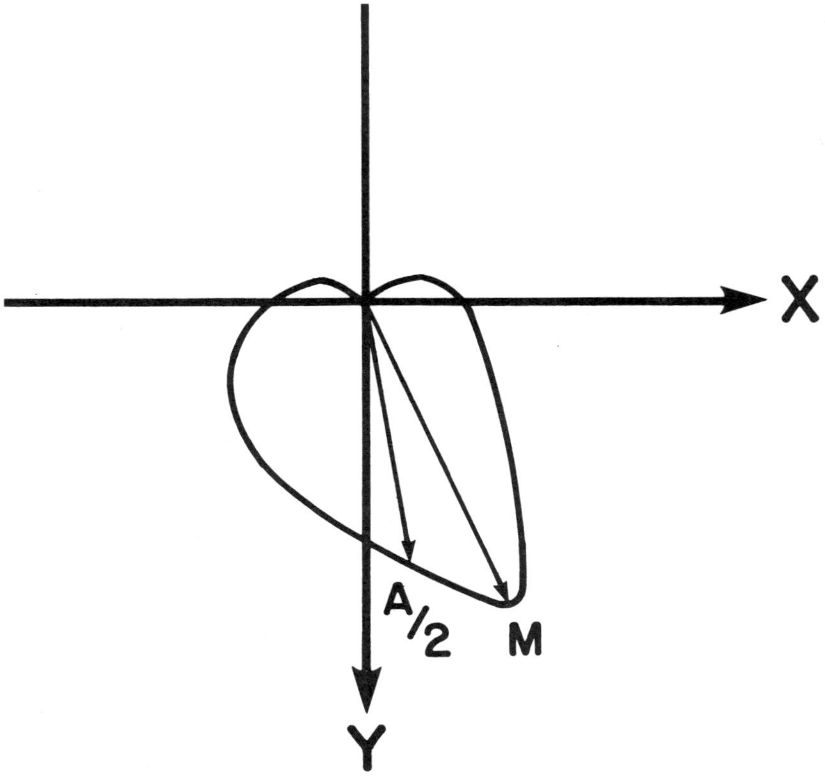

Figure 2-46 The major (i.e., largest) vector in this frontal plane loop is indicated by M. The mean electrical axis is represented by the vector dividing the area enclosed by the loop in half (A/2).

As would be expected, the P loop is directed inferiorly, anteriorly, and to the left in a normal individual. The QRS loop shows the same sequential age-related changes as are seen on the scalar EKG (see Fig. 2-19—2-22). Initial forces due to septal depolarization are directed anteriorly, superiorly, and slightly to the right in normal individuals of all ages. The major forces are also directed anteriorly and rightward in the newborn infant, and the sequence of loop rotation is clockwise in the horizontal plane (Fig. 2-19). With advancing age the loop shifts progressively to the left with the horizontal direction of rotation becoming a figure-of-eight (initially counterclockwise, terminally clockwise). In older children and adults the major portion of the QRS loop lies in the left, posterior, inferior quadrant, and the horizontal loop rotates entirely counterclockwise (Fig. 2-22). Timing marks are spaced more closely at the beginning and end of the loop, reflecting a slower spread of the excitation wave at these times. Terminal forces not uncommonly are again slightly rightward but are usually posterior rather than anterior and are directed superiorly in the frontal plane.

The T loop like the P loop is less well understood than that due to QRS forces. Like the scalar T wave, it is directed to the left and anteriorly at birth and moves progressively toward the left, posterior quadrant in the first week of life. After early childhood its orientation is far more variable.

Ventricular Hypertrophy

Right Ventricular Hypertrophy

In the newborn infant, right ventricular hypertrophy is again a diagnosis on the basis of increased magnitude of forces which are basically normally directed (Fig. 2-47A). In the older child, progressive change in the direction of forces occurs with increasing severity. Mild right ventricular hypertrophy may be manifested solely by some increase in terminal forces which are directed to the right and usually posteriorly as shown in Fig. 2-47B.

As the severity of hypertrophy increases, major forces are directed progressively toward the right and anterior (Fig. 2-47C). Initial forces generally remain normal, and the loop begins to rotate in a normal counterclockwise manner and swings back in a clockwise direction toward the right. In more severe hypertrophy, initial forces are also altered and are directed to the left and frequently posteriorly so that the entire loop rotates clockwise with major forces toward the right and anterior (Fig. 2-47D). Repolarization abnormalities are reflected in a T loop which is directed opposite to the QRS.

Left Ventricular Hypertrophy

The newborn will manifest his left ventricular hypertrophy by relative deficiency of rightward forces and a QRS loop oriented further to the left and more posteriorly than is normal for age. The initial forces remain normal and loop rotation is counterclockwise (Fig. 2-48). In the older child the diagnosis is based on increased magnitude of the major vector, which is often deviated somewhat more posteriorly as hypertrophy increases in severity. With severe hypertrophy there may be some deviation of initial forces more posteriorly with progressively greater magnitude of the major vector. Horizontal loop rotation is normal (i.e., counterclockwise) in this age group.

Some investigators in the area of spatial (three dimensional) vectorcardiography feel that the maximal spatial voltage to the left or right may be a more accurate reflector of left or right ventricular hypertrophy respectively. Spatial voltage is calculated as follows:

$$\text{Spatial voltage} = \sqrt{x^2 + y^2 + z^2}$$

where x, y, and z represent the instantaneous voltage magnitude in leads x, y, and z, respectively. The maximal such value directed to the left or right is the maximal spatial voltage. Since this determination may require computation of a number of sequential points, it becomes somewhat tedious and is done far more easily with the aid of a computer. Some workers have found good correlation between the maximal spatial voltages and left or right ventricular peak systolic pressures in congenital aortic or pulmonic stenosis.

Combined Ventricular Hypertrophy

Criteria for hypertrophy of one ventricle are generally clear with overtly increased or upper limits of normal voltage in the opposite direction. Increased magnitude of the initial forces during the first 10-20 msec of the QRS complex is frequently seen. One may see a loop with two major vectors, both of which are of increased magnitude. Alternatively, combined ventricular hypertrophy may be represented by a nearly round or "fat" loop in at least two planes (Fig. 2-49).

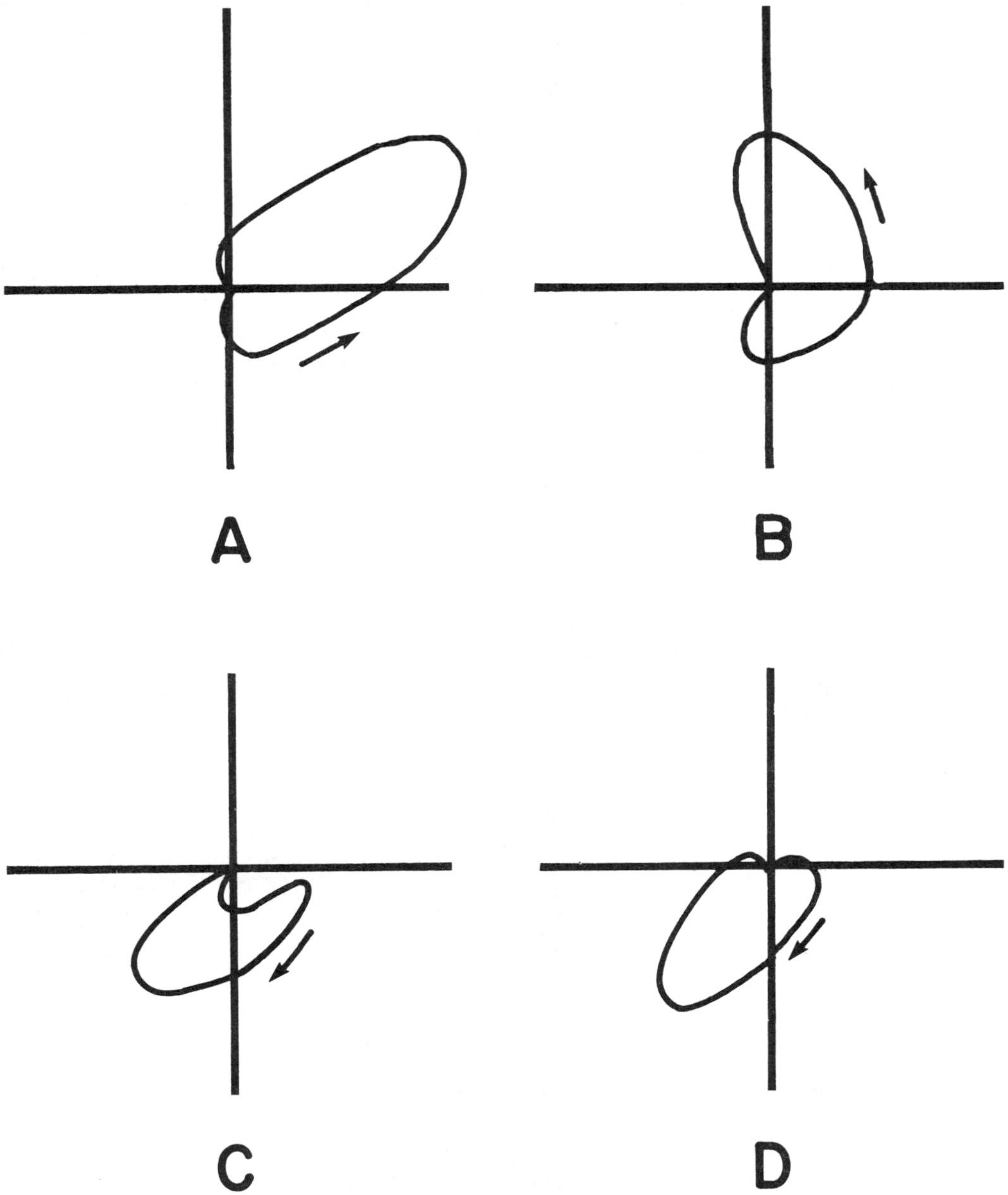

Figure 2–47 Horizontal plane loops in right ventricular hypertrophy. (A) Normal horizontal loop in an older child with the predominant forces oriented leftward and posteriorly. The arrow indicates the direction of loop rotation. (B) With mild degrees of right ventricular hypertrophy, there is a shift in the terminal forces toward the right. (C) In more severe degrees of hypertrophy the initial forces are directed normally, but the loop is oriented anteriorly and rightwards with clockwise rotation of the major portion of the loop. (D) In severe cases, the initial forces are also altered and are directed leftwards with clockwise rotation of the entire loop.

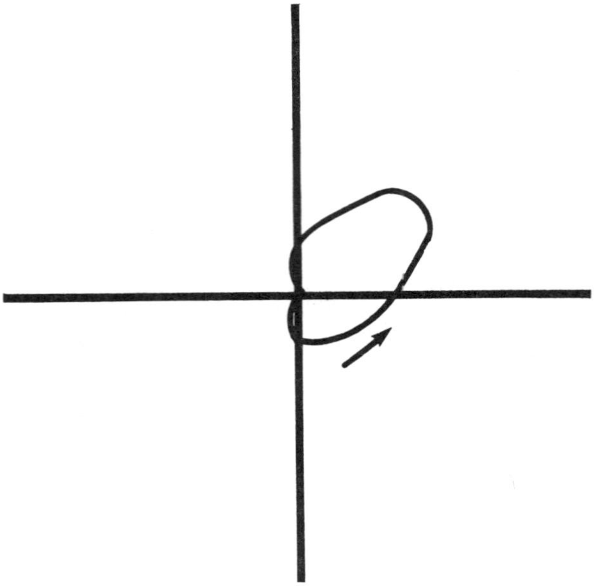

Figure 2–48 Horizontal loop in a newborn with left ventricular hypertrophy. Vector magnitudes are basically normal, but the loop is oriented predominately leftwards and posteriorly with counterclockwise rotation and thus is more mature than expected for age.

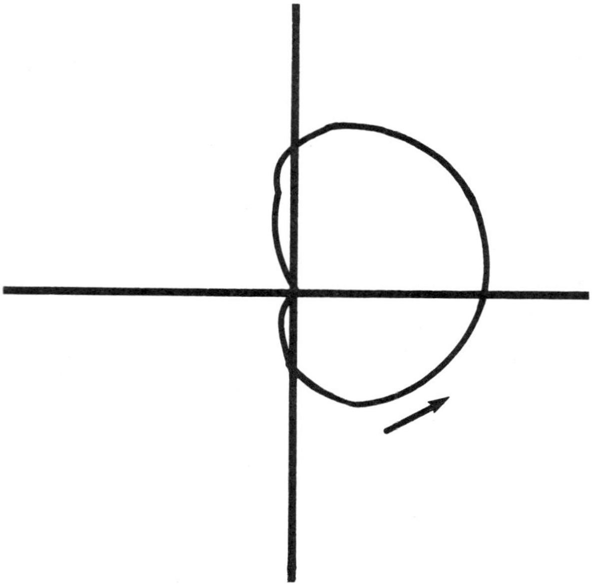

Figure 2–49 A "fat" loop is seen in the horizontal plane with prominent anterior and posterior forces indicative of combined ventricular hypertrophy.

Abnormalities in the Sequence of Ventricular Excitation

Right Bundle Branch Block

Initial and major QRS forces are normally directed for age, but there is a prominent terminal limb directed to the right and usually anteriorly in right bundle branch block as shown in Fig. 2-50. Close spacing of the terminal time dots reflects the slow spread of the excitation wave.

The magnitude of these terminal forces is not useful in evaluation of associated ventricular hypertrophy. There are other features more easily recognizable on the vectorcardiogram than on the scalar EKG which may be of value. Figure 2-51 shows the tracing in a patient with combined right bundle branch block and right ventricular hypertrophy. Initial forces are normal, but the major portion of the loop rotates clockwise and is oriented anteriorly to the E point before terminating in the conduction delay. Associated left ventricular hypertrophy may be suggested by increased magnitude of leftward forces.

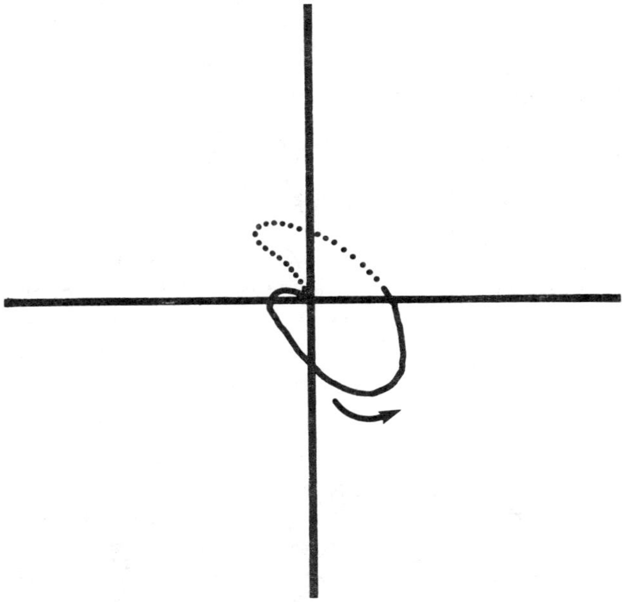

Figure 2-50 Horizontal plane loop in right bundle branch block. Initial forces and body of the loop are normal in direction and magnitude, but there is a prominent terminal limb directed rightward and anteriorly with marked slowing as indicated by the closely spaced time dots.

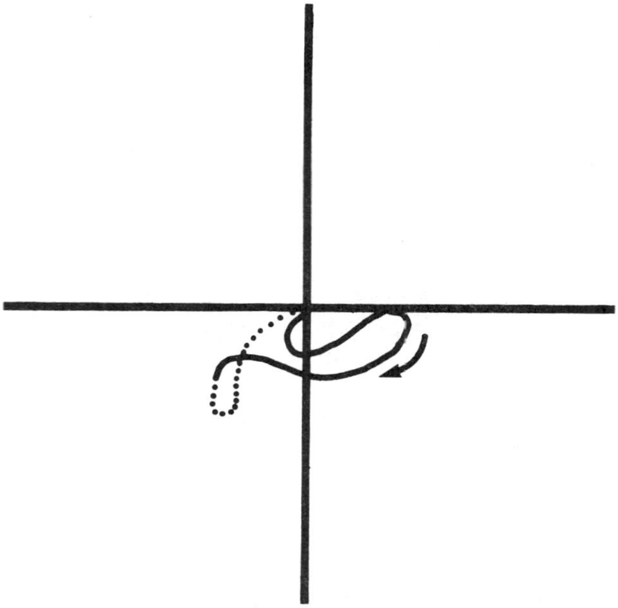

Figure 2–51 When right ventricular hypertrophy is associated with right bundle branch block, the horizontal loop may show abnormal anterior orientation and predominant clockwise rotation indicative of the hypertrophy as well as the terminal conduction delay.

Left Bundle Branch Block

Left bundle branch block is manifested by a relatively narrow QRS loop directed strongly leftward and posteriorly. Timing dots are closely spaced throughout the entire loop, in keeping with the concept that this is a conduction delay involving the total QRS complex. Initial forces are directed more posteriorly than normal.

Of more interest in pediatrics is left anterior fascicular block which is easily recognized on the VCG. Initial inferior rightward direction of initial forces and the overall left axis deviation are shown in Fig. 2-52, together with the counterclockwise rotation of the frontal plane loop. Changes due to ventricular hypertrophy may be recognized.

Preexcitation

In the WPW type of preexcitation, the delta wave is seen as abnormal slowing of the initial portion of the loop directed either anteriorly (type A) (Fig. 2-53) or leftward and posteriorly (type B). The major QRS vector is concordant with the delta wave in most cases of preexcitation without severe associated congenital heart disease. The presence of discordancy (e.g., anterior delta wave with posterior major vector) suggests a complicated abnormality. The T loop is commonly discordant with the major forces and the delta wave.

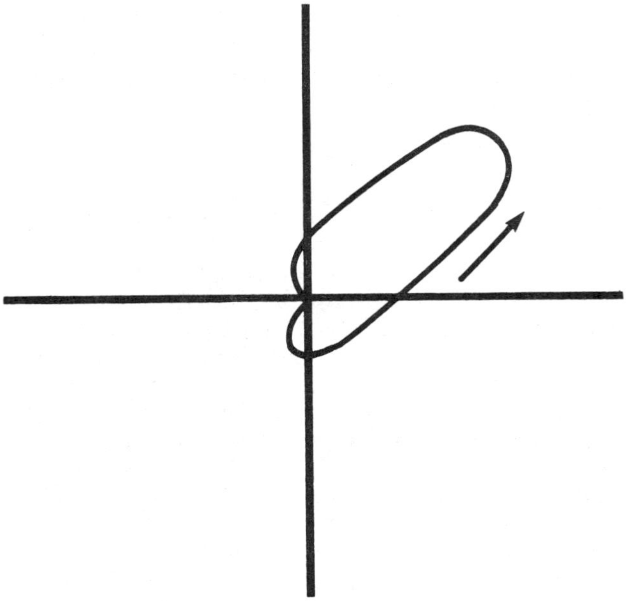

Figure 2-52 Frontal plane QRS loop in left anterior fascicular block. The initial forces are directed rightward and inferiorly with the body of the loop deviated leftwards and superiorly. The direction of loop rotation is counterclockwise as indicated by the arrow.

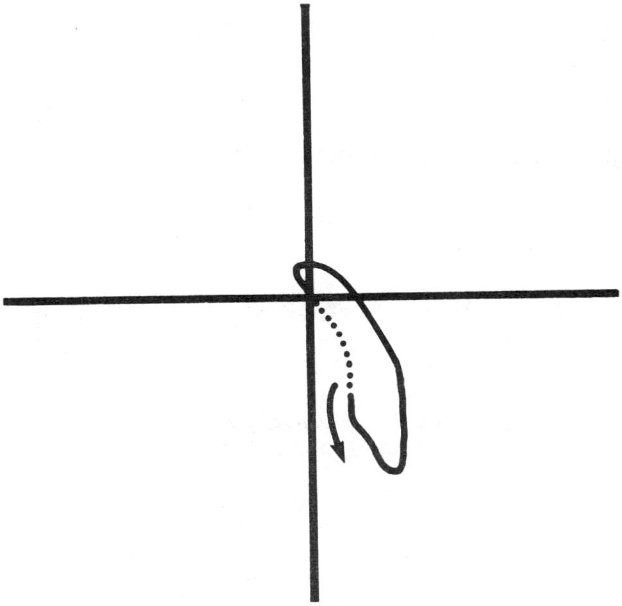

Figure 2-53 Horizontal loop in type-A WPW. Marked slowing of the initial forces equivalent to the delta wave on the scalar EKG. Initial forces are oriented anteriorly as the major portion of the remainder of the loop.

Radiographic Evaluation

The analysis of the heart on the chest radiograph should be systematic. Table 2-9 outlines the suggested approach.

Cardiac Size

The determination of the cardiothoracic ratio is an acceptable simple method for evaluation cardiac size. This is accomplished by relating the largest transverse diameter of the heart to the widest internal diameter of the chest (Fig. 2-54). A cardiothoracic ratio of 0.5 or less is considered within normal limits. In the newborn, however, a cardiothoracic ratio of 0.55 on a supine inspiratory film is acceptable. This ratio should not be the sole determinant of cardiac enlargement since the heart may appear normal in the PA projection yet the lateral film may disclose abnormalities. These measurements are also influenced by the phase of the cardiac cycle (systole, diastole) and by the phase of respiration.

Cardiac Silhouette, Chamber Enlargement

This section outlines the various structures that form the cardiac borders in the posteroanterior and lateral projections. The following are outlined in the posteroanterior projection of a normal 6 year old (Fig. 2-55A).

On the Left from Top to Bottom

1. The curve of the aortic arch (Ao)
2. The main pulmonary artery (PA)
3. The left atrial appendage (LAA) (not always visualized)
4. The sweeping long curve of the left ventricle (LV) (which also makes up the cardiac apex)

Table 2-9 Steps in Evaluating the Chest X-Ray in Relation to Heart Disease

Heart size
Specific chamber enlargement
Pulmonary vascularity
Type: Arterial, venous, lymphatics
Status: Increased, normal, decreased
Location of the aortic arch (right, left)
Cardiac and abdominal situs
Lung parenchyma and bony thorax
Ask for the presence or absence of cyanosis

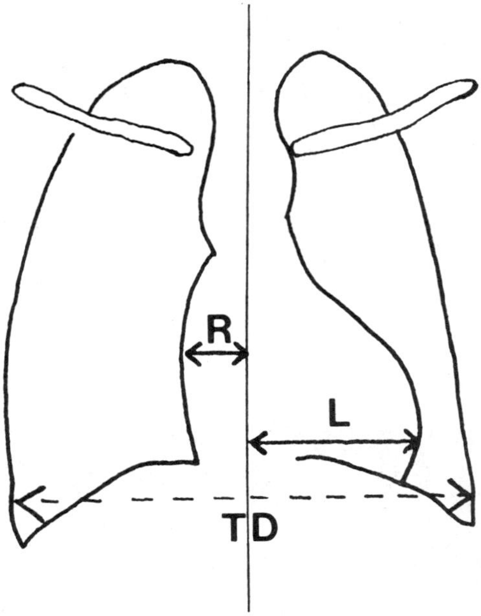

$$CT = \frac{R + L}{TD}$$

Figure 2–54 Determination of the cardiothoracic (CT) ratio. R - maximal cardiac dimension to the left of the midline, L - maximal cardiac dimension to the left of the midline, TD - transverse dimension at the widest expansion of the bony chest. The cardiothoracic ratio is obtained by entering these parameters in the above formula. (Reproduced with permission from Rabinowitz J, Pediatric Radiology, 1978, J. B. Lippincott Co., Philadelphia.)

On the Right from Top to Bottom

1. The superior vena vava (SVC) presents as a vertical shadow.
2. The right atrium (RA).
   Note: The right ventricle is located anteriorly and is not border-forming in this projection. The aortic knob is usually inconspicuous in children. However, the position of the arch can be determined by the displacement of the trachea. This is always positioned opposite the aortic arch; the tracheal air column is deviated to the right. The descending aorta may be seen in the left paraspinal area.

Lateral Projection (Fig. 2–55B)

Anterior Border

The right ventricle (RV) in this projection is the anterior border-forming structure. It lies adjacent to the lower third of the sternum and is surrounded superiorly by the retrosternal clear space. In the infant, however, the thymus is still enlarged and normally occupies and obliterates this space.

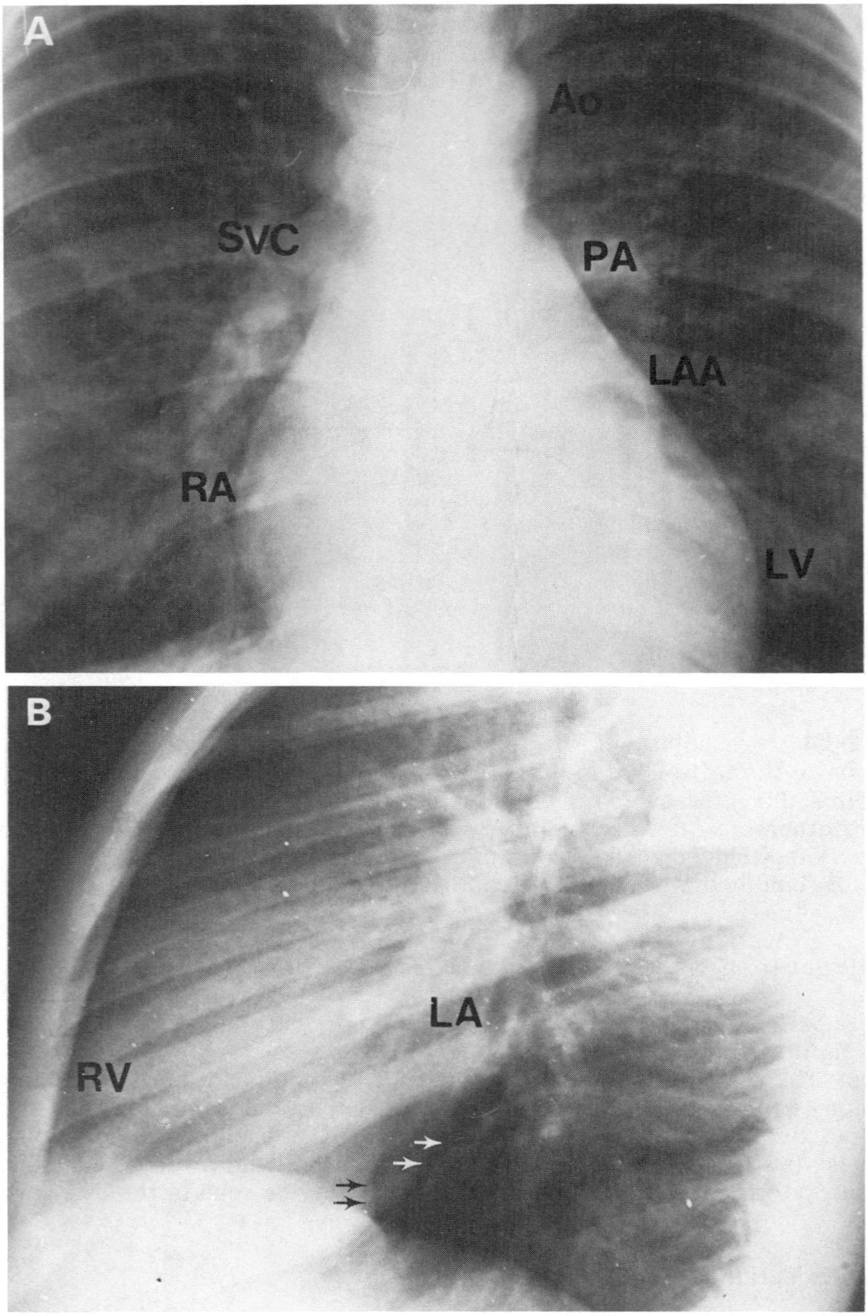

Figure 2-55 (A) Posteroanterior view of the chest of a normal 6-year-old. Ao - aorta, PA - pulmonary artery, LAA - left atrial appendage, LV - left ventricle, SVC - superior vena cava, RA - right atrium (see text). (B) Lateral projection of the same patient. The posterior border of the left ventricle (white arrows) is seen clearly just beyond the IVC (black arrows). The right ventricle (RV) is contiguous with the lower third of the sternum. LA - left atrium.

Posterior Border

The posterior-inferior border of the heart is formed by the left ventricle (LV) above which lies the border of the left atrium (LA). The inferior vena cava as it reaches the right atrium is easily identified as a vertical curvilinear density, extending posteriorly through the diaphragm. The posterior cardiac border normallly does not protrude significantly beyond it.

Specific Chamber Enlargement

Right Atrial Enlargement (Fig. 2-58)

Right atrial enlargement is indicated by an increased prominence of the right atrial border on the frontal projection.

Left Atrial Enlargement (Fig. 2-56A)

When the left atrium enlarges, it causes many alterations within the cardiac contour as well as to various adjacent structures. For example:

1. A double-density outline is observed on the right side of the heart. The inner linear density is usually the border of the left atrium as it expands to the right. The outer density represents the right atrium.
2. The carinal angle is widened when the left atrium expands superiorly and elevates the left main bronchus.
3. The left atrial appendage becomes more prominent and bulges selectively on the frontal projection.
4. In the lateral projection the left atrium enlarges posteriorly. This (Fig. 2-56B) displaces the left main bronchus superiorly and indents the anterior margin of the neighboring esophagus. The latter is best demonstrated when the esophagus is filled with barium.

Left Ventricular Enlargement (Figs. 2-56, 2-57)

1. The cardiac apex enlarges downward and laterally (down and out) on the frontal plane.
2. In the lateral projection there is significant posterior displacement of the LV border beyond the IVC shadow. The border of the heart approaches the vertebral column.

Right Ventricular Enlargement (Figs. 2-58, 2-59)

1. The apex of the heart is elevated in the frontal projection and often assumes a smaller radius of curvature (Fig. 2-58).
2. Anteriorly, the RV border impinges on and fills in the retrosternal clear space (Fig. 2-59).
   Note: It is important to remember that the right ventricle has no visible borders on the frontal projection. It is a common error to mistake a prominent right atrial border for the right ventricle.

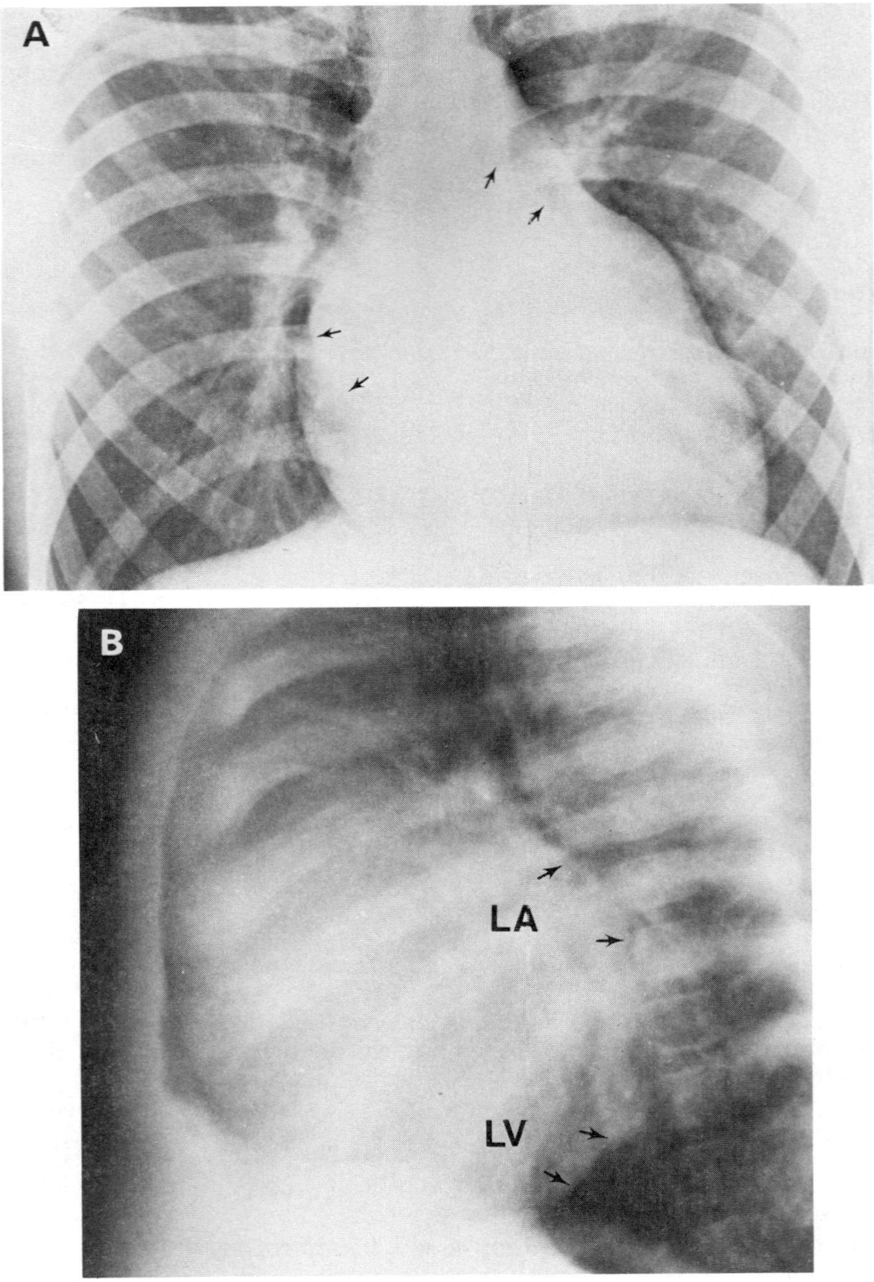

Figure 2–56 (A) Chest radiograph of mitral stenosis and insufficiency showing moderate cardiomegaly, with massive left atrial enlargement as evidenced by an enlarged LAA, elevated left mainstem bronchus, and a double density (arrows). Also note LV dilatation as manifested by downward displacement of the cardiac apex. (B) Large ventricular septal defect. The enlarged left atrium (LA) is seen pushing the left bronchus posteriorly. The left ventricle (LV) is protruding posteriorly beyond the IVC.

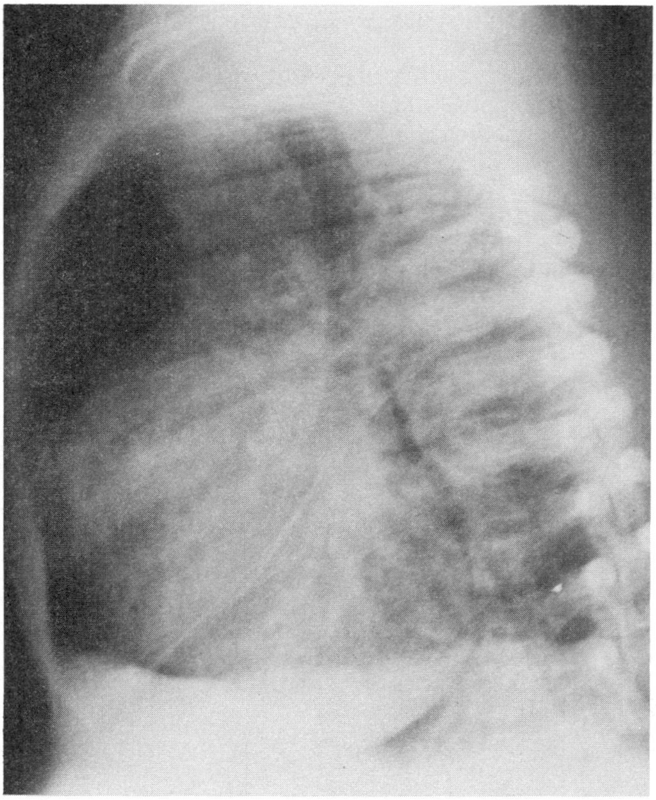

Figure 2-57 Chest film of a 2-year-old. The greatly enlarged left ventricle extends posteriorly to reach the vertebral bodies.

Pulmonary Vessels

The pulmonary vasculature consists of arteries, veins, and lymphatics with the arteries and to some extent the veins forming the major part of the hilum (Figs. 2-60, 2-61).

As the pulmonary arteries branch, they can be seen both longitudinally and on end. If one divides the pulmonary lung field into three vertical sections, central, medial, and lateral, the pulmonary arteries will be best seen in the medial and central lung fields (Figs. 2-60, 2-61). They taper progressively toward the periphery and are normally not too apparent in the more lateral lung fields. The pulmonary veins are less well defined than the arteries, and in the region of the hilum are lower in position and more horizontally directed than the arteries. Under normal circumstances the lymphatics are not seen.

Increased arterial flow is recognized when the arteries appear enlarged and extend into the lateral third of the lung field (Figs. 2-50B, 2-61B). More vessels are seen on end and are often larger than the bronchus they accompany. In the older erect patients there is also evidence of redistribution of flow. Ordinarily because of the hydrostatic pressure, the pulmonary arteries are more distended in the lung bases than in the apices. If there is increased pulmonary arterial flow, the partially collapsed vessels of the lung apices offer the least resistance to additional flow. Thus, a small shunt produces the greatest change in the lung apices.

Decreased arterial blood flow is suspected when the hilum appears small and the remaining lung fields appear empty and devoid of pulmonary vessels (Fig. 2-60C). The vessels themselves are small and thin.

Venous and lymphatic engorgement is associated with pulmonary venous hypertension of variable causes. In this state the margins of the pulmonary vessels are hazy and indistinct. The haziness often involves the entire lung (Fig. 2-62). Dilated lymphatics appear as short horizontal linear densities within the outer inferior lung fields. These are the classic Kerley B lines. Central lymphatics, Kerley A lines, radiate as thin linear densities toward the hilum. Pleural effusion associated with wet fissures is another feature (Fig. 2-62). The classical fluffy, butterfly distribution of pulmonary edema seen in the adult is rarely encountered in the pediatric age group.

In the presence of severe obstruction to the pulmonary arterial blood flow or in the absence of the pulmonary arteries, bronchial arteries provide an alternate route for pulmonary blood supply. These vessels present a lacy pattern throughout the lung fields. An important radiologic feature is an empty hilum that is produced by the small or absent pulmonary arteries. The bronchial vessels arise

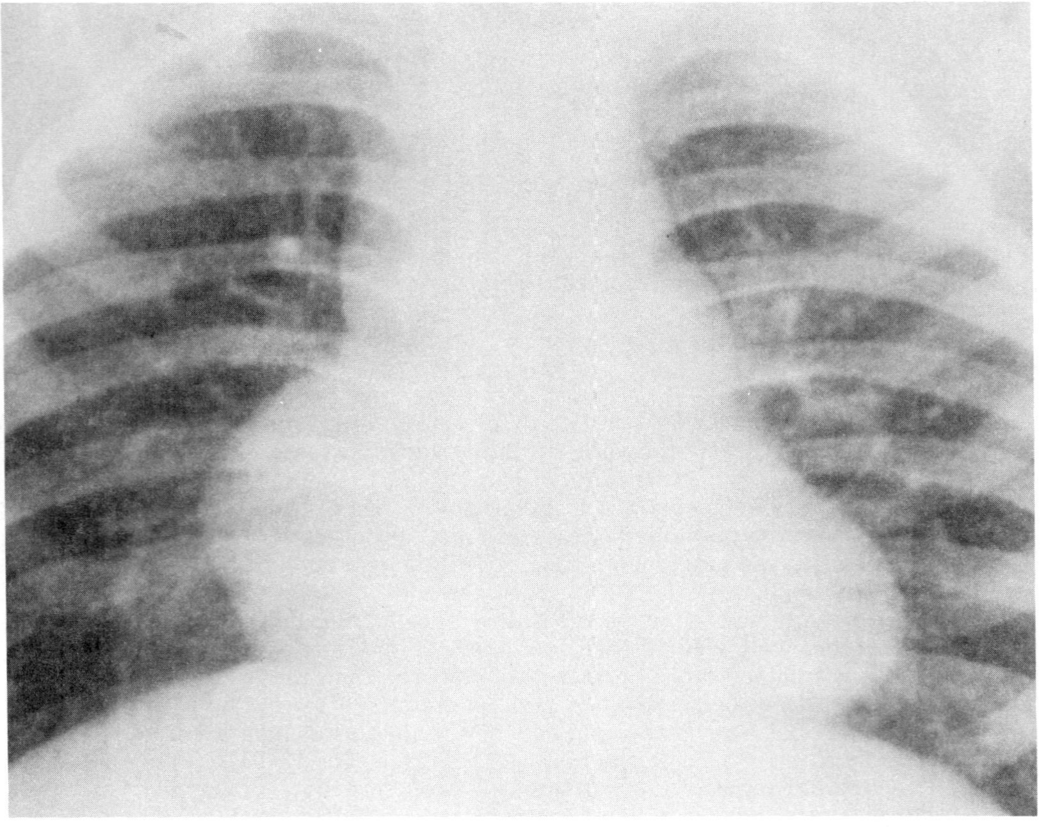

Figure 2–58 Pulmonary stenosis. A 3-month-old with cardiomegaly and right ventricular enlargement manifested by a definite elevation of the apex. The right atrium is enlarged, and the main pulmonary artery segment is prominent.

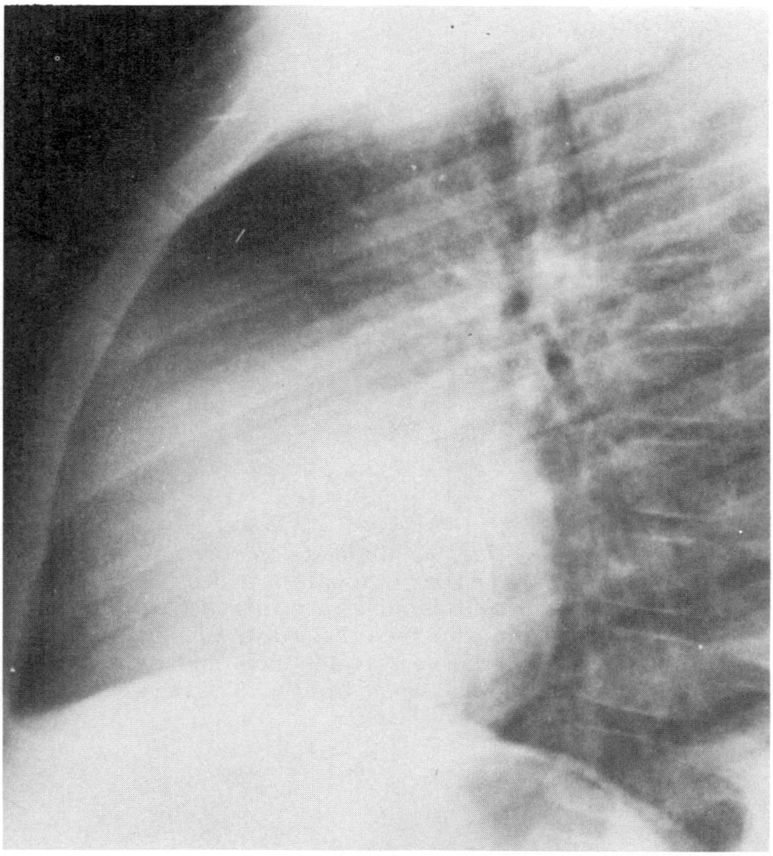

Figure 2-59 Chest film of a patient with both left and right ventricular enlargement. The retrosternal space is impinged upon by the anteriorly enlarged right ventricle.

from the descending aorta and, therefore, present higher in the hilum than the pulmonary vessels (Fig. 2-63).

Severe pulmonary arterial hypertension associated with increased pulmonary vascular resistance is recognized by the extremely dilated central pulmonary arteries that narrow abruptly beyond the central subdivision (Fig. 2-64). This is referred to as pruning.

Cardiac Situs

It is always necessary to determine the cardiac and abdominal situs, especially when cardiac malposition is encountered. The following nomenclature can be used.

Abdominal situs solitus: liver on the right, stomach on the left
Abdominal situs inversus: liver on the left, stomach on the right
Abdominal situs indeterminate: usually a midline stomach and liver

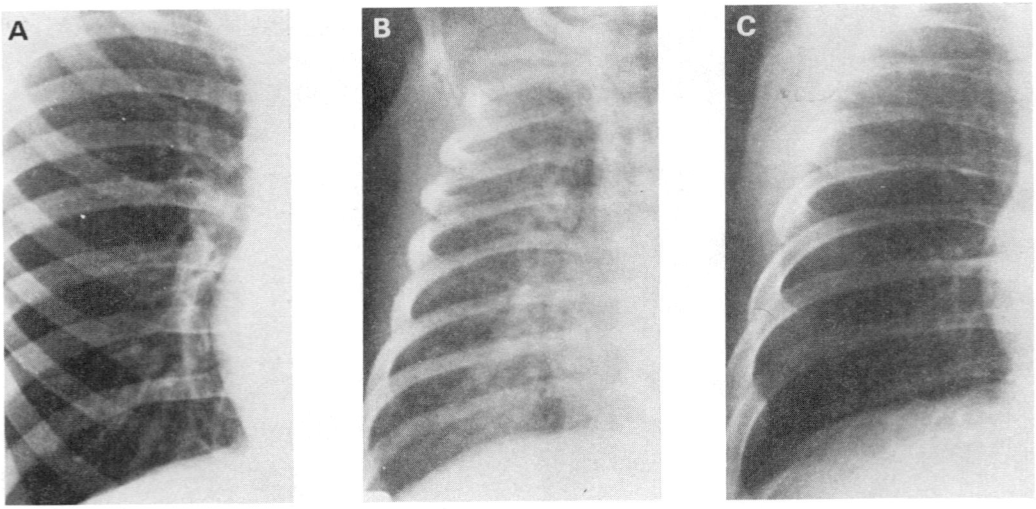

Figure 2-60 Hilar vessels. (A) Normal hilum is composed of branching pulmonary arteries, veins, and bronchi that taper gradually toward the periphery. (B) Shunt vasculature (VSD). The lung fields demonstrate increased pulmonary blood flow. The central vessels are large and well seen through the lung fields. Note the many vessels on end. The borders of the vessels are hazy and fuzzy because of superimposed interstitial edema caused by heart failure. (C) Decreased pulmonary blood flow with few if any identifiable vessels.

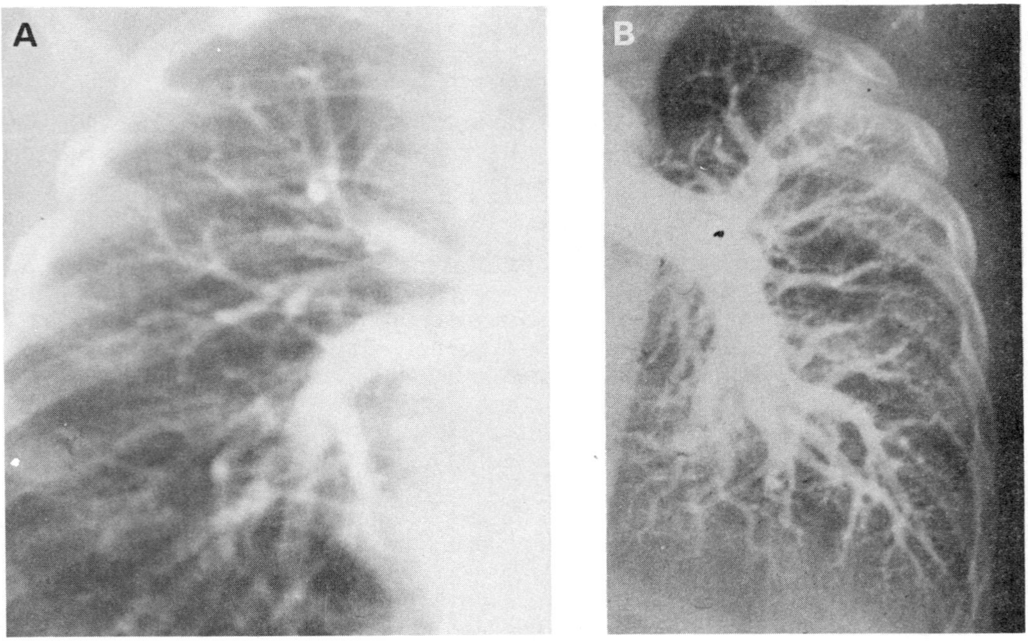

Figure 2-61 (A) Normal pulmonary angiogram with gradual branching pattern of the vessels. (B) The pulmonary arteries of a patient with shunt vascularity demonstrate numerous tortuous vessels extending within the peripheral lung fields.

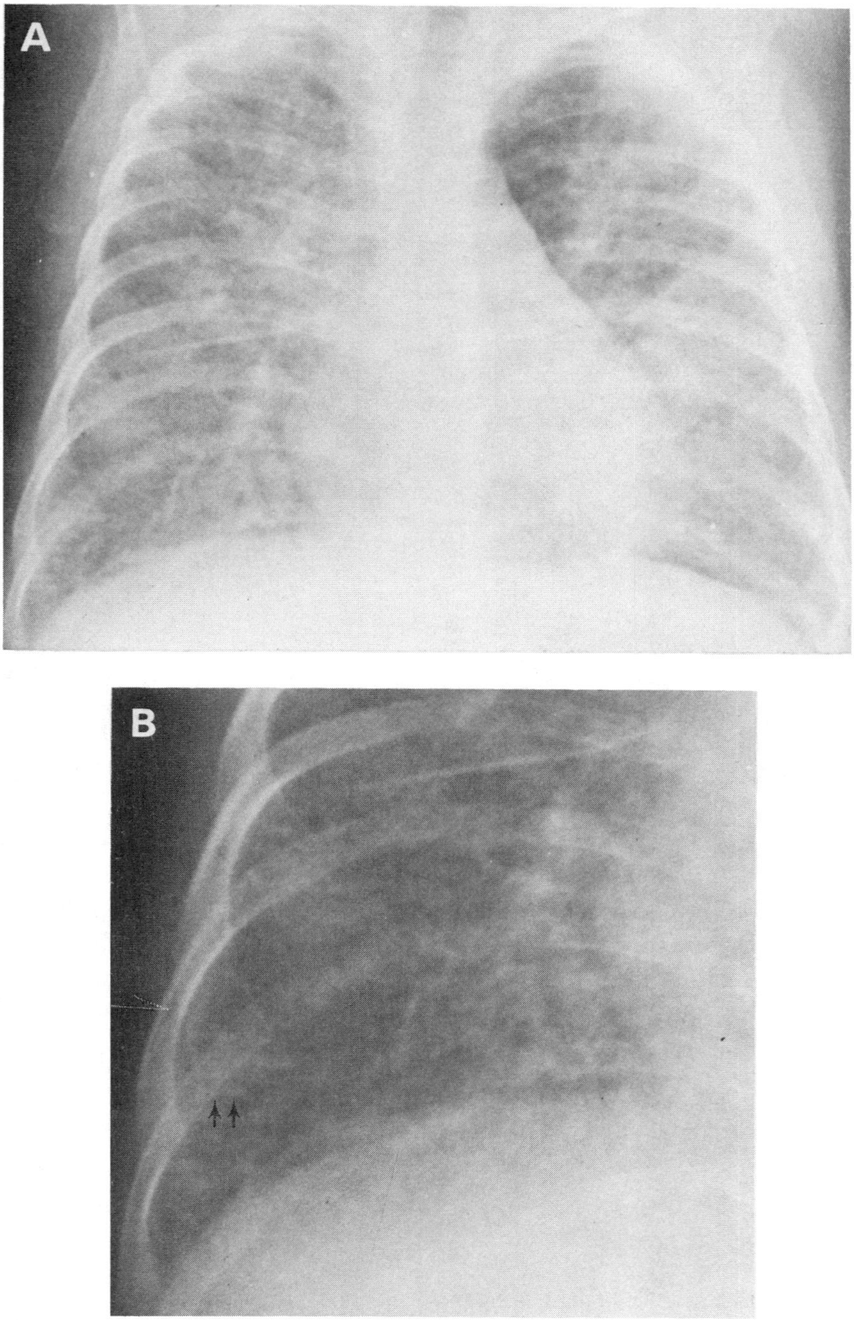

Figure 2–62 (A) Pulmonary venous obstruction. The lung fields are hazy and the fissures are wet. Kerley B lines are present within the outer lower lung fields. (B) Closeup of the right lower lung field. Arrows mark a Kerley B line.

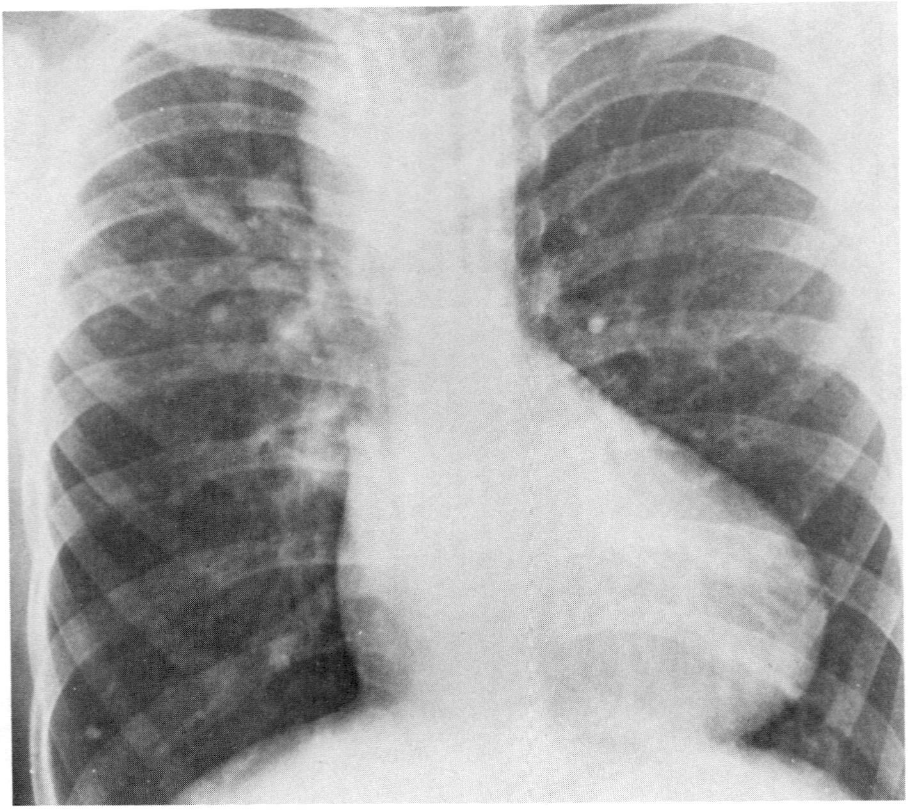

Figure 2–63 Truncus arteriosus (type IV). There are no identifiable pulmonary arteries. The vessels at the right hilar area are large, multiple tortuous bronchial arteries. No single main pulmonary artery is present. The bronchial vessels arise high from the aorta.

Stating only the cardiac situs (dextrocardia, levocardia) and the abdominal situs avoids the cumbersome and confusing classification of dextroversion, dextroposition, and so forth (Figs. 2-65, 2-66).

Dextrocardia can be either primary or secondary to volume changes. The latter may occur in association with a hypoplastic right lung (Fig. 2-66) and manifests smaller intercostal spaces and increased density in the right hemithorax due to the mediastinal shift and hypoplastic lung. The opposite lung field by contrast is hyperinflated.

Bony Thorax

Any extracardiac structural abnormality that may shed light on a probable diagnosis should be noted. For example, severe pectus excavatum, straight back syndrome, and severe scoliosis can modify the observed cardiac silhouette in both size and shape. Moreover, abnormalities of the ribs, vertebrae, and sternum are associated with various syndromes that include cardiac disease (e.g., vertebral anomalies with the VaTER syndrome). Increased vertical diameter of the lumbar vertebrae when associated with a bifid manubrium are strongly suggestive of

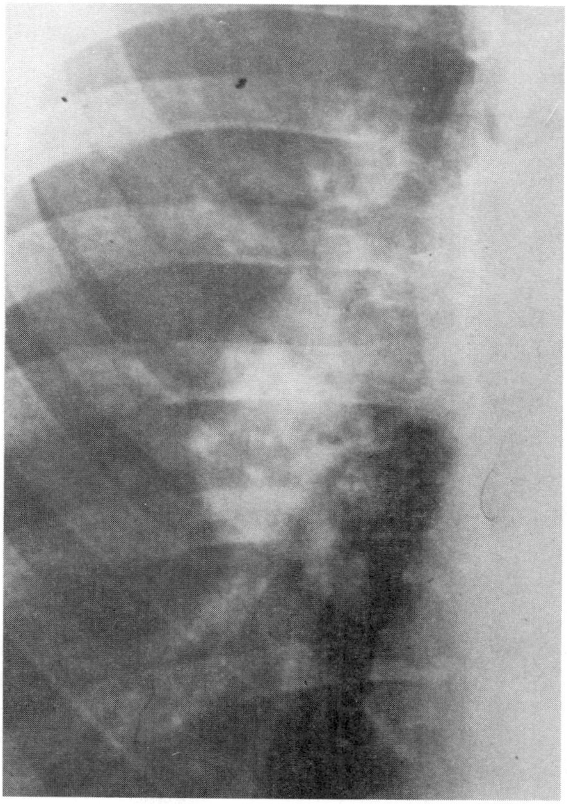

Figure 2–64 Pulmonary arterial hypertension associated with elevated pulmonary vascular resistance. The right pulmonary artery is markedly dilated. Note the sudden pruning of the vessel.

Down syndrome. Notching of the fourth to eighth ribs is associated with coarctation of the aorta (Fig. 2-67).

Abnormality of the ribs related to previous cardiac surgery should be observed. A left thoracotomy is usually performed for ductal ligation, banding of the main pulmonary artery, and coarctectomy. Occasionally subclavian artery to pulmonary artery shunt is also performed on the left. Right-sided thoracotomies are performed for creation of aortopulmonary shunts and atrial septectomy for transposition of the great vessels.

The Systematic Approach

The outline in Table 2-9 provides the reader with a basic guideline for evaluating the cardiac status on chest x-ray. After analyzing the features in a systematic manner, it becomes possible to further categorize the cardiac lesions into major groups (Table 2-10). In general, congenital heart disease is divided into two major categories: acyanotic and cyanotic heart disease. These are further subdivided into two subgroups, one associated with increased pulmonary arterial vascularity and the other with decreased or normal pulmonary arterial vascularity.

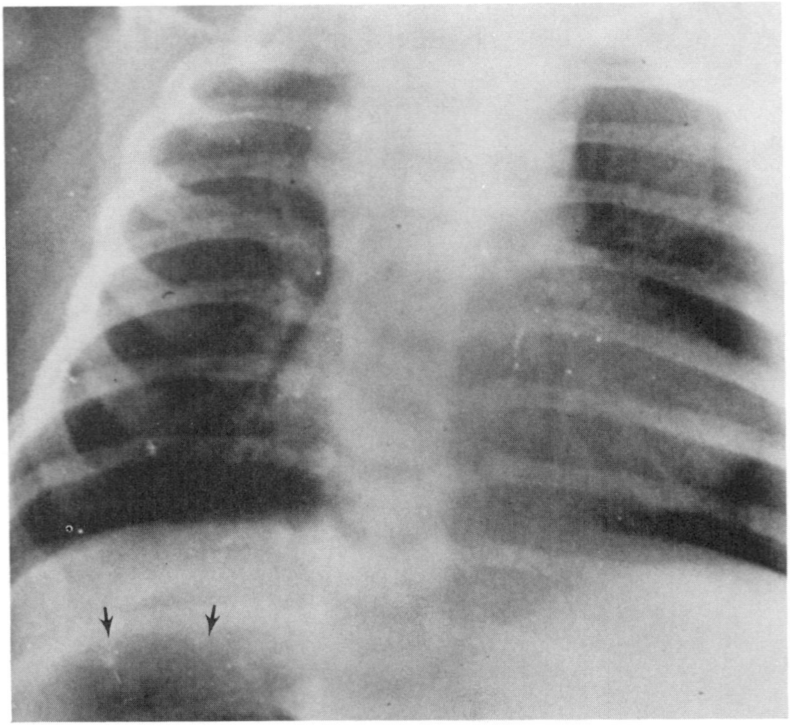

Figure 2-65 Chest radiograph of a newborn manifesting levocardia and abdominal situs inversus. The stomach is on the right (arrow). The elevated apex on the left indicates right ventricular enlargement.

Since both cyanotic and acyanotic congenital heart disease can be associated with increased pulmonary arterial vessels, the presence or absence of clinical cyanosis must be known in order to even begin to consider a proper differential diagnosis. For example, x-ray findings of normal size heart with increased pulmonary arterial blood flow in a cyanotic patient belongs to category I.b in Table 2-10. Specific chamber enlargement, clinical presentation, and physical examination help establish a specific diagnosis.

Phonocardiography

The recording of heart sounds and associated events in a visual presentation has been in use for many years. From the beginning it has generated a steadily increasing breadth of knowledge regarding heart sounds and murmurs. In the last few years with highly sophisticated instrumentation, the phonocardiogram, particularly when combined with high-fidelity recordings of intracardiac pressure, has altered some of the traditional concepts about the origin of these events. The monograph by Leon and Shaver (listed in the bibliography) is a compendium of excellent papers in this area.

The other obvious advantage of this type of presentation is in teaching students about cardiac examination. For the novice the auscultatory exam becomes more meaningful when combined with the visual. This concept has been put to use in the development of several types of teaching aids allowing the student to see and hear simultaneously.

Equipment

Because of the frequency-response characteristics necessary for proper recording of heart sounds, optical recorders are preferred to those using some type of mechanical stylus. As a minimum and suitable for only basic teaching, two channels of recording are required, consisting of a phonochannel and a channel for recording the electrocardiogram for timing purposes. Variable high- and low-frequency cutoff controls should be incorporated. For more sophisticated studies, multiple channels are utilized, generally consisting of an electrocardiogram, two phonocardiogram channels (with different filter settings), and a channel for recording either peripheral vascular pressure or the displacement characteristics of the cardiac apex (apexcardiogram). It should be possible to monitor the recording visually on an oscilloscope as well as to listen with attached earphones. A variety of pickup microphone designs are available that in their simplest form consist of either bell or diaphragm chest pieces of appropriate size which can be coupled to a transducer capable of converting pressure energy to electrical energy.

A diagramatic example of a typical recording is shown in Fig. 2-2. The first heart sound is seen as consisting of two to four recordable components occurring approximately at the time of the QRS complex. The second and third components are of greater intensity and are the only ones generally audible. The two components of the second sound can be readily seen occurring shortly after the T wave on the EKG. If a carotid arterial pulse wave is recorded, the aortic component of the second sound coincides with the dicrotic notch on the pressure tracing, and the same is true of pulmonic component if an appropriate tracing from the pulmonary artery is available. Precise evaluation of the splitting of the second sound and its

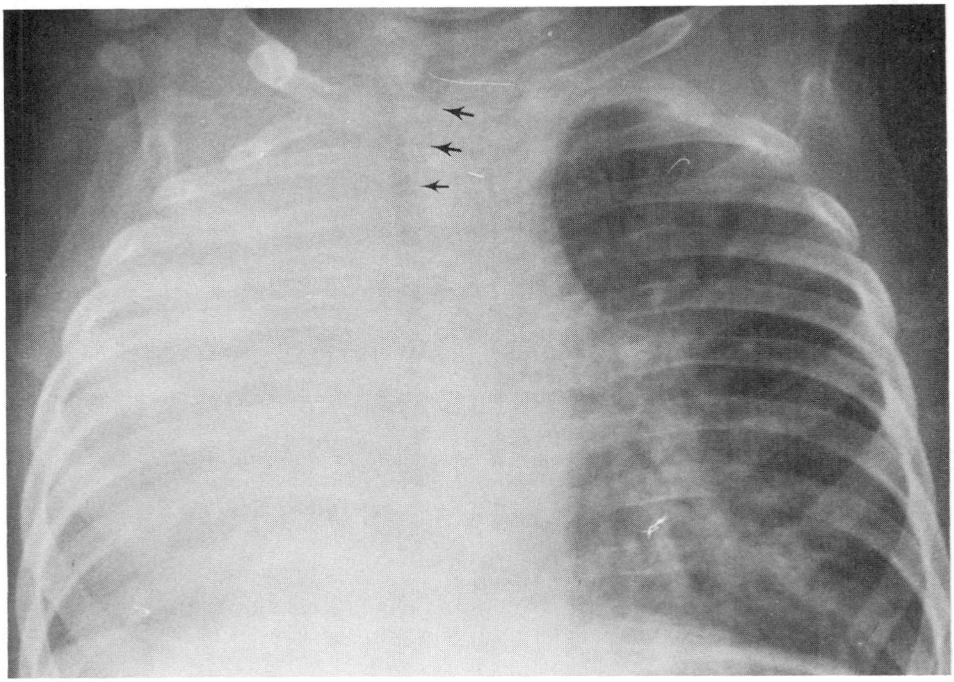

Figure 2-66 A cyanotic infant with situs solitus (stomach on the left) and dextrocardia secondary to hypoplastic right lung. Note the small intercostal spaces on the right and the hyperinflated lung on the left. The trachea is pulled to the right (arrows). The heart borders cannot be distinguished from the adjacent hypoplastic lung.

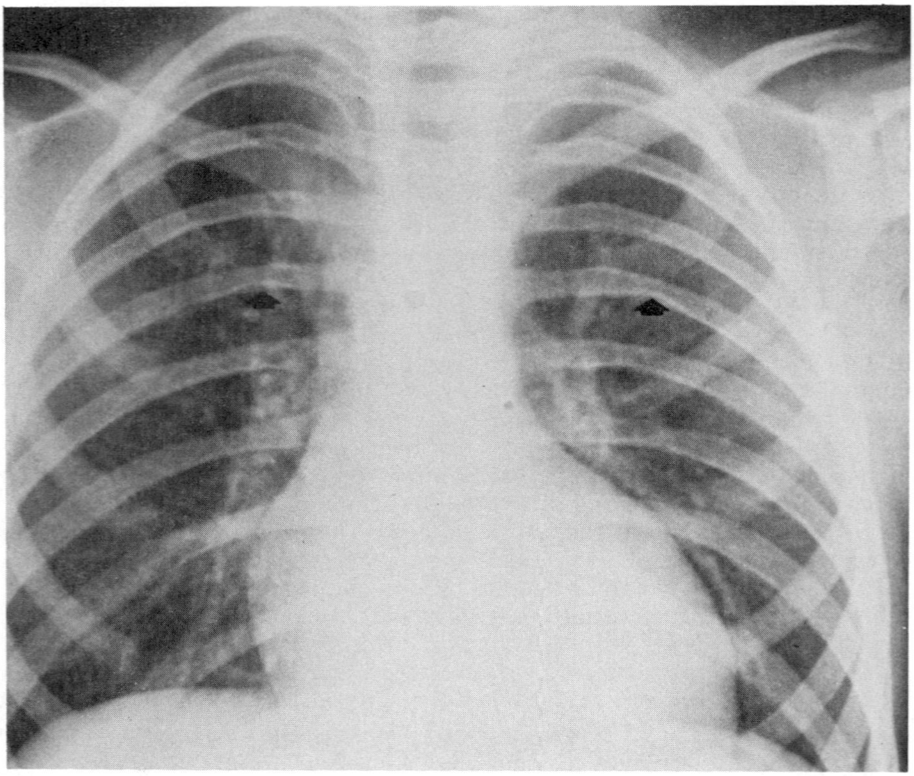

Figure 2-67 Coarctation of the aorta associated with rib notching (arrows).

Table 2-10 Categories of Heart Disease

According to the findings from Table 2-9, the following categories apply

I. *Cyanotic Heart Disease*
   a. With increased pulmonary blood flow
   b. With decreased pulmonary blood flow

II. *Acyanotic Heart Disease*
   a. With increased pulmonary blood flow
   b. With normal pulmonary blood flow

behavior with respiration are possible. The third sound is a low-frequency event following S_2. Its identity can be confirmed by simultaneous recording of the apexcardiogram since the third sound coincides with the peak of the wave due to rapid ventricular filling. The fourth sound is also a low-frequency event occurring after atrial depolarization. Although not audible in normal patients, it has been occasionally picked up on the phonocardiogram.

Precise evaluation of all of the characteristics of heart murmurs mentioned in the section on physical examination is often difficult in young children because of the physiologic tachycardia which is present. A great deal of clarification can be obtained from the phonocardiogram, particularly regarding the location of the murmur within the cardiac cycle, timing of onset, termination, and the contour of the murmur. Examples are seen in Fig. 2-68 - 2-71.

Phonocardiography by no means replaces auscultation in the hands of the experienced examiner and should not be regarded as a tool to detect events which cannot be heard with the stethoscope. Much skill is required to select proper recording frequencies to maximally bring out desired events and reduce artifact. Improperly used, it can be more confusing than helpful. In the routine practice of pediatric cardiology, it is a less important diagnostic modality than others discussed in this chapter, but its role in teaching and investigation remains unchallenged.

Exercise Testing

Although utilized for many years in the evaluation of adults with suspected coronary artery disease, exercise testing as a diagnostic tool in the pediatric patient has come into its own in the last few years. In part its utilization has awaited the development of exercise modalities suitable for use in children and for analysis of types of problems which they present. There are several general areas where exercise testing may be of value in investigation of a patient.

1. Evaluation of total pump function (i.e., determination of the heart's ability to meet demands for increased output)
2. Evaluation of selected hemodynamic aspects (e.g., change in the gradient across the stenotic valve with exercise)
3. Evaluation of myocardial blood supply
4. Evaluation of arrhythmias

Evolution of exercise testing as an investigative tool and as a useful modality in patient care has progressed nearly simultaneously. The clinician may seek the answer to several types of questions through exercise.

1. The detection of unrecognized cardiac disease: This is of limited value in children with the exception of arrhythmias (v.i.). It may, however, be of value in the opposite sense, that is, in the exclusion of cardiac problems when the patient presents with a multiplicity of vague symptoms.
2. Evaluation of severity of a lesion where other diagnostic modalities are of limited precision and/or reliability: As an extension of this concept, it would be useful in certain patients in arriving at a decision regarding surgery.
3. Planning allowable exercise in children with persistent or unremiable cardiac defects.
4. Assessing the functional results of surgery.
5. Provoking suspected arrhythmias or evaluating the effect of exercise on proven ones.

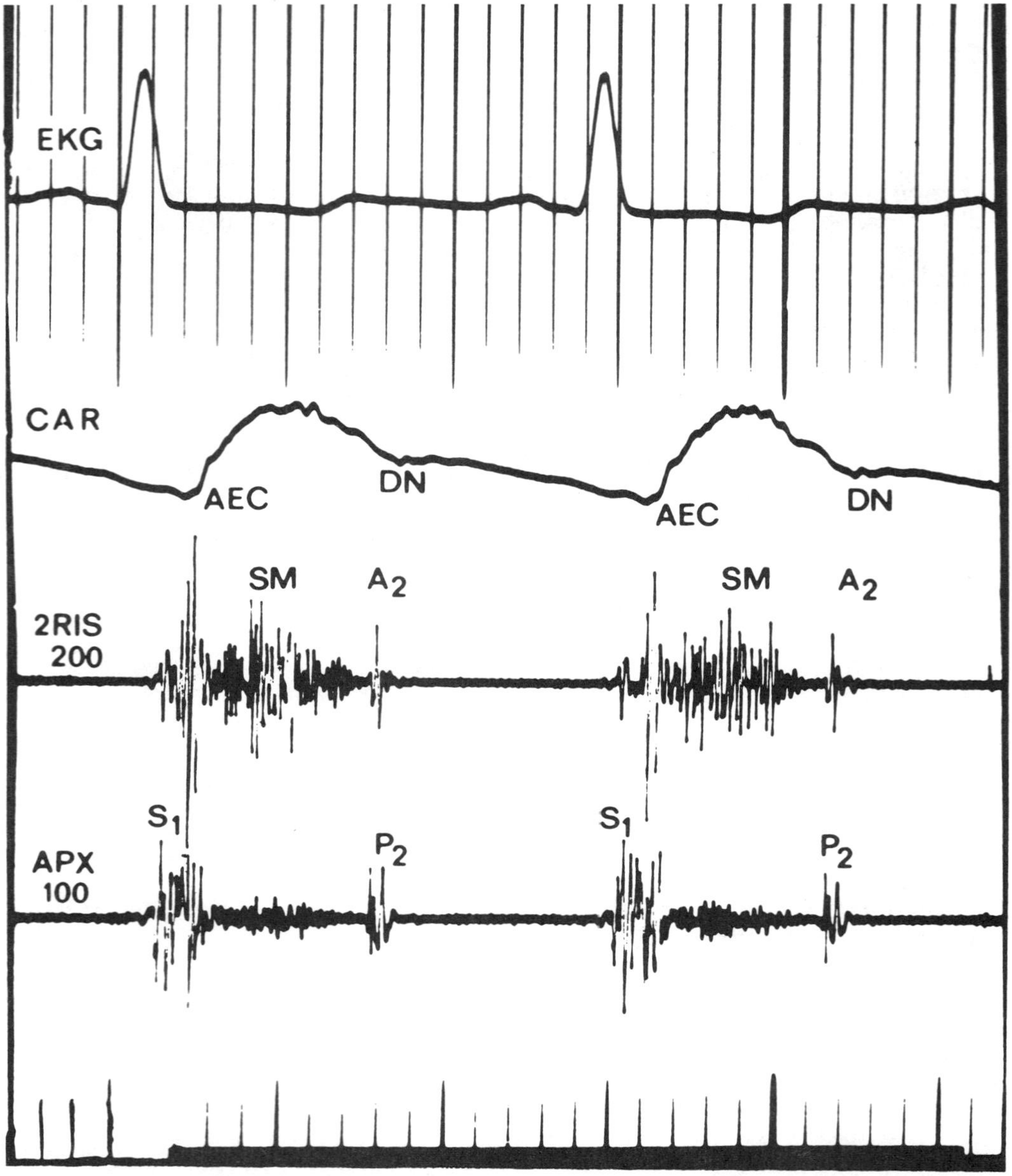

Figure 2-68 Electrocardiogram, carotid arterial pulse tracing (CAR) and simultaneous phonocardiograms recorded at the second right intercostal space (2RIS) and apex (APX) in a patient with congenital aortic stenosis. The numbers at the left of the phonocardiograms represent the upper frequency filter limit. An aortic ejection click (AEC) is synchronous with the rise in the carotid pulse tracing and the aortic component of S_2 (A2) coincides with the dicrotic notch (DN). There is a diamond-shaped ejection murmur recorded best at the upper right sternal border. Both the aortic and pulmonic (P2) components of S_2 are noted at the apex. (Reproduced with permission from Nades AS, Fyler DC, Pediatric Cardiology, 3rd ed., 1972, W. B. Saunders Co., Philadelphia.)

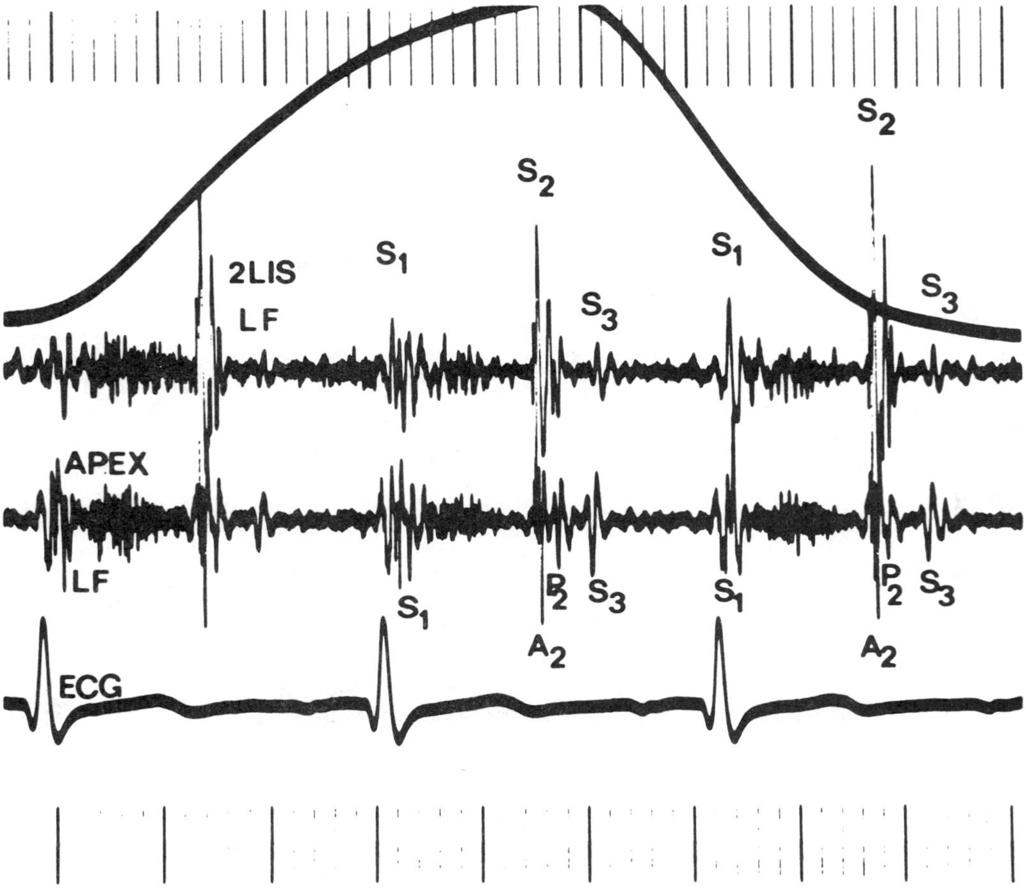

Figure 2-69 Phonocardiograms at the second left intercostal space and apex in a patient with gallop rhythm. Low-frequency third heart sound (S_3) is best recorded at the apex. Respiration is indicated by the curve at the top of the figure. (Reproduced with permission from Nades AS, Fyler DC, Pediatric Cardiology, 3rd ed., 1972, W. B. Saunders Co., Philadelphia.)

Methods

A number of different techniques for the administration, monitoring, and evaluation of exercise performance exists, and these will vary with the institution as well as with the age of the patient and type of information desired. One should not forget the value of a carefully taken history in the assessment. Historically, the technique developed by Masters, consisting of repetitive ascents of a small step-stool was one of the first to be widely used, but was difficult to quantitate precisely.

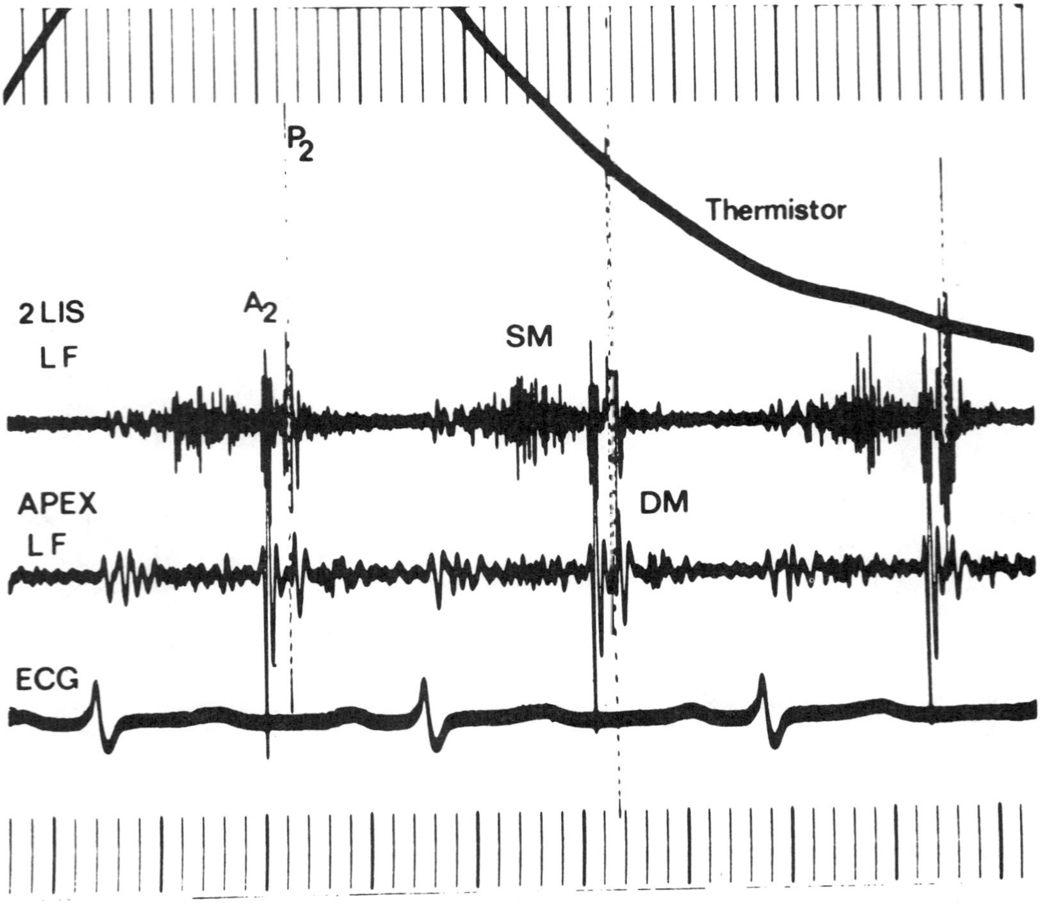

Figure 2–70 Low-frequency phonocardiograms recorded at second left intercostal space and apex in a child with an atrial septal defect. There is a diamond-shaped systolic ejection murmur recorded best at the upper left sternal border and a short early diastolic murmur (DM) best detected at the apex. Second heart sound is widely split and shows little variation with respiration (curve marked thermistor). (Reproduced with permission from Nades AS, Fyler DC, Pediatric Cardiology, 3rd ed., 1972, W. B. Saunders Co., Philadelphia.)

Body Position

Supine

Supine exercise is generally performed with a pedal-type ergometer mounted horizontally and is most widely used for the assessment of selected hemodynamic parameters in the catheterization laboratory. It is perhaps more easily utilized in this context than upright exercise but is of limited value in small children who are often sedated and/or have difficulty in reaching the pedals.

Upright

It does not seem clear whether this position is any more accurate, but intuitively it appears more physiologic since most exercise is performed in the upright position. The stroke volume as well as rate are adjusted to provide increased cardiac output in contrast to the supine position where rate alone is involved. Most laboratories use a motor-driven treadmill or a bicycle ergometer. Both methods allow incremental increases in exercise workload. The treadmill has the disadvantage of being potentially dangerous for small children who may fall off if the device is started abruptly or if they become fatigued. The bicycle ergometer,

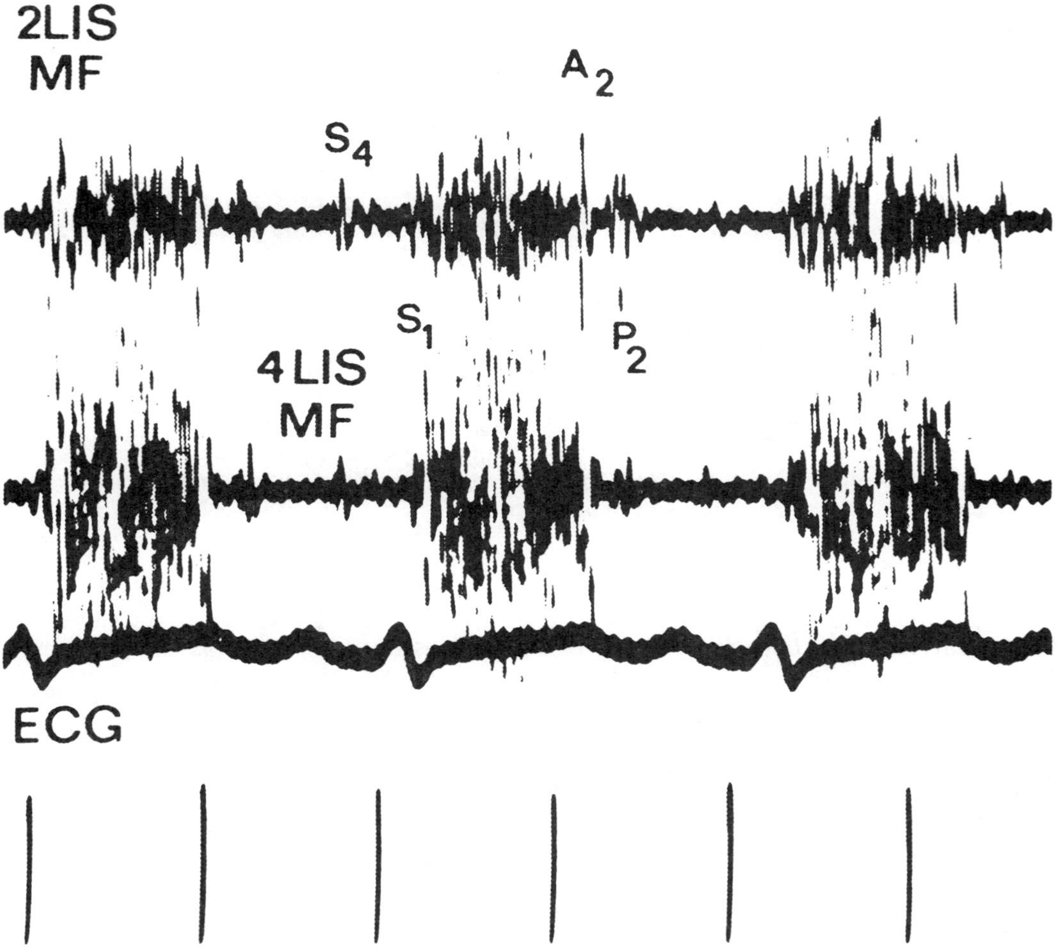

Figure 2-71 A medium-pitch holosystolic murmur is recorded primarily at the fourth left intercostal space in a child with ventricular septal defect. Note that the murmur begins with S_1 and virtually obliterates the aortic component of S_2 at the area of maximal intensity. The fourth heart sound (S_4) is recorded following the P wave of the EKG. (Reproduced with permission from Nades AS, Fyler DC, Pediatric Cardiology, 3rd ed., 1972, W. B. Saunders Co., Philadelphia.)

on the other hand, is readily accepted by children, and models are available which can accommodate small body sizes.

Exercise Programs

All programs have in common a low initial workload with increases in predetermined increments. The absolute work levels and rate at which they are increased will vary with the size of the patient and with the type of testing device. Most laboratories utilizing the bicycle ergometer in studying children start with a workload of 100 kg/m/min.

Parameters Evaluated

Total Pump Function (Work Capacity)

1. *Measurement of cardiac output:* This is the ultimately desirable parameter for the evaluation of the overall pumping capacity of the heart but generally requires invasive techniques, making it a particularly difficult to utilize in young children. Methods making use of the indirect Fick principle with rebreathing or utilizing inhalation of other gases have been developed but are complicated and are appropriate to the research laboratory.
2. *Cardiac rate:* This is the easiest parameter to measure but has not been sufficiently sensitive to allow evaluation of cardiac function.
3. *Maximum oxygen consumption:* Maximum oxygen consumption is a relatively good estimator of oxygen delivery to the tissue, but its value in children with congenital heart disease has not yet been proven.
4. *Maximum endurance:* Comparison of maximum workload and duration achieved with available standards for children is easily carried out and appears of great promise in assessing cardiac work capacity.

Selected Hemodynamic Parameters

For the most part, selected hemodynamic parameters have been applied to evaluation of the change in the pressure gradient across a stenotic valve with exercise and, therefore, have been utilized in the catheterization laboratory. Difficulties in applicability to children have been mentioned previously. Attempts have been made to simulate exercise pharmacologically or electrically in ways which would not require patient cooperation, but their value has been limited. Atrial pacing has been shown to be of little use in this regard. Isoproterenol infusion has been utilized in some centers for years, but its relationship to spontaneous exercise has been uncertain. Recent studies have carefully correlated the two modes and offer some promise of increased applicability of such pharmacologic maneuvers. Changes in chamber volumes and in myocardial contractility can be assessed only by complicated methodology suitable at the present time for research but not clinical use.

Electrocardiographic Changes

1. *Ischemic changes:* Detection of ischemic depression of the ST segment was the first use of exercise testing and is a routine technique in adult cardiology. As discussed later, certain congenital cardiac defects interfere with myocardial perfusion, and this type of evaluation may be of great use in assessing the severity of such abnormalities.

2. *Rhythm changes:* The EKG is monitored for appearance or disappearance of arrhythmias with exercise or for evaluation of rate response in selected abnormalities (v.i.).

Clinical Applications

Evaluation of Symptoms

Assessment of exercise capability is helpful in two situations encountered commonly in children: those patients who present with symptoms apparently out of proportion to the cardiac findings and in the evaluation of chest pain.

A history of easy fatigability and inability to participate in physical activities is frequently obtained in situations where the remainder of the cardiovascular evaluation suggests that the symptoms are not of cardiac origin. This is no problem if the child clearly does not have cardiac abnormality, but in the presence of apparently mild congenital heart defects may be somewhat more difficult to assess. Objective measurement of maximum work capacity can clarify the confusion very rapidly. Likewise, we have encountered frequent referrals for evaluation of chest pain, primarily during early adolescent years. In most instances a careful history will establish a pattern of benign idiopathic chest pain (see Chap. 1). A history of exercise-induced pain is of somewhat more concern and may warrant evaluation of maximum endurance together with an exercise electrocardiogram.

Assessment of Severity of Selected Lesions

A relatively good idea of the severity of most congenital and acquired heart defects in children can be obtained from the evaluation of the history, physical examination, electrocardiogram, and x-ray. A particular problem is encountered with congenital aortic stenosis, since it is well recognized that there is a tendency for progressively increasing severity with growth, and severe degrees of obstruction may be seen with essentially no abnormalities other than the presence of the murmur. Likewise, increasing severity may not be accompanied by other changes. This has committed most children with this abnormality to serial catheterizations, and for this reason widespread efforts have been made to find methods of noninvasive evaluation which are more precise. The increased ventricular wall tension seen in more severe degrees of aortic stenosis may interfere with myocardial perfusion, and it has been known for a number of years that ischemic ST-T changes on the EKG may be precipitated by exercise. More recently, the correlation with cardiac catheterization results has suggested that such changes are generally seen when the transvalvular gradient exceeds 50 torr (Fig. 2-72). Other studies have shown similar findings in patients with aortic regurgitation, but correlation of severity has not been carried out. Exercise testing may be extremely useful in following such patients and may reduce the need for cardiac catherization.

Proper timing of the cardiac surgery for maximum preservation of myocardial function remains an unanswered question in virtually all congenital heart lesions. As techniques of exercise testing allow for ready determination of total pump function and selected aspects of ventricular function, they may be of some value in determining the proper time for surgical intervention.

Evaluation of the Postoperative Patient

In the past, attempts at quantitative evaluation of patients following surgery have generally been limited to performing cardiac catheterizations in those in

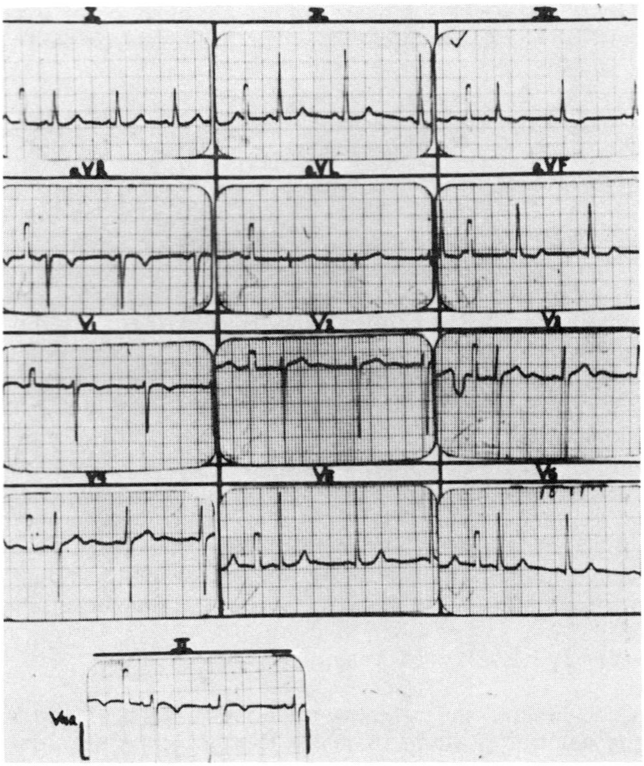

Figure 2-72A A 13-lead EKG in a 12-year-old boy with moderate congenital valvular aortic stenosis. Mildly excessive leftward-posterior QRS forces suggest the presence of left ventricular hypertrophy (see Fig. 2-72B).

whom there is overt evidence of a residual defect. More recently, exercise testing, particularly involving measurement of cardiac output, has cast serious doubt on the concept of total correction of even the simplest defects. Cardiac output response to exercise has been found to be subnormal in such lesions as atrial septal defect, ventricular septal defect, and tetralogy of Fallot. The full significance of these findings and their implication for the future life of the patient remain unclear at this time, and much more investigation in this area is needed.

Evaluation of Arrhythmias

Premature beats, particularly of ventricular origin, are commonly seen in children and may occur with alarming frequency. If there is no underlying heart disease, the vast majority of these will be alleviated when tachycardia is induced by exercise. Such an evaluation is important because exercise elimination of these beats generally indicates a benign prognosis (see Figs. 27-5 and 27-9). Another area for exercise investigation would be in patients where sinus node dysfunction or abnormalities of atrioventricular conduction are present. Bradycardia is the rule in these patients, and assessment of the degree to which the ventricular rate can accelerate with exercise would be an important factor in planning further therapy. Exercise may be used in an attempt to provoke an

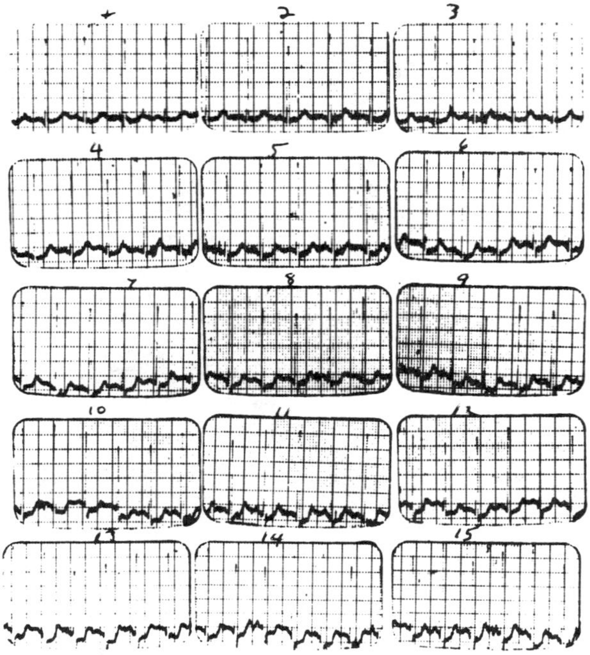

Figure 2-72B Exercise electrocardiogram from the same patient. Numbers at the top of each strip indicate the duration of exercise in minutes. There is a significant horizontal depression of the ST segment indicative of at least a moderate degree of obstruction. Gradient across the aortic valve at catheterization proved to be 70 mmHg.

arrhythmia where the history is suggestive but resting tracings have failed to demonstrate any problem.

Of increasing importance in the last 2-3 years is the utilization of exercise testing in an effort ot provoke arrhythmias in the postoperative patient. Episodes of sudden death occasionally occurring several years after apparently successful surgery for some of the congenital heart defects have precipitated this concern. Sudden death has been reported in patients following surgery for tetralogy of Fallot or congenital aortic stenosis. Studies performed to date have suggested that premature ventricular contractions or runs of ventricular tachycardia during or immediately following exercise have an ominous prognosis. As with the assessment of myocardial function in the postoperative patient, the evaluation of arrhythmias is in its infancy, and much additional work needs to be done.

Echocardiography

Echocardiography has proven to be one of the most rewarding techniques yet developed for noninvasive evaluation of the heart. Although the basic principles of reflected ultrasound have long been known, it is only relatively recently that refinement in instrumentation and technique has made cardiac ultrasound an indispensible and widely available diagnostic tool. It is beyond the scope of this chapter to discuss the physical principles of ultrasound or to discuss the instrumentation. However, the following brief summary of the basic principles of echocardiography is necessary for understanding the technique and its application.

M-Mode Echocardiography

M-mode echocardiography utilizes a single beam of ultrasound (2.25 - 7.5 mHz) generated by a crystalline transducer placed on the chest wall. After a short transmission, the transducer acts as a receiver listening for returning sound or echoes. Echoes are reflected from any interface between material having different densities (muscle, blood, valves, lungs, chest wall). The returning sound energy is then converted to an electrical impulse which can be displayed and recorded on a strip chart. The motion of the cardiac structure in the line of the transducer beam can be shown on one axis, and time can be displayed on the other axis (Fig. 2-73). Thus, motion in respect to time can be visualized permitting assessment of the range and velocity of motion of various cardiac structures. The transducer is positioned perpendicular to the chest wall along the left sternal border in a position at which the anterior mitral valve leaflet is well seen (Fig. 2-73, position 2). From this position the transducer is pivoted in various directions so as to visualize serially the cardiac structures of interest (Fig. 2-73).

Mitral Valve

Motion of the mitral valve has been well defined since it is the easiest cardiac structure to be visualized and was the first one to be identified. The motion pattern of both the normal and abnormal valve has been correlated with specific events occurring in systole and diastole (Fig. 2-74). At the onset of diastole, the valve leaflets rapidly move in opposite direction to the point of maximum opening (d-e). Thereafter, the leaflet rapidly, then slowly, moves toward a position of midclosure during ventricular filling (e-f). With atrial systole, a transient reopening motion occurs (a-point) closely coinciding with a fourth heart sound, following which the leaflets rapidly move to the final point of closure (c-point), marking the onset of ventricular systole. The leaflets maintain their closed position during systole with gradual anterior motion terminating at the next point of diastolic opening (d-point).

Specific abnormal patterns of motion have been identified for many conditions affecting the mitral valve (Fig. 2-75). More commonly encountered problems include mitral stenosis (diminished E-F slope, abnormal anterior diastolic motion of the posterior leaflet, multiple dense mitral echoes suggesting calcification) (Fig. 2-75A). Mitral valve prolapse is easily demonstrable on the M-mode echocardiogram. A spectrum of M-mode patterns has been described. Late systolic posterior displacement of the posterior and often anterior mitral valve leaflet is most confirmatory. Holosystolic hammocking is less often convincing unless the hammocking exceeds 2 mm. In patients who do not have a clear prolapse on the M-mode echocardiogram, two-dimensional echocardiography (2-D) may provide further confirmation.

High-frequency diastolic vibrations of the anterior leaflet of the mitral valve are often seen with aortic regurgitation (Fig. 2-75C). The occurrence of this finding seems more related to the direction of the regurgitant jet rather than to the degree of aortic regurgitation.

Systolic anterior motion (SAM) of the mitral valve is seen in obstructive cardiomyopathy (Fig. 2-75D). This is usually associated with a thick flat septum without similar hypertrophy of the posterior left ventricular wall. The degree of impingement of the mitral valve on the septum during systole correlates with the presence or absence of obstruction.

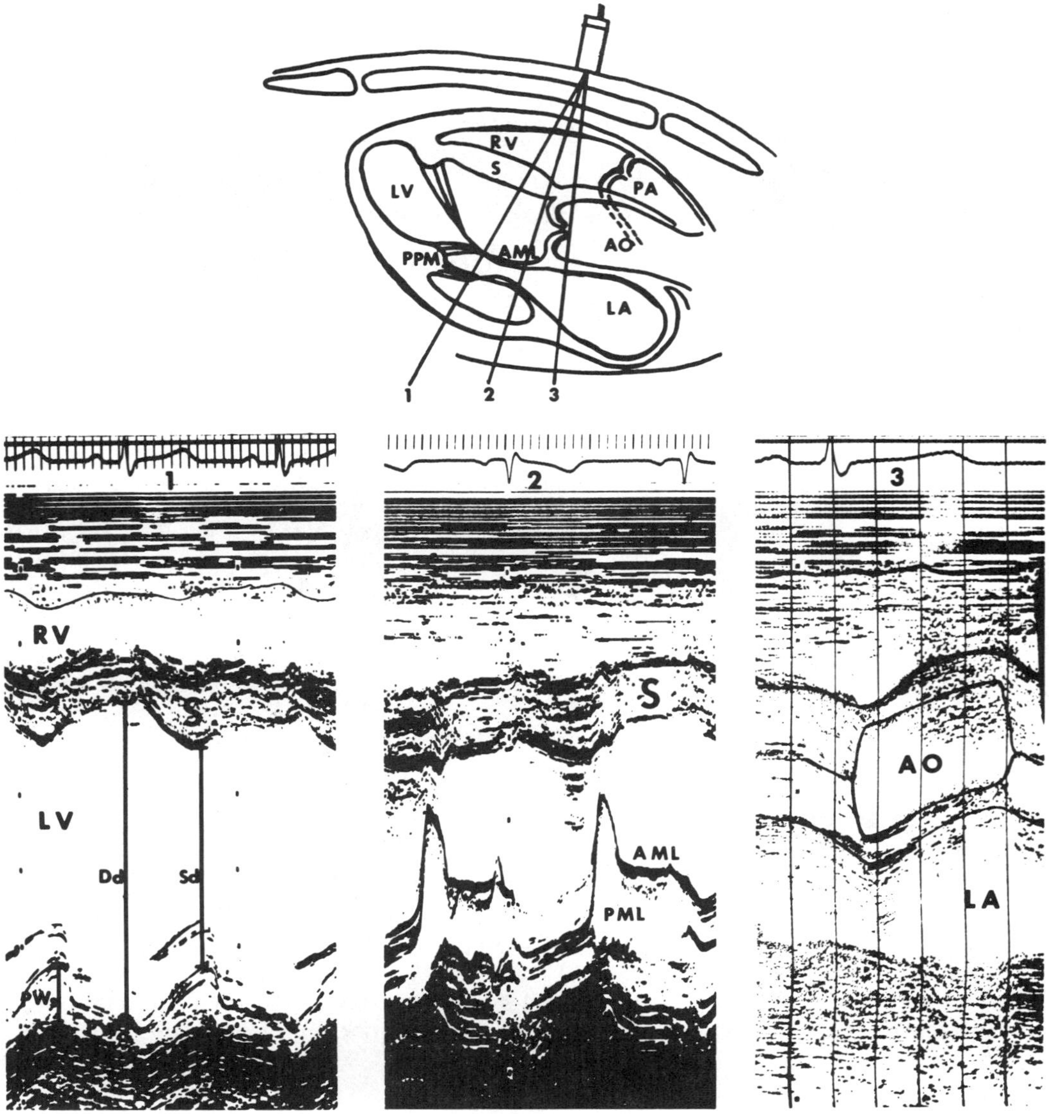

Figure 2–73 Pivoting the transducer on the chest wall can direct the sound beam through different cardiac structures. In panel 1, the beam is directed toward the apical region, intersecting in succession the chest wall, right ventricular wall, right ventricular cavity (RV), ventricular septum (S), left ventricular cavity (LV), and left ventricular posterior wall (PW). Directing the beam more cephalad (panel 2) identifies the anterior and posterior mitral leaflets (AML, PML) and chordal attachments. Further cephalad orientation (panel 3) projects the sonic beam through the aortic root (Ao) with the left atrial cavity (LA) lying posteriorly. The aortic valve cusps open and close in boxlike fashion. Note that the aortic root lies posterior to the septal plane. The posterior aortic wall is continuous with the mitral annulus and the anterior aortic wall continuous with the ventricular septum.

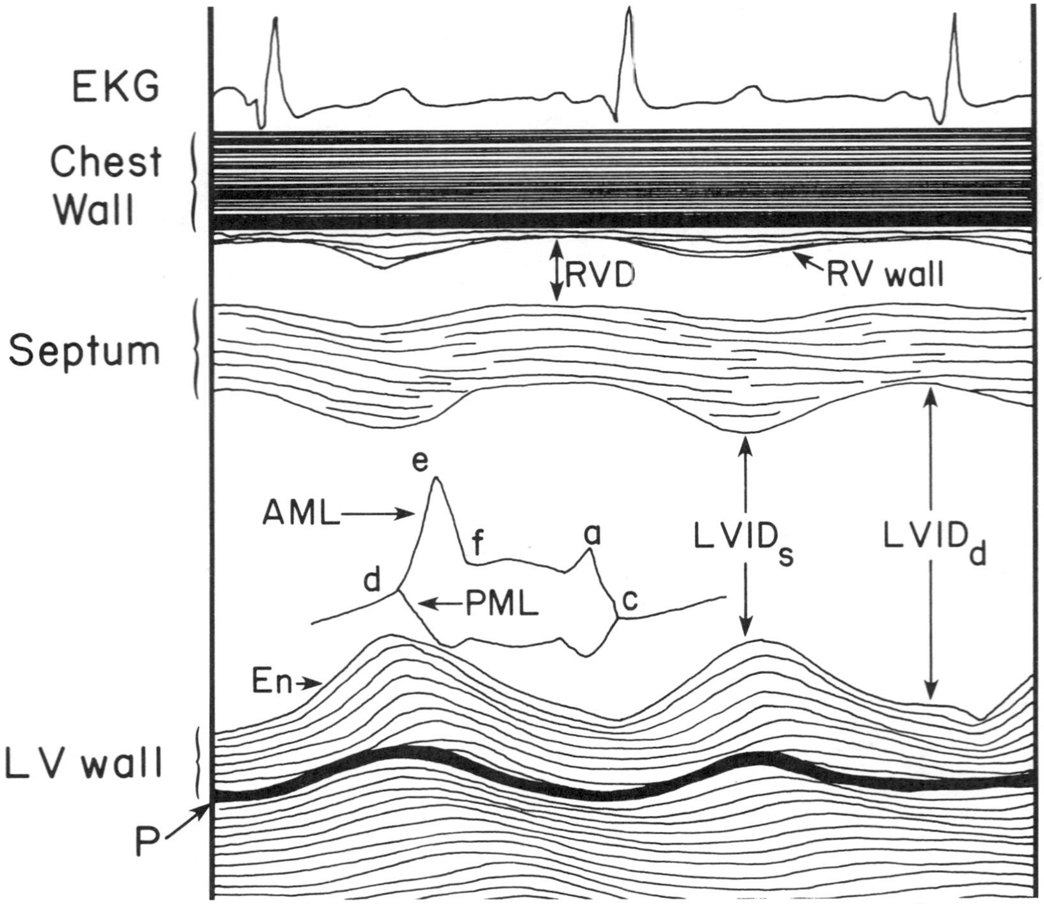

Figure 2-74 Ventricular chamber dimensions and normal mitral valve motion as determined from echocardiogram. RVD - right ventricular dimension. $LVID_s$ - left ventricular systolic dimension. $LVID_d$ - left ventricular diastolic dimension, En - endocardium, AML - anterior mitral leaflet, PML - posterior mitral leaflet, P - pericardium. See text for discussion of normal mitral motion.

Aortic Valve

The echocardiogram of the aortic root is recognized by the characteristic undulating systolic-diastolic parallel motion of the anterior and posterior aortic walls. Typically, two of the three aortic valve cusps can be identified opening in boxlike fashion during systole and closing in the midline of the confines of the aortic root (Fig. 2-73, panel 3; Fig. 2-76). The relationship of the septum to the anterior margin of the aorta can be demonstrated by scanning the mitral valve all the way to the aorta. The septum is then seen continuous with the anterior wall of the aorta, whereas the anterior leaflet of the mitral valve is continuous with the posterior wall of the aorta.

Aortic stenosis is suggested by significant eccentricity of the diastolic closure line and multiple dense valve echoes (Fig. 2-76B). Supravalvular aortic stenosis has been identified by narrowing of the supravalvular area with normal cusp motion.

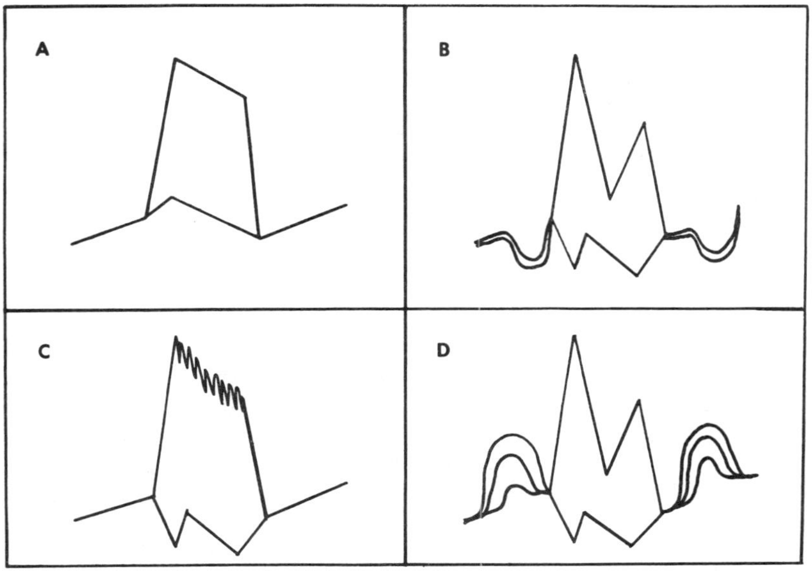

Figure 2–75 Examples of various abnormal mitral valve motion patterns. (A) Stenotic mitral valve. Note diminished early diastolic closure motion of anterior leaflet ("flat" E–F slope) and abnormal anterior diastolic motion of posterior leaflet paralleling that of the anterior leaflet. (B) Mitral valve prolapse. Abrupt posterior motion of the valve in mid and late systole with multiple closure lines. (C) Vibrations of the anterior leaflet of the mitral valve resulting from aortic regurgitation. (D) Systolic anterior motion (SAM) of the mitral valve as seen in asymmetric septal hypertrophy (hypertrophic subaortic stenosis or obstructive cardiomyopathy).

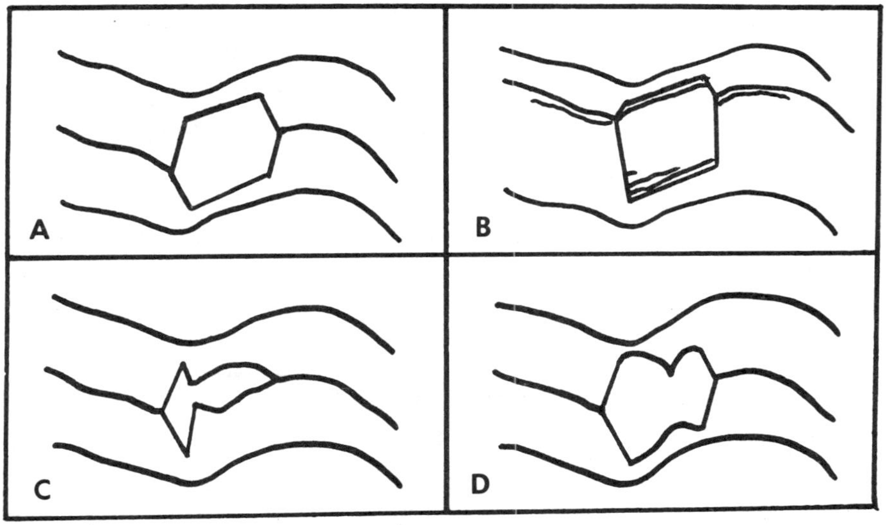

Figure 2–76 Examples of aortic valve motion patterns. (A) Normal aortic valve. (B) Eccentric diastolic closure line of the aortic cusps seen in bicuspid aortic valve. (C) Early systolic closure of the aortic cusps seen in discrete subvalvular aortic stenosis. (D) Midsystolic closure of the aortic valve as seen in obstructive hypertrophic cardiomyopathy.

Discrete subvalvular stenosis results in subvalvular narrowing, systolic fluttering of the cusp, and an early systolic closing motion (Fig. 2-76C). The latter may also be seen in hypertrophic subaortic stenosis, although the partial closure occurs slightly later in systole, and a prominent late systolic opening motion is present (Fig. 2-76D). Aortic regurgitation may be associated with prominent diastolic vibration of the valve.

Pulmonic Valve

The pulmonic valve is somewhat more difficult to record because of anatomic considerations, and frequently only the posterior cusp is clearly defined. A characteristic presystolic downward motion (A wave) of the pulmonic valve occurs following atrial contraction, and the diastolic closure line normally slopes downward (Fig. 2-77A). Pulmonic stenosis results in an exaggerated A wave (see Fig. 2-77B), while pulmonary hypertension flattens or reverses the diastolic slope, may eliminate the A wave, and produces a midsystolic closing motion of the cusp (Fig. 2-77C).

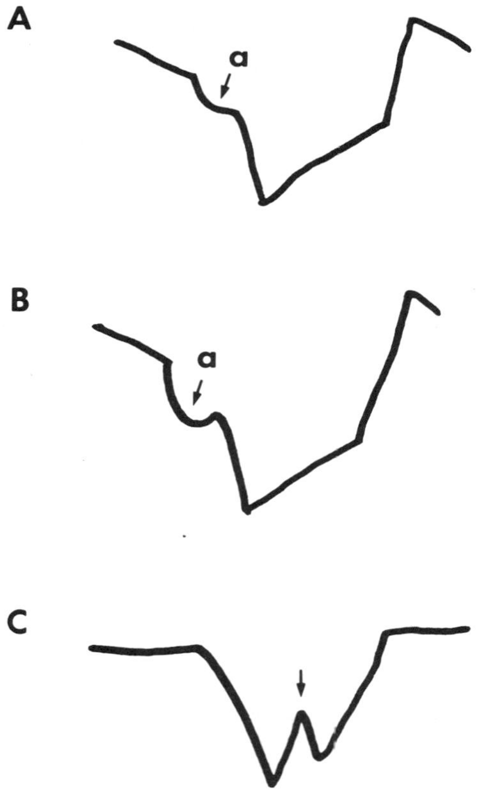

Figure 2-77 Examples of pulmonic valve motion patterns. (A) Normal pulmonic valve with a normal A wave. (B) Exaggerated A wave in pulmonic valvular stenosis. (C) Absent A wave, diastolic flattening, and midsystolic closure (arrow) in pulmonary hypertension.

Tricuspid Valve

The tricuspid valve has been studied less extensively, but is fairly easy to record in children. Its motion resembles that of the mitral valve. Abnormalities of motion have been defined in the Ebstein malformation where late closure is highly characteristic. Wide excursions and flattening of the diastolic closure slope are also seen. Other abnormalities of tricuspid valve motions are seen in tricuspid stenosis, pulmonary regurgitation, and atrioventricular canal defect.

Right Ventricular Volume Overload

The lesions most often associated with right ventricular volume overload are secundum-type atrial septal defect, ostium primum defect, total anomalous pulmonary venous drainage, pulmonic regurgitation, and tricuspid regurgitation. The two echocardiographic features classically associated with right ventricular volume overload are increased right ventricular dimensions and abnormal septal motion (Fig. 2-78).

Normally the ventricular septum moves posteriorly (away from the transducer) during systole, towards the left ventricular wall to effect left ventricular emptying (Fig. 2-79). Paradoxical septal motion exists when the septum moves anteriorly (synchronous with the left ventricular wall) during systole. In between these two extremes, the motion may be flat and is called intermediate. The proper recording of septal motion is attained when the tip of the mitral valve and the chordae are just showing.

The mitral valve echo is an important distinguishing feature between ostium secundum and primum defect (Fig. 2-78). In ostium secundum defect the mitral valve echo appears normal, whereas in ostium primum defect the mitral valve echo is grossly abnormal (Fig. 2-78B). There are multiple echoes during systole and diastole, and the valve strikes the interventricular septum in diastole. If the dominant lesion is a left-to-right shunt at the atrial level, the left atrium is not enlarged.

Left Ventricular Volume Overload

Left ventricular volume overload is produced by aortic and mitral regurgitation, patent ductus arteriosus, or by ventricular septal defect as well as congestive cardiomyopathy or heart failure.

Aortic regurgitation results in dilated left ventricle, but normal left atrium (Fig. 2-80). There is usually diastolic fluttering of the mitral valve. In contrast, in mitral regurgitation both left atrium and left ventricle are enlarged (Fig. 2-81). Evaluation of the atrial dimensions on serial examination is quite useful in assessing the progression of the disease.

Ultrasound has been extremely useful in assessing the left-to-right shunting through the patent ductus arteriosus in premature infants. The increased left-atrium-to-aortic ratio appears to correlate with the amount of pulmonary blood flow and, therefore, the degree of left-to-right shunt. (Fig. 7-9, Chap. on PDA).

In congestive cardiomyopathy (Fig. 2-82) both the left atrium and left ventricle are large; however, contractility is diminished as well as mitral valve excursion during diastole. This is in contrast to mitral regurgitation where both these chambers are enlarged, but the left ventricle is hyperdynamic.

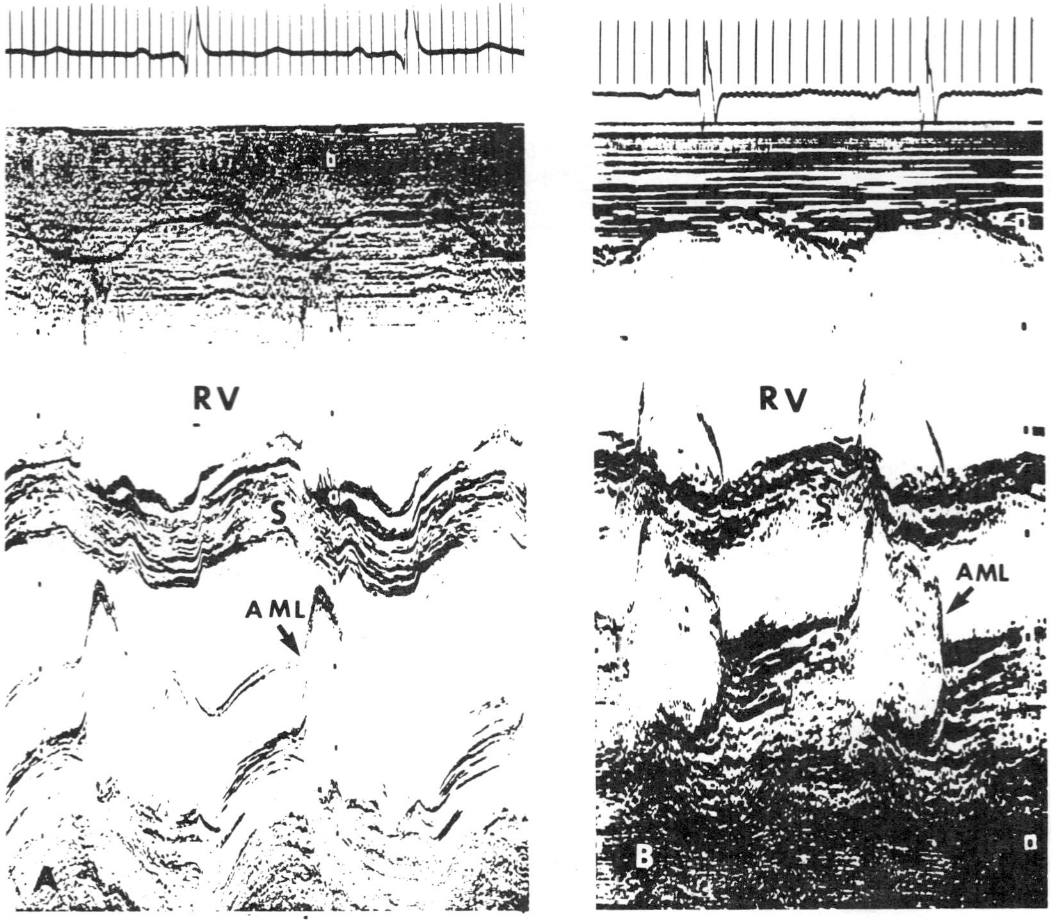

Figure 2-78 Right ventricular volume overload. (A) Atrial septal defect 2°. The right ventricle is enlarged; there is paradoxical septal motion. (B) Ostium primum defect. The findings are the same as above. The anterior mitral valve echo is abnormal, exhibting multiple systolic and diastolic echoes. During diastole the anterior mitral valve leaflet appears to go through the septum. RV - right ventricle, S - septum, AML - anterior mitral leaflet.

Left Ventricular Outflow Obstruction

In this category we include aortic valvular stenosis, subvalvular stenosis, and hypertrophic obstructive cardiomyopathy. The main echocardiographic findings in aortic valvular stenosis are:

1. Multiple diastolic echoes of the aortic valve
2. Eccentric aortic closure line
3. Increased thickness of the septum and free wall of the left ventricle
4. Increased shortening fraction of the left ventricle

Shortening fraction has the highest correlation with the aortic valve gradient measured at the time of catheterization. In patients with a shortening fraction, equal to or less than 40%, the gradient was always less than 45 mmHg; however, if the shortening fraction was larger, there was a great chance for a gradient to be over 70 mmHg. In addition, left ventricular end-systolic wall thickness and left ventricular end-systolic cavity dimension derived from echo measurements are used in the following formula to estimate left ventricular systolic pressure (LVSP) (Fig. 10-5).

$$\text{LVSP} = 225 \times \frac{\text{Left ventricular end-systolic wall thickness}}{\text{Left ventricular end-systolic cavity dimension}}$$

The left ventricular pressure derived this way in children with aortic stenosis correlates well with the left ventricular pressure determined at cardiac catheterization.

Obstruction to the left ventricular outflow from discrete subaortic membrane or obstructive cardiomyopathy has distinct echocardiographic findings. These findings were briefly mentioned in a previous section of this chapter (Fig. 2-76).

Cyanotic Congenital Heart Disease

Echocardiogram has been most useful in the neonatal period, enhancing our ability to diagnose or exclude congenital heart disease. It is impossible in this format to enumerate and illustrate the various lesions in this category. This

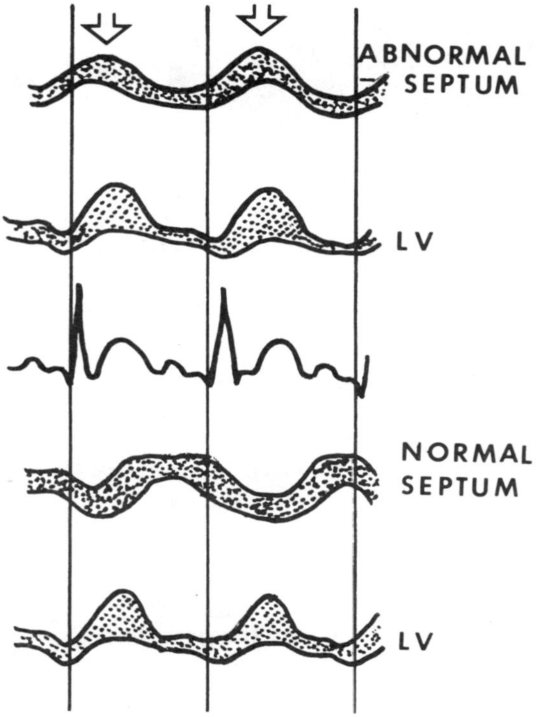

Figure 2-79 Patterns of septal motion. See text for explanation.

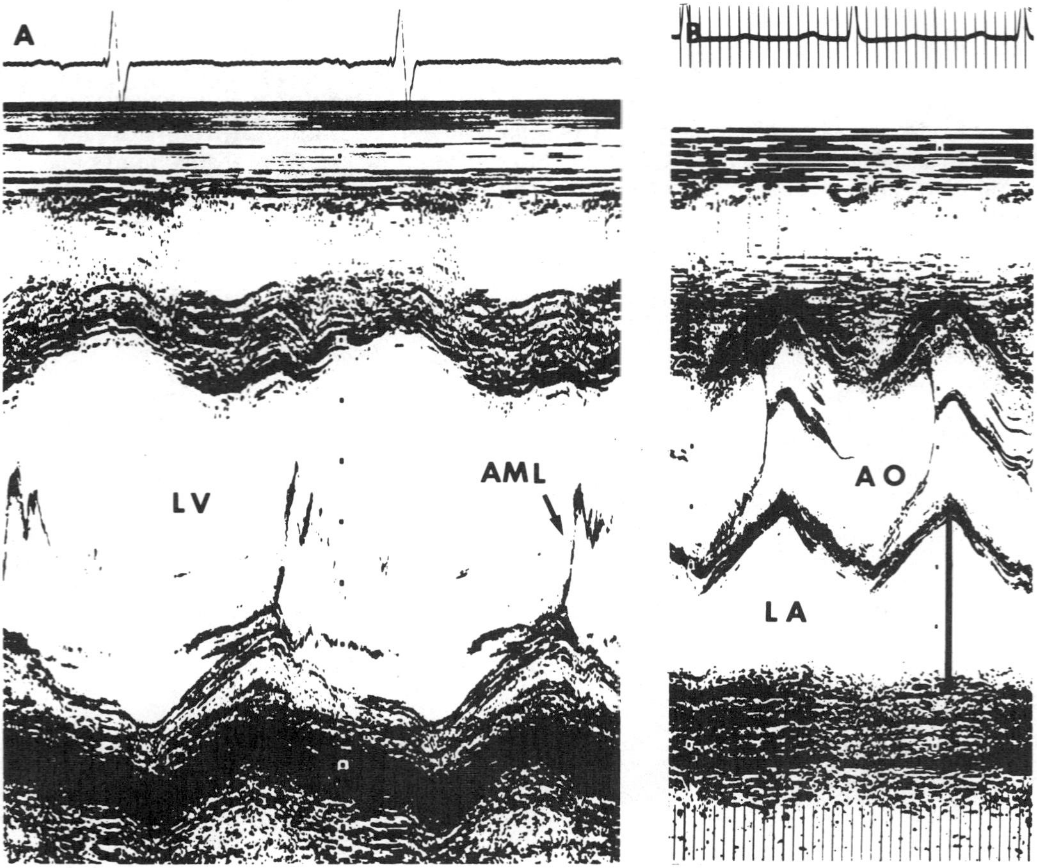

Figure 2-80 Echocardiogram of a 12-year-old with aortic regurgitation. The left ventricle is enlarged. The left atrium, however, is of normal size. LV - left ventricle, Ao - aorta, LA - left atrium, AML - anterior leaflet of the mitral valve.

technique has been most useful in demonstrating overriding of the aorta in tetralogy of Fallot, confirming the suspicion of a single ventricle by demonstrating absent ventricular septum. It is most reliable in diagnosing hypoplastic left heart, demonstrating absent or slitlike left ventricular cavity, and minute aorta. Most cyanotic heart diseases in the newborn are better diagnosed with a 2-D echocardiogram.

Assessment of Left Ventricular Function

The M-mode echocardiogram remains the best noninvasive tool for assessing left ventricular function, contractility, dimension, and thickness.

Shortening Fraction (SF)

The shortening fraction of the left ventricle is a measure of its contractility. It represents the ratio of the difference of the end-diastolic dimension (Dd) and the end-systolic dimension (Ds) over the end-diastolic dimension (Fig. 2-73).

$$SF = \frac{Dd - Ds}{Dd} \times 100$$

The end-diastolic dimension is measured at the onset of the QRS. The end-systolic dimension is measured at the nadir of posterior motion of the interventricular septum when septal motion is normal. These measurements should be performed at the mitral chordal level (Fig. 2-73, between positions 1 and 2). The normal shortening fraction varies between 28 and 38%.

Shortening fraction appears to be the most reliable index of left ventricular function. A single value, however, is of limited use in assessing ventricular performance. Serial evaluation provides a more reliable indication of relative change in myocardial performance. The shortening fraction is usually decreased in the poorly compensated ventricle, regardless of the cause of the dysfunction: pressure or volume overload, or primary myocardial disorder. Conversely, left ventricular shortening fraction increases in compensated ventricular overload (e.g., aortic regurgitation, aortic stenosis, or even hypertrophic cardiomyopathy).

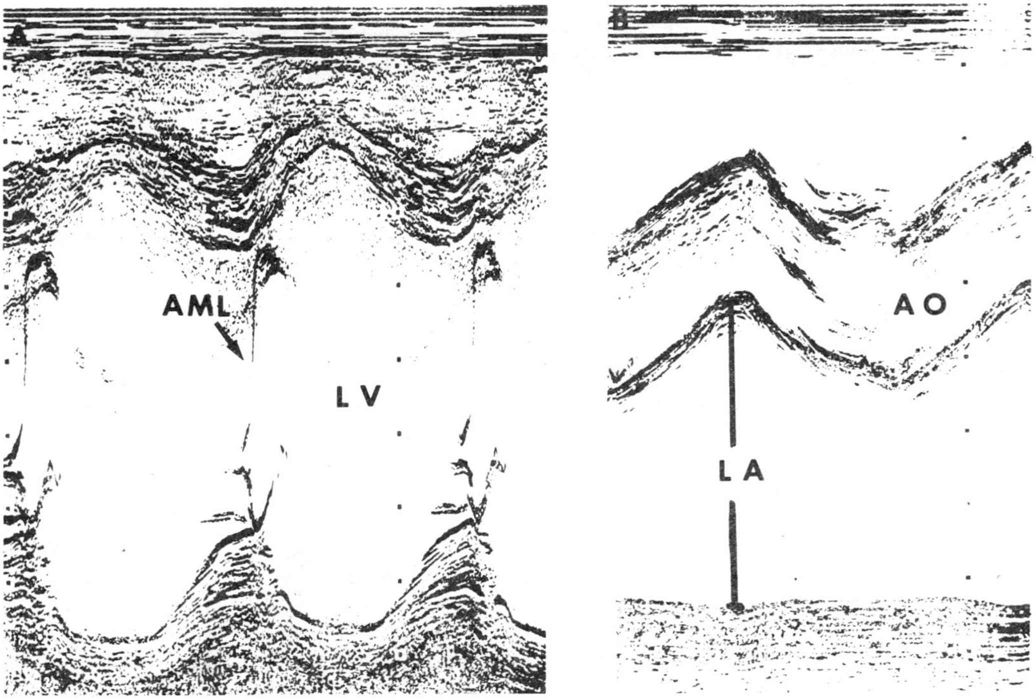

Figure 2-81 Echocardiogram of a patient with rheumatic mitral regurgitation. Note the large hyperdynamic LV and the markedly enlarged left atrium. LA - left atrium, LV - left ventricle, Ao - aorta, S - septum, AML - anterior leaflet of the mitral valve.

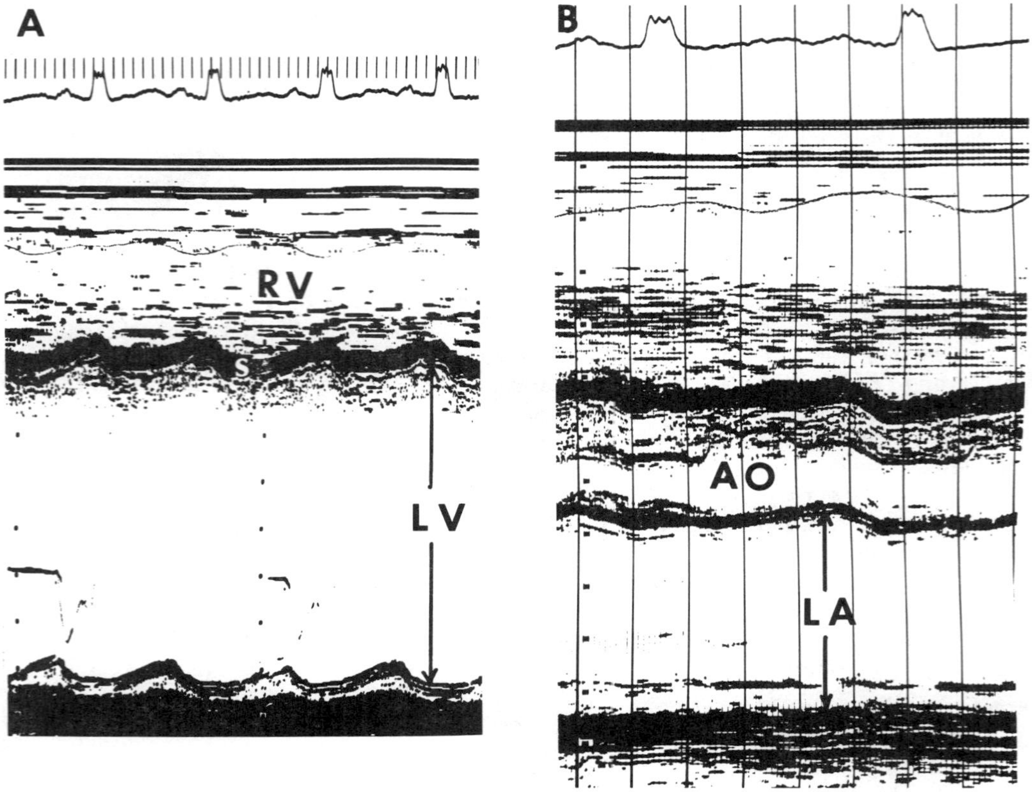

Figure 2-82 Echocardiogram of a patient with dilated cardiomyopathy. Note the dilated left ventricle, decreased contractility, normal aorta, but enlarged left atrium. The shortening fraction is 20%. LV - left ventricle, LA - left atrium, Ao - aorta, S - septum, RV - right ventricle.

Adriamycin Toxicity

Adriamycin is a most useful chemotherapeutic agent in the treatment of malignant tumors. However, there is a dose-dependent cardiomyopathy which manifests as decreased voltage in the electrocardiogram and cardiac failure. Once cardiac failure has developed, the mortality is in the range of 75%.

In an attempt to identify the patients at risk, the shortening fraction was found to be the most useful parameter of left ventricular function to monitor. A greater than 5% decrease in shortening fraction is indicative of significant myocardial changes. In a large series reported by Meyer, 44% of the patients developed signs of adriamycin toxicity (a shortening fraction under 28%), but only 4% developed severe congestive cardiomyopathy (a shortening fraction under 15%). In asymptomatic patients with evidence of progressive cardiac dysfunction, cessation of adriamycin therapy alone resulted in improved function. It is our practice to obtain an echocardiogram before beginning adriamycin therapy, before each additional treatment, and 2-3 months after cessation of adriamycin therapy.

Systolic Time Intervals

The systolic time interval (STI) of a ventricle includes the preejection period (PEP) and the ventricular ejection time (VET) (Fig. 2-83). The PEP is measured from the onset of the Q wave of the electrocardiogram to the opening of the semilunar valve. VET is measured from cusp opening to cusp closure. The effect of the heart rate can be minimized by deriving a ratio of PEP/VET. The normal value for the right ventricle (RPEP/RVET) is 0.24 (range 0.16-0.30) and for the left ventricle (LVEP/LVET) is 0.35 (range 0.30-0.39).

Several factors influence the duration of PEP and VET. These are: (1) preload, (2) contractile state of the myocardium, and (3) afterload or sequence and rate of ventricular conduction. In the presence of decreased myocardial contractility, as the ventricular performance diminishes, the PEP lengthens and VET shortens, thereby producing an elevated PEP/VET ratio.

Changes in afterload can cause an increase or decrease in systolic time intervals. Reduction in afterload such as large aortic runoff (PDA) causes reduction in PEP and, therefore, reduction in the ratio (assuming the contractility is normal). When afterload is elevated such as in pulmonary or systemic hypertension, the PEP lengthens, the VET shortens, and the ratio increases. The application of RPEP/RVET has become useful in assessing the pulmonary artery diastolic pressure. There is a good correlation between the right ventricular STI and pulmonary artery diastolic pressure measured at cardiac catheterization. Of patients with a ratio of 0.30 or less, 95% have pulmonary artery diastolic pressure of less than 30 mmHg.

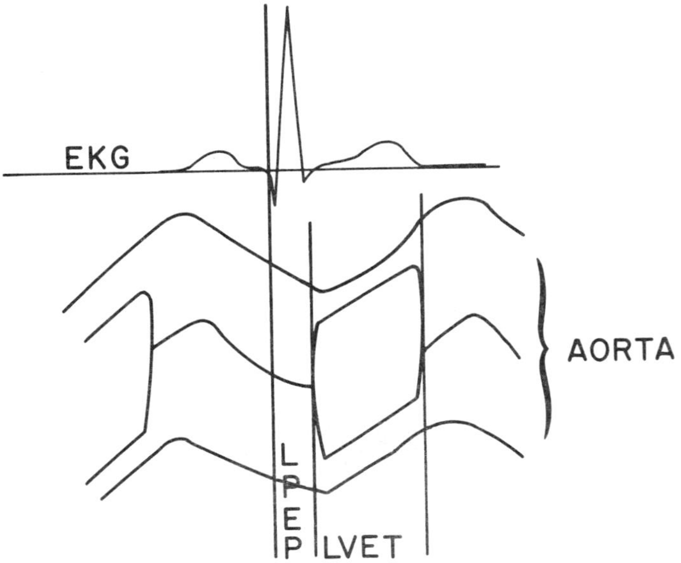

Figure 2-83 Method for determining left ventricular systolic time intervals from echocardiographic recording of aortic valve. Preejection period (LPEP) is measured from the Q wave of the electrocardiogram to the opening of the valve. Left ventricular ejection time (LVET) is the interval from opening to closing of the valve. These and the ratio, LPEP/LVET, are indicators of ventricular function.

Two-Dimensional Echocardiography

Two-dimensional (2-D) ultrasonic imaging of the heart has enormously increased our appreciation of spacial orientation of cardiac structures. At the present time there are three methods of two-dimensional real-time imaging. These are: (1) mechanical sector scanner, (2) multielement linear array, and (3) electronic sector scanner or phased-array system.

The mechanical scanner consists of a single crystal transducer made to oscillate rapidly by means of an electric motor through a 30-60° arc. The disadvantages of this system are the narrow angle and the noise and vibrations which may be uncomfortable and scare the young child. More recently, a wide-angle (80-90°) mechanical sector scanner, utilizing multiple rotating crystals, has been developed which overcomes most of these problems.

Since all echoes start at the transducer face and fan out, the result will be a cone-shaped sector with maximal line density at the top of the cone and decreased line density at the bottom of the cone due to the fanning effect. It is difficult to display the true information content of the pictures generated by these systems in still illustrations since the 2-D is a dynamic examination of images displayed rapidly enough to give the effect of a motion picture. Abnormalities of shape or motion pattern of either walls or valvular structure are much more easily detected when the examination is reviewed in real time. Permanent recording can be made on videotape, and single frames can be printed on Polaroid film.

The information obtained depends on the orientation of the transducer. Many views of the heart and great vessels are possible with different transducer positions. The following are the most commonly employed views (Fig. 2-84).

1. The long-axis view or sagittal plane
2. The short-axis view or transverse plane
3. The apical four-chamber view
4. The subxiphoid approach (four-chamber view)
5. The suprasternal notch approach

The Long-Axis Plane

The long-axis plane is displayed as a sagittal section of the heart viewed from the left side of the supine patient. The left ventricle inflow and outflow regions can be viewed as well as a portion of the right ventricle. The septal motion is clearly seen, and the aortic valve motion is identified. The left atrium lies behind the aorta. This view provides dynamic assessment of the mitral valve and aortic motion as well as the presence or absence of subvalvular or supravalvular aortic stenosis.

The Short-Axis Plane

The short-axis plane is obtained by rotating the transducer 90° clockwise from the long-axis plane. The circular aortic valve with its three cusps is visualized with a crescent-shaped right ventricular outflow tract above it (Fig. 2-85C). Angulating the transducer superiorly, one can visualize the pulmonic valve superiorly and to the left of the aortic. The pulmonic trunk can be followed up to its division into the right and left pulmonary arteries, just posterior to the aorta (Fig. 2-85D). Again, the circular left atrium is seen posterior to the aorta. By angulating the transducer downward, the left ventricle is transected at the level of the mitral valve which is seen as a "fish mouth" surrounded by the left ventricular myocardium (Fig. 2-85B). Further downward angulation along the left ventricular axis permits visualization of the papillary muscles and the left ventricular apex (Fig. 2-85A).

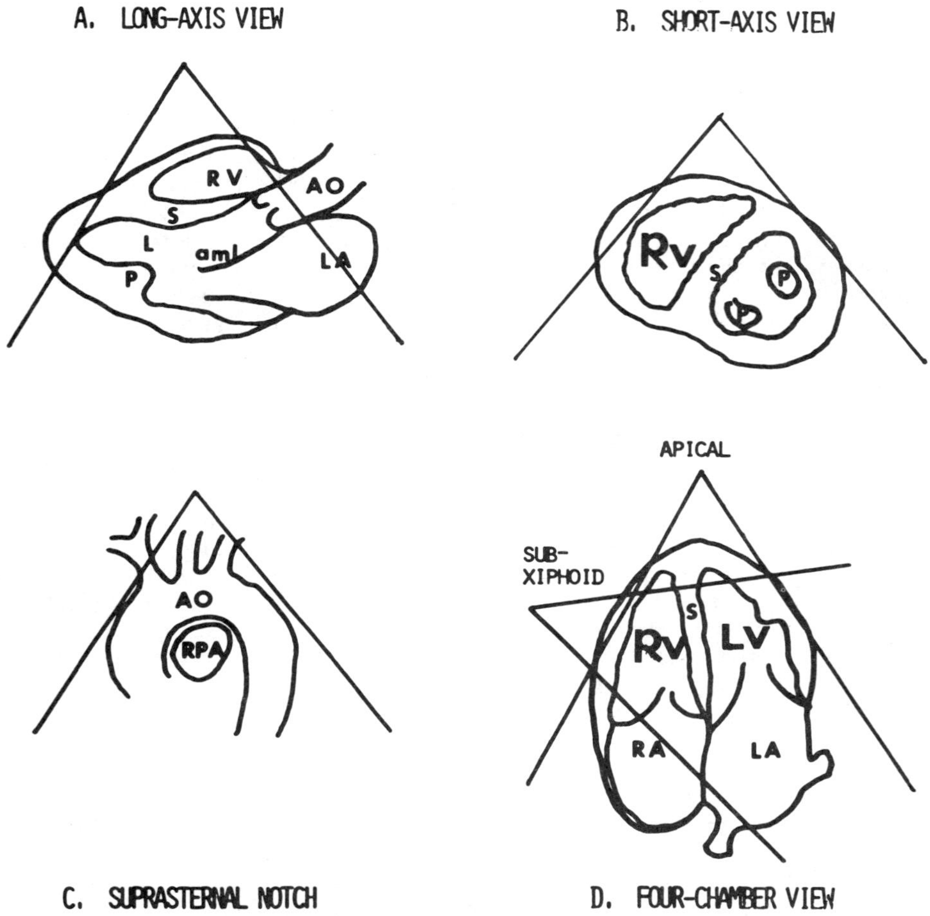

Figure 2-84 Diagram showing the transducer position used to obtain: (A) long-axis view, (B) short-axis view, (C) suprasternal view, and (D) four-chamber view. RV - right ventricle, LV - left ventricle, RA - right atrium, LA - left atrium, S - septum, Ao - aorta, RPA - right pulmonary artery, aml - anterior mitral valve, P - papillary muscle.

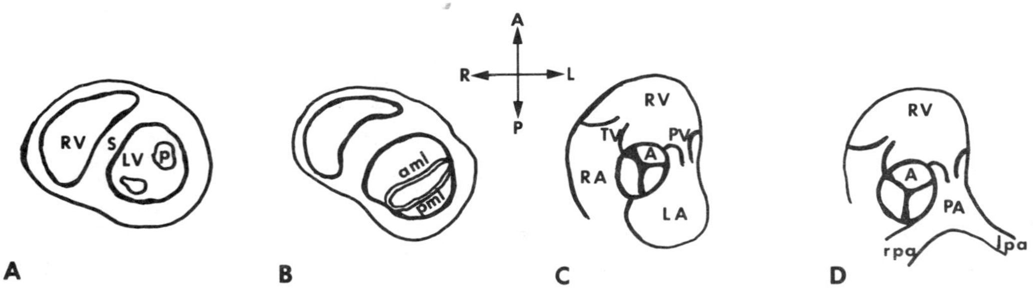

Figure 2-85 Schematic drawing of the images obtained from four levels of the short-axis view. (A) Through the left ventricle (LV), right ventricle (RV), and papillary muscle (P). (B) Through the anterior leaflet of the mitral valve (aml) and posterior leaflet (pml). (C) At the level of the aorta (A) with the right ventricular outflow (RV) and pulmonary valve (PV). (D) The pulmonary artery (PA) is seen branching (lpa and rpa).

Four-Chamber Views (Apical, Subxiphoid)

The four chamber view from the apex provides a unique image of ventricular and atrial anatomy. As shown in Figure 2-84D, the view provides a picture of all four chambers of the heart at one time. The image can be displayed on the screen in various ways depending on the equipment used and the transducer (Fig. 2-86). In our machinery the image seen in Fig. 2-86A and B, can be obtained by simply rotating the transducer 180°. Some of the machines are equiped with the possibility of rotating the image 180° without moving the transducer and, therefore, displaying it on the screen as an angiogram (Fig. 2-86C). This view provides an excellent visualization of the ventricular and atrial septae and the central fibrous body where both AV valves insert. The primum portion of the atrial septum and the upper portion of the ventricular septum are well seen; thus, this view is helpful for the diagnosis of endocardial cushion defect.

By shifting the transducer to the subxiphoid area, the ultrasound is more perpendicular to the ventricular and secundum atrial septum; therefore, it provides better images of these two structures (Fig. 2-86). It provides an excellent view of the secundum atrial septal defect and septal tears following balloon septostomy. Slight angulation of the transducer towards the outflow tract provides good image of the membranous ventricular septum and outflow tract. In infants with transposition of the great vessels, an outflow view of the left ventricle will demonstrate the bifurcation of the pulmonary artery (Fig. 2-89). The subxiphoid approach also permits the visualization of the inferior vena cava entering the right atrium, therefore aiding in the diagnosis of cardiac malposition.

Suprasternal Notch Approach

From this approach, by angulating the transducer in the direction of the aortic arch, the ascending aorta, the brachiocephalic vessels, and the aortic arch can be visualized. The images appear as a lateral aortic angiogram (Fig. 2-84C). The right pulmonary artery is cut transversely and seen immediately under the aortic arch. With proper angulation, the superior vena cava and the innominate vein can also be seen.

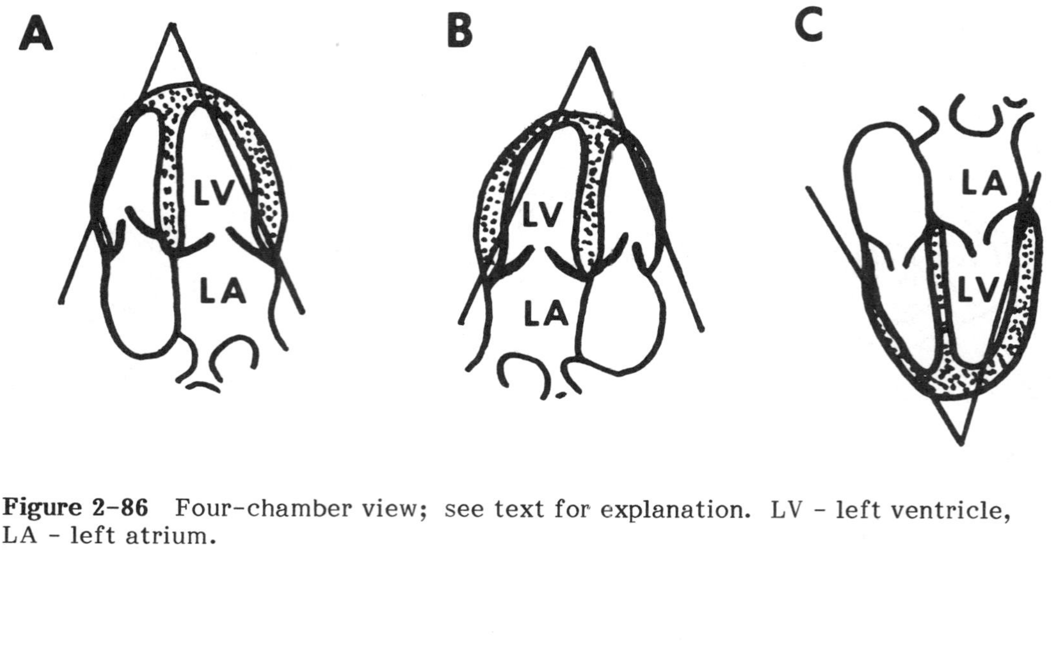

Figure 2-86 Four-chamber view; see text for explanation. LV - left ventricle, LA - left atrium.

Two-Dimensional Applications

The greatest contribution of pediatric echocardiography has been in the neonatal period. This technique permits us to study sick neonates at the bedside with minimal disturbance of their environment. It may allow the differentiation of sick infants with heart disease from their equally sick counterparts without structural cardiac anomalies.

Newborn in Shock

The echo has been useful in diagnosing hypoplastic left heart syndrome and, therefore, obviating the necessity for cardiac catheterization. With combined aortic and mitral atresia, and intact ventricular septum, the aortic root is small or absent. The mitral valve echo is distorted, and the posterior ventricle is small, while the right ventricle and pulmonary artery are markedly enlarged. In contrast, in patients with critical aortic stenosis the aortic root is nearly normal in size, and the left ventricle is thick and smaller than normal; the aortic valve is generally thickened.

Cyanotic Newborn

Cyanotic infants can be divided into two groups according to the appearance of the pulmonary vascularity on the chest radiograph.

Decreased Pulmonary Blood Flow

Decreased pulmonary blood flow generally implies obstruction at the pulmonary valve or tricuspid valve area, such as pulmonary atresia with intact ventricular septum or with VSD and tricuspid atresia. Other possibilities include transposition of the great vessels or single ventricle, both with severe pulmonary outflow obstruction. Tricuspid atresia is suggested when only the mitral valve echo is identified. The right ventricle as well as the pulmonary artery are small, and the subxiphoid view identifies a septum secundum defect. In pulmonary atresia the pulmonary echo is distorted, the right ventricle is small, but occasionally it may be quite large depending on the presence of tricuspid regurgitation. Severe tetralogy of Fallot is easily diagnosed by visualizing the ventricular septal defect, large overriding aorta, and small pulmonary artery (Fig. 2-87). This is best seen in the long-axis view.

Increased Pulmonary Blood Flow

The common lesions of increased pulmonary blood flow are transposition of the great vessels, single ventricle, and truncus arteriosus, type I. The most common cyanotic congenital heart disease is transposition of the great arteries. The ability of the 2-D echocardiography to assess the relationship of the great arteries is particularly useful. Normally, in the short-axis view the aorta appears as a circle and the pulmonary artery wraps around it anteriorly and to the right (Fig. 2-85C,D). In transposition of the great arteries, the aorta is anterior, and both arteries appear as circles one behind the other (Fig. 2-88). Slight superior and inferior angulation of the transducer demonstrates the posterior vessels to be the pulmonary artery bifurcating superiorly and originating from the left ventricle inferiorly. This abnormal origin can easily be shown from the subxiphoid approach (Fig. 2-89). This view is also excellent in assessing the results of the atrial balloon septostomy. The

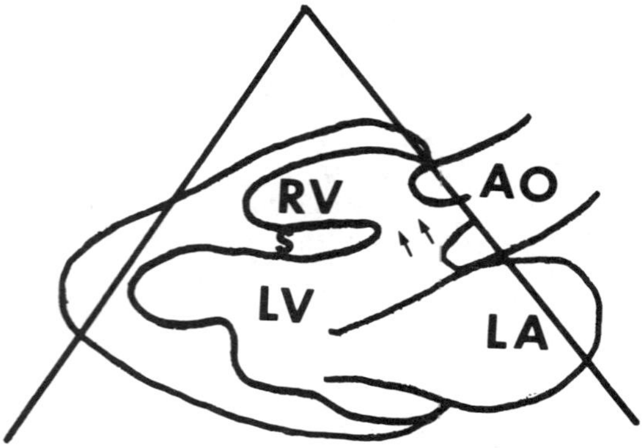

Figure 2–87 Tetralogy of Fallot. Long-axis view demonstrates the ventricular septal defect (arrows) and the large aorta overriding the septum.

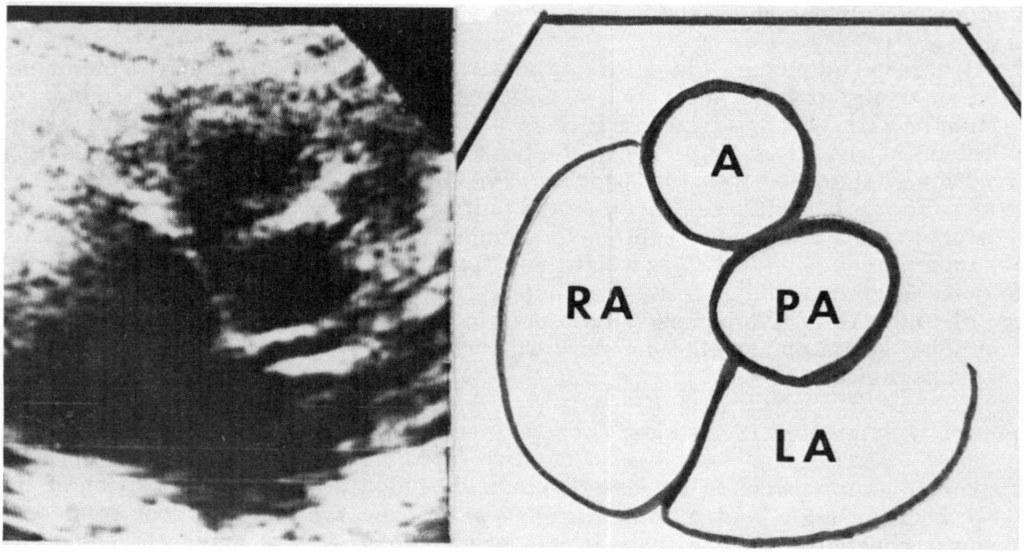

Figure 2–88 Transposition of the great arteries; short-axis view through the semilunar valves. The aorta (A) is anterior and the pulmonary artery (PA) is posterior. RA - right atrium, LA - left atrium.

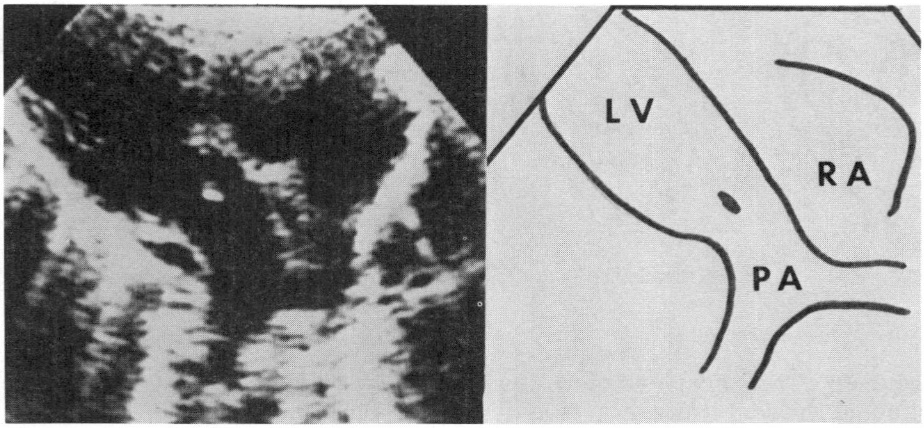

Figure 2-89 Transposition of the great arteries; subxiphoid view with slight angulation of the transducer towards the left ventricular (LV) outflow tract demonstrates the origin of the pulmonary artery (PA) from the left ventricle and its bifurcation.

infants with a single ventricle can be identified by the lack of ventricular septum in the short-axis and four-chamber view. The four-chamber view is excellent for visualization of the AV valve, excluding the possibility of an atretic valve. The infants with truncus arteriosus, type I, show a large overriding trunk over a large ventricular septal defect. The pulmonary valve is absent and, therefore, cannot be visualized in the short axis.

Infants and Children

Atrial Septal Defect

The M-mode echocardiogram is an excellent modality for diagnosing right ventricular volume overload. The 2-D echo, however, has a unique ability to visualize the atrial septum clearly and to differentiate between septum primum and secundum defects. The best view is the subxiphoid approach where one sees the ostium secundum defect in the upper part of the septum and the ostium primum defect just above the mitral and tricuspid attachments (Fig. 2-90). In the latter case, the valvular attachment is abnormal with absence of the atrioventricular septum. The ventricular septum is usually intact; however, in complete endocardial cushion defect there is VSD, ASD primum defect, and confluence of the atrioventricular valves (Fig. 2-91). Similarly, as previously mentioned, this approach is useful in assessing the adequacy of balloon atrial septostomy.

Ventricular Septal Defect

Ventricular septal defects are well visualized from the subxiphoid or apical approach (Fig. 2-92). Small defects may not be visualized, and aneurysms of the membranous septum are also easily detected.

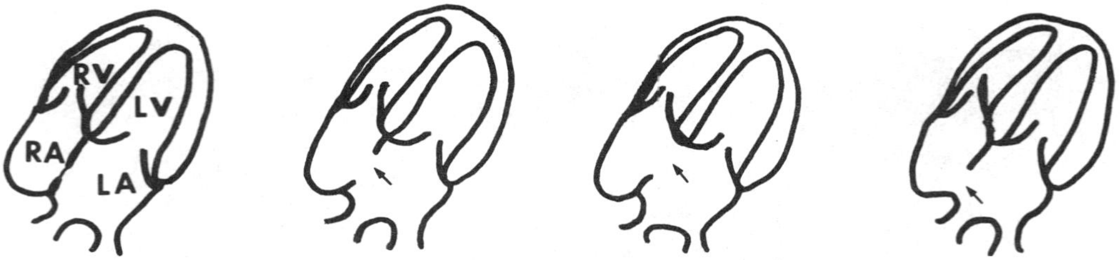

Normal — Secundum ASD — Primum ASD — Sinus Venosus ASD

Figure 2–90 The subxiphoid view illustrating the normal anatomy of the interatrial septum and the features characteristic of secundum, primum, and sinus venosus defect.

Ventricular Outflow Obstruction

The long-axis view of the left ventricular outflow tract and the ascending aorta is essential for adequately localizing the site of obstruction. Discrete subaortic obstruction can usually be differentiated from muscular hypertrophic stenosis. In hypertrophic subaortic stenosis the ventricle is thickened and hypercontractile with cavity obliteration during systole. There is also abnormal anterior systolic mitral motion. On the other hand, in discrete subaortic stenosis, the membrane can easily be seen. The aortic valve in valvular aortic stenosis appears thickened and domed with restricted opening excursion. Supravalvular narrowing can also be seen in this view (Fig. 2-93). Coarctation of the aorta can be visualized from the suprasternal approach.

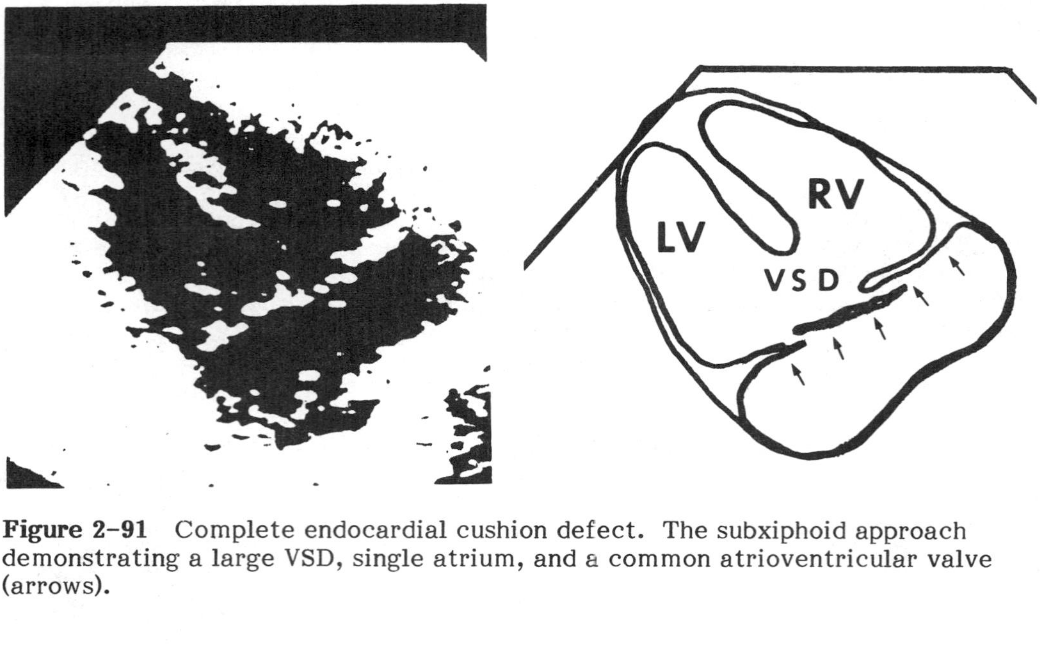

Figure 2–91 Complete endocardial cushion defect. The subxiphoid approach demonstrating a large VSD, single atrium, and a common atrioventricular valve (arrows).

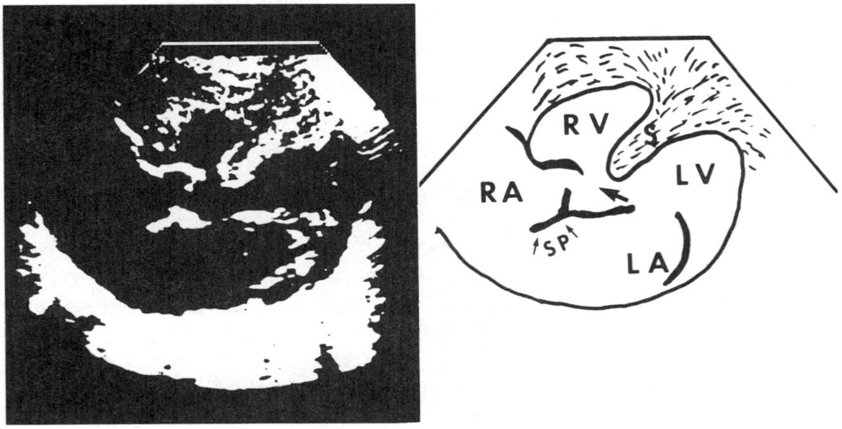

Figure 2-92 The subxiphoid approach showing a large ventricular septal defect (arrow). There is also an atrial septal defect secundum type. The septum primum (SP) is well visualized.

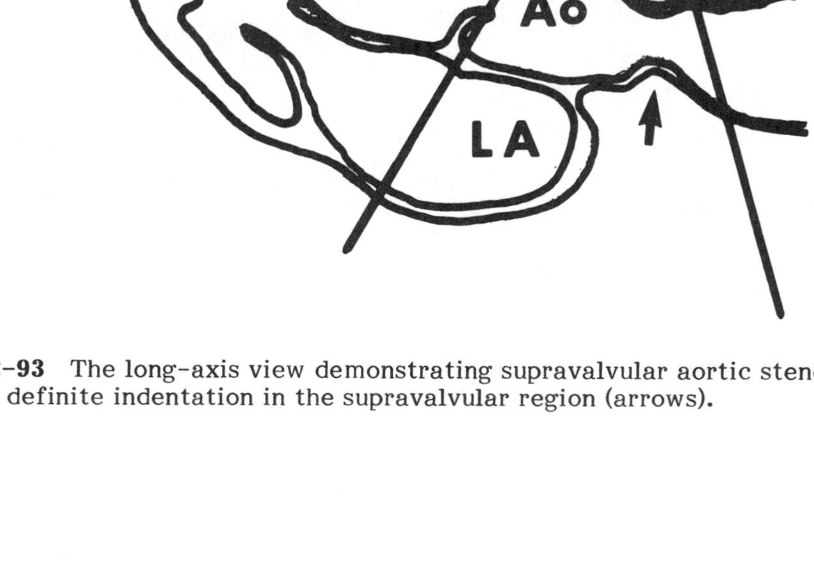

Figure 2-93 The long-axis view demonstrating supravalvular aortic stenosis. There is definite indentation in the supravalvular region (arrows).

Diagnosis of pulmonic stenosis is possible by directing the echo beam along the long axis of the pulmonic artery. The pulmonic valve is usually seen opening rapidly with the leaflets parallel to the pulmonary artery. In pulmonic stenosis, however, the leaflets are domed, and the movement is restricted, allowing for better visualization of the valve.

Other Applications

In children who present with a cardiomyopathic picture, the 2-D echo is useful in assessing the cardiac morphology, the pattern of contractility, and the presence or absence of intracardiac clots (Fig. 2-94). Certainly intracardiac masses such as myxoma or vegetations are easily seen and diagnosed. The yield of detecting vegetations with the 2-D echo is much improved over the M-mode system.

Attempts should be made to visualize the origin of the coronary arteries. Absence of the left coronary artery orifice may suggest its anomalous origin from the pulmonary artery. Recently, the ability to visualize the coronary arteries has enhanced the detection of coronary aneurysms and dilatation associated with Kawasaki disease (Fig. 21-7).

Contrast Echo Examination

The sudden injection of dextrose and water, blood, or saline into a peripheral or central line produces microcavitation at the end of the catheter. These microcavitations have different density than the surrounding blood, reflecting the ultrasound and are, therefore, visualized as a cloud of echoes on the oscilloscope. This technique is quite useful in the diagnosis of neonates with respiratory distress and cyanosis. In several of these patients, contrast studies from the umbilical venous catheter revealed large right-to-left shunting at the atrial level, accounting for the cyanosis. The four-chamber view is the best view for demonstrating these shunts.

In prematures with suspected patent ductus arteriosus, a forceful injection of 1 cc of dextrose and water into the aortic catheter (assuming the catheter tip is above the diaphragm) will demonstrate left-to-right shunting at the ductal level.

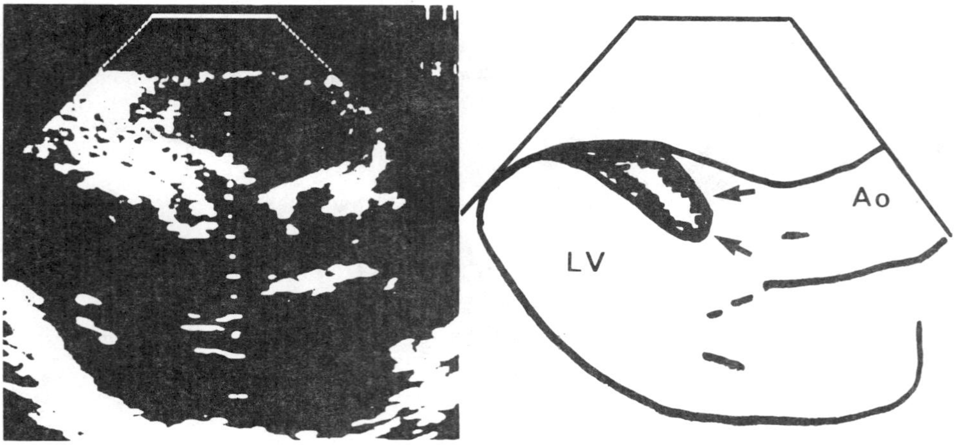

Figure 2-94 The long-axis view of a patient with severe dilated cardiomyopathy. There is a fingerlike protrusion (arrows) attached to the septum which represents intracardiac clot. This was confirmed at autopsy.

This is readily observed utilizing the short-axis view at the plane of the great vessels where the aorta and pulmonary artery are simultaneously visualized. The contrast does not appear in the circular aorta since this is the ascending aorta, but is visualized in the pulmonary artery (via the patent ductus arteriosus). We have been using this technique following open heart surgery where right and left atrial lines are left in place for monitoring purposes. Utilizing the four-chamber view, injecting 1 cc of glucose and water into the left atrial line, the contrast can demonstrate the presence or absence of residual ventricular or atrial septal defects.

Bibliography

Chang S: M-Mode Echocardiographic Techniques and Pattern Recognition, Lea & Febiger, Philadelphia, 1976.

Ellison RD, Restieaux NJ: Vectorcardiography in Congenital Heart Disease, W.B. Saunders Co., Philadelphia, 1972.

Feigenbaum H: Echocardiography, 3rd ed., Lea & Febiger, Philadelphia, 1981.

Glanz S, Helenbrand WE, Berman MA, Talner NS: Echocardiographic assessment of the severity of aortic stenosis in children and adolescents. Am J Cardiol 38: 620-625, 1976.

Godfrey S: Exercise Testing in Children, W.B. Saunders Co., Ltd., London, 1974.

Goldberg SJ: Exercise in Cardiac Patients, in Heart Disease in Infants, Children, and Adolescents, Moss AJ, Adams FH, Emmanouilides GG (eds.), 2nd ed., Williams and Wilkins Co., Baltimore, 1977.

Goldberg SJ, Allen HD, Sahn DJ: Pediatric and Adolescent Echocardiography, 2nd ed., Year Book Medical Publishers, Chicago, 1980.

Gramiak R, Waag RC: Cardiac Ultrasound, C.V. Mosby Co., St. Louis, Mo., 1975.

Gutgesell HP, Paquet M: Atlas of Pediatric Echocardiography, Harper & Row Publishers, Hagerstown, Md., 1978.

Henry WL: Evaluation of older children and adults with congenital heart disease by M-mode and cross-sectional echocardiography, in Roberts WC (guest ed.), Congenital heart disease in the adult, in Brest AN (ed.), Cardiovascular Clinics. F.A. Davis, Philadelphia, 1979.

Henry WL, Marin BJ, Griffith JM: Cross-sectional echocardiography in the diagnosis of congenital heart disease. Identification of the relation of the ventricle and great arteries. Circulation 56:267, 1977.

Henry WL, et al.: Report of the American Society of Echocardiography Committee on nomenclature and standards in two-dimensional echocardiography, Am Heart Assoc Scientific Sessions, Anaheim, Ca., Nov. 1979. Circulation 62:212-217, 1980.

Hurst JW, Logue RB, Schlant RC, Wenger NK: The Heart, 3rd ed., Physical Examination, pp. 147-289, McGraw-Hill Book Co., New York, 1974.

Kotler MN, Mintz GS, Segal BL, Parry WR: Clinical uses of two-dimensional echocardiography. Am J Cardiol 45:1061, 1980.

Leon DF, Shaver JA: Physiologic Principles of Heart Sounds and Murmurs, American Heart Association, New York, 1975.

Liebman J: Electrocardiography, in Heart Disease in Infants, Children, and Adolescents, Moss AJ, Adams FH, Emmanouilides GG, 2nd ed., Williams and Wilkins Co., Baltimore, 1977.

Liebman J, Downs TD, Priede A: The Frank and McFee Vectorcardiogram in Normal Children, pp. 483-559, Vectorcardiography 2, by Hoffman I, Hamby RI, Glassman E, North-Holland Publishing Co., Amsterdam, 1971.

Meyer RA, Kaplan S: Echocardiography in the diagnosis of hypoplasia of the left or right ventricle in the neonate. Circulation 46:55, 1972.

Meyer RA: Pediatric Echocardiography, Lea & Febiger, Philadelphia, 1977.

Nadas AS, Fyler DC: Pediatric Cardiology, 3rd ed., Electrocardiography, Chapter 3, pp. 36-76; The Vectorial Approach, Chapter 4, pp. 77-87; Phonocardiography, Chapter 5, pp. 88-108, W.B. Saunders Co., Philadelphia, 1972.

Ongly PA: Phonocardiography, in Heart Disease in Infants, Children, and Adolescents, Moss AJ, Adams FH, Emmanouilides GG, 2nd ed., Williams and Wilkins Co., Baltimore, 1977.

Park MK, Guntheroth WG: How to Read Pediatric ECG's, Year Book Medical Publishers, Chicago, 1981.

Rushmer RF: Cardiovascular Dynamics, 4th ed., Chapter 11, pp. 411-445, Cardiovascular Sounds, W.B. Saunders, Philadelphia, 1976.

Sapin SO: Vectorcardiography, in Heart Disease in Infants, Children, and Adolescents, Moss AJ, Adams FH, Emmanouilides GG, 2nd ed., Williams and Wilkins Co., Baltimore, 1977.

Tajik AJ, et al.: Two-dimensional real-time ultrasonic imaging of the heart and great vessels. Technique, image orientation, structure identification, and validation. Mayo Clinic Proc 53:271-303, 1978

Travel ME: Clinical Phonocardiography and External Pulse Recording, 2nd ed., Year Book Medical Publishers, Inc., Chicago, 1972.

Weissler AM, Lewis RP, Leighton RF: The systolic time interval as a measurement of left ventricular performance in men, in Yu PN, Goodwin F (eds.), Progress in Cardiology, Lea & Febiger, Philadelphia, 1972.

Williams RG, Tucker CR: Echocardiographic Diagnosis of Congenital Heart Disease, Little, Brown & Co., Boston, 1977.

Chapter 3

CARDIAC CATHETERIZATION

Purposes

Of paramount importance in the field of pediatric cardiology, cardiac catheterization is an invasive procedure with very definite risks and should be treated with respect. It is undertaken when the information to be provided is of importance and not simply for idle curiosity.

1. Evaluation of anatomy and identification or exclusion of associated lesions

What is the defect?

2. Assessment of hemodynamics (severity)

How bad is it?

3. Evaluation of complex arrhythmias through electrophysiologic studies

Risks

Potential complications will vary with the age of the patient, type of procedure, nature of the lesion, and experience of the operator. Although in older children potentially dangerous or life-threatening complications should occur in less than 1% of all cases, a number of problems may occur.

Arrhythmias

Premature ventricular contractions occur in virtually 100% of all studies. Short runs of ventricular tachycardia are not infrequent but are of more concern since they may lead to ventricular fibrillation. These occur when ventricular endocardium is stimulated with the catheter tip or when an injection of contrast material is made too close to the endocardium. Supraventricular premature beats and tachyarrhythmias are somewhat less frequent, but may be seen for the same reasons. Atrioventricular conduction defects may be induced through excessive vagal discharge at any stage of the procedure or by direct trauma to the atrioventricular (AV) node. It is essential that every laboratory carrying out such procedures have a fully equipped emergency cart with all equipment necessary for cardiopulmonary resuscitation as well as an appropriate supply of antiarrhythmic drugs. A DC defibrillator-cardioverter must always be available.

Reduction in Cardiac Output

Reduction in cardiac output is most often the result of excessive stress on a severely diseased myocardium, with further impairment of myocardial contractility. Most common precipitating factors are excessive administration of fluids or contrast material. Arrhythmias may, of course, have the same result. Cardiac output may also be dangerously reduced if a stenotic valve becomes obstructed with the catheter or in some patients following injection of contrast medium into the pulmonary artery in the presence of severely elevated pulmonary vascular resistance. Deterioration of myocardial function may be difficult to recognize in the catheterization laboratory in milder degrees, thus, at the first signs of trouble function may actually be so impaired as to be difficult to manage and to constitute a serious threat to life. The study will usually have to be terminated at this point. The risk of this problem can be reduced by paying careful attention to the recognition of impaired myocardial performance and optimizing medical management prior to the study. When the nature of the problem and/or the lack of response to medical therapy dictate that catheterization must be done in the presence of significant myocardial impairment, the increased risk may have to be accepted, but should be explained to the patient or family carefully. Extreme care must be paid to fluid load, and the volume of contrast agent must be kept to the minimum necessary to obtain the information sought. *Perforation of the heart* or major vascular structures should be exceedingly rare when the procedure is performed by an experienced cardiologist.

Arterial Hypoxemia

Most frequently the result of the excessive use of sedation with resultant hypoventilation, arterial hypoxemia may also be seen in children with right-to-left shunts and obstruction to pulmonary blood flow (e.g., tetralogy of Fallot) if systemic vascular resistance is lowered. Increased right-to-left shunt and progressive hypoxemia may result and occasionally precipitate a hypoxic spell. The use of sedative agents which dilate the systemic vascular bed such as chlorpromazine is to be avoided in such children.

Vascular Complications

The vascular complication of major concern is arterial occlusion following retrograde left heart study. Incidence of this problem can be reduced by attention to technique as described subsequently. The newborn presents special problems since he is generally quite sick when undergoing catheterization, being in significant congestive heart failure or having profound arterial hypoxemia. He is also less tolerant of any manipulation. Careful monitoring for the development of hypothermia and/or acidosis is a must. Constant monitoring of rectal temperature is undertaken, and the infant is studied while being warmed by an external heating device, usually a water-filled heating pad or radiant warmer. The myocardium is also far more subject to catheter perforation at this age, and extreme care in catheter manipulation is essential. Because of the small vessel size, vascular complications are also more frequent. The study should be performed without unnecessary delays, and both the volume of blood removed for determinations of oxygen saturation and the volume of fluid infused vigorously monitored.

Equipment

The procedure is performed under fluoroscopy utilizing an image-intensifier system to reduce radiation exposure. The fluoroscopic image is most conveniently viewed on a TV monitor mounted as to be moved easily into suitable position. Transducers, generally of the strain-gauge type, are utilized for pressure recording, and their signals together with an electrocardiographic signal are fed into a multichannel optical recorder which provides both real-time viewing as well as a permanent record. For pediatric work, a system for biplane angiocardiography is essential. Ideally both biplane cine and serial film are available, especially if the lab is to be used for both cardiac and vascular work. Recent advances in cineangiocardiography (v.i.) require filming in projections which cannot be achieved with fixed anteroposterior (AP) and lateral biplane systems without extremely difficult repositioning of the patient. This is very time-consuming and may be impossible in larger patients. For this reason, the x-ray tubes and image intensifiers should be mounted on biplane C or U arms which allow rotation into all projections without having to move the patient. An instant-replay system, either videotape or videodisc, should be available for each plane of cineangiocardiography. A device for measuring oxygen saturation is also necessary. In most laboratories the time-consuming Van Slyke technique of determining oxygen content has been replaced by the utilization of photometric oximetry for measuring saturation. The latter is sufficiently accurate and has the advantage of being rapidly performed and utilizing a minimal amount of blood. A blood gas analyzer should be readily accessible. One or more methods for measuring cardiac output as discussed subsequently should also be in use.

Techniques

Although young infants are routinely studied without any form of premedication, some type of sedation is generally needed in children to allay anxiety and restlessness. We most frequently employ a combination of sedatives known as the DPT mixture (also lytic cocktail or Toronto mixture) as follows.

Meperidine (Demerol) 0.5-1.0 mg/lb
Promethazine hydrochloride (Phenergan) 0.25 mg/lb
Chlorpromazine (Thorazine) 0.25 mg/lb

As mentioned previously, chlorpromazine is generally omitted when the diagnosis of tetralogy or a hemodynamically similar lesion is suspected and the dose of promethazine hydrochloride (Phenergan) increased proportionately. Because of a somewhat erratic response to this mixture, we have been more recently studying particularly anxious children utilizing either ketamine or a mixture of fentanyl and droperidol (Innovar). Whenever possible the child is breathing room air, although severely cyanotic infants or those in profound failure generally receive oxygen supplementation.

Right Heart Catheterization

In the majority of instances the catheter is introduced into a femoral vein utilizing the percutaneous technique originally described by Seldinger. After the vein is entered with a short-bevel needle, a flexible guidewire is advanced through the needle for a short distance up the vein. The needle is withdrawn, and a thin-wall sheath as illustrated in Fig. 3-1 advanced over the wire into the vein. This

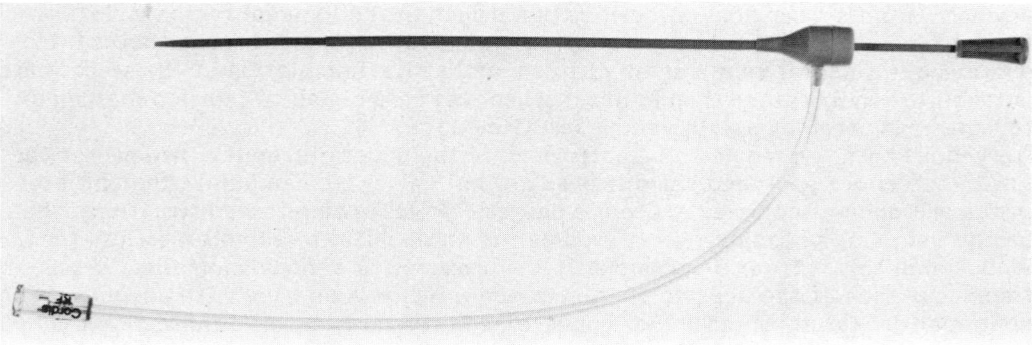

Figure 3-1A Venous sheath for catheter introduction. The sheath with its tapered inner cannula is inserted into the vein over a guidewire, following which the wire and inner cannula are removed, the outersheath remaining in the vein. The clear plastic side arm facilitates flushing of the sheath and removal of clots.

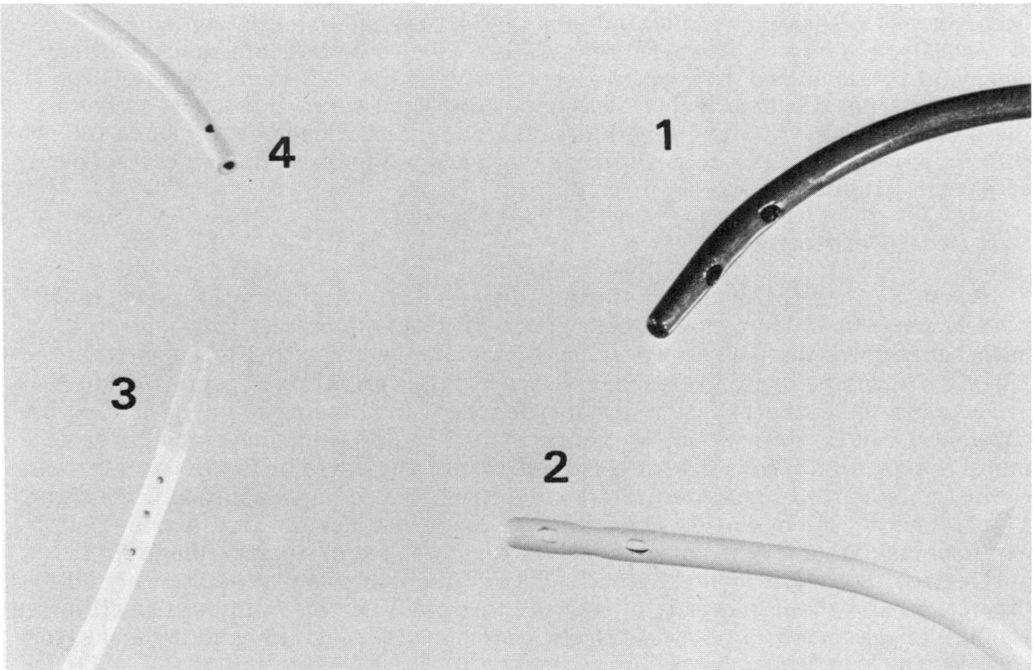

Figure 3-1B Representative catheter types (numbered clockwise, starting at upper right-hand corner). (1) Tapered tip with end-hole and proximal side holes (Gensini type). Can be introduced percutaneously over a guidewire without utilization of a sheath. (2) Closed-end with proximal side holes (NIH). Of primary value in angiocardiography since closed-end reduces risk of catheter recoil and/ or intramyocardial injection of contrast agent. A good general all-purpose catheter for sampling and pressure recording as well. (3) Balloon-tip (closed-end) catheter with proximal side holes. A flow-directed catheter useful for difficult manipulations and in angiocardiography. (4) End-hole catheter with two proximal side holes. Of primary value in obtaining pulmonary arterial wedge pressure.

sheath will permit the utilization of a wide variety of catheters. Occasionally in newborn infants a surgical cutdown is performed in the inguinal region isolating the saphenous vein. Should the saphenous vein prove too small for catheter introduction, the femoral vein may be utilized and, at the completion of the study, care is taken to repair rather than ligate it whenever possible since ligation may lead to significant problems with venous insufficiency.

Venous cutdown may also be performed in the upper extremity. We prefer the lower-extremity approach since it is somewhat easier to manipulate the catheter in the presence of complex anatomic defects. In less complicated situations, the basilic vein may be isolated as it crosses the antecubital fossa and the catheter introduced in this manner. Occasionally the presence of venous anomalies, in particular absence of the hepatic portion of the inferior vena cava with azygous continuation, force utilization of upper-extremity veins in small infants, and in this event the axillary vein may be exposed. Such an approach requires precise surgical dissection to avoid injury to the surrounding nerve trunks.

The catheter is passed proximally to the right atrium and, if anatomic abnormalities are not too complex, it is easy to direct the tip medially crossing the tricuspid valve and then superiorly to enter the pulmonary artery. Another advantage of the lower-extremity approach is that, if the foramen ovale is patent, the catheter can be easily manipulated into the left atrium and left ventricle. This is generally the case in newborn infants. It may also be possible to cross other abnormal communications such as a ventricular septal defect or patent ductus arteriosus from this approach. Pressures and oxygen saturation are recorded in the pulmonary artery, right ventricle and atrium, and venae cavae. Once the procedure is completed the catheter and sheath are withdrawn and hemostasis easily effected by digital pressure.

Left Heart Catheterization

When the foramen ovale is patent, right and left heart catheterization may both be performed from the venous approach. If a balloon-tip, flow-directed catheter is used, the aorta may frequently be entered from the left ventricle. When the foramen ovale is closed, left heart catheterization is performed by introducing the catheter into a peripheral artery and passing it retrograde across the aortic valve. Here again, we generally utilize percutaneous entry into a femoral artery. If there is a severe coarctation of the aorta or if the catheter cannot be manipulated across the aortic valve from the femoral approach, the right brachial artery is employed. One must, of course, be certain that an aberrant right subclavian artery is not present. In the presence of mirror-image right aortic arch, the left brachial artery is used. The artery is exposed by careful dissection, and the catheter is introduced through an arteriotomy. In small infants the axillary artery may be used. Great care must be taken in handling any artery in order to prevent circulatory impairment following completion of the study. Retrograde passage of the catheter across the mitral valve into the left atrium is difficult, although it may occasionally be accomplished utilizing special catheters. More frequently when a retrograde left heart study is performed, left atrial pressure is measured by recording a pulmonary arterial wedge pressure. This is obtained by passing an end-hole catheter as far distally in either pulmonary arterial tree as possible until an atrial waveform (v.i.) and fully saturated blood are obtained. If there is no obstruction to pulmonary venous return, the wedge pressure gives an accurate reflection of left atrial pressure.

There is a small but definite risk of arterial thrombosis following retrograde arterial procedures. This can be reduced if arterial catheter time is kept to a minimum and care paid to not utilizing a catheter of such a size that it severely impedes flow into the distal artery. Both catheters are kept filled with a solution of heparinized dextrose and water and, in the case of the arterial catheter, when pressure monitoring is not actually being carried out this solution is infused slowly through the catheter to minimize fibrin deposits on the catheter tip. Prior to removal of the percutaneously inserted catheter, a small blood sample is forceably withdrawn in an effort to remove any fibrin adherent to the holes in the catheter tip. The catheter is then removed and blood is allowed to spurt from the puncture site for two or three beats to flush any fibrin that might be adherent to the artery at this point. Hemostasis then is easily affected by digital pressure. Following reports of reduced arterial complications with systemic heparinization, we have begun injecting 50 U/kg of heparin through the venous catheter at the time the arterial puncture is performed. This has virtually eliminated the incidence of diminished pulses or overt arterial occlusion in our laboratory, and to date we have had no problems with postcatheterization hemostasis. Removal of the catheter from a brachial artery is followed by flushing the vessel with heparinized saline and the passage of a Fogarty arterial embolectomy catheter into both proximal and distal arterial segments. With the balloon gently inflated, the catheter is withdrawn, removing any fibrin clot adherent to the vessel wall. The arteriotomy is then repaired with interrupted sutures utilizing either 6-0 or 7-0 size.

Catheter Types

The great variety of catheter types far exceeds the space available to discuss them in a book of this type. In general they fall into several broad groups each of which has certain advantages (Fig. 3-1B).

End-Hole Catheters

As the name implies, the catheter lumen opens at the distal tip, with or without additional side holes over a short distance proximally. In some models the distal tip is tapered so that the catheter may be introduced percutaneously by passing it directly over a guidewire without the use of an additional sheath. Likewise, flexible guidewires can be utilized where necessary to aid manipulation into difficult areas such as across the aortic valve. The presence of an end-hole is mandatory for measuring pulmonary arterial wedge pressure. Catheters of this type which are to be used for angiocardiography have several side holes as well, but the presence of an end-hole still increases the degree of catheter recoil during contrast injection and also the risk of intramyocardial injection of contrast material.

Closed-End Catheters (NIH Type)

Closed-end catheters are equipped with four to six side holes located near the distal tip. Although they are a good general all-purpose catheter, they offer specific advantages in the area of angiocardiography as the problems mentioned previously are less likely.

Flow-Directed Catheters

Flow-directed catheters are generally constructed as a double-lumen model with one lumen communicating with a balloon at the tip. The balloon can be inflated with air or carbon dioxide and the catheter floated into some difficult locations along lines of blood flow. Some models have a second lumen opening at the distal tip of the catheter and are used primarily for pressure monitoring, being particularly adaptable to obtaining pulmonary arterial wedge pressure. Of particular value in the pediatric field are flow-directed angiographic catheters in which the balloon is at the distal tip with side holes proximal. Development of materials which withstand pressure well has allowed production of catheters with two lumena and thin walls which will accommodate a good rate of flow of contrast medium. Not only do they have the advantages of flow direction but, with the catheter positioned in either ventricular apex, the balloon can be inflated during angiocardiography and held in a relatively stable position with arrhythmias minimized. Still other models with three to four lumena have been developed for special purposes, such as thermodilution cardiac output determination. One final type of balloon-tip catheter is included with this group, although it was not designed as a flow-directed catheter. This type is constructed with a stronger balloon at the tip and designed for performance of balloon atrial septostomy as discussed under transposition of the great arteries.

Electrode Catheters

Several varieties of electrode catheters exist with one to six electrodes at intervals at and proximal to the catheter tip. A lumen for pressure and oxygen monitoring is usually present but is generally small. Wires imbedded in the catheter wall attach the electrodes to connectors at the proximal end from which the electrical signal can be transmitted to the recorder. They are used primarily for the recording of intracardiac electrophysiologic events and also in shunt detection following hydrogen inhalation (v.i.).

Manometer-Tipped Catheters

Extremely small pressure-sensitive transducers have been incorporated in cardiac catheters, and their utilization provides extremely high-fidelity recordings of pressure events.

Directly Measured Hemodynamic Parameters

Pressure

Pressure monitoring is essential, not only to the hemodynamic evaluation of a given lesion, but also to catheter manipulation. The position of the catheter tip is recognized by a combination of the fluoroscopic image and the pressure waveform recorded. Typical atrial, ventricular, and arterial waveforms are shown in Fig. 2-2 and normal values listed in Table 3-1. The multichannel photographic recorders used in cardiac laboratories have the capability of inserting a square wave calibration signal at the end of the pressure tracing. The accuracy of this calibration wave can be checked periodically using a mercury manometer. Pressure is typically recorded in all cardiac chambers and arteries entered. Only the phasic pressure wave is recorded in the ventricles, whereas both phasic and mean pressure are obtained in atria or arteries. The latter is electronically derived by the recorder. The possibility of stenosis of one of the cardiac valves is best evaluated by either withdrawing the catheter across the valve with continuous-pressure recording (e.g., pulmonary artery to right ventricle) or by simultaneously recording pressures on both sides of the valve utilizing two catheters.

Table 3-1 Normal Intracardiac Pressures (mmHg or torr)

	Phasic	Mean
Right atrium	A = 5-10 V = 4-8	2-6
Right ventricle	15-25/2-6	—
Pulmonary artery	15-25/8-12	10-16
Left atrium	A = 6-12 V = 8-15	5-10
Left ventricle	90-110/6-12	—
Aorta	90-110/65-75	70-80

Oxygen Saturation

As previously mentioned, oxygen saturations are most often measured by photoelectric techniques, and a wide variety of instruments are available. The presence of a left-to-right shunt can be recognized by a stepup in oxygen saturation within the right heart or pulmonary artery, whereas a right-to-left shunt would be indicated by a decrease in saturation of samples obtained from the left heart or aorta. Saturation values are also utilized in the calculation of cardiac output and shunt volumes.

Derived Hemodynamic Data

Cardiac Output

A time-honored method of measuring cardiac output utilizes the Fick principle.

$$\text{Cardiac output (l/min)} = \frac{\text{Oxygen consumption}}{\text{Arteriovenous difference in oxygen content}}$$

$$\text{Cardiac output} = \frac{\text{Oxygen consumption (cc/min)}}{(O_2\text{sat arterial} - O_2\text{sat mixed venous}) \times O_2 \text{ capacity} \times 10}$$

Oxygen carrying capacity may be measured directly using special instruments or more often is estimated by multiplying the patient's hemoglobin times a factor of 1.34. Oxygen consumption may be determined by collecting the total volume of expired air in a bag. This is somewhat difficult in small children, and several methods exist for measuring the oxygen content of expired air obtained by pulling room air through a hood in which the patient is breathing. Tables of basal rates of oxygen consumptions in unsedated children exist, but their use gives rise to significant error as these values bear little relation to the oxygen consumption of children in the catheterization laboratory, particularly when one considers the effects of stress, hypoxia, and so forth. Indicator dilution techniques may also be utilized (v.i.).

Calculation of Shunts

Systemic blood flow (Qs) is synonymous with cardiac output and is calculated as mentioned utilizing the saturation from the pulmonary artery as the mixed venous if there is no left-to-right shunt. If a shunt is present, the mixed venous sample may be obtained from the right atrium or, if the shunt is at that level, from the venae cavae using a weighted average.

$$\frac{3\,(\text{SVC saturation}) + 1\,(\text{IVC saturation})}{4} \qquad \text{or}$$

$$\frac{1\,(\text{SVC saturation}) + 2\,(\text{IVC saturation})}{3}$$

during exercise.

Comparison with the normal in patients of different size is best obtained by expressing the systemic blood flow as the index:

$$\text{Systemic index (l/min/m}^2) = \frac{\text{Qs (l/min)}}{\text{Body surface area (m}^2)}$$

Pulmonic blood flow (Qp) is calculated in a similar manner as follows.

$$\text{Qp} = \frac{\text{Oxygen consumption}}{(\text{O}_2\text{sat pulm. venous} - \text{O}_2\text{sat pulm. art.}) \times \text{O}_2 \text{ capacity} \times 10}$$

Pulmonary venous blood may also be obtained from pulmonary wedge position, left atrium, or systemic artery if there is no right-to-left shunt. This flow may also be normalized for body size as shown.

In addition to determining the flow through systemic and pulmonary vascular beds, one may also calculate the effective or true pulmonary blood flow, that is, the flow through the pulmonary vascular bed due to systemic venous return.

$$\text{Qp eff.} = \frac{\text{Oxygen consumption}}{(\text{O}_2\text{sat pulm. venous} - \text{O}_2\text{sat mixed venous}) \times \text{O}_2 \text{ capacity} \times 10}$$

The mixed venous samples are obtained from right atrium or venae cavae as discussed. The total left-to-right shunt may be computed as:

$\text{Left} \rightarrow \text{right}_T = \text{Qp} - \text{Qp eff}$ and total right to left:

$\text{Right} \rightarrow \text{left}_T = \text{Qs} - \text{Qp eff}$

In this manner bidirectional shunts can be quantitated and the net shunt determined.

$$\text{Left} \rightarrow \text{right}_N = (\text{left} \rightarrow \text{right}_T) - (\text{right} \rightarrow \text{left}_T) = Qp - Qs$$

$$\text{Right} \rightarrow \text{left}_N = (\text{right} \rightarrow \text{left}_T) - (\text{left} \rightarrow \text{right}_T) = Qs - Qp$$

Of somewhat more practical value in the assessment of intracardiac shunts is the pulmonary-to-systemic-flow ratio (Qp/Qs) which in the absence of shunts should equal 1. Calculation of a Qp/Qs greater than 1 would indicate the presence of a net left-to-right shunt, whereas a value less than 1, a net right-to-left shunt. If oxygen consumption is not measured, this ratio can still be determined from oxygen saturations as follows.

$$Qp/Qs = \frac{\dfrac{\text{Oxygen consumption}}{(O_2\text{sat pulm. venous} - O_2\text{sat pulm. art.}) \times O_2 \text{ capacity} \times 10}}{\dfrac{\text{Oxygen consumption}}{(O_2\text{sat art} - O_2\text{sat mixed venous}) \times O_2 \text{ capacity} \times 10}}$$

$$Qp/Qs = \frac{O_2\text{sat art} - O_2\text{sat mixed venous}}{O_2 \text{ sat pulm. venous} - O_2 \text{ sat pulm. art.}}$$

Vascular Resistance

Resistance can be estimated using an application of Ohm's law to fluid dynamics.

$$\text{Resistance} = \frac{\text{Pressure}}{\text{Flow}}$$

Although resistance across any portion of the circulatory system could be calculated in this manner, it is primarily applied to resistance across the systemic or pulmonary arterial bed as follows.

$$\text{Pulmonary vascular resistance (PVR)} = \frac{\bar{P}_{pa} - \bar{P}_{pv}}{Qp}$$

where $\bar{P}_{pa}$ = mean pulmonary arterial pressure

$\bar{P}_{pv}$ = mean pulmonary venous pressure

$$\text{Systemic vascular resistance (SVR)} = \frac{\bar{P}_{Ao} - \bar{P}_{ra}}{Qs}$$

where $\bar{P}_{Ao}$ = mean aortic pressure

P_{ra} = mean right atrial pressure

If standard units of pressure and flow as discussed are utilized, the units of vascular resistance will be mmHg/l/min or so-called relative resistance units. These units are simple conceptually but do not represent true resistance units if resistance is measured directly rather than calculated. When measured directly, resistance is expressed as absolute resistance units or dynes second-centimeters^{-5}. Relative resistance units can easily be converted to absolute by multiplying the former by a correction factor of 80. The practice of calculating total pulmonary or systemic resistance by dividing the respective mean arterial pressures by flow is to be condemned since serious error is introduced if either atrial pressure is elevated. As discussed in the next chapter, one is frequently concerned with alterations in the pulmonary or systemic arterial bed secondary to cardiac abnormalities, and assessment of these changes requires determination of the pulmonary or systemic vascular resistance.

Valve Areas

Although subject to some error in application, calculation of valve areas utilizing the formulas developed by Gorlin is useful as a general index of valvular stenosis. The formulas basically relate the pressure gradient and flow across the valve. Cardiac output must be precisely quantitated for these calculations to have any degree of reliability. In addition, they are based on forward flow across the valve, and considerable error is introduced if regurgitation is present.

$$\text{Mitral valve area} = \frac{\text{Mitral valve flow}}{31\sqrt{\bar{P}_{pv} - \bar{P}_{lvd}}}$$

$$\text{Mitral valve flow} = \frac{\text{Qs (cc/min)}}{\text{Diastolic filling period (sec/min)}}$$

where $\bar{P}_{pv}$ = mean pulmonary venous or left atrial pressure during diastole

$\bar{P}_{lvd}$ = mean left ventricular diastolic pressure

As generally applied, left atrial and left ventricular pressures are recorded simultaneously at equal gain, and the mean diastolic gradient across the valve is obtained following integration of the area between the two pressure curves. Details of how this is carried out are discussed in the work by Yang et al. (see bibliography). The diastolic filling period is the number of seconds per minute occupied by diastole and is obtained by measuring directly from the pressure tracings. Tricuspid valve area is calculated using the same formula. Normal mitral valve area in adults is between 4 and 6 cm^2.

The formula for calculation of aortic or pulmonic valve area is:

$$\text{Aortic (or pulmonic) valve area} = \frac{\text{Aortic valve flow}}{44.5\sqrt{\bar{P}_{lvs} - \bar{P}_{Aos}}}$$

$$\text{Aortic valve flow} = \frac{\text{Qs (cc/min)}}{\text{Systolic ejection period (sec/min)}}$$

where $\bar{P}_{lvs}$ = left ventricular systolic mean pressure and

$\bar{P}_{Aos}$ = aortic systolic mean pressure

The mean systolic ejection gradient is best obtained by integration of the area between simultaneously recorded ventricular and arterial curves. The systolic ejection period is measured directly from the pressure tracings as previously mentioned.

Pulmonic blood flow, if different from systemic, is utilized when calculating pulmonic valve area. In adults, normal aortic valve area is 3-4 cm^2, and a value less than 0.8 cm^2 indicates critical stenosis. In children, a valve area of less than 0.5-0.8 cm^2/m^2 body surface area is critical.

Angiocardiography

Although most of the simple defects can be evaluated relatively adequately with measurement of pressures and flows alone, the visualization of structure has been the thing that has made possible surgical approaches to the more complicated defects. Additional valuable information is provided regarding the simple defects as well, and at the present time angiocardiography is an integral part of the catheterization procedure in virtually all studies. With the development of improved catheters and radiographic techniques, highly selective studies are now possible to demonstrate virtually all parts of the circulatory system.

Contrast Materials

Visualization of the heart or vessels must be achieved by the injection of a liquid which is opaque to the x-ray beam. This injection may be into any of the cardiac chambers or any blood vessel, depending on the type of information needed. There are many types of contrast agents available, all of which are complicated organic iodide molecules. The sodium salts of these molecules are less viscous and, therefore, more easily injected, but have a greater toxic effect on the myocardium. The more commonly used preparations are a combination of the sodium and meglumine salts of diatrizoic acid. As any of these solutions are quite viscous, injection by hand is difficult unless a very large catheter is utilized since the injection must be rapid if adequate visualization is to be achieved. Some type of automatic pressure injector is usually employed.

The usual dose of contrast agent employed is 1.0-1.5 cc/kg per injection, with slightly smaller volumes being required for vascular procedures. The total dose per procedure does not exceed 3-5 cc/kg except in rare instances where the importance of the information justifies the slightly increased risk and where there has been a sufficient period of time between injections.

Risks

Angiocardiography adds a slight amount of increased risk to the catheterization procedure due totally to the contrast agent, either by virtue of the chemical effects on the circulation or to injection in an undesirable location. Severe allergic reactions, even to the point of anaphylactic shock may occur, but are fortunately rare. The conscious patient should be warned to expect a generalized sensation of warmth lasting approximately 30 sec following the injection. Cardiac output is increased, and in some patients with a diseased myocardium the ventricular end-diastolic pressure may be inordinately elevated for a number of minutes after the injection. This has been utilized by some as a rough indicator of myocardial function and should be monitored carefully in any patient with reduced function in whom multiple injections are required. Severe pulmonary vasospasm has been observed in patients with elevated pulmonary vascular resistance. Accordingly, right heart injections should be made with caution in patients with significant pulmonary hypertension and are probably contraindicated when severe pulmonary vascular obstructive disease occurs in the absence of a congenital heart defect (so-called primary or idiopathic pulmonary hypertension).

Injection of the contrast agent directly into the myocardium from an inappropriately positioned catheter may provoke severe arrhythmias, including ventricular fibrillation, or may result in myocardial rupture. Extracardiac or extravascular injection secondary either to myocardial rupture or cardiac perforation carries not only the risk of bleeding but also the rapid accumulation of fluid in the area of extravasation since all of the contrast agents are extremely hypertonic. This is of extreme importance with an intrapericardial injection. The degree of bleeding into the pericardium may be minimal, particularly if the catheter perforation has occurred in the ventricle, but subsequent accumulation of fluid may be of sufficient magnitude to produce tamponade; thus, the patient must be watched carefully over a period of several hours. Since these agents are all excreted by the kidneys, they must be used with extreme care where renal dysfunction is present, and they have also been known to further reduce renal function or cause renal shutdown. The extreme hypertonicity of these agents produces a significant osmotic diuresis which may result in dehydration in infants. Studies in newborn animals have demonstrated intracranial hemorrhage following intravenous injections of contrast agents and other hyperosmolar solutions secondary to brain shrinkage and tearing of bridging veins. Great care must be taken to maintain adequate hydration during the postcatheterization period, especially in infants and when large volumes of contrast agent have been employed.

Radiographic Techniques

Either 35-mm motion picture (cineangiocardiography) or serial large-film changers are employed. In the latter instance the changer should be capable of maximum filming rates of 6-12 frames/sec. In pediatric studies, biplane filming is highly desirable, both to give a more nearly three-dimensional appreciation of complicated anatomy and to obtain the most information with the least amount of contrast agent. Modern equipment allows rotation of both tubes through an almost limitless range of projections while maintaining orientation through a fixed cardiac isocenter. In this manner, the heart can be imaged from almost any point on the surface of a sphere surrounding it. This type of approach has markedly increased understanding of congenital defects, over and above what could be learned from traditional AP, lateral, and oblique views alone. The most useful of these new angled or axial views have been the hepatoclavicular, long-axial oblique, and craniocaudad AP. The hepatoclavicular or four-chamber view is a left anterior oblique projection combined with 40-45° of craniocaudad angulation. All four chambers are displayed without overlapping. The atrial and ventricular septa are seen in profile as are both AV valves. It is especially useful for visualizing defects of the atrial and posterior ventricular septa, the left ventricular outflow tract, aorta, and left pulmonary artery. Endocardial cushion defects are especially well imaged. The long-axial oblique allows visualization of the anterior septum. Excellent imaging of the right ventricular outflow tract, pulmonary valve, and arteries may be achieved in the AP projection with 45° of craniocaudad angulation. Pulmonary venous drainage is well delineated, and atrial septal defects are seen almost as well as in the hepatoclavicular view.

Cineangiocardiography has the advantage of being more rapidly carried out than large-film techniques and instantly available for review with simultaneous recording on videotape. This technique is best for evaluating dynamic events such as valve motion and ventricular function as well as for detecting small shunts. Prior to the development of axial cineangiocardiography, biplane large-film techniques tended to give a better appreciation of spatial relationships. This advantage no longer exists, and cine techniques are the ones employed in most pediatric laboratories.

Indicator Dilution Curves

Although variable in application, all indicator dilution curves have in common the injection of some type of foreign substance into the circulation with detection at a remote point. They are used primarily in the quantitation of flow rates or in detection of shunts. In general there are three classes of indicator substances.

1. Foreign gases (e.g., hydrogen or krypton)
2. Dyes
3. Temperature

Foreign Gas Curve

Foreign gas curves are used for the detection and localization of left-to-right shunts with hydrogen being the most commonly employed. The gas is injected into the pulmonary veins by having the patient inhale it from a bag, and is detected where desired by a platinum-tipped electrode catheter. Upon being absorbed in the blood, the gas rapidly dissociates into hydrogen ion (H^+) and induces a voltage change upon contacting the platinum electrode.

The electrode catheter is connected so as to record an intracardiac electrocardiogram which is taken at low gain and slow paper speed. The voltage change induced by the H^+ produces a pronounced shift in the baseline and the appearance time, that is, time between injection and the baseline shift is utilized in shunt detection. For example, a normal appearance time in the absence of a shunt with the catheter tip positioned in the right heart is 6-10 sec, whereas positioning the electrode in the pulmonary wedge position gives a virtually instantaneous appearance time. In the presence of a ventricular septal defect there would be shunting of the hydrogen ion into the right heart, and a rapid appearance time of 1-2 sec would be recorded if the catheter tip were positioned in the right ventricle or pulmonary artery, whereas the appearance time would be normal in the right atrium or at any point further proximally (Fig. 3-2). The technique is easily applied even in sleeping children and has the advantage of detecting tiny shunts. The gas is, however, highly explosive and must be stored and handled with care.

Dye Dilution Curves

Dye dilution curves are colored substances, and their appearances are detected by a change in optical density at an appropriate wavelength for the substance as blood is continuously drawn through a photoelectric cuvette. Indocyanine green is the most commonly employed and has its peak spectral absorption at 800-810 nm in blood. The dye can be injected at any point within the circulatory system and detected at any other point desired. Multiple catheter techniques may be employed, allowing detection at two or more points simultaneously. Dye dilution curves may be employed qualitatively for localization of shunts in either direction

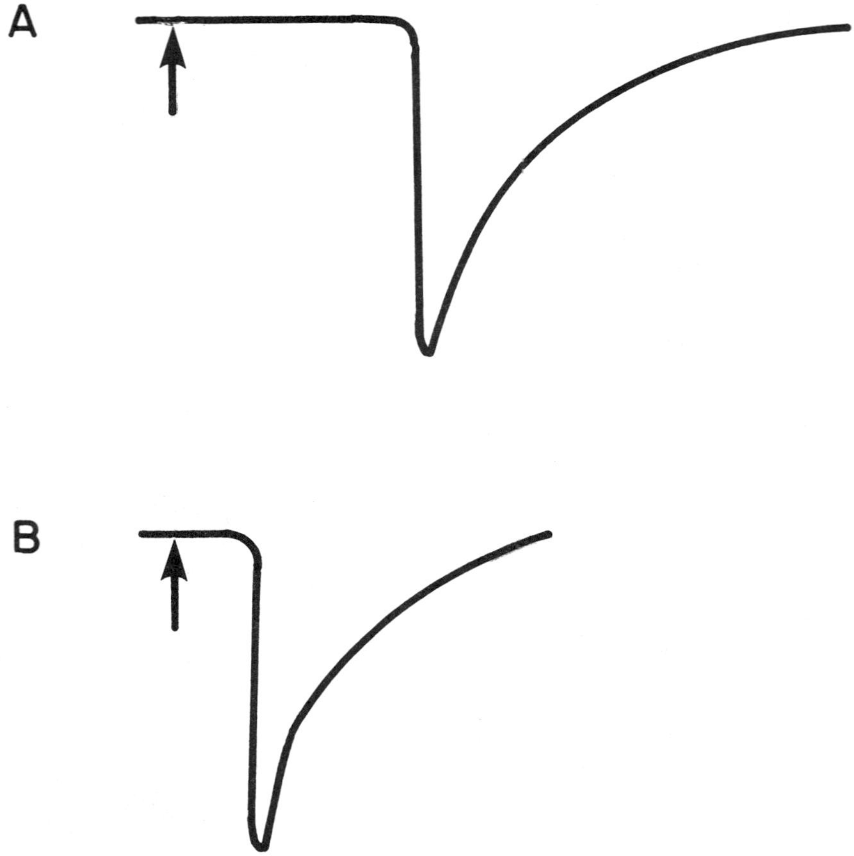

Figure 3-2 Hydrogen inhalation curves. Curve A was recorded with the platinum electrode in the right atrium and curve B with the tip in the right ventricle in a patient with a VSD. The time of hydrogen inhalation is indicated by the arrows. The baseline deflection indicating the detection of hydrogen by the catheter tip occurs significantly earlier in curve B, consistent with a left-to-right shunt at the ventricular level.

or quantitatively for measurement of blood flow. When utilized for determination of cardiac output, injection is usually made into the pulmonary artery and detected by withdrawal from the aorta or peripheral artery. As blood containing the bolus of dye is drawn through the densitometer, a typical waveform as shown in Fig. 3-3A, is recorded. This is characterized by a nearly vertical rise and exponential decay and a low-amplitude, secondary deflection due to recirculation. The curve can be calibrated for dye concentration and, if no shunts are present, integration of the area under the curve allows easy calculation of the cardiac output.

A variety of online microcomputers are available which will compute the cardiac output within 5 sec of recording the curve and make the technique far simpler. By modification of the basic method, shunts can also be quantitated. The mathematical basis for indicator dilution curves and the methodology of calculating flows and shunts are beyond the scope of this book but are well discussed in the references in the bibliography at the end of this chapter. If a sterile withdrawal system is used, the blood withdrawn may be reinfused at the end of each recording. The volume required for each curve may be as much as 15-20 cc, limiting its application in small infants who cannot stand volume shifts of this magnitude.

Without calibration, indocyanine green curves may be utilized to detect and localize shunts in either direction. The time of injection is recorded by a marking switch, and the appearance time as well as configuration of the curve is noted. In the presence of the left-to-right shunt, injection of dye into the right heart with sampling from a systemic artery shows a normal appearance time and a delayed downslope (Fig. 3-3B). In the presence of a very large left-to-right shunt, the upstroke may be reduced in amplitude and somewhat slow. The delayed downslope is due to the fact that a certain proportion of the dye returning to the left heart from the lungs recirculates with the shunt and is delayed in reaching the point of detection. The same waveform will be recorded regardless of the location of the left-to-right shunt and regardless of where the dye is injected into the right heart. Thus, the location of the left-to-right shunt could not be defined in this manner. If, however, injection is made in the left heart, with arterial sampling the delayed downslope will be seen only if the injection is made at the level of or proximal to

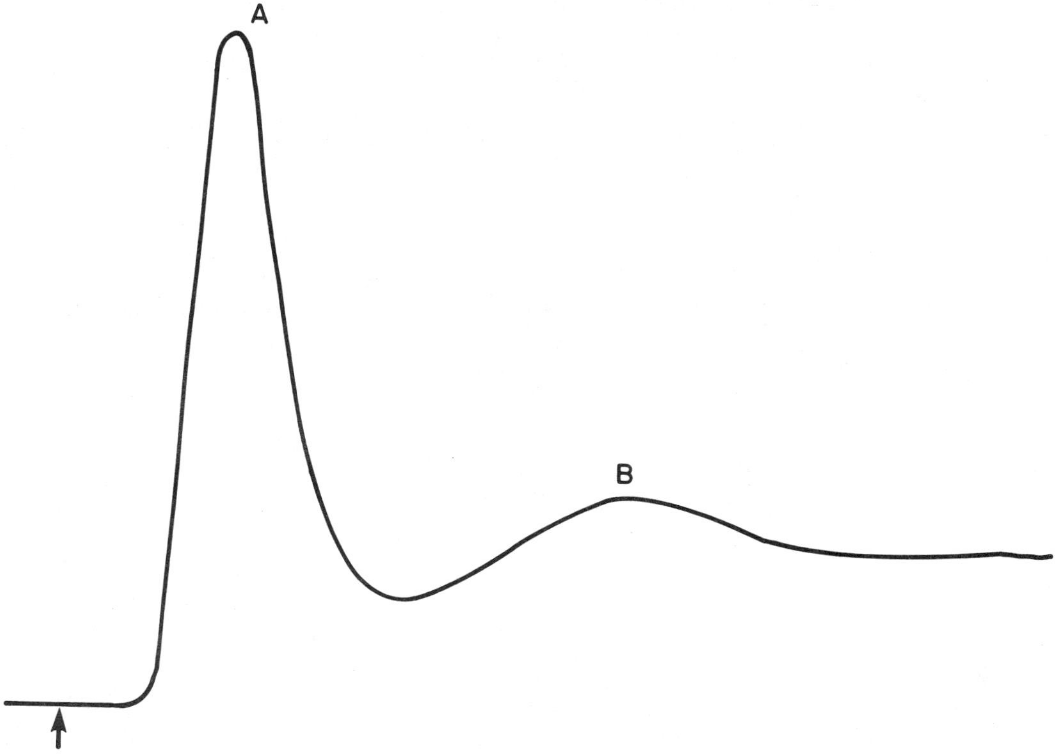

Figure 3-3A Normal indocyanine green curve following injection into the MPA with sampling from the femoral artery (FA). The horizontal axis is time (increasing to the right). The point of injection is indicated by the arrow. Peak A represents the appearance of dye having passed through the lungs, left heart, and aorta, whereas peak B is a recirculation hump (see also B and C).

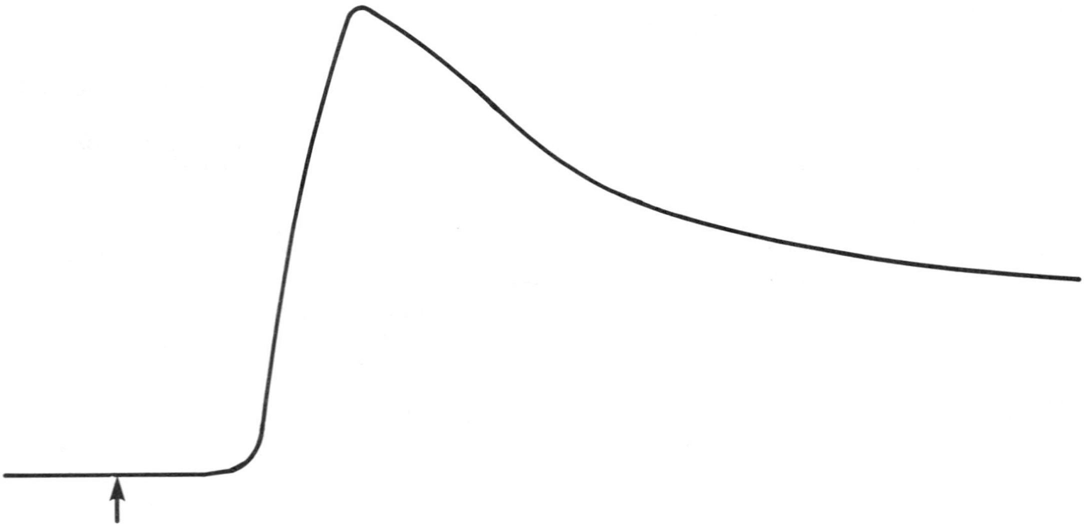

Figure 3-3B Indocyanine green curve in the presence of a left-to-right shunt. Following injection into the main pulmonary artery, the appearance time may be normal or somewhat delayed, with a decreased rate of rise of the initial peak and a delayed downslope due to repetitive recirculation through the shunt (also see A and C).

the shunt. For example, injection into left ventricle or left atrium in a patient with a ventricular septal defect would give the typical wave contour of left-to-right shunt, whereas injection into the aortic root would record a normal curve. Appearance time would be quite rapid with left heart injection. Alternatively, left heart injection with right heart sampling could be utilized to locate left-to-right shunts.

In the presence of a right-to-left shunt, injection of dye into the right heart at or proximal to the location of the shunt will produce a rapid appearance time with an initial early peak due to the shunt and secondary peak due to dye which has normally passed through the lungs (Fig. 3-3C). Injection distal to the point of the shunt would be normal. Thus, right-to-left shunts can be detected and localized in this manner, whereas left heart injection and arterial sampling would be of no value. In the presence of a bidirectional shunt, the curve would be a combination of the above (Fig. 3-3C).

Temperature

The temperature technique employs a negative temperature change as the indicator and is used for determination of cardiac output. Generally one catheter is employed. The ones in common use are flow-directed with a balloon at the distal tip and usually two separate openings, one at the tip for pressure recording and blood sampling and one more proximally for injection of cold saline. A thermistor is mounted on the catheter several centimeters distal to the injection port. This distance must be of sufficient length to allow complete mixing of the indicator with the blood and sufficiently short to minimize heat loss through the vessel wall. The presence of significant shunts results in variable mixing of the indicator with blood or in the loss of indicator, reducing the accuracy of the

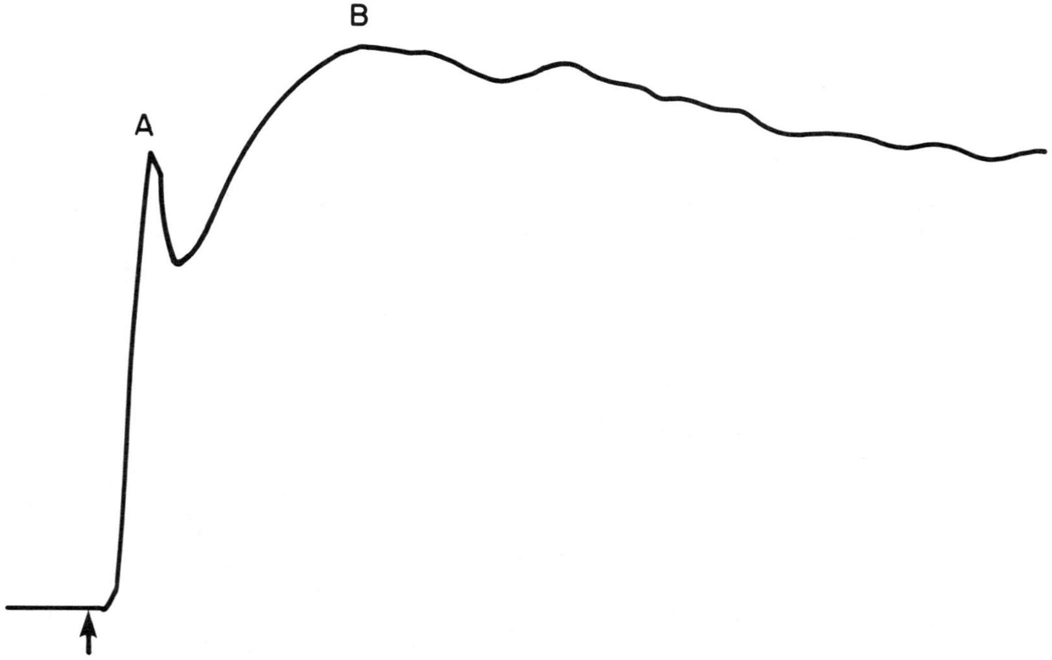

Figure 3–3C Indocyanine green curve from a patient with a VSD and bidirectional shunting. Following injection of dye into the right ventricle, as indicated by the arrow, there is a rapid appearance of dye in the peripheral artery with an early peak (A). This is due to right-to-left shunt. The secondary peak (B) is due to dye passing normally through the lungs and left heart; delayed downslope is the result of the left-to-right shunt (see also A and B).

technique. A waveform is recorded, and blood flow can be computed using standard indicator dilution mathamatics. All of the commercially available devices rapidly compute and display flow in digital format. A high degree of correlation with both Fick and dye dilution methods has been achieved, and the technique is applicable even in small infants. It is quick and easy to use and can be repeated as rapidly as desired.

His Bundle Recording

Although intracardiac electrocardiography recordings have been obtained for many years, it is within the last 10–15 years that special catheters and techniques have been developed to allow recordings of potentials from points along the normally silent conduction system. Depending upon the information desired, one or more catheters with two to six electrodes each may be used. A multiple-channel recorder is necessary to allow simultaneous recording of two or three surface electrocardiogram leads and two or more intracardiac channels.

A normal tracing is shown in Fig. 3-4, with primary deflections due to polarization of low atrium, His bundle, and ventricle. Occasionally, potentials from the atrioventricular node or the bundle branches may also be detected. Measurement of the interval between onset of the P wave and the low atrial deflection (PA

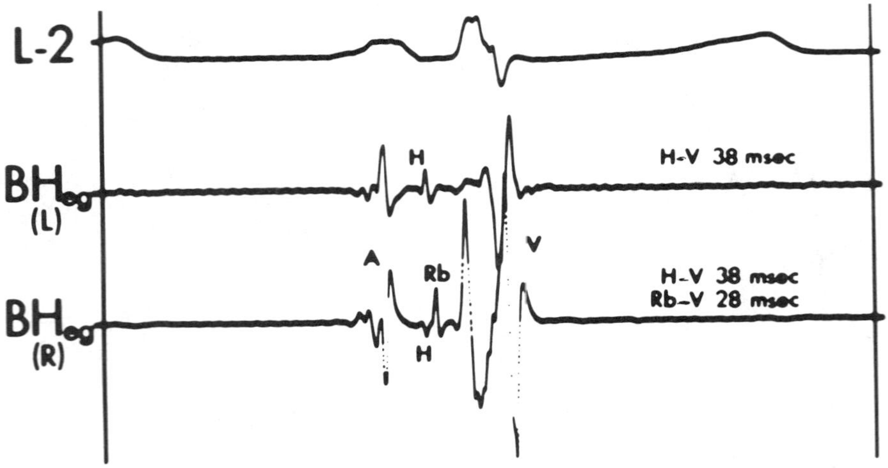

Figure 3–4 Simultaneous recording of EKG lead II and bipolar intracardiac EKGs obtained from the left and right side of the interventricular septum, respectively. Atrial excitation recorded by the intracardiac catheters is indicated by A and coincides with the P wave of the surface electrogram. His bundle excitation potential is labeled H, and ventricular depolarization is indicated by V. The right heart catheter records a potential (Rb) from the right bundle branch. The HV interval represents time passage of excitation wave through the distal conduction system. (Reproduced with permission from Narula, OS, His Bundle Electrocardiography and Clinical Electrophysiology, 1975, F. A. Davis, Philadelphia.)

interval) allows estimation of intraatrial conduction, whereas the interval from atrial deflection to His bundle deflection (AH interval) measures AV nodal delay. Conduction through the bundle branch-Purkinje system is evaluated by the interval from His bundle deflection to ventricular deflection interval (HV interval). Multiple-channel recordings when combined with intracardiac pacing at various sites have immeasurably increased the understanding of mechanisms of tachyarrhythmias, bundle branch disorders, preexcitation, and virtually all types of rhythm and conduction disorders.

Evaluation of Cardiac Function

Evaluation of cardiac function is also a new area, with multiple techniques developed within the last 10 years in an attempt to assess the functional state of the myocardium and to provide quantitative information which can be compared with that obtained in muscle physiology laboratories. In general, techniques fall into two areas, those related to pressure determinations and those related to volume determinations. The former involves primarily the rate of development of tension and related parameters such as the first derivative of the ventricular pressure curve, dP/dT. Results are somewhat difficult to interpret because of the sensitivity of this type of measurement to cardiac rate, volume (preload), and pressure (afterload). Pressure-related parameters, therefore, have limited applicability to the individual patient and are primarily utilized in investigative approaches. On the other hand, measurement of volume of all four cardiac chambers from the angiocardiogram has progressed to a high degree of sophistication. For the most part, biplane angiocardiographic techniques are required with calibration for magnification. Appropriate mathematical formulas are available for the conversion of measurements from the angiocardiogram to chamber volume. For instance, end-systolic and end-diastolic volume of a ventricle could be determined, and one could then calculate:

$$\text{Stroke volume (cc/beat)} = \text{(end-diastolic volume)} - \text{(end systolic volume)}$$

$$\text{Ejection fraction} = \frac{\text{Stroke volume}}{\text{End-diastolic volume}}$$

$$\text{Cardiac output} = \text{stroke volume} \times \text{heart rate.}$$

Other parameters such as the rate of myocardial fiber shortening can also be computed. The ejection fraction which normally in children is 0.6-0.63 is a useful parameter, and low values indicate a significant degree of reduced myocardial function.

As computer techniques are applied to the catheterization laboratory, the amount of information obtained is increasing. Instantaneous determination of cardiac volumes and function parameters on a beat-to-beat basis may be possible. The future in this area is extremely promising.

Bibliography

Grossman W: Cardiac Catheterization and Angiography, 2nd ed., Lea and Febiger, Philadelphia, 1980.

Nadas AS, Fyler DC: Pediatric Cardiology, 3rd ed., Chap. 6, pp. 109-137, W. B. Saunders, Philadelphia, 1972.

Narula OS: His Bundle Electrocardiography and Clinical Electrophysiology, F. A. Davis, Philadelphia, 1975.

Rudolph AM: Congenital Disease of the Heart, Chap. 4, pp. 49-167, Year Book Medical Publishers, Inc., Chicago, 1974.

Wood EH: Symposium on Use of Indicator Dilution Techniques in the Study of the Circulation, American Heart Association, New York, 1962.

Yang SS, Bentivoglio LG, Maranhao V, Goldberg H: From Cardiac Catheterization Data to Hemodynamic Parameters, F. A. Davis, Philadelphia, 1972.

Zimmerman HA: Introvascular Catheterization, 2nd ed., Charles C Thomas, Springfield, Illinois, 1966.

Part II

BASIC PRINCIPLES

Chapter 4

GENERAL CONCEPTS OF NORMAL AND ABNORMAL CARDIOVASCULAR FUNCTION

Elements of the System

Basically the cardiovascular system can be considered as a complex control system designed to maintain adequate blood flow to the numerous tissue vascular beds under diverse conditions of loading or stress. Reduced to its basic elements it consists of the following components.

1. A pump
2. A network of nonrigid pipes of variable capacity
3. Control mechanisms

An alteration in any of these elements will effect not only its function but that of the others.

Determinants of Pump Function (Fig. 4-1)

Any deviation of the cardiovascular system from its equilibrium state can be considered as affecting one or more of the following parameters which are the basic factors determining the ability of the heart to function as a pump.

1. Preload
2. Afterload
3. Inotropic state
4. Heart rate

Preload (Fig. 4-2)

Defined by muscle physiologists as the load at which muscle begins to develop tension, preload in the intact heart is related to end-diastolic muscle fiber tension, hence to end-diastolic fiber length. It has been known for many years that the muscle fiber whose resting tension (i.e., length) is increased will, upon stimulation, develop increased force of active contraction which is proportional to the increase in fiber length up to a point beyond which further increases in length will reduce the fiber's ability to develop tension. This, of course, is the classic Frank-Starling relationship. In terms of the intact heart, an acute increase in end-diastolic volume (e.g., sudden increase in blood volume or acute valvular regurgitation) will

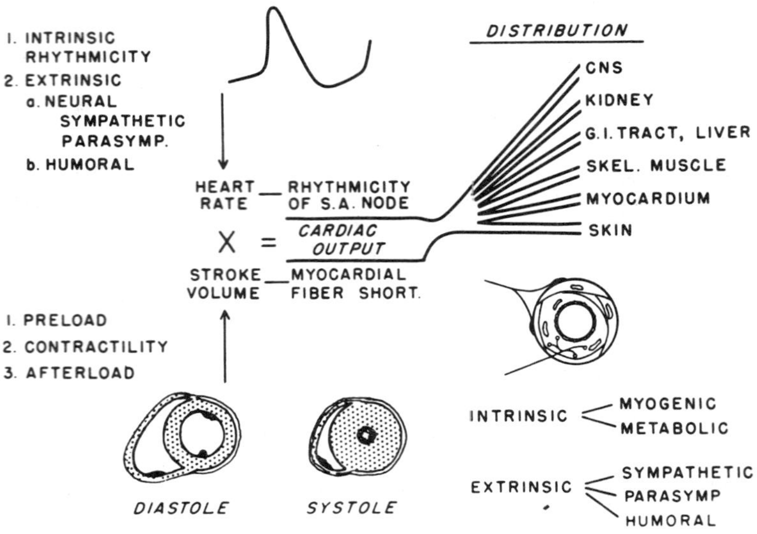

Figure 4-1 Schematic representation of the circulation. Cardiac output is determined by heart rate and stroke volume as illustrated in the center of the figure. Heart rate is a function of the automaticity of the sinoatrial node, whereas stroke volume is a function of degree of myocardial fiber shortening. The principal determinants of heart rate and stroke volume are listed at the left of the figure. Distribution to the various peripheral vascular beds is indicated in the upper right corner. This distribution is governed primarily by the resistance arterioles, illustrated in the lower right, together with factors which act to control these vessels. (Reproduced with permission from New England Journal of Medicine, 290: 1124, 1974.)

produce an increase in systolic pressure, rate of pressure rise, velocity of fiber shortening, and stroke volume. Acute preload changes, therefore, have a positive effect and result in increased output.

Chronic ventricular dilatation does not appear to operate in the same manner, that is, through the Frank-Starling mechanism. As dilatation progresses, the sarcomeres (contractile units of the muscle fiber) reach their maximal functional length (approximately 2.2 μm) early, and further dilatation is due to either an increase in size of myocardial cells or the number of sarcomeres. Unless the stress-producing ventricular dilatation is so severe as to produce congestive heart failure, the performance of each contractile unit is normal. At an increased end-diastolic volume, however, the ventricle is able to develop a large stroke volume with a lesser degree of fiber shortening and, therefore, without an increase in the performance of each contractile unit. The ventricular compliance or distensibility tends to remain normal since conditions which produce increased ventricular filling do not result in significant thickening of the ventricular wall, thus the increased diastolic filling of the ventricle is accomplished without any significant increase in filling pressure unless dilatation is severe. Because of its thinner wall, the right ventricle has a greater complaince than the left, at least after the first few months of life. If a significant amount of edema and/or fibrosis of the myocardium develops, ventricular compliance will be compromised and filling pressure increased. This could result in the development of pulmonary or systemic venous hypertension even though the degree of ventricular dilatation is unchanged.

Afterload

Afterload is defined as tension in the ventricular wall during the shortening or ejection phase of the cardiac cycle. Changes in afterload are basically those of pressure loading or increased impedance to ventricular ejection. As these changes develop acutely, there is a decrease in performance of each contractile unit with an increase in ventricular pressure, decrease in the degree and velocity of wall shortening and, therefore, a decrease in stroke volume and cardiac output. In order to compensate for the decreased contractile unit performance, myocardial hypertrophy develops in the chronic or steady state. In this manner, the performance of the intact pump may be maintained even though that of each component part is reduced. In the intact animal, an increase in afterload usually results in the shifting of blood volume out of systemic venous reservoirs and an increase in ventricular size. In either the acute or chronic state such a volume shift may aid in maintaining the stroke volume of the ventricle. It is, however, not seen early in the course of the chronically increased afterload in the pediatric patient.

Inotropic State (Fig. 4-3)

The inotropic state or contractility of the myocardium is the ability of the fibers to contract independent of loading conditions; thus, regardless of other factors, an increase in contractility will produce an increase in the velocity and degree of contraction and, therefore, an increase in stroke volume and cardiac output. In response to adverse loading conditions, compensatory changes in

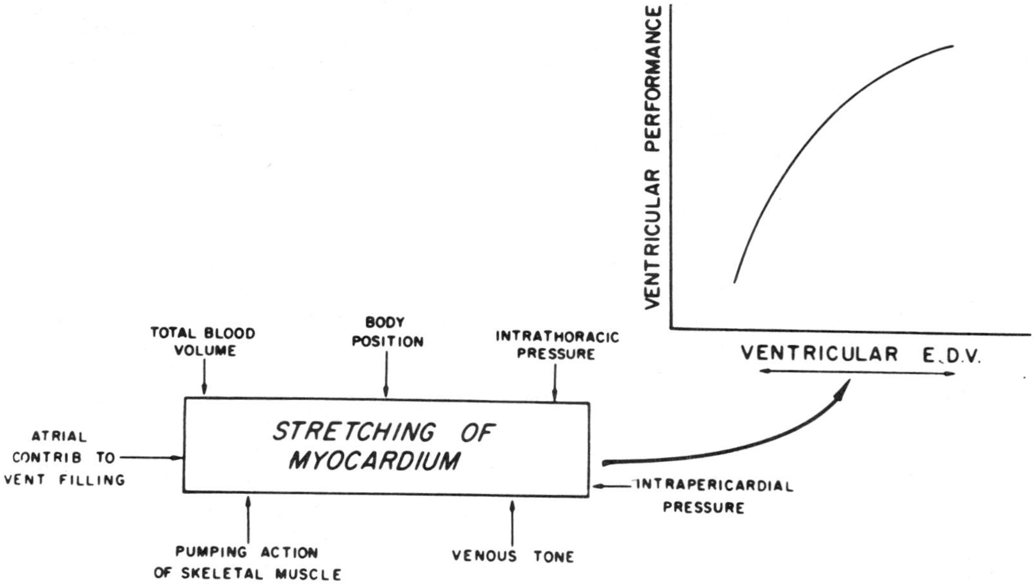

Figure 4-2 The relationship between ventricular end-diastolic volume and ventricular performance is shown by the classic Frank-Starling curve in the upper right-hand corner. Factors affecting the end-diastolic volume are shown in the lower left-hand portion of the figure. (Reproduced with permission from Braunwald E, Ross J, Sonnenblick EH, Mechanisms of Contraction of the Normal and Failing Heart, 2nd ed., 1976, Little, Brown and Co., Boston.)

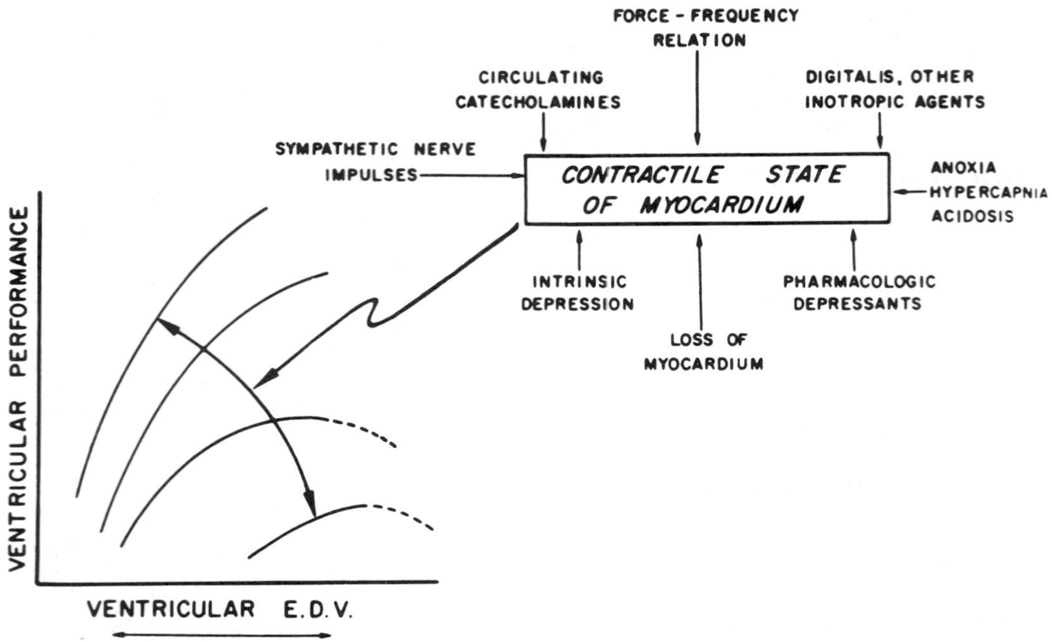

Figure 4–3 Alterations in myocardial contractility may act to increase or decrease the ventricular performance at a given end-diastolic volume as shown by this family of Frank-Starling curves. If contractility is decreased, the curve is shifted downwards and to the right as shown. Determinants of myocardial contractility are shown in the upper right-hand corner. (Reproduced with permission from Braunwald E, Ross J, Sonnenblick EH, Mechanisms of Contraction of the Normal and Failing Heart, 2nd ed., 1976, Little, Brown and Co., Boston.)

contractility may be brought about by action of the sympathetic nervous system and circulating catecholamines as well as by certain drugs such as digoxin or isoproterenol. On the other hand, depression of myocardial contractility is basic to the state known as congestive heart failure (q.v.) and may result from excessively severe loading conditions as well as from myocardial inflammation, certain storage diseases, cardiomyopathies, or myocardial ischemia.

Heart Rate

As long as ventricular filling is maintained, an increase in cardiac rate will produce a proportionate increase in cardiac output. Thus, changes in rate are a key mechanism for increasing output under such conditions as exercise. In addition to this straightforward effect on cardiac output, there is evidence of an increase in myocardial contractility at increased heart rate.

The Pipes

The complex network of tubing which delivers blood to and returns it from the tissue cells is not a rigid passive system, but rather an active one with two parameters which can be controlled: resistance and capacitance. The resistance of both the pulmonary and systemic vascular beds is primarily a function of the small muscular arteries (precapillary sphincters). An increase in vasoconstriction tone in these vessels results in a decrease in lumen size and an increase in the resistance to flow through that portion of the vascular bed. These precapillary sphincters are capable of responding to a variety of stimuli including intralumenal pressure, neural control, metabolic factors, and so forth. Such resistance alterations are extremely important in regulating the volume of flow through the multiple branches of the systemic vascular bed. The capacitance of the vascular system, on the other hand, is primarily a function of the systemic veins which are capable of contracting or dilating to produce significant volume shifts into or out of the heart as previously discussed. This constitutes a major element in the maintenance of ventricular filling under various conditions of stress.

Control Mechanisms

The basic elements of any control system are illustrated in Fig. 4-4. Regulation of the cardiovascular system involves monitoring numerous parameters including flow, blood pressure, tissue metabolic demands, and so forth, and instituting appropriate adjustments in cardiac output and distribution of blood flow to respective vascular beds. Thus, a large number of detection and feedback mechanisms are involved and interact in a complicated manner. The mechanisms which provide feedback control to the heart and blood vessels include:

1. *Neural regulation:* Neural regulation is mediated through the autonomic nervous system. Resting control of the heart is under vagal regulation with the sympathetic system involved only when there is a demand for increased output or regional vasoconstriction.
2. *Humoral factors:* There are numerous circulating substances such as catecholamines or vasoactive polypeptides which may act on the heart to control rate and/or contractility or on blood vessels to change resistance. Some locally produced vasoactive substances may also play a role.
3. *Intrinsic mechanisms:* Some of the direct effects of loading conditions on the myocardium have already been mentioned. In addition, changes in vasomotor tone may occur in direct response to varied stretch.

Regulation of Cardiac Output

With the maintenance of adequate tissue flow to meet metabolic demands as the ultimate goal, cardiac output can be regulated by changes in rate or stroke volume. The former is a major factor increasing cardiac output during exercise and is primarily under control of the autonomic nervous system.

Regulation of Stroke Volume

Changes in stroke volume can be affected by altering any of the following parameters.

Afterload

Any decrease in impedance to ventricular ejection such as generalized diminution of systemic vascular resistance should theoretically improve cardiac output. In the clinical situation, a decrease in cardiac output evokes exactly the opposite response, namely, increased resistance in most of the branches of the systemic vascular bed in an effort to redistribute flow to vital organs. Thus, as a physiologic

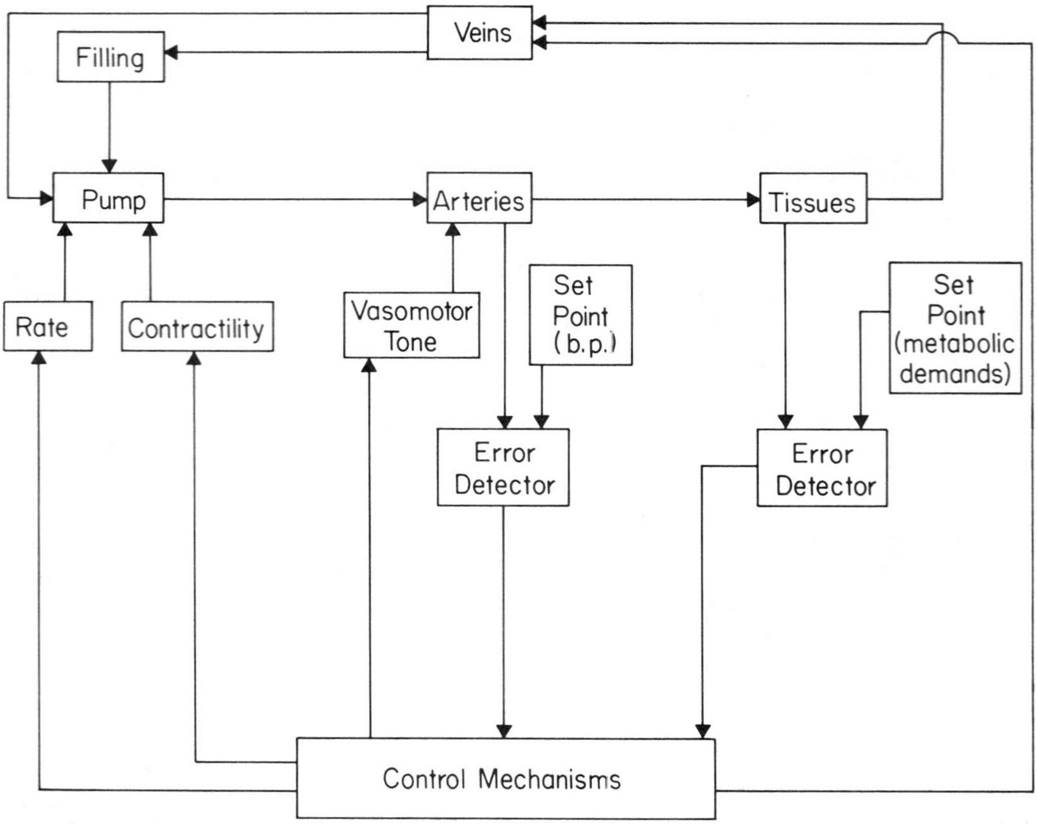

Figure 4–4 Schematic representation of the circulation as a control system. Two possible control mechanisms are illustrated. Peripheral arterial baroreceptors constantly compare arterial blood pressure with the desired level (i.e., the set point), and any significant deviation from the desired level may activate control mechanisms, resulting in changes in vasomotor tone in various peripheral vascular beds, in myocardial contractility, or in cardiac rate. Ventricular filling can also be altered by volume shifts into and out of peripheral venous reservoirs. Any significant variation in delivery of oxygen and/or nutrients in relation to tissue metabolic demands may activate similar control mechanisms to alter cardiac output or peripheral vascular distribution.

control mechanism, decreases in ventricular afterload do little to aid in the maintenance of cardiac output. This is a fruitful area for therapeutic investigation, and several agents directed toward afterload reduction are already in clinical use.

End Diastolic Volume

Acute increases in ventricular end-diastolic volume will act to increase stroke volume and cardiac output through altered preload as previously discussed. A similar improvement in the degree and velocity of fiber shortening is not seen in chronic ventricular dilatation, rather the geometry of the dilated ventricle allows stroke volume to be maintained with a lesser degree of fiber shortening. Shifts of volume into and out of venous reservoirs in response to acute demands constitute an important mechanism for altering preload control of cardiac output. Total blood volume may also be increased, primarily through renal mechanisms. In addition to dynamic effects of changing venous reservoir capacitance, other factors which have a direct effect upon ventricular end-diastolic volume include body posture, intrathoracic and intrapericardial pressure, and effects of atrial contraction.

Alterations in Inotropic State

Physiologic changes in contractility are primarily mediated via the sympathetic nervous system or more slowly by circulating catecholamines. The force frequency relationship by which myocardial contractility is increased at increasing cardiac rate may also play a slight role in the regulation of cardiac output. However, changes in the inotropic state of the myocardium are not operative to any significant degree in milder states of increased cardiac output; increases in rate and end-diastolic volume are the primary regulating factors in such circumstances.

Control of Blood Flow Distribution

Under conditions of increased demand in localized portions of the systemic circuit or when pump output is reduced, a major redistribution of blood flow can be effected to meet the increased demands and to maintain the necessary supply to critical organs such as the brain. This redistribution is effected through changes in vasomotor tone in the precapillary resistance vessels. Although not operative to any significant degree in the maintenance of basal vasomotor tone, the sympathetic nervous system and/or circulating catecholamines are the primary factors responsible for increasing local vascular resistance in less critical portions of the systemic circulation. In addition, vascular supply to some organs (e.g., the kidney) is capable of intrinsic autoregulation. The postulated mechanism of this type of control is illustrated in Fig. 4-5. The nature of the metabolic vasodilator substances is not totally clarified; various vasoactive polypeptides and/or tissue hypoxia may be involved.

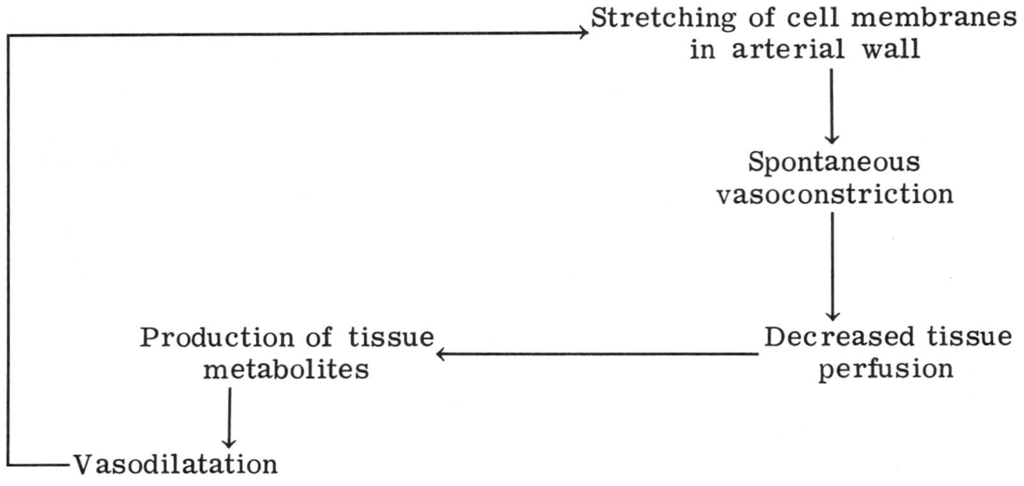

Figure 4-5 Mechanism of intrinsic vascular autoregulation.

Alterations in Pump Function

Stresses on the myocardium secondary to congenital or acquired heart disease in children are usually complex and involve more than one of the determinants of function discussed previously.

Volume Loading

In left-to-right shunts or valvular regurgitation, the affected ventricle must eject an increased stroke volume consisting of the normal (effective) flow to the lungs or body plus the shunt or regurgitant flow. The end-diastolic volume of that ventricle is increased, but in general not rapidly enough to utilize the Frank-Starling relationship. If contractility remains normal, the same degree of myocardial fiber shortening at the larger end-diastolic volume will result in a greater stroke volume. Wall tension is increased, resulting in an increased afterload and some degree of myocardial hypertrophy. On the other hand, the low resistance pathway to ventricular ejection produced by the shunt or regurgitation reduces afterload and acts to improve myocardial performance. If shunt or regurgitant flow is sufficiently severe, however, effective forward flow may not be achieved, and congestive heart failure results.

Pressure Loading

Semilunar valvular stenosis or hypertension (systemic or pulmonary) increases ventricular afterload and consequently decreases performance of the individual contractile units. If the resultant hypertrophy is severe, reduced ventricular compliance may significantly increase filling pressures leading to signs of pulmonary or systemic venous hypertension in spite of effective forward flow. In severe degrees of pressure overloading, myocardial perfusion may be interfered with, leading to fibrosis and further impairment of compliance and contractility.

Primary Endomyocardial Disorders

A number of lesions such as endocardial fibroelastosis, myocarditis, cardiomyopathies, and so forth, act primarily to decrease the inotropic state of the myocardium and generally lead to congestive failure. Little compensation is achieved by hypertrophy although some improvement may result from the previously described effects of increased end-diastolic volume.

Congestive Heart Failure

Congestive failure is defined as a state of impaired cardiac function in which the heart is unable to pump blood at a rate commensurate with requirements of metabolizing tissues. Basically, this may result from one or more of the following abnormal states.

1. An extremely rapid or slow heart rate: Ventricular filling impaired in the former and the maximum cardiac output limited in the latter.
2. Impaired ventricular filling: As seen for example, in mitral stenosis or constrictive pericarditis.
3. Severe impairment of myocardial performance: Assessment of the primary mechanism involved is of critical importance as the treatment will vary accordingly. Drugs designed to improve myocardial contractility would be of

little value if ventricular filling is impaired. More frequently in pediatric patients, severe pressure or volume loading lesions or primary myocardial diseases will result in depression of the inotropic state. In some patients the compensatory mechanisms discussed previously (increased end-diastolic volume, myocardial hypertrophy, and increased sympathetic discharge or catecholamine release) will improve myocardial performance, and an adequate output is maintained, at least under basal conditions. In more severe lesions, however, such compensation may be ineffective, and typical manifestations of congestive failure will result.

The primary myocardial alteration in congestive failure is a depression in contractility. If the end-diastolic fiber length in the failing heart is decreased, myocardial performance diminishes. Thus, the failing heart is operating on the ascending limb of a depressed myocardial function curve (Fig. 4-3). The biochemical mechanisms for this decreased contractility are not yet clear. Abnormalities of production and/or storage of high-energy phosphate do not appear to be responsible. A decrease in myofibrillar adenosine triphosphatase (ATP-ase) has been found which suggests a role for reduced utilization of energy stores. Also noted has been a decreased uptake of calcium by the sarcoplasmic reticulum which may result in less calcium being available for contraction. Adrenergic support for the failing myocardium is defective with decreased norepinephrine stores present in the myocardium. Circulating levels of catecholamines are increased but do not fully compensate. Parasympathetic control of the sinus node discharge rate is decreased in an effort to maintain output through cardiac rate. The complexity of the interrelated responses to congestive failure is illustrated in Fig. 4-6.

The PQR Concept

Basic to the understanding of many forms of congenital heart disease, especially when a communication exists between systemic and pulmonary circulations, is the relationship between pressure, flow, and resistance. This is expressed mathematically by a modification of Ohm's law.

$$\text{Flow (Q)} = \frac{\text{Pressure (P)}}{\text{Resistance (R)}}$$

When a communication exists, flow will go preferentially along the line of least resistance. Resistance to flow may occur at any of several points along the flow pathway. The basic principles are best understood through an analysis of a common example, the ventricular septal defect.

In the presence of the ventricular septal defect, the left ventricle faces two pathways for ejection of its stroke volume: into the systemic bed and through the defect. In the uncomplicated defect, flow through the ventricular septal defect is from left ventricle to right ventricle and is referred to as a left-to-right shunt. The resistance opposing the flow into the systemic circulation (systemic vascular resistance or SVR) originates in the precapillary arterioles. For all practical purposes the shunt flow (through the ventricular septal defect) meets resistance at the defect and in the pulmonary vascular bed (PVR). When the ventricular septal defect is small, it presents a resistance to flow which exceeds SVR, and the left ventricular output goes preferentially to the systemic vascular bed with only a small left-to-right shunt. A large amount of pressure energy is expended in producing the small amount of flow across the resistance of the small ventricular

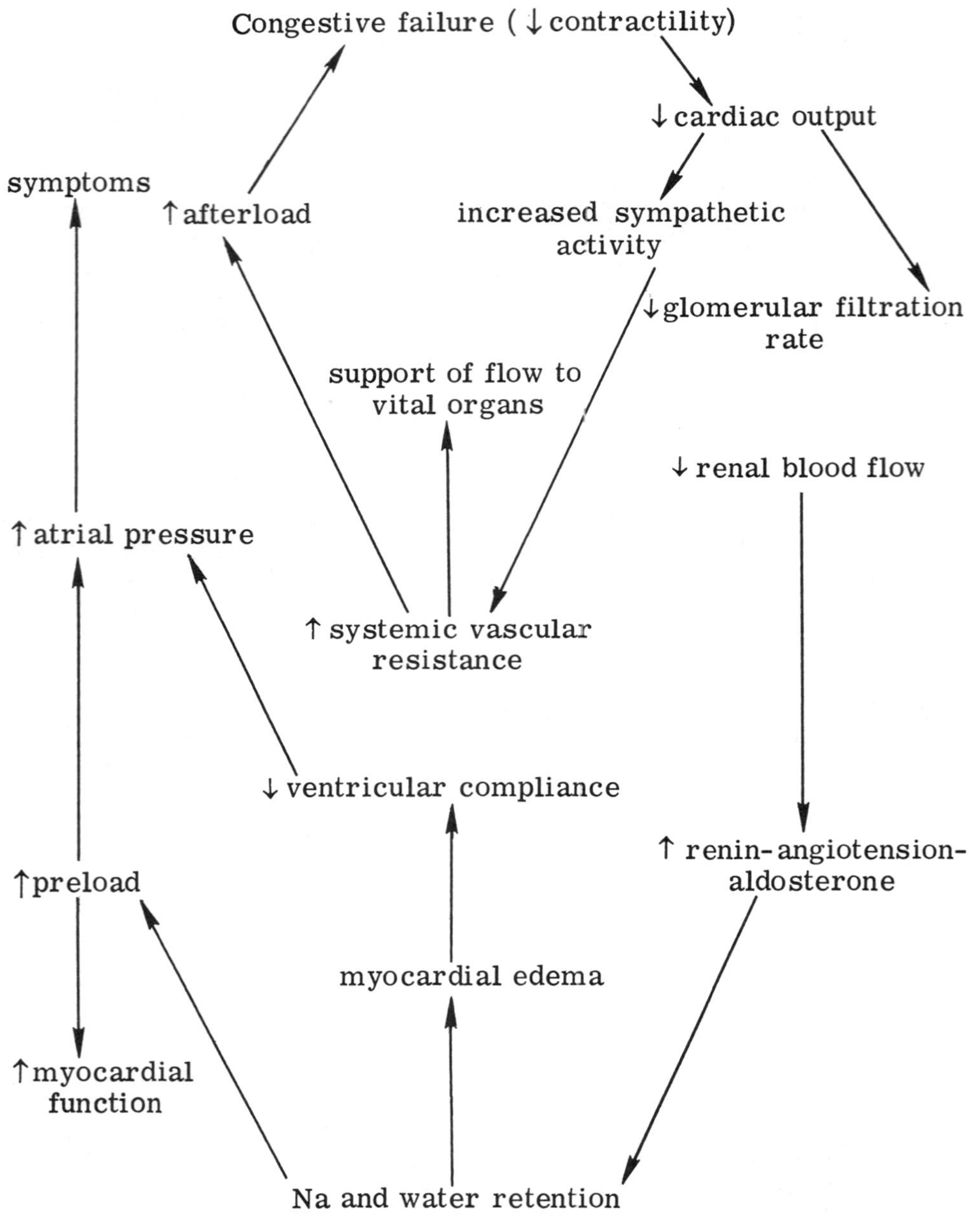

Figure 4-6 Interrelated responses to congestive heart failure.

septal defect; thus, left ventricular pressure is not transmitted to the right heart, and the pressure in the right ventricle and main pulmonary artery remains normal. Since there is only a modest increase in pulmonary flow (Qp), volume loading of the left ventricle as determined by the pulmonary venous return is small.

The pressure developed in the nonfailing left ventricle remains within the limits imposed by SVR, and increased pressure is not the usual method by which larger left-to-right shunts are produced. Rather, increasing the size of the ventricular septal defect produces less resistance to flow; if the size of the defect is approximately equal to the aortic valve area, it is essentially nonobstructive. In the large defect, the left-to-right shunt volume is determined by the PVR which is the only resistance opposing that flow. If PVR is low relative to SVR, there will be a large shunt and consequently significant volume loading of the left ventricle. In the majority of patients with a large ventricular septal defect, PVR does not decrease below the normal range, therefore, an increased pulmonary arterial pressure is required to propel the large pulmonary blood flow. This pressure is developed by the left ventricle and right ventricle acting together as a common ejectile chamber. Such high-flow (Qp), low-resistance (PVR) pulmonary hypertension is referred to as hyperkinetic or dynamic (Fig. 4-7).

Thus, pulmonary hypertension is an obligatory finding when there is a large communication at ventricular or great artery level. It is of extreme importance in evaluating the defect to decide the degree to which increased PVR is contributing to the pressure elevation, as the clinical course and possibly surgical closure of the defect are markedly effected. The status of the pulmonary vascular bed in the fetus and the changes in the normal transitional circulation are discussed in the next section of this chapter. In addition to vasoconstriction in the arterioles, PVR may be increased by greater thickness of the walls of the small arteries and arterioles with encroachment upon the lumen, referred to as pulmonary vascular obstructive disease (PVOD). In earlier stages, thickening of the media is followed

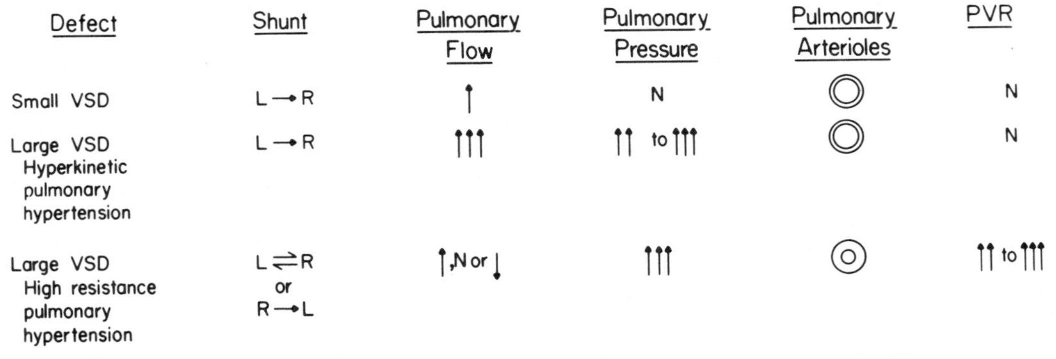

Figure 4-7 The relationship between pressure, flow, and resistance is illustrated in the example of the ventricular septal defect as discussed in the text. In the small defect, the pulmonary arterial pressure and resistance (PVR) are normal. There is a small left-to-right shunt and slight increase in pulmonary flow. Pulmonary hypertension accompanies the presence of a large defect, but if the pulmonary vascular resistance is normal, there will be a large left-to-right shunt and large pulmonary blood flow (hyperkinetic pulmonary hypertension). On the other hand, if pulmonary arteriolar vasoconstriction or pulmonary vascular obstructive disease narrows the precapillary resistance vessels producing high pulmonary vascular resistance, the shunt will be bidirectional or dominant right to left with appropriate alterations in pulmonary blood flow.

by intimal hyperplasia and fibrosis. In far-advanced PVOD there is thrombosis and ultimately necrotizing arteritis. Factors which initiate the sequence of pulmonary vascular obstructive disease are not fully understood. Progressive PVOD is by no means present in every patient with a large ventricular septal defect. It would appear that PVOD develops in patients with an underlying, perhaps genetically determined, predisposition (i.e., a hyperreactive pulmonary vascular bed).

Elevation of PVR will reduce pulmonary blood flow and, therefore, the volume of the left-to-right shunt. As the pulmonary vascular resistance approaches and/or exceeds systemic vascular resistance, an increasing degree of bidirectional shunting will develop, progressing to a dominant right-to-left shunt (so-called Eisenmenger physiology). Volume loading of the left ventricle will decrease, leaving pressure loading of the right ventricle as the primary hemodynamic stress. In many infants elevated PVR begins as failure of complete involution of the high-resistance fetal pulmonary vessels (v.i.) so that PRV remains elevated from birth, and a large left-to-right shunt never develops. In some, however, PVR decreases significantly over the first 2-4 months of life with a large left-to-right shunt and frequently congestive heart failure, and then a subsequent increase in pulmonary vascular resistance and development of pulmonary vascular obstructive disease occur. Such an infant may seem to improve as volume loading and congestive heart failure are relieved; tragically the prognosis is worse since a PVR/SVR greater than 0.7 is generally associated with high surgical mortality for closure of the ventricular septal defect and with irreversible PVOD in the survivors.

The relationship between pressure flow and resistance is applicable to all physiologic and pathologic cardiovascular states and is basic to understanding of all congenital lesions. In analyzing any congenital heart defect, one must look at the pressure relationships and identify sources of resistance to flow. Thus in classic tetralogy of Fallot (q.v.), pressure in right ventricle, left ventricle, and aorta are identical, and flow through the septal defect is right to left because the resistance imposed by the pulmonic stenosis exceeds SVR.

Fetal and Transitional Circulation

The fetus, with all of its respiratory functions as well as input of nutrients and waste elimination carried out at a point remote from the body, has different circulatory needs than the extrauterine infant. Highly oxygenated blood must still be delivered to the brain, but this blood returns to the right atrium (from the placenta) rather than to the left. For maximal efficiency, blood with the lowest-oxygen content should be routed to the placenta. The fetal circulation has several unique features which allow this to be carried out.

1. The placenta
2. The presence of shunt pathways
3. Low levels of pulmonary blood flow

The major hemodynamic effect of the placenta on fetal circulation is due to its function as a low-resistance "arteriovenous malformation" containing a large volume of blood. Its presence in the systemic circulation results in a level of SVR lower than that seen postnatally. This low resistance serves to route the high flows necessary for respiratory and metabolic function through the placenta.

Three shunt pathways are present prior to birth, each with a different purpose.

1. Foramen ovale
2. Ductus arteriosus
3. Ductus venosus

The foramen ovale is an opening in the interatrial septum so constructed as to function as a one-way valve allowing flow from right atrium to left atrium. Because of the anatomic relationship between the foramen ovale and the inferior vena cava (IVC) a major portion of the venous return from that vessel is directed into the left atrium. The oxygen content of this blood, consisting in part of blood returning from the placenta, is significantly higher than that returning from superior vena cava (SVC). In this manner maximum oxygen delivery to the ascending aorta and to the brain is effected. Venous return to the SVC together with coronary sinus return and a portion of the IVC blood enter the right ventricle and pulmonary artery. In the absence of respiratory function, circulatory requirements of the lungs are limited to those necessary for growth and maintenance of cell function and are, therefore, quite low. It is also desirable to direct this poorly oxygenated blood away from the lungs so that the blood delivered to the brain by the left ventricle is not reduced in oxygen content. The ductus arteriosus connecting the main pulmonary artery and descending aorta provides such a bypass pathway.

Limitation of pulmonary blood flow to low levels is facilitated by the elevated pulmonary vascular resistance characteristic of the fetus. This high resistance results from a combination of arteriolar vasoconstriction and increased thickness of the medial layer of these vessels, resulting in a reduced lumen diameter. As a result, PVR exceeds SVR in the fetus, and right ventricular output is directed preferentially into the ductus arteriosus and descending aorta. This increase in medial thickness and, therefore, in pulmonary vascular resistance increases with gestational age and is somewhat less well developed in the premature infant.

The overall structure of the fetal circulation is depicted diagrammatically in Fig. 4-8. In essence, the ventricles are connected in parallel, both ejecting into the systemic circulation. The resistance (afterload) faced by the right ventricle is higher than that faced by the left and higher than that present after neonatal circulatory adjustments are complete. Physiologic right ventricular hypertrophy results, and by the third trimester of pregnancy the right ventricular mass dominates that of the left ventricle. The ductus venosus serves to direct umbilical venous flow into the inferior vena cava, bypassing the high-resistance hepatic vascular bed.

The fetal myocardium presents a peculiar problem which may extend over to the newborn period. There are fewer sarcomeres per unit mass and a higher water content than will be true later. As a result, less active tension is generated by contraction making the fetal myocardium a less effective pump. Myocardial compliance is reduced with greater resting tension for a given end-diastolic volume. Similarly, studies of the fetal lamb have indicated poor control mechanisms. Sympathetic innervation of the heart is incomplete at term and may have less effect on rate or contractility changes in response to stress. The degree of innervation varies with the species studied, and information in the human fetus is lacking. An increase in cardiac output in response to an acute increase in preload has not occurred in some studies, indicating that the Frank-Starling mechanism is inoperative. More recent work has, however, suggested that it may play a role. Regulation of cardiac output in the fetus appears to be primarily through alteration in rate, although the myocardium is responsive to circulating catecholamines.

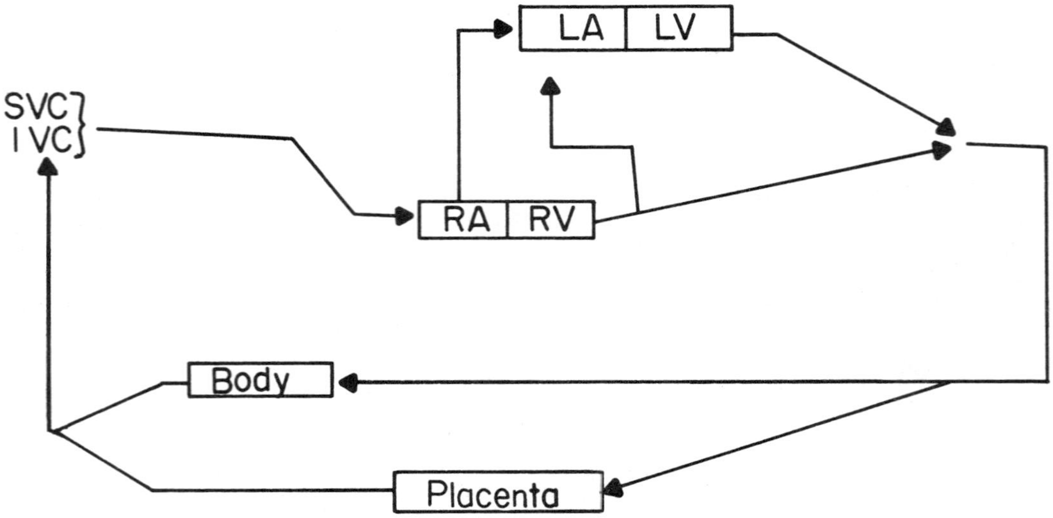

Figure 4-8 Schematic representation of the fetal circulation. Right and left ventricles eject in parallel into the systemic circulation. Direct shunting of blood from right atrium to left atrium through the foramen ovale and a small pulmonary blood flow are shown. Systemic blood flow is distributed to the body and placenta in almost equal proportions.

These factors are of great concern in relation to the newborn's ability to deal with congenital heart defects, but as mentioned the degree to which they place him at greater risk is not clear.

Neonatal Circulatory Adjustments

Following birth, a number of major hemodynamic changes occur, some rapidly and some over a period of weeks to months. The exact sequence of these changes is not well worked out and probably varies between individuals. Ligation of the umbilical cord acutely elevates systemic vascular resistance and to some degree systemic arterial and left ventricular pressure. There is a marked decrease in circulating blood volume and, therefore, in venous return to the right atrium. This results in a decrease in right atrial pressure and in the degree of shunt via the foramen ovale.

With onset of respiration and the resultant increase in arterial pO_2, vasodilatation in the pulmonary vascular bed occurs, precipitously decreasing pulmonary vascular resistance (Fig. 4-9) and pulmonary artery pressure. Pulmonary blood flow rapidly increases, and the increase in pulmonary venous return to the left atrium elevates pressure in that chamber, functionally closing the foramen ovale. A transient reversal of flow through the PDA (i.e., left-to-right shunt) secondary to the reduction in PVR frequently occurs, further increasing pulmonary venous return.

Functional closure of the ductus arteriosus occurs by way of vasoconstriction within the first 10-15 hr. All the factors producing this constriction are not yet understood, but it appears clear that the primary stimulus is the increase in arterial pO_2. Autonomic control does not appear to be involved in this process. The extent to which circulating or locally produced vasoactive substances are involved

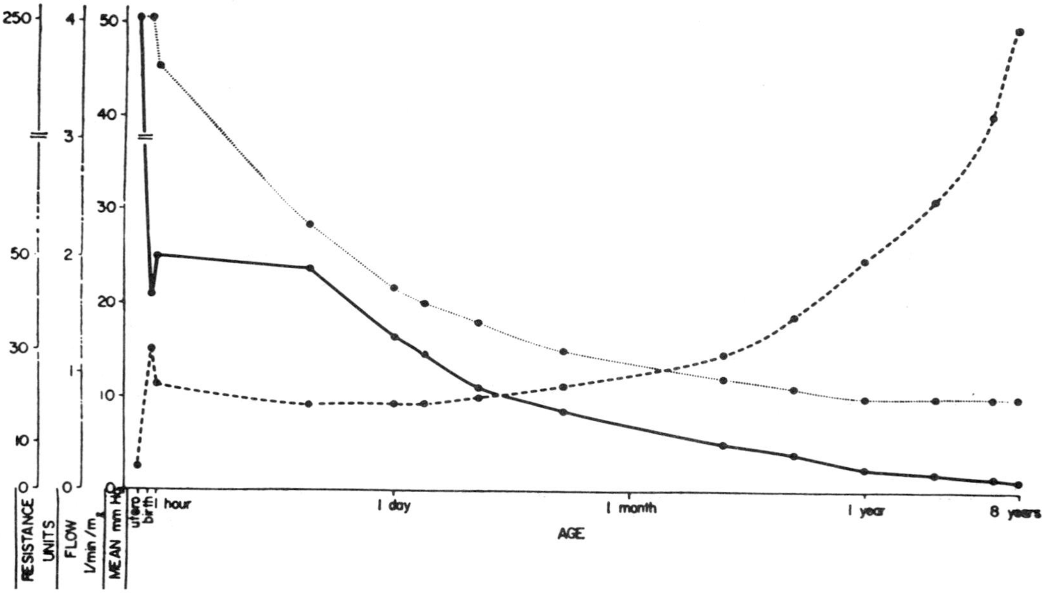

Figure 4–9 Changes in pulmonary vascular resistance (solid line), pulmonary arterial pressure (dotted line), and pulmonary arterial blood flow (dashed line) with increasing age. The immediate decrease in pulmonary vascular resistance with the onset of respiration is accompanied by an increase in blood flow and gradual decline in pulmonary arterial pressure. (Reprinted with permission from Rudolph AM, Normal and Abnormal Respiration in Children, Report of the 37th Ross Conference on Pediatric Research, Fomon SJ, Columbus, Ohio, Ross Laboratories, 1961, p. 67.)

has not been clarified. Prostaglandins (PG) of the E series (especially PGE_2) apparently act to maintain ductal patency in utero, but are ineffective at postnatal levels of oxygen tension. This action on the ductus is being applied in the presurgical palliation of cyanotic congenital heart defects with reduced pulmonary blood flow in the newborn (q.v.). Ductal constriction in response to oxygen is less pronounced in the premature and is partially responsible for the high incidence of patent ductus arteriosus in these infants.

With functional closure of the ductus arteriosus, conversion to a postnatal circulation arrangement in which the ventricles are connected in a series is complete (Fig. 4–10). The ductus venosus closes within the first days of life, but the mechanism by which this is initiated is unknown. Little hemodynamic change is effected by this closure.

Certain stresses can partially delay or reverse this transition. The most potent of these is hypoxemia which may result in dilatation of the ductus arteriosus and profound pulmonary vasoconstriction. In its more severe form this pathophysiologic state is being referred to as the persistent fetal circulation syndrome and is characterized by patent ductus arteriosus, high pulmonary vascular resistance, and pulmonary hypertension. A right-to-left shunt through a PDA and often in addition through the foramen ovale are present, resulting in greater hypoxemia, and a vicious circle is set up which may be difficult to reverse. Therapeutic

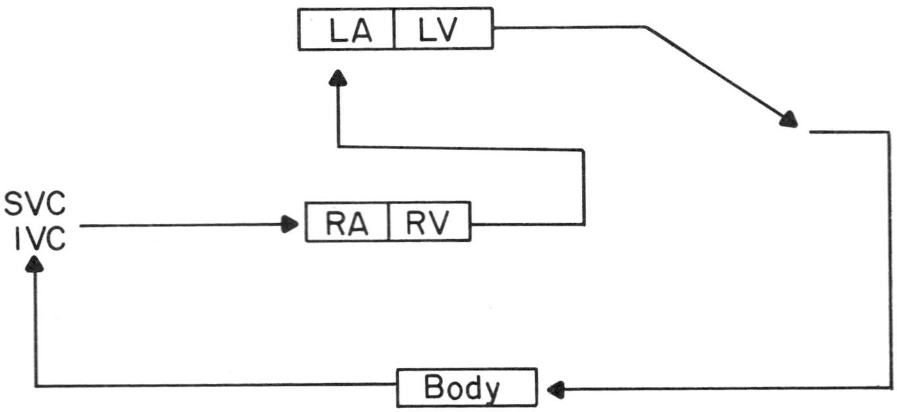

Figure 4–10 Schematic representation of the circulation after neonatal transitional changes are completed. The two ventricles are now connected in series through the pulmonary vascular bed.

efforts are directed at the pulmonary problem producing the hypoxemia and toward attempts at dilatation of the pulmonary bed. Tolazoline has been of some value in alleviating the latter.

Some of the circulatory adjustments characterizing the transitional period may not be complete for several weeks or longer. Fibrous obliteration of the ductus arteriosus is progressive over the first month of life, but anatomic sealing of the foramen ovale is much more gradual and may be incomplete in as many as 25% of otherwise normal adults. The decline in pulmonary vascular resistance which began with vasodilatation is completed by gradual decrease in medial thickness. There is a steady increase in left ventricular mass due to the increased systemic vascular resistance, and from an EKG standpoint this ventricle tends to dominate the right within 1–2 years; however, a typical adult pattern may not be achieved for a decade or more.

Cyanosis

The presence of visible cyanosis reflects the presence of at least 5 g% reduced hemoglobin in the systemic capillaries. This may or may not be due to systemic arterial hypoxemia. A significant reduction in cardiac output as with severe congestive failure or constriction of cutaneous vessels following exposure to cold will produce a slowing of flow through the skin capillaries and increased oxygen extraction. If a sufficient amount of hemoglobin is reduced, cyanosis is seen. This is referred to as peripheral cyanosis and is characterized by a normal arterial pO_2 with a wide arteriovenous oxygen difference and by relief of cyanosis following correction of the primary cause.

Central cyanosis is the result of arterial hypoxemia which may be due to pulmonary or cardiac disease. As mentioned in Chap. 1, determination of arterial blood gasses is mandatory when cyanosis is noted, especially in the newborn where other differentiating features may be obscure. Although both impaired ventilation of alveoli and impaired diffusion of oxygen from alveoli to capillaries may result in pulmonary venous and systemic arterial desaturation, the types of pulmonary problems which produce cyanosis, especially in the young infant, generally have a component of hypoventilation with an elevated arterial pCO_2. The arteriovenous oxygen difference is usually normal in the absence of associated cardiac problems. Central cyanosis due to cardiac disease is the result of an admixture of pulmonary and systemic venous blood, and pulmonary venous saturation is normal. Examination of arterial blood gases reveals a decreased pO_2 and a pCO_2 which is normal or somewhat reduced if hyperventilation is present. In general, the degree of hypoxemia due to cyanotic congenital heart disease varies inversely with volume of pulmonary blood flow. One exception is complete transposition of the great arteries (q.v.) in which condition pulmonary venous blood, although well saturated and of normal-to-increased volume, may not be able to gain access to the aorta.

In many cases, particularly in the newborn, differentiation between causes of central cyanosis may be difficult. The cardiac examination is often normal even in the presence of severe congenital heart disease. Pulmonary disease producing cyanosis usually causes radiographic changes, but problems in interpretation of the newborn x-ray are well recognized. Delineation of the etiology is generally facilitated by having the infant breathe 100% oxygen. In most instances of hypoxemia on the basis of pulmonary disease, significant rise in arterial pO_2 will occur, usually to levels in excess of 200-250 torr. If a definite increase in pO_2 is not seen, positive-pressure ventilation or increased end-expiratory pressure may be added and may be necessary to improve systemic oxygenation in some cases of pulmonary disease. This should be attempted only in qualified neonatal intensive care units. Infants in less sophisticated facilities must be transferred promptly if there is no improvement on 100% oxygen alone. Little change in arterial pO_2 occurs in most cases of cardiac right-to-left shunting. Profound hypoxemia due to congenital heart disease in the young infant is usually the result of markedly decreased pulmonary blood flow or poor venoarterial mixing as in transposition of the great arteries. In any case, an increased concentration of inspired oxygen is of little benefit. There are a number of cyanotic congenital heart lesions which are characterized by increased pulmonary blood flow and unrestricted admixture of pulmonary and systemic venous flows (so called admixture lesions; e.g., single ventricle, truncus arteriosus, etc.). Here cyanosis is less severe, and there may be a significant increase in arterial pO_2 with oxygen; however, levels of 200-250 are not exceeded. Because cyanosis is so mild as to often go unrecognized, these lesions less often present in the newborn period. Persistent pulmonary vasoconstriction with right-to-left shunting through a patent ductus arteriosus or foramen ovale (v.s.) may also cause severe hypoxemia and considerable confusion as mentioned previously. In some of these cases, simultaneous measurement of pO_2 from radial and umbilical arteries will reveal a lower pO_2 in the lower half of the body secondary to ductal shunting. A therapeutic trial of tolazine may produce significant improvement in a few infants. Occasionally cardiac catheterization may be required to exclude congenital heart disease.

Hematologic Aspects

In the presence of anemia, cyanosis may be difficult to recognize since a greater degree of desaturation is required to reduce a sufficient amount of hemoglobin. Thus, it is important to follow the hematologic picture carefully in all children with cyanotic congenital heart disease. If the hemoglobin and hematocrit are normal in the cyanotic child over 3 months of age, anemia is present and should be evaluated and treated promptly. The reduced oxygen-carrying capacity of anemic blood may intensify hypoxemia-related symptoms. Return of hemoglobin to more appropriate levels may intensify the cyanosis but reduce the symptoms.

The usual hematological response to chronic hypoxia is polycythemia, the degree of which varies inversely with arterial pO_2. There is an increased demand for iron and, if dietary supply is inadequate, body stores may be exhausted. Thus, iron deficiency is a common cause of anemia. On the other hand, marked polycythemia may be equally detrimental. Elevations of hematocrit in excess of 65% are associated with a rapid increase in blood viscosity. Microcirculatory sludging and hypoxic infarcts, especially of the brain, are potential complications. It must be kept in mind, however, that cerebral infarcts are also seen in the presence of anemia and are probably even more common when the hematocrit is low. Severe polycythemia with a hematocrit in excess of 70-75% is best treated by surgical intervention to increase the arterial saturation. If this is not feasible, periodic phlebotomy with isovolumic replacement with plasma or albumen may temporarily alleviate symptoms. A rebound increase in hematocrit will occur, and such treatment must be repeated.

Hypoxic Spells

Children with the cyanotic congenital heart lesions characterized by decreased pulmonary blood flow may occasionally experience episodes of hyperpnea and deepening cyanosis which may begin abruptly and are potentially life-threatening. These are also known as anoxic spells or paroxysmal hyperpnea. The typical picture is that of a child between 3-5 months of age who, usually a few minutes after awakening, begins to hyperventilate. Respiratory rate may be rapid or relatively slow, deep, and sighing. At times these spells are preceded by crying or defecation but not infrequently are unassociated with any definable precipitating factor. The child becomes progressively more cyanotic, with the episode lasting from a few minutes to several hours. Milder episodes may terminate spontaneously; more often, specific intervention is required. If not aborted, the spell may progress rapidly to coma, convulsions, and death.

There have been a number of theories regarding the etiology of these spells, one of which has been spasm of the pulmonic infundibulum in patients with tetralogy of Fallot, with increased right-to-left shunting through the ventricular septal defect and a decrease in arterial pO_2. Response to treatment with propanolol suggests that this mechanism may be operative in some patients but cannot be the only factor as spells are also seen in patients who do not have a subpulmonic infundibulum, such as in pulmonic atresia or truncus arteriosus with reduced pulmonary blood flow. Another pathophysiologic sequence has been based on the observation that arterial pO_2 in this group of patients is higher when asleep. Upon awakening, the increase in cardiac output increases venous return to the right ventricle (Fig. 4-11). When resistance to flow into the pulmonary bed is fixed, as it is in this group of lesions, with a large communication between right ventricle and systemic circulation, increased right-to-left shunting must occur with a further decrease in arterial pO_2. If arterial chemoreceptors have not adjusted to waking levels of pO_2, this increased shunting may increase hyperpnea, which in turn may decrease systemic vascular resistance and increase venous return to the right heart through an increased pressure gradient between intra- and extrathoracic veins. A further increase in right-to-left shunting occurs, and a vicious circle is set up. Tachyarrhythmias, both atrial and ventricular, have been found to initiate spells, as well as any stimulus which decreases systemic vascular resistance. For the latter reason we avoid the use of chlorpromazine in sedative mixtures for cardiac catheterization of patients with tetralogy of Fallot.

Treatment can be based on understanding of these mechanisms (Table 4-1). Squatting or assuming a knee-chest position will decrease systemic venous return

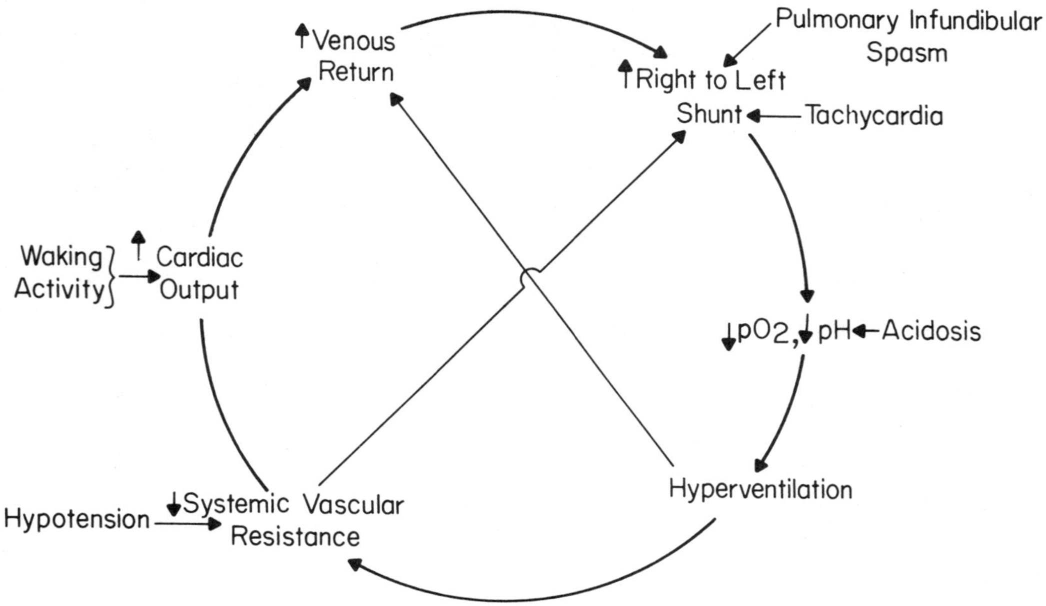

Figure 4-11 Postulated mechanisms in hypoxic spells. The episode can be viewed as a vicious circle initiated by activity and increasing cardiac output with subsequent sequence of changes as shown. Other factors affecting the sequence at various points are indicated on the periphery.

Table 4-1 Treatment of Hypoxic Spells

Therapy	Action
Knee-chest position	Decreased venous return; increased systemic resistance
Oxygen	Reduced hypoxemia (limited value)
Morphine	Decreased hyperventilation
Bicarbonate	Reduced acidosis
Phenylephrine angiotensin	Increased systemic resistance
Correct anemia	Where indicated, increased tissue oxygen delivery
Correction of pathological tachyarrhythmias	May abort spell
Surgery	Increased pulmonary blood flow, elimination of hypoxemia

and may increase systemic vascular resistance somewhat; both changes will decrease right-to-left shunting and improve the arterial pO_2. This is the basis for squatting as a learned adaptation in these patients. Parents can be taught to utilize this at home at the first sign of hyperventilation. The young infant can be more easily placed in this position by holding him over the parent's shoulder (in the burping position) and flexing his thighs against his abdomen. Oxygen should be administered, although its value is limited by the ability of reduced pulmonary blood flow to pick it up. The other traditional method of therapy is morphine, which probably acts by depressing respiratory center responsiveness to signals from the chemoreceptors. The usual dose is 0.1-0.2 mg/kg of body weight. Arterial gases should be obtained, and bicarbonate administered since acidosis rapidly develops and will serve to perpetuate the spell. If there is no response to this treatment, an infusion of a systemic vasopressor such as norepinephrine, phenylephrine, or angiotensin should be started. With the increase in systemic vascular resistance and blood pressure that results, right-to-left shunting will be reduced and pulmonary blood flow improved. As mentioned, propanolol may be of benefit in those patients in whom infundibular spasm is operative. Such patients may be difficult to recognize in advance, and propanolol requires caution in administration if a vasopressor is being concurrently administered. An EKG should be obtained, and any ectopic tachycardia treated as this alone may terminate the spell. Digoxin is potentially dangerous, however, as it may produce infundibular spasm in susceptible patients. If significant anemia is noted, packed cell transfusion may also be rapidly therapeutic. Correction of anemia is more often of value in preventing further episodes.

An occasional patient will fail to respond to any of these measures, and emergency surgical intervention is necessary. The choice between a palliative systemic-to-pulmonary arterial anastomosis and open heart surgery will depend upon the ability of the surgical team.

It is important to remember that the onset of episodes of paroxysmal hyperpnea indicates hemodynamic deterioration which is generally progressive at a variable rate. Any such spell is potentially fatal. Although spells may occasionally be prevented by the correction of anemia or by the chronic administration of propanolol, they are generally an indication to proceed with appropriate surgical therapy of the underlying defect.

Bibliography

Braunwald E, Ross J, Sonneblick EH: Mechanisms of Contraction of the Normal and Failing Heart, 2nd ed., Little, Brown and Company, Boston, 1976.

Guntheroth WG, Morgan BC, Mullins GL: Physiologic Studies of Paroxysmal Hypernea in Congenital Heart Disease, Circulation 31:70, 1965.

Morgan BC, Guntheroth WG, Bloom RS, Fyler DC: A Clinical Profile of Paroxysmal Hypernea in Cyanotic Congenital Heart Disease, Circulation 31:66, 1965.

Nadas AS, Fyler DC: Pediatric Cardiology, 3rd ed., Chapter 14, pp. 293-316, General Principles, W. B. Saunders, Philadelphia, 1972.

Rudolph AM: Congenital Disease of the Heart, Chapters 1-3, pp. 1-48, Chapter 5, pp. 168-185, Year Book Medical Publishers, Inc., Chicago, 1974.

Part III

CONGENITAL
CARDIOVASCULAR
ABNORMALITIES

Chapter 5

ATRIAL SEPTAL DEFECT

In this chapter abnormal interatrial communications of the ostium secundum and sinus venosus types are discussed. Defects of the atrial septum associated with abnormal development of septum primum and endocardial cushions are discussed in Chap. 8.

Incidence

Atrial septal defect is a common lesion observed in approximately 10% of patients with congenital heart disease. Associated partial anomalous pulmonary venous connection is found in 9% of all reported cases.

Embryological and Anatomic Considerations

Separation of the right and left atrium starts with the downward growth of the septum primum from the roof of the common atrium (Fig. 5-1). Prior to complete fusion of the septum primum with the endocardial cushions, perforations appear in the upper part of the septum to form the ostium secundum, allowing for the mandatory right-to-left shunt necessary in fetal life.

A second septum (septum secundum) developing to the right of the septum primum grows downward and anteriorly and assumes a crescent shape which partially covers the hole in the septum primum. Atrial septal defects of the ostium secundum variety could, therefore, be due to either too large an ostium secundum or inadequate development of the septum secundum (Fig. 5-1D, E; Fig. 5-2). Defects in the posterior-superior portion of the atrial septum immediately underneath the superior vena caval junction are called sinus venosus defects (Fig. 5-2). These are often associated with partial anomalous venous drainage into the superior vena cava.

Incompetence of the foramen ovale is occasionally encountered in infancy and is mostly related to lesions associated with left atrial overload (Fig. 5-1F). Increased left atrial volume or pressure could cause prolapse of the valve of the foramen ovale into the right atrium, allowing shunting to occur.

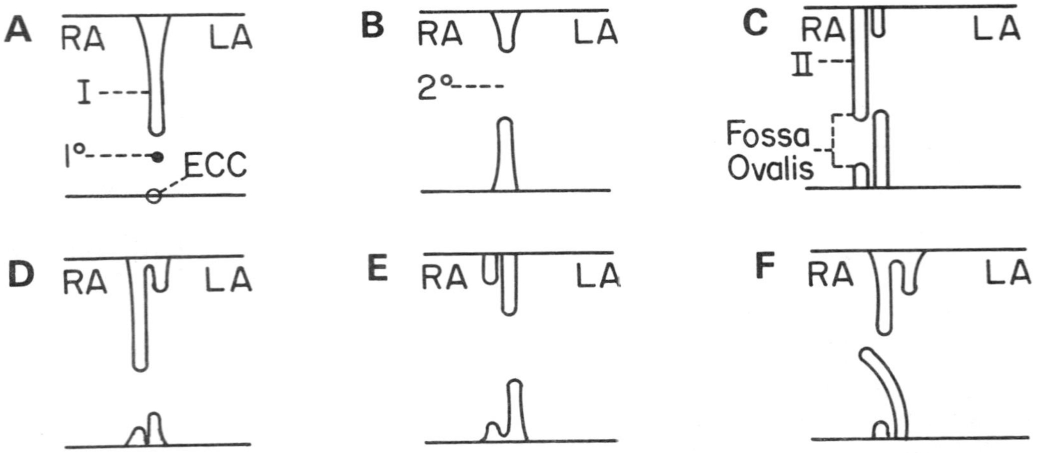

Figure 5–1 Diagrammatic portrayal of the embryological development and defects of the atrial septal (RA and LA, right and left atrium, respectively; 1°-ostium primum, I-septum primum, 2°-ostium secundum, II-septum secundum, ECC-endocardial cushion). (A) Septum primum growing toward the endocardial cushion to close ostium primum. (B) Septum primum complete, ostium secundum is formed. (C) Septum secundum developing to overlap ostium secundum. (D) ASD secundum type due to large ostium secundum. (E) ASD secundum type due to inadequate development of septum secundum. (F) Prolapsed valve of the foramen ovale.

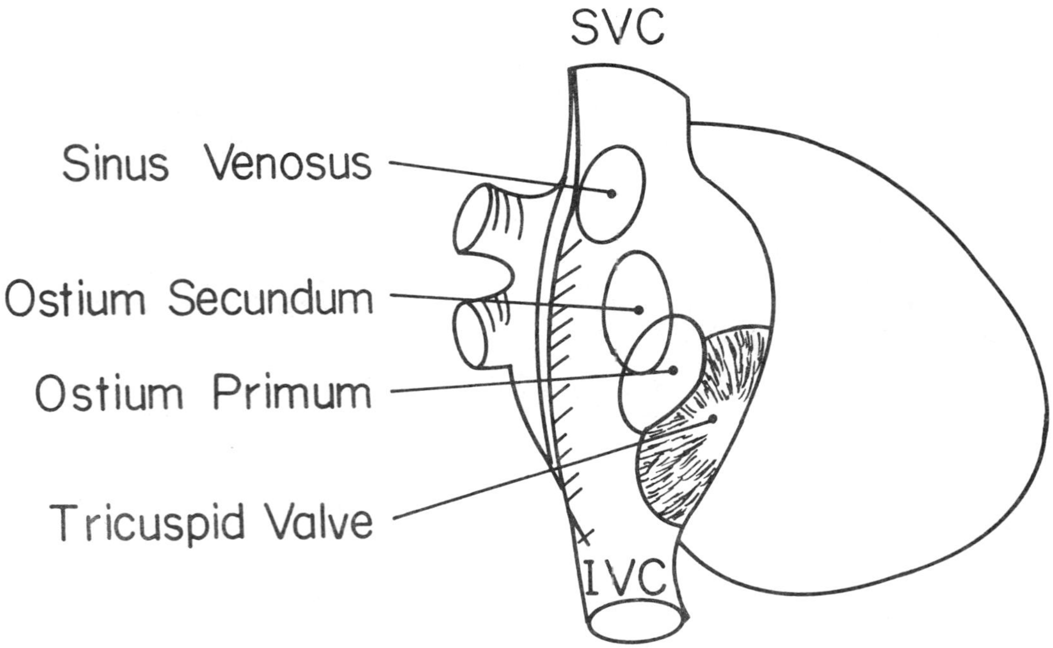

Figure 5–2 Diagram showing the most common types of ASD. The right atrial wall is removed, and the interatrial septum is visualized. Sinus venosus defect is located adjacent to the SVC. Ostium secundum defect occurs at the midpoint of the atrial septum. Ostium primum defect appears just above the tricuspid valve.

Hemodynamic Considerations

Normally, left atrial pressure is higher than right, and in the presence of an atrial septal defect (ASD) the net direction of blood flow is left to right. In many patients with large ASD there is some degree of right-to-left shunting from the inferior vena cava following the fetal pathway; however, for all practical purposes, the direction of flow in an uncomplicated ASD is left to right. Consequently, the right atrium, ventricle, and pulmonary artery have to accommodate not only the systemic venous return, but also the shunt across the defect and, as a result, these structures are dilated (Fig. 5-3). The degree of dilatation is primarily determined by the volume of the left-to-right shunt.

The volume of left-to-right shunt depends on the size of the defect and the relationship of systemic to pulmonic vascular resistance or right ventricular compliance. A reduction in pulmonary resistance or right ventricular pressure is associated with increased left-to-right shunt. The large volume load appears to be handled well by the right ventricle for many years without the development of right heart failure. The large pulmonary blood flow under low pressure does not produce the same risk of pulmonary vascular disease as with ventricular septal defect (VSD) and patent ductus arteriosus (PDA). Pulmonary vascular disease is, therefore, rarely seen in children. It is more common beyond the fourth decade and, once established, is usually progressive.

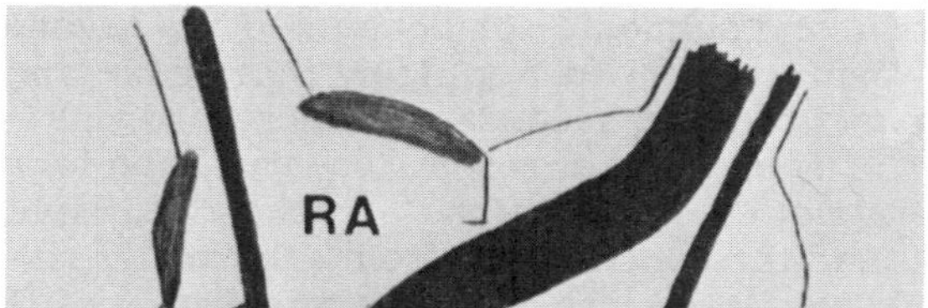

Figure 5-3 Schematic representation of a heart with ASD. The arrows indicate the flow of blood. RA - right atrium, RV - right ventricle, MPA - main pulmonary artery, LA - left atrium, LV - left ventricle, Ao - aorta.

Manifestations

History

Children with ASD are usually asymptomatic with a murmur discovered on routine physical examination. This murmur might be misdiagnosed as functional if the significance of the associated findings, such as abnormal second sound, EKG, or x-ray, is not recognized. Some observers support the concept that the full left-to-right shunt evolves slowly; therefore, the findings are often missed early in childhood. Symptomatology of ASD ranges from none-to-easy fatigability and rarely right heart failure. Contrary to prior belief, an increasing number of infants with ASD and congestive heart failure have been reported.

Physical Examination

Growth is usually not seriously affected, although the patient may appear thin. Precordial bulge and a right ventricular impulse are often associated with a large shunt. The first heart sound is normal, although prominence of the tricuspid component has been described. The second heart sound is widely split without evidence of respiratory variation (fixed splitting) (Fig. 5-4). This fixed splitting is one of the most important diagnostic tools differentiating atrial septal defect from physiologic ejection murmur and from wide but variable splitting associated with right bundle branch block.

Normally, the aortic and pulmonic components of the second heart sound are narrowly split during expiration. Wider splitting that occurs in inspiration is due to delay in the pulmonary closure, secondary to increased right ventricular stroke volume (see Chap. 2). The absence of respiratory variation in patients with ASD is related to the interatrial communication. The right ventricle fills from the right and left atrium, and the contribution from each varies reciprocally with the phase of respiration. The normal inspiratory augmentation of the right ventricular filling is nullified by an equal diminution in the left-to-right atrial flow. The result is no change in right ventricular stroke volume in inspiration as compared to expiration and, therefore, fixed splitting. Infants with documented moderate-sized ASD might not exhibit this wide splitting. This is probably related to the fast heart rate and respiration.

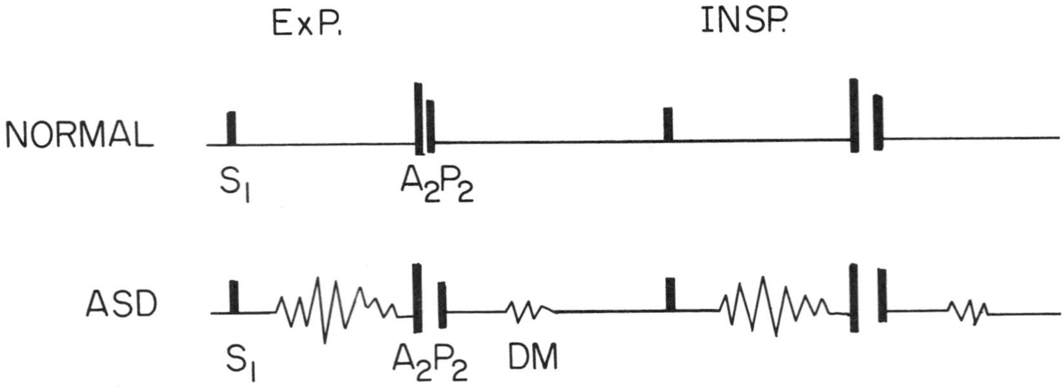

Figure 5-4 Phonocardiogram of a normal patient and a patient with ASD. Note the wide fixed splitting of the second heart sound in the patient with ASD. There is also a systolic ejection murmur and a diastolic rumble (DM). (For explanation see text.)

An ejection systolic murmur is heard at the upper left sternal border originating from large flow across the pulmonic valve. In the presence of a large left-to-right shunt, there is a low-frequency, early diastolic murmur (rumble) at the tricuspid area. This flow rumble is heard when the pulmonary-to-systemic-flow ratio is more than 2:1.

Electrocardiogram

The electrocardiogram usually shows right axis deviation with a frontal axis of +90–+180°. There is mild right ventricular hypertrophy usually manifested by increased rightward terminal forces (Fig. 5-5). There is a typical rsR' in the right precordial leads associated with a larger than normal S wave in the left precordial leads. A significant degree of right ventricular hypertrophy is unusual in patients with uncomplicated septum secundum defects. It is more often found in infants with significant atrial septal defect (Fig. 5-6) or associated pulmonic stenosis and, in older patients, with pulmonary hypertension.

Echocardiogram

In the presence of a large left-to-right shunt, the echocardiogram demonstrates increased right ventricular dimension and paradoxical septal motion. These are nonspecific findings associated with right ventricular volume overload (Fig. 5-7).

Radiological Evaluation

The cardiac enlargement is often related to the size of the left-to-right shunt. The right-sided chambers, as well as the main pulmonary artery, are dilated (Figs. 5-8, 5-9). The pulmonary arterial circulation is increased, mainly at the hilar region.

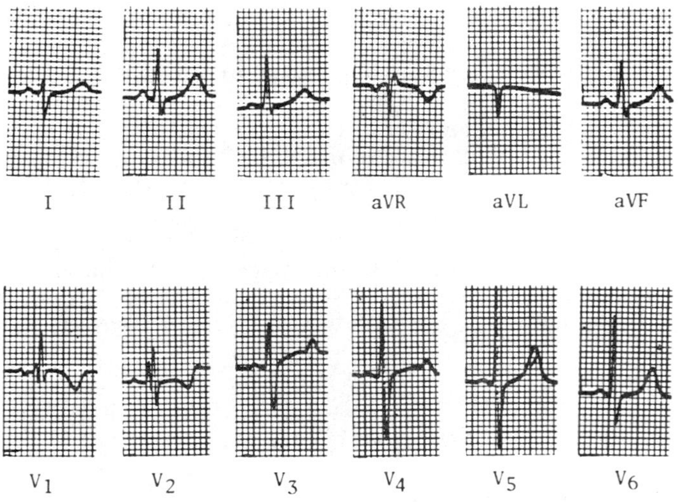

Figure 5-5 Electrocardiogram of a 10-year-old girl with secundum atrial septal defect. The frontal plane QRS axis is +110° with right ventricular hypertrophy.

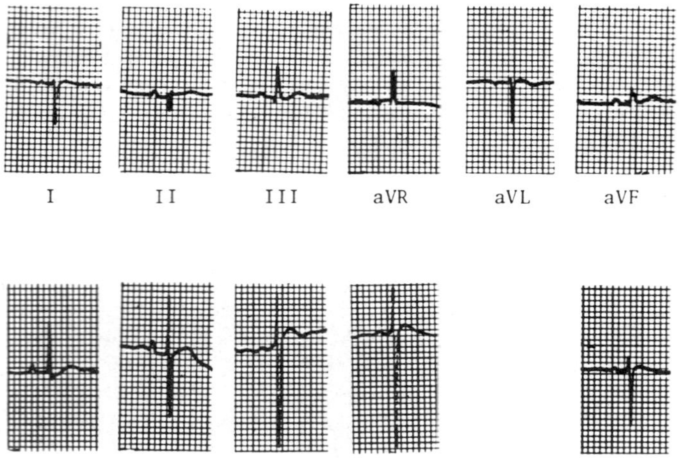

Figure 5-6 Electrocardiogram of a 1-month-old child with a large ASD. The QRS axis is approximately +170° with evidence of right ventricular hypertrophy.

Cardiac Catheterization

1. The most obvious finding is increased oxygen saturation in the right atrium as compared with the superior vena cava. The inferior vena caval saturation can be elevated due to reflux of oxygenated blood from the right atrium; therefore, comparing right atrial and inferior vena caval saturations for the purpose of diagnosis may be erroneous. Quantitating the shunt may be difficult when the right pulmonary veins drain anomalously into the superior vena cava.
2. In the large ASD the right atrial pressure characteristically exhibits an M-shaped curve related to the prominent V wave.
3. Right-sided pressures are usually normal. Systolic gradients up to 20 mmHg across the pulmonic valve are frequently encountered and related to excessive flow.
4. The catheter usually passes easily across the atrial septal defect into the left atrium.
5. Main pulmonary artery angiogram in the posteroanterior projection demonstrates the left-to-right shunt. When the contrast medium returns from the lung to the left atrium, the atrial septum is poorly defined with immediate opacification of the right atrium. Partial anomalous pulmonary venous connection cannot always be excluded although imaging in the hepatoclavicular projection or the AP projection with elevation of the head and thorax (see Chap. 12) may clarify the pulmonary venous connection. This may also be diagnosed utilizing selective right or left pulmonary angiograms or indicator dilution curves.

Differential Diagnosis

Although a large ASD can be diagnosed by clinical examination, EKG, and roentgen manifestations, there are several situations that may be confusing.

Functional Murmur

The systolic ejection murmur of an ASD may be difficult to differentiate from an innocent murmur. Wide fixed splitting of the second sound, abnormal EKG, and x-ray are helpful. In the presence of the small ASD this differentiation might not be possible.

Mild Pulmonic Stenosis

Mild pulmonic stenosis produces an ejection systolic murmur similar to an ASD. The second heart sound is not widely split and exhibits respiratory variation.

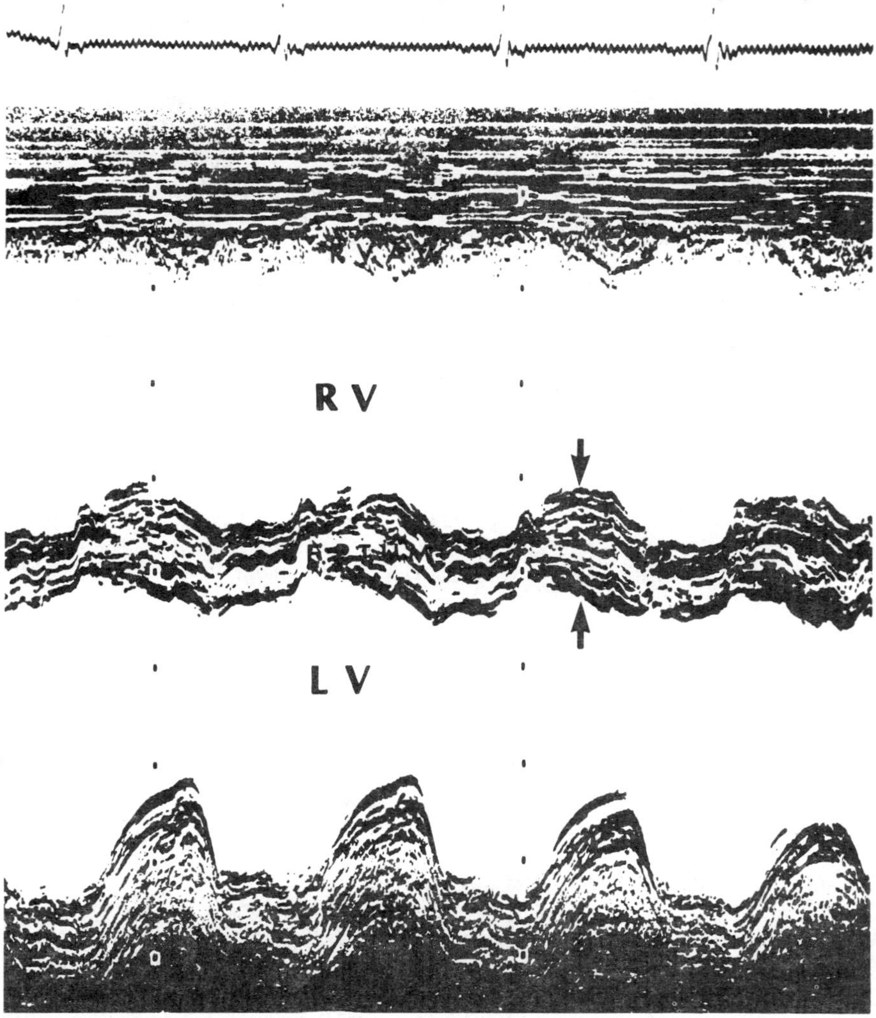

Figure 5-7 Echocardiogram of a patient with ASD 2° demonstrating large right ventricle (RV) and paradoxical septal motion (arrows). The septum moves principally anteriorly during systole. LV - left ventricle. (See Fig. 2-74 for normal echo.)

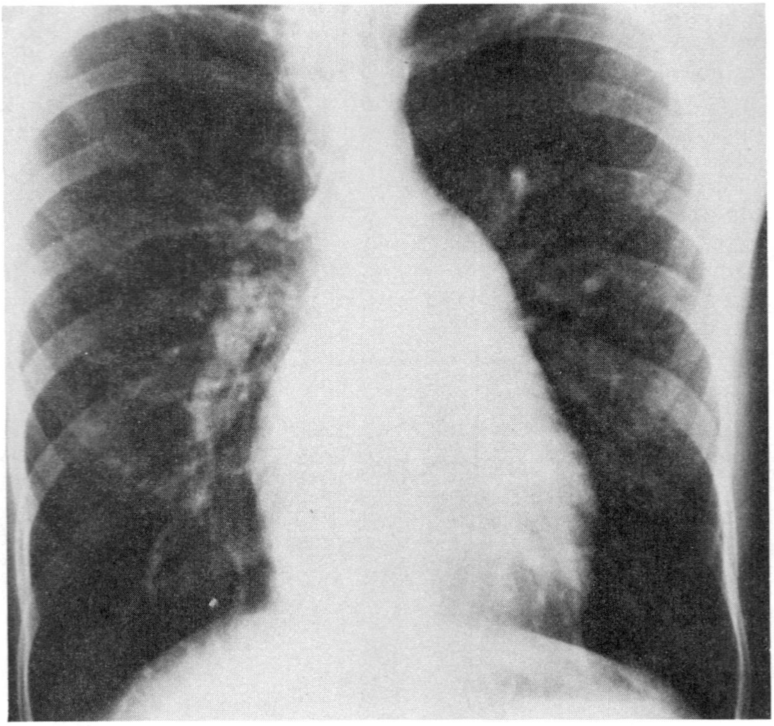

Figure 5-8A Chest radiograph of a 10-year-old with a large atrial septal defect. Note the large main pulmonary artery and increased pulmonary arterial circulation seen mainly at the right hilum.

A systolic ejection click is seldom heard in ASD but almost always in valvular pulmonic stenosis.

Ostium Primum Defect and Common Atrium

In ostium primum defect and common atrium, the clinical findings may be indistinguishable from secundum ASD. In the ostium primum defect there may, however, be an additional systolic murmur of mitral insufficiency. The EKG of patients with ASD secundum type exhibit right axis deviation, whereas the endocardial cushion defects manifest a left superior axis in the frontal plane.

Total Anomalous Pulmonary Venous Connection

Total anomalous pulmonary venous connection rarely may produce a clinical picture identical to a large ASD. The cyanosis may be so minimal that it is not appreciated. If the pulmonary veins drain into the vertical vein, there may be a so-called "snowman" sign on the chest roentgenogram (see Chap. 17). Cardiac catheterization is necessary to establish the diagnosis.

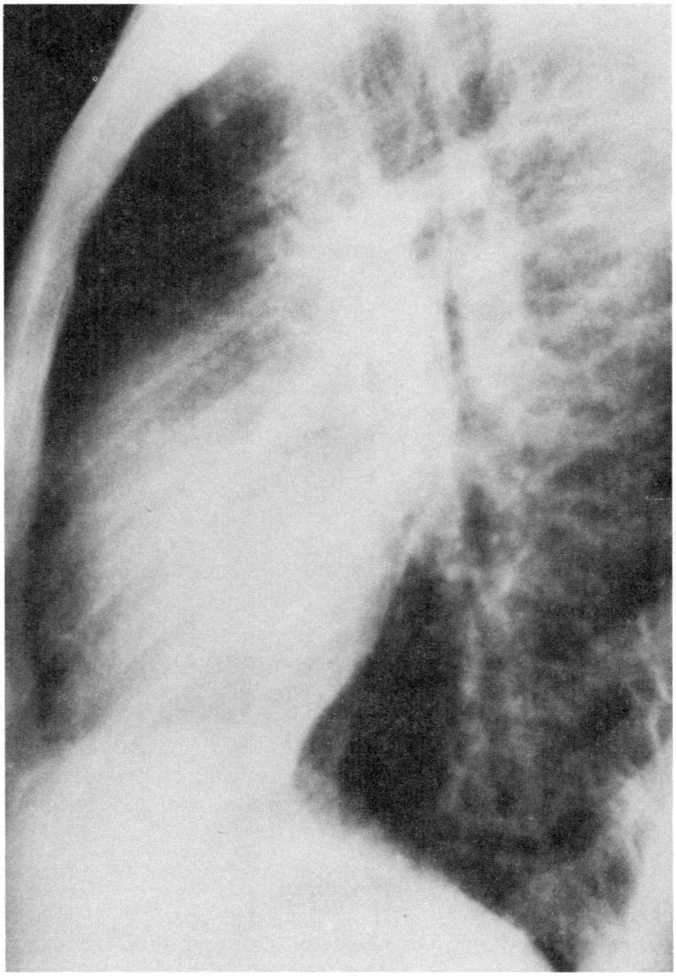

Figure 5–8B Chest radiograph of a 10-year-old with a large atrial septal defect. The lateral projection showing encroachment of the retrosternal space by an enlarged right ventricle.

Course and Prognosis

As a rule, ASD is well tolerated in infancy and childhood. Occasionally a large ASD might cause congestive heart failure in infancy and require surgical intervention. The main reason for closing the defect in early childhood is to prevent the later development of pulmonary vascular disease, right heart failure, and atrial arrhythmias. Pulmonary hypertension is rare in childhood but is present in 10% of patients under 40 years and in 50% above that age. Bacterial endocarditis is a rare occurrence. The results of surgery are gratifying with return of most parameters to normal.

Mitral valve prolapse has been reported in a third or more patients with ostium secundum atrial septal defect. This lesion is occasionally detected prior to surgery; however, it may not manifest itself until several years postrepair. The effect of this abnormality on the natural history of the atrial septal defect is not

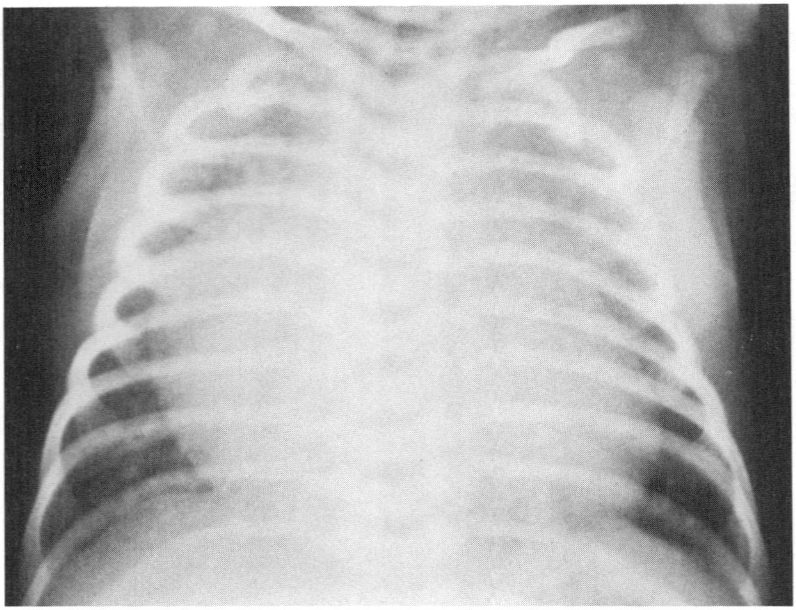

Figure 5-9 Chest radiograph of a 3-week-old with atrial septal defect and congestive heart failure. There is marked cardiomegaly, large right atrium, and increased pulmonary circulation.

yet known. In adults, however, this lesion may lead to progressive mitral insufficiency, bacterial endocarditis, severe arrhythmia, and sudden death.

Treatment

Most patients are asymptomatic and require no special treatment. In the presence of heart failure, however, the standard approach is indicated. Patients with a large, uncomplicated, left-to-right shunt with pulmonary-to-systemic-flow ratio of at least 1.5:1.0 are candidates for surgical closure. This is usually done prior to entering school. Associated partial anomalous pulmonary venous return can be corrected at that time. Patients with associated pulmonary hypertension and increased pulmonary vascular resistance should be studied carefully to determine operability.

Bibliography

Dushane JW, Weidman DW, Brandenburg RO, Kirklin JW: Differentiation of inter-atrial Communications by Clinical Methods: Ostium Secundum, Ostium Primum, Common Atrium and Total Anomalous Pulmonary Venous Connection. Circulation 21:363, 1960.

Hoffman JIE, Rudolph AM, Danilowicz D: Left to Right Atrial Shunts in Infants. Am J Cardiol 30:868, 1972.

Nakamura FF, Hauck AJ, Nadas AS: Atrial Septal Defect in Infants. Pediatr 34:101, 1964.

Radtke WE, Tajik AJ, Gav GT, Scattenberg TT, Giuliani ER, Tancredi RG: Atrial Septal Defect: Echocardiographic Observations. Ann Int Med 84:246, 1946.

Victorica BE, Elliot LP, Gessner IH: Ostium Secundum Atrial Septal Defect Associated with Balloon Mitral Valve in Children. Am J Cardiol 33:668, 1974.

Zaver AG, Nadas AS: Atrial Septal Defect—Secundum Type. Circulation 32:III-24 Supplement, December, 1965.

Chapter 6

VENTRICULAR SEPTAL DEFECT

Incidence

Ventricular septal defect is the most common congenital heart defect, accounting for 20% of all congenital cardiac malformations. The incidence of isolated ventricular septal defect (VSD) is 2/1000 live births and is evenly distributed between the two sexes. VSD is frequently found in association with other cardiac malformations, such as truncus arteriosus, tetralogy of Fallot, and so forth.

Embryological and Anatomic Considerations

Formation of the interventricular septum depends upon the normal embryological development of three structures in addition to formation of the muscular septum inferiorly. These are the endocardial cushions, the growth of the fibrous tissue at the crest of the interventricular septum, and the downward growth of the conotruncal ridges. Most ventricular septal defects are probably the result of maldevelopment of one or more of these structures. When viewed from the right ventricular septal surface, the interventricular septal defects can be classified according to their location (Fig. 6-1).

1. Membranous defect: This is the most common defect connecting the inflow portion of the right ventricle with the subaortic portion of the left ventricle.
2. Muscular defect: Located lower down in the ventricular septum between the muscular trabeculae.
3. Supracristal defect: Located above the crista supraventricularis under the pulmonic valve.
4. Endocardial cushion defect: Ventricular septal defect of the endocardial cushion variety will be discussed in Chap. 8.

The anatomy of the conduction system and its relationship to the defect is of great surgical importance. In membranous ventricular septal defect, the bundle of His runs along the posteroinferior aspect of the defect. Supracristal and muscular defects are not in such close proximity to the conduction system which is, therefore, less vulnerable during surgical correction.

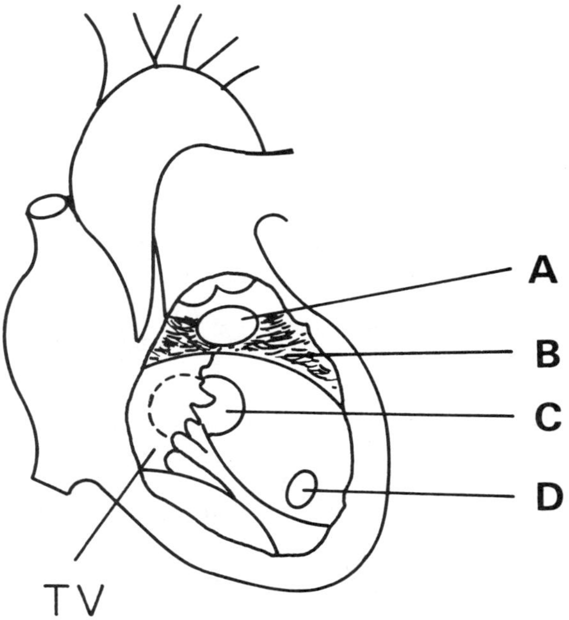

Figure 6-1 Anatomical position of ventricular septal defects as viewed from the right septal surface. TV - tricuspid valve. (A) Supracristal defect located just under the pulmonic valve. (B) Crista supra ventricularis. (C) Membranous defect. (D) Muscular defect.

Hemodynamic Considerations

All ventricular septal defects can be classified into four main groups according to their hemodynamic presentation.

1. Isolated small ventricular septal defect with normal pulmonary vascular resistance
2. Moderate ventricular septal defect with normal pulmonary vascular resistance
3. Large ventricular septal defect with dynamic pulmonary hypertension
4. Large ventricular septal defect with pulmonary hypertension and elevated pulmonary vascular resistance

The hemodynamic effect of the ventricular septal defect is not related to the anatomic location, but rather to the size of the defect and the relative systemic and pulmonic vascular resistances.

At birth, systemic and pulmonary vascular resistance are equal (Fig. 6-2A). With expansion of the lungs, the pulmonary vascular resistance drops slowly to the adult level by a few weeks of age. When pulmonary pressure is lower than systemic pressure, a left-to-right shunt is established through the anatomical communication. The full magnitude of the shunt is manifest only when pulmonary vascular resistance reaches its lowest level (see Fig. 6-2B). As a consequence, infants with large ventricular septal defect do not become symptomatic during the first few weeks of life.

Under normal conditions, the lung has a large vascular reserve capacity, namely, not all vessels are open at the same time. Under conditions of increased flow,

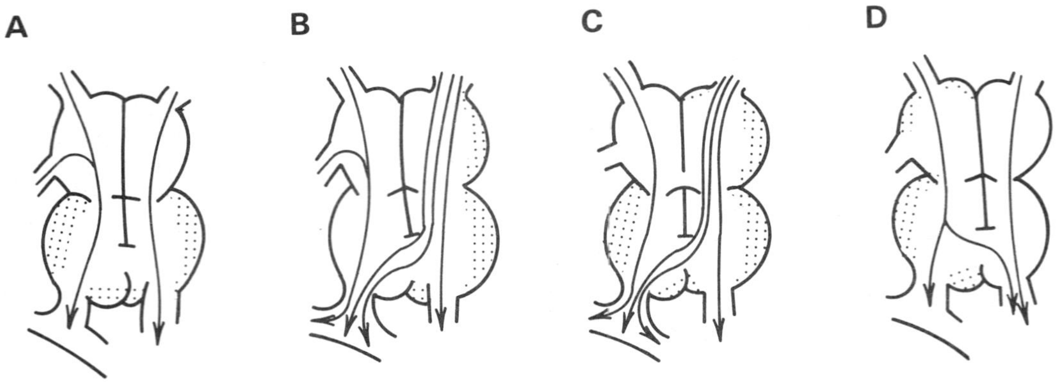

Figure 6–2 (A) Newborn, equal resistance in both pulmonic and systemic circulation. No shunt. (B) As pulmonic resistance drops, a large left-to-right shunt is established. Left ventricular and left atrial dilatation and hypertrophy develop. The RV muscle mass has regressed to normal. (C) Large left-to-right shunt with dynamic pulmonary hypertension and biventricular hypertrophy. (D) Pulmonary hypertension with increased resistance. Right-to-left shunt. The left ventricular dilatation and hypertrophy have regressed. There is now right ventricular and right atrial hypertrophy.

which occurs with exercise or left-to-right shunt, an additional increment in pulmonary artery pressure could distend and open closed vessels held in reserve. In face of a sizable shunt all vessels are open, and the pulmonary vascular reserve capacity would be eliminated or absent. All vasoconstrictive stimuli such as acidosis or hypoxemia will then cause pressure elevation and subsequent right ventricular hypertrophy (see Fig. 6–2C). Persistent pulmonary hypertension may in due time cause damage to the pulmonary vessels. This process is progressive, leading to irreversible arterial damage, with marked narrowing of the lumen, an overall decrease in the cross-sectional diameter of the pulmonary tree and, therefore, increased pulmonary vascular resistance. Associated with these changes is an increased pulmonary pressure and, therefore, increase in workload on the right ventricle, decrease in the left-to-right shunt, and eventually development of right-to-left shunt and cyanosis (see Fig. 6–2D).

Small Ventricular Septal Defect

The small defect offers large resistance to the flow of blood, resulting in a small left-to-right shunt. Trivial ventricular septal defect has been historically designated as Roger's disease.

Clinical Features

These patients are found to have a murmur shortly after the neonatal period. This murmur is quite loud but is unassociated with any cardiac symptomatology. On physical examination there is normal growth and development. The cardiac examination reveals normal vital signs. The heart sounds are usually normal. A systolic thrill at the lower left sternal border is palpable in approximately 80% of patients. This is associated with a grade IV/VI harsh, holosystolic murmur heard best at the same location radiating horizontally (Fig. 6-3A). There is no diastolic murmur and usually no other associated abnormal findings. Electrocardiogram and chest x-ray are usually within normal limits.

Cardiac Catheterization

A small stepup of oxygen saturation may be demonstrated at the right ventricular level. Often this is not appreciable, and more sophisticated means, such as dye dilution curves or hydrogen electrodes, are necessary to detect the presence of a left-to-right shunt. Injection of contrast material into the left ventricle may document a small shunt across the interventricular septum.

Differential Diagnosis

The lesions to be considered are pulmonic valvular or infundibular stenosis and mitral regurgitation. Valvular pulmonic stenosis can usually be distinguished on the basis of the location and quality of the murmur. The murmur is an ejection type, located at the second left intercostal space, radiating toward both lung fields and accompanied by an ejection systolic click and right ventricular hypertrophy on the electrocardiogram.

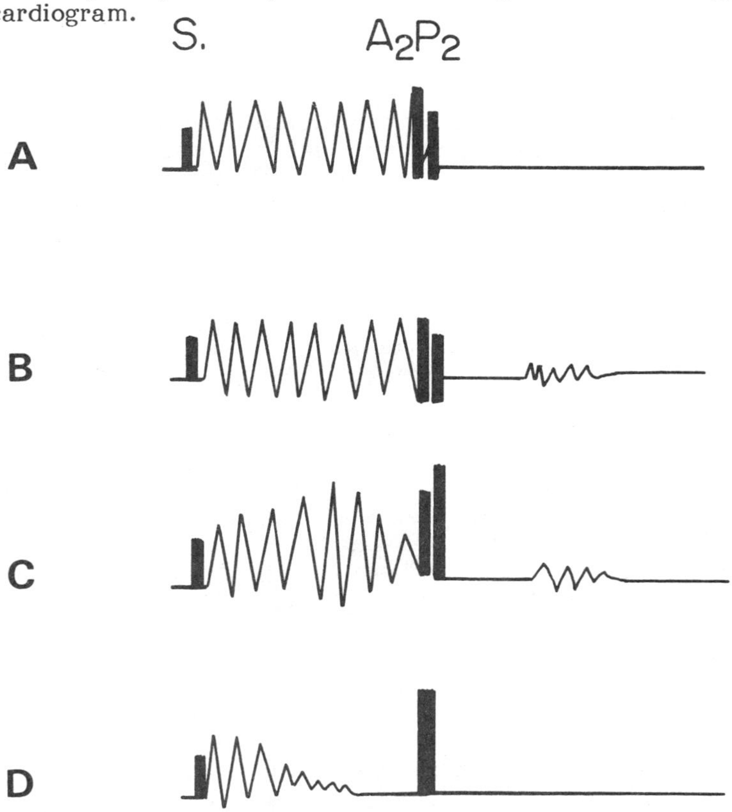

Figure 6-3 Phonocardiogram of the various hemodynamic stages of ventricular septal defect (for explanation see text). (A) Small ventricular septal defect. (B) Large ventricular septal defect. (C) Large ventricular septal defect with dynamic pulmonary hypertension. (D) Large ventricular septal defect with increased pulmonary vascular resistance.

Infundibular pulmonic stenosis might be difficult to differentiate. There is no ejection systolic click. The murmur occupies most of systole and is often associated with a systolic thrill at the midleft sternal border. Right ventricular impulse and EKG evidence of right ventricular hypertrophy are suggestive of a right-sided lesion.

Mitral regurgitation is associated with a holosystolic, blowing murmur heard best at the apex radiating toward the left axilla. Tricuspid insufficiency, although rare, should also be considered. It presents with a holosystolic murmur at the lower-left sternal border. The intensity of the murmur might increase with inspiration.

Moderate-Size Defect with Normal Pulmonary Vascular Resistance

In the presence of a moderate-size defect and normal pulmonary vascular resistance, there is a large left-to-right shunt, resulting in a large pulmonary blood flow and pulmonary venous return to the left heart (see Fig. 6-2B). The left atrium and ventricle dilate and hypertrophy in order to accommodate and propel the large volume.

Clinical Features

Due to the normal postnatal hemodynamic evolution, these children are initially asymptomatic. As the magnitude of the shunt increases, they become more symptomatic and a few eventually develop congestive heart failure. A typical history is a 2-3-month-old child with frequent colds and congestion. He is tachypneic, sweats profusely, and has difficulty in feeding.

Physical Examination

These children usually manifest some failure to thrive; the weight is affected more than the height. They are acyanotic, tachypneic, and tachycardic with subcostal retractions and nasal flaring.

The overactivity of the left ventricle is reflected as a palpable thrust laterally and inferiorly displaced. A systolic thrill may be palpable at the lower left sternal border. The first and second heart sounds are normal. A gallop rhythm is often present. A loud holosystolic murmur is best heard at the lower left sternal border but radiates widely and can also be heard at the back (see Fig. 6-3). The large pulmonary venous return to the left atrium creates an early diastolic murmur as it flows through the mitral valve into the left ventricle (see Figs. 6-2B, 6-3). In the face of congestive heart failure the liver is enlarged, and auscultation of the lungs may reveal scattered rales and expiratory wheezes. Fluid retention is manifested as periorbital edema. Pedal edema is not common in this age group.

Chest x-ray demonstrates cardiomegaly with left ventricular and left atrial enlargement and increased pulmonary vascularity (Fig. 6-4A). The electrocardiogram reflects the basic hemodynamic disturbance, namely, left ventricular and, possibly, left atrial hypertrophy (Fig. 6-5A). Typically there are large inferior forces in the limb leads (large R in II, III, and AVF) and left precordial leads. The large left precordial Q wave reflects septal hypertrophy and left ventricular volume overload.

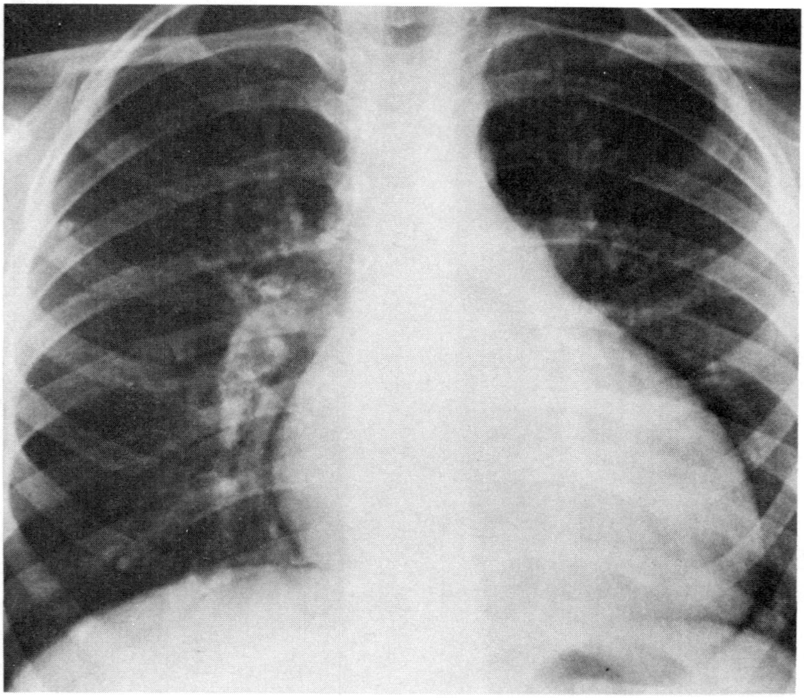

Figure 6-4A Radiograph of an 8-year-old with moderate-size ventricular septal defect and normal pulmonary artery pressure. Note the cardiac enlargement, left ventricular enlargement, and increased pulmonary vascular markings.

Cardiac Catheterization

The diagnosis of a large ventricular septal defect is based on the demonstration of a large oxygen stepup in the right ventricle, as compared with the right atrium, reflecting the large shunt of oxygenated blood into the right ventricle. The pulmonary venous blood is often mildly desaturated, due to pulmonary edema. The pressure in all chambers is normal, but the left ventricular end-diastolic pressure may be elevated, especially in the presence of congestive heart failure. Occasionally the catheter can be manipulated from the right ventricle into the left ventricle or aorta through the defect. Left ventricle or main pulmonary artery angiogram in the left anterior oblique or hepatoclavicular projections will demonstrate the presence of the ventricle septal defect and its relative location.

Differential Diagnosis

These patients should be differentiated from others with large left-to-right shunts. In the acyanotic group, the main lesions to be considered are patent ductus arteriosus and endocardial cushion defect. Patent ductus arteriosus can be distinguished by the presence of bounding pulses and a continuous murmur at the left infraclavicular area and back. The EKG is not helpful since it also shows left ventricular hypertrophy. The chest x-ray in patent ductus may show a large aorta.

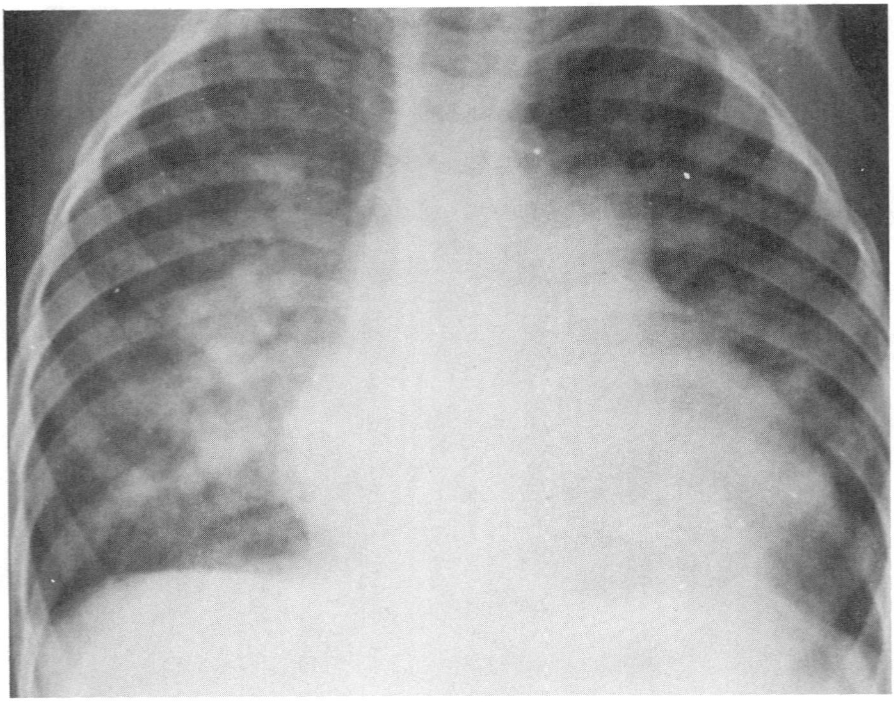

Figure 6-4B A 3-month-old with large ventricular septal defect, dynamic pulmonary hypertension, and congestive heart failure. There is cardiomegaly, prominent main pulmonary artery segment, increased pulmonary vascularity. There is obliteration of the right costophrenic angle with fluid and evidence of pulmonary edema.

Endocardial cushion defect, including left-ventricular-to-right-atrial shunts is usually present in 50% of those with Down syndrome who have congenital heart disease. The clinical examination may be identical to that of ventricular septal defect. The EKG exhibits left axis deviation.

Large Ventricular Septal Defect and Dynamic Pulmonary Hypertension

In large ventricular septal defect and dynamic pulmonary hypertension, the patient exhibits a large left-to-right shunt and close approximation of the right ventricular and pulmonary arterial systolic pressure to systemic arterial pressure (Fig. 6-2C). The elevated right-sided pressure results in right ventricular pressure overload.

Manifestations

The history is quite similar to that of the preceding group. The patients are, however, sicker and become symptomatic sooner. The failure to thrive may be more profound. Physical examination reveals a poorly developed child who often has a chest deformity, secondary to the large heart. The apical thrust is often accompanied by a visible xiphoid impulse. A thrill is palpable in about half of these patients. Auscultation differs only by the presence of a loud pulmonic component at the second sound reflecting a high pulmonary arterial pressure (see Fig. 6-3C). A systolic murmur may often be ejection type rather than holosystolic. Signs of congestive heart failure are usually present.

The electrocardiogram shows biventricular hypertrophy and, often, left atrial enlargement (see Fig. 6-5B). The chest radiograph reveals an enlarged heart involving both ventricles and left atrium. The main pulmonary artery and its branches are dilated (see Fig. 6-4B).

Cardiac Catheterization

A large left-to-right shunt at the ventricular level is demonstrated by an increase in the right ventricular oxygen content. It is usually easy to manipulate the catheter from the right ventricle into the aorta via the defect. Left atrial pressure may be elevated, and the pulmonary artery pressure is elevated and may approach systemic arterial pressure. Calculated pulmonary vascular resistance is usually low with a pulmonic-to-systemic-resistance ratio of less than 0.5 in most children.

Cineangiocardiogram at the left ventricle in left anterior oblique or hepatoclavicular projection is best for demonstrating the size and location of the defect. An aortic injection is also recommended to exclude the association of a patent ductus arteriosus.

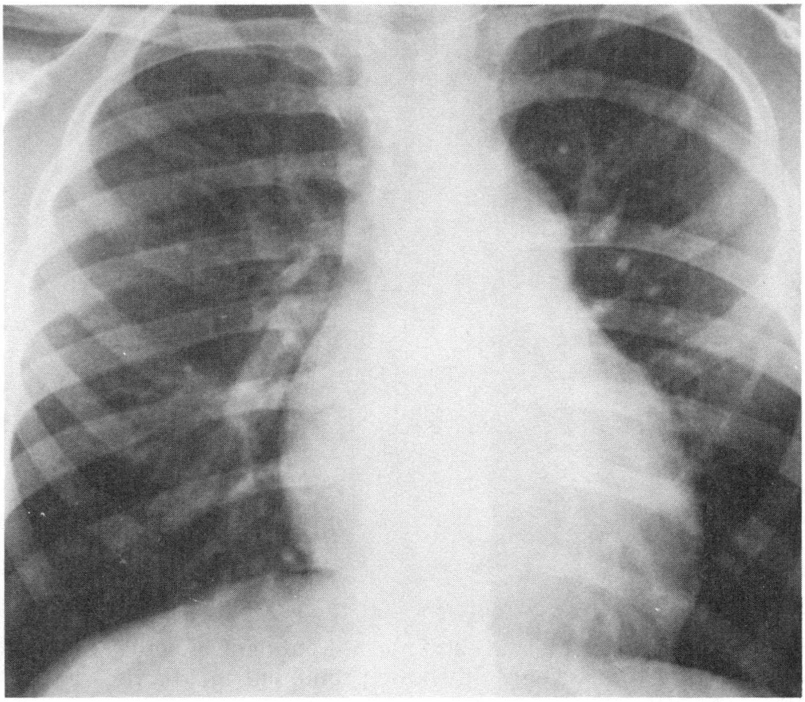

Figure 6-4C An 8-year-old with large VSD and markedly elevated pulmonary vascular resistance. Note the normal heart size and markedly enlarged main pulmonary artery. The right pulmonary artery is enlarged with an abrupt cutoff or pruning typical of pulmonary hypertension with increased resistance.

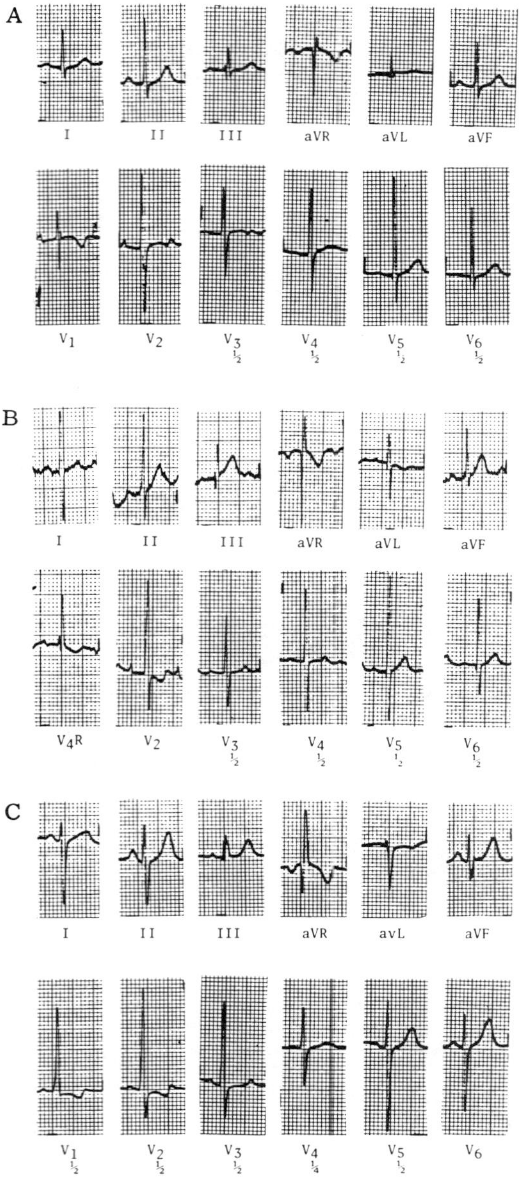

Figure 6–5 (A) Moderate-size VSD and normal pulmonary artery pressure. The electrocardiogram of this 4-year-old shows prominent left ventricular forces. (B) Large VSD and dynamic pulmonary hypertension in a 7-month-old. There is evidence of biventricular hypertrophy and suggestion of left atrial enlargement. (C) Electrocardiogram of a 6-year-old with ventricular septal defect and markedly increased pulmonary vascular resistance. Right axis deviation and severe right ventricular hypertrophy are present.

Patients with admixture cyanotic lesions, such as single ventricle and truncus arteriosus with large pulmonary blood flow, are often indistinguishable from patients with large ventricular septal defect and congestive heart failure. The diagnosis must often be established by cardiac catheterization.

Large Ventricular Septal Defect with Increased Pulmonary Vascular Resistance

Some patients with a large ventricular septal defect and dynamic pulmonary arterial hypertension eventually develop progressive pulmonary vascular obstruction, and 20% become inoperable between 1 and 7 years of age. Rarely does this process occur in infancy in patients who seem to have vascular obstructive disease from the start, never having been through the dynamic phase.

Manifestations

Most patients pass through the dynamic stage of the disease with evidence of a large left-to-right shunt (see Fig. 6-2B, C), congestive heart failure, and recurrent respiratory illness. With the onset of increased pulmonary vascular resistance or obstructive disease, the pulmonary flow decreases with resulting symptomatic improvement (see Fig. 6-2D). There is a decreased incidence of pulmonary infection, tachypnea, tachycardia, and decreased exercise tolerance.

These patients usually exhibit growth retardation. There is no cyanosis observed early in the course, although it may become apparent later. The left ventricular impulse is less prominent. A strong right ventricular impulse is observed at the xiphoid area, accompanied by a palpable second heart sound. On auscultation, the first heart sound may be accentuated, and the second heart sound is booming and often single (see Fig. 6-3D). The thrill is no longer present, and a systolic ejection murmur is best heard along the lower left sternal border. There are usually no diastolic murmurs; however, in the presence of severe pulmonary vascular obstruction, a pulmonary regurgitant murmur may be audible.

The electrocardiogram shows progressive right axis deviation, and a decrease in the left ventricular forces concomitant with increased right ventricular forces (see Fig. 6-5C). Right atrial enlargement is occasionally present. The transition from biventricular hypertrophy to right ventricular hypertrophy reflects the decrease in the magnitude of the left-to-right shunt and increased right-sided pressures.

The changes seen in the physical examination and electrocardiogram are reflected in the chest radiograph (see Fig. 6-4C). There is diminution in the overall cardiac size and regression of the left ventricle and left atrium. The right ventricle becomes dominant, and the pulmonary blood flow decreases peripherally with marked dilatation of the main pulmonary artery and its central branches. This discrepancy in size between central and peripheral vessels is termed pruning.

Cardiac Catheterization

The salient features are pulmonary hypertension without evidence of a sizable left-to-right shunt. There might, however, be a small right-to-left shunt present. The magnitude of either shunt relates to the relationship between pulmonary and systemic resistances. Left ventricular angiogram demonstrates a small or no shunt across the ventricular septal defect. The peripheral pulmonary arteries are markedly tortuous, typical of pulmonary hypertension with increased resistance (see Fig. 2-64).

Whenever pulmonary hypertension with increased pulmonary vascular resistance is documented, the pulmonary vascular reactivity should be tested. This can be accomplished by inhalation of 100% oxygen or by injecting vasodilators such as tolazoline into the pulmonary artery. If the pulmonary vasculature is still reactive, it will dilate, producing increased left-to-right shunt and/or a drop in the pulmonary artery pressure. In the presence of irreversible changes, this does not occur.

Differential Diagnosis

All lesions associated with a large pulmonary blood flow, with the exception of simple ASD, might potentially produce pulmonary hypertension and should be considered. These include:

1. Patent ductus arteriosus
2. Endocardial cushion defect
3. Truncus arteriosus
4. Single ventricle
5. Transposition of the great arteries
6. Double-outlet right ventricle

An electrocardiogram suggesting superior left axis in the frontal plane is suggestive of endocardial cushion defect. However, when pulmonary arterial hypertension is established, the primary diagnosis may not be apparent, and cardiac catheterization is indicated.

Echocardiographic Findings

The ventricular septal defect is uncommonly imaged directly utilizing M-mode techniques. Rather, the study reflects the volume of the left-to-right shunt. Findings may be completely normal with small defects. With moderate-to-large left-to-right shunts there is dilatation of left atrium and left ventricle in proportion to the degree of increase in pulmonary venous return. Left ventricular hypertrophy is not usually detected. Indices and left ventricular performance are usually normal to slightly increased deflecting the effects of volume loading. Diminished or decreasing indices of performance constitute an ominous prognostic sign, indicating the need for definitive medical or surgical intervention. In the presence of pulmonary hypertension there may be some dilatation of the right ventricle and thickening of the right anterior wall. Changes in the pulmonary valve waveform (flattening of the diastolic flow, disappearance of the A dip) as well as an increase in the right ventricular pre-ejection period/right ventricular ejection time (PEP/RVET) ratio will reflect increase in pulmonary vascular resistance. Findings on two-dimensional echocardiography are similar, although it is possible to more frequently visualize the ventricular septal defect in this manner.

Course and Prognosis

Patients with small ventricular septal defect are usually asymptomatic. It is estimated that approximately 50% of all small defects close spontaneously within 10 years. There are several different mechanisms by which the VSD might close. The most common is probably by growth and hypertrophy of the muscular portion of the septum around the defect. Apposition of the septal leaflet of the tricuspid valve against the defect and aneurysm of the membranous septum have also been implicated. Patients who are symptomatic within the first year of life usually enter the second and third functional subgroups previously mentioned. With proper medical and surgical management, the mortality rate is 5% among this group. Those who survive the first 1 or 2 years of life may improve symptomatically, in relation to dimunition of the left-to-right shunt. The following mechanisms are postulated.

1. Decrease in the size of the defect.
2. Development of pulmonary infundibular obstruction. Hypertrophy of the crista supraventricularis causes right ventricular outflow obstruction, with increased resistance to right ventricular ejection and, thereby, a dimunition in the left-to-right shunt.
3. Development of pulmonary vascular obstruction.

Some patients remain, however, in chronic congestive heart failure with failure to thrive. These are the patients whose left ventricle never seems to be able to cope adequately with the tremendous volume overload imposed on it. They continue to have elevated left ventricular end-diastolic, left atrial, and pulmonary capillary pressure which results in pulmonary hypertension.

By far, the poorest long-term prognosis is that of the 10% in whom there is progressive pulmonary vascular obstruction. Fifty percent of the patients with a large ventricular septal defect and dynamic pulmonary hypertension ultimately develop pulmonary vascular obstructive disease. Only 10%, however, develop it in late infancy or early childhood, and only 1% have obstructive disease from birth. Chronic congestive heart failure and pulmonary hypertension are the two leading causes of death in patients with ventricular septal defect. The former is more common in infancy, and the latter becomes more probable after adolescence. Bacterial endocarditis is a major risk, especially in the patients with small VSD. This is not a common occurrence in childhood, the peak incidence occurring during the third and fourth decade.

Treatment

In summary, the natural history of ventricular septal defects is such that the majority of small defects close spontaneously, and the large defects may decrease in size. Pulmonary vascular changes may develop within the first 6-12 months and, in the presence of large defects, may be quite advanced by 2-3 years of age. These principles serve as a guide to caring for patients with VSD.

1. *Small VSD:* These children are essentially asymptomatic and do not require medical or surgical intervention. It is important, however, to maintain antibiotic treatment for the prevention of bacterial endocarditis during periods of potential bacteremia such as dental procedures or abdominal surgery.

2. *Moderate-size defect with normal pulmonary vascular resistance:* The medical treatment of the patient in congestive heart failure consists of fluid restriction, diuretics, digitalization, increased ambient oxygen, if necessary, and placing the baby in an infant seat or elevating the head of the crib. The majority of patients respond favorably to medical management. Once the failure is under control, we routinely catheterize these infants in order to define the hemodynamic abnormality. If the pulmonary artery pressure is less than 50% of systemic, there is minimal risk for developing pulmonary vascular disease. With the passage of time, the VSD often decreases in size, and they become asymptomatic. At 4-5 years of

age, if the VSD still appears to be large, they are subjected to repeat cardiac catheterization followed by elective surgery. There are a few patients, however, who remain in intractable congestive failure and require surgical intervention in infancy. Banding of the pulmonary artery used to be the procedure of choice before the refinement of cardiopulmonary bypass and the introduction of hypothermia. It should still be performed in centers where this expertise is not available. Main pulmonary artery banding increases right ventricular outflow resistance and thereby decreases the left-to-right shunt. Patients with pulmonary artery banding should, at a later stage, have primary closure of the VSD with removal of the band. It is not recommended to delay the final surgery for many years since occasionally the band may cause permanent residual constriction of the pulmonary artery, requiring further repair. Direct closure of the VSD using cardiopulmonary bypass and hypothermia is now the initial procedure of choice in most centers.

3. *Large VSD with dynamic pulmonary hypertension:* The medical approach to these patients is similar to that outlined in the previous category. It is important to emphasize, however, that the patients with pulmonary hypertension and mildly pulmonary vascular resistance should be carefully followed for signs of increasing resistance. If the failure is controlled, growth is adequate, and there are no indications of increased pulmonary vascular resistance, they should be recatheterized at approximately 2 years of age to reassess the hemodynamic status. If dynamic hypertension is still present, surgery is then indicated in order to prevent progressive pulmonary vascular disease. The surgical risk for primary closure of the defect is approximately 5-15%. Lower vascular resistance, large flow, and weight above 30 lb influence the prognosis favorably.

4. *Large VSD with increased pulmonary vascular resistance:* The patient with elevated pulmonary vascular resistance who responds favorably to oxygen inhalation and vasodilators (tolazoline) should be promptly operated, with the possibility of postsurgical regression of the vascular changes. When pulmonary vascular resistance is high and irreversible, the patient should be considered inoperable. If the VSD is surgically closed, the high-pulmonary resistance interferes with pulmonary blood flow and, secondarily, with systemic blood flow, whereas when the VSD is left open, there is no difficulty maintaining systemic blood flow. With progressive disease manifested by right-to-left shunt, cyanosis, and polycythemia, the treatment is symptomatic to prevent hyperviscosity.

Ventricular Septal Defect with Aortic Regurgitation

The incidence of aortic insufficiency associated with VSD is 2.5%. In Japan, where supracristal ventricular septal defect is prevalent, the incidence of associated aortic regurgitation is higher.

Pathology and Etiology

The majority of cases are associated with a small subpulmonic VSD which is in close association with the right coronary cusp of the aortic valve. It is believed that this area of the septum is essential for support of the aortic valve leaflet.

The main factors influencing the prolapse of the aortic cusp into the right ventricle are the mechanical lack of support to the valve and associated hemodynamic changes. During systole, the velocity of blood streaming through the high VSD pulls the cusp with it towards the right ventricle and, during diastole, the intra-aortic pressure forces the unsupported cusp down, leading to regurgitation (Fig. 6-6).

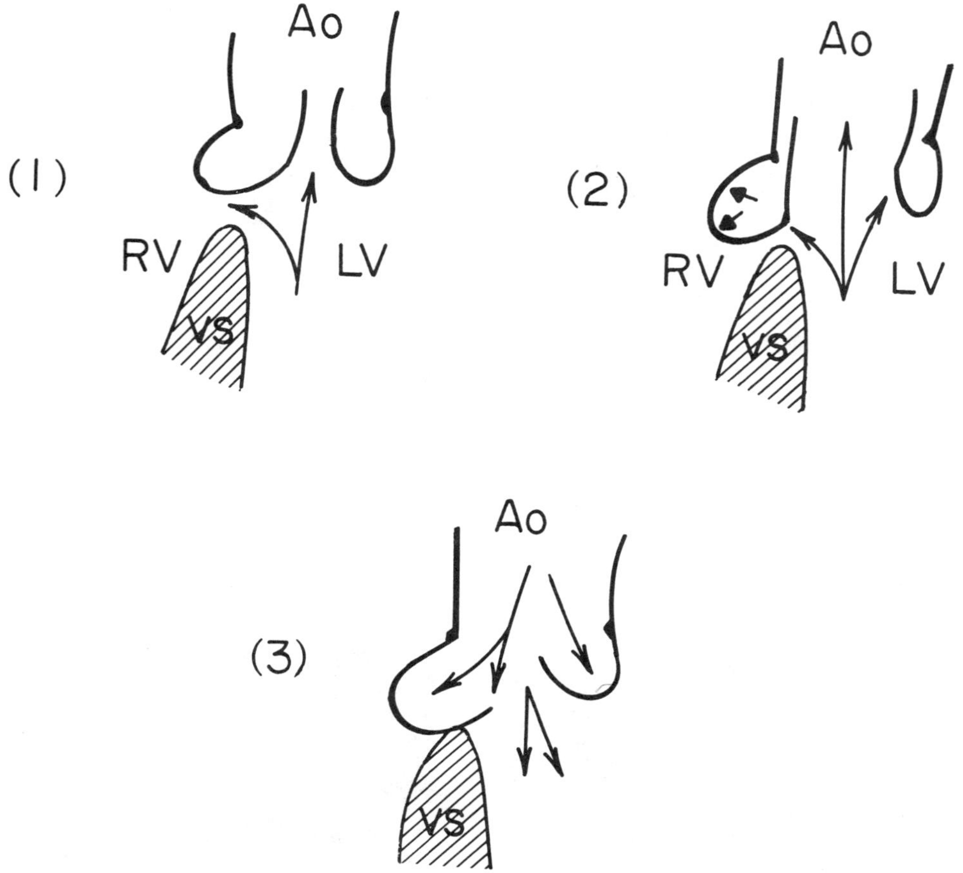

Figure 6-6 Ventricular septal defect with aortic regurgitation. (1) Early systole: The right aortic cusp is drawn down into the right ventricle by the shunted blood through the VSD. (2) Midsystole: The aortic flow pushes the unsupported cusp further out into the right ventricle. (3) Diastole: The aortic pressure forces the free edge of the elongated cusp down. This occludes the VSD but renders the valve incompetent.

Clinical Features

Aortic regurgitation associated with VSD can occur at any time; however, most patients are diagnosed before the age of 8 years. Since the VSD is usually small, the clinical symptoms largely depend upon the degree of aortic regurgitation. The physical examination discloses a VSD murmur associated with an early diastolic decrescendo murmur at the left sternal border. The pulses may be normal or bounding. The diastolic blood pressure may be reduced, and there may be evidence of left ventricular enlargement, depending upon the severity of the aortic involvement.

Echocardiographic Findings

Echocardiographic manifestations of left-to-right shunt at ventricular level will be present to variable degree, depending upon the volume of the shunt.

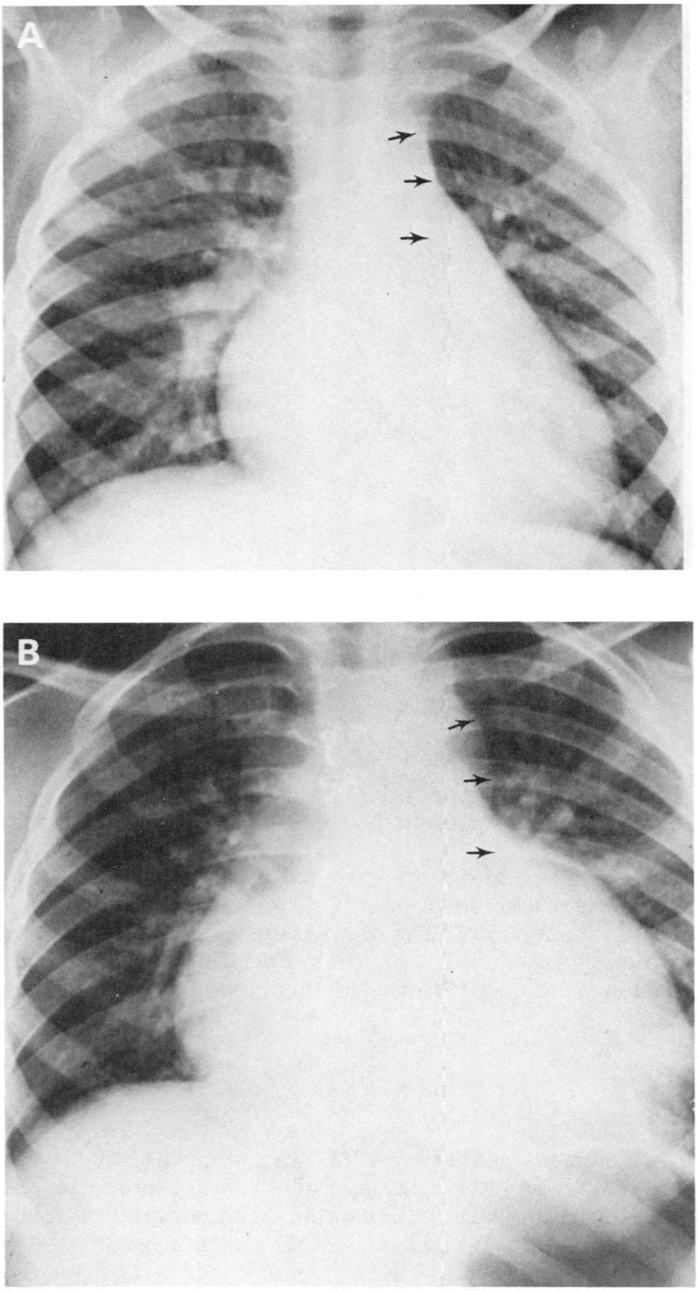

Figure 6–7 (A) A 4-year-old boy with small supracristal ventricular septal defect and aortic regurgitation. Note the cardiomegaly, left ventricular enlargement, and a dilated tortuous aorta (arrows). Pulmonary vascularity is increased. (B) The same patient 3 years postclosure of the VSD and aortic valve plication with obvious worsening of the aortic regurgitation. There is massive cardiomegaly with normal pulmonary vascular markings. The dilated aorta is again seen (arrows).

Diastolic fluttering of the anterior mitral leaflet and occasionally of the interventricular septum may be seen with moderate or severe degrees of regurgitation. The anatomy of the aortic valve and the degree of prolapse may be well visualized by two-dimensional technique.

Chest X-Ray

The chest x-ray shows a variable degree of left ventricular dilatation as well as dilatation and tortuousity of the aorta (Fig. 6-7). The electrocardiogram likewise reflects the degree of aortic insufficiency with increasing left ventricular hypertrophy. This is often progressive (Fig. 6-8).

Course and Prognosis

Keane et al., studying the natural history of the disease, concluded that:

1. In patients with VSD and aortic regurgitation, the aortic lesion is the primary handicap, since the VSD is usually small.
2. Closure of VSD alone was of more benefit to patients with subpulmonic defect.
3. Patients with severe aortic regurgitation should be treated surgically by closing the VSD and repairing or replacing the aortic valve.
4. Mild aortic incompetence tends to remain stable under medical treatment.
5. There is a relatively high incidence of bacterial endocarditis (8%).

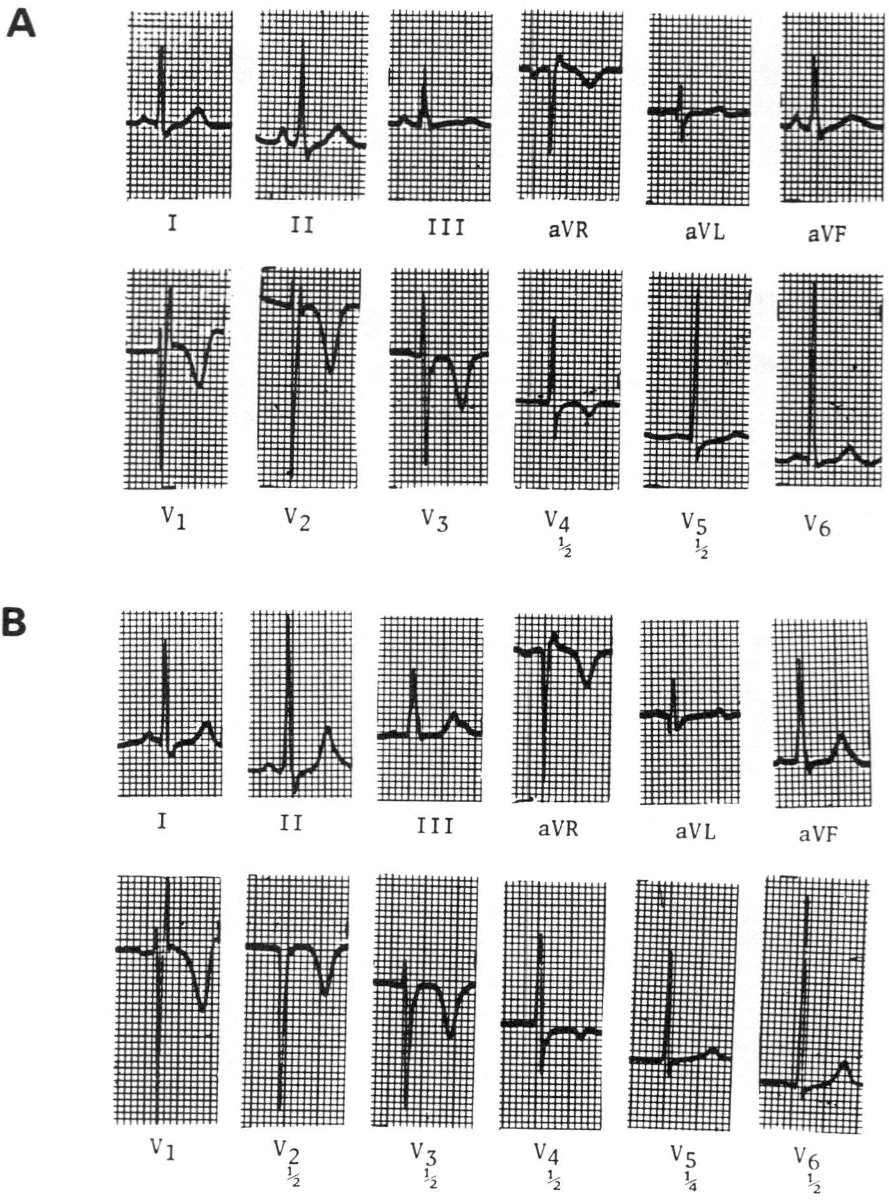

Figure 6–8 (A) Small ventricular septal defect associated with moderate aortic insufficiency in a 4-year-old. There are prominent left ventricular forces. (B) The same patient 3 years postclosure of VSD and aortic valvuloplasty. There is clinical evidence of progression of the aortic regurgitation. The electrocardiogram shows marked increase in the left ventricular forces seen both in the precordial and inferior leads.

Bibliography

Allen HD, Anderson RC, Noren GR, Moller JH: Postoperative follow-up of patients with ventricular septal defect. Circulation 50:465, 1974.

Bloodfield DH: The natural history of ventricular septal defect in patients surviving infancy. Circulation 29:914, 1964.

Glasser SP, Cheitlin MD, McCarty RJ, Haas JH, Hall RJ, Mullins CE: Thirty-two cases of interventricular septal defect and aortic insufficiency. Am J Med 53:473, 1972.

Hoffman JIE, Rudolph AM: The natural history of ventricular septal defect. Am J Cardiol 16:634, 1965.

Keane JF, Plauth WA, Nadas AS: Ventricular septal defect with aortic regurgitation. Circulation 56: Suppl I, 1-72, 1977.

Ritter DH, Feldt RH, Weidman WH, Dushane JW: Ventricular septal defect. Circulation 32:III-42 Supplement, December, 1965.

Tatsuno K, Konno S, Ando M, Sakakibara S: Pathogenetic mechanism of prolapsing aortic valve and aortic regurgitation associated with ventricular septal defect. Anatomical, angiographic and surgical considerations. Circulation 48:1028, 1973.

Ysui H, Yashitoshi M, Miyamoto AT, Kato H, Takeda Y, Tokunaga K, Tasaki H, Tomoike H: Ventricular septal defect: selection of patients and timing for surgery. Am Heart J 93:40, 1977.

Chapter 7

PATENT DUCTUS ARTERIOSUS

Incidence

Isolated patent ductus arteriosus (PDA) is the second most common congenital heart defect and is seen in 12-15% of all patients.

Embryological and Anatomic Considerations

The ductus arteriosus connects the pulmonary artery with the aorta just distal to the left subclavian artery (Fig. 7-1). Embryologically, the ductus arteriosus represents persistence of the sixth aortic arch or, specifically, that portion of the sixth aortic arch that connects the left main pulmonary artery and the aorta. Prenatally, the ductus functions to bypass the nonaerated lung, redirecting the pulmonary artery blood into the descending aorta (Chap. 4). The mechanism of ductal constriction is not completely understood. The ductus has a larger medial circulatory smooth muscle component as compared with the aorta or pulmonary artery. The smooth musculature is reactive to various stimuli, and its active constriction initiates normal ductus closure after birth. This process leads to a physiologic closure, whereas complete anatomic closure occurs at 1-6 weeks of age. Prior to complete anatomic closure, the ductus can intermittently open and close in response to various stimuli.

It is known that the ductal tissue constricts in response to oxygen, acetylcholine, and bradykinin. There is also evidence that indomethacin, which is a potent prostaglandin synthetase inhibitor, can constrict the ductus. Prostaglandin found in fetal ductal tissue is believed to be the mediator responsible for keeping the ductus patent during fetal life. Administration of this substance has proven successful in keeping the ductus open in the immediate postnatal period.

Persistent Patency of the Ductus Arteriosus

Little is known about the reasons for persistent patency of the ductus. Intrauterine rubella infection is often associated with PDA and peripheral pulmonic stenosis. This may be related to the viral infection and secondary replacement of the muscular media with fibrotic tissue. PDA also occurs with increased frequency at high altitudes and is believed to be due to chronic hypoxia. It is also a common associated defect with coarctation of the aorta, ventricular septal defect, and endocardial cushion defect.

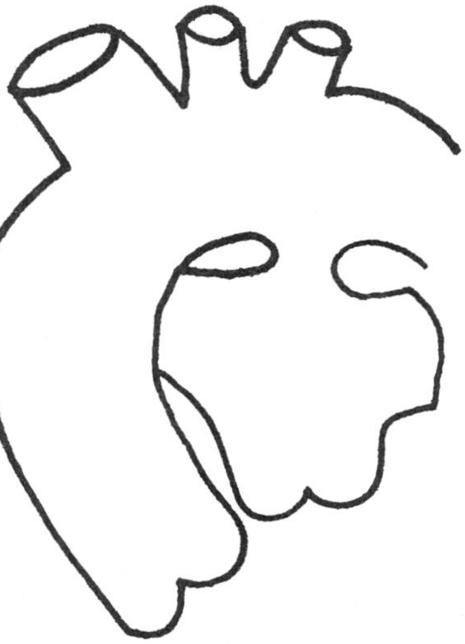

Figure 7-1 A drawing illustrating a patent ductus arteriosus connecting the pulmonary artery and the aorta just beyond the left subclavian artery.

Clinical Categories

The hemodynamic alterations of persistent PDA are related to the size of the ductus, the relationship between systemic and pulmonary resistance, and myocardial function.

Small Ductus Arteriosus

As pulmonary vascular resistance declines in the first few weeks of life, a left-to-right shunt through the ductus is established since there is a continuous pressure gradient between the aorta and pulmonary artery. The shunt occurs during both systole and diastole. The pulmonary flow and, consequently, venous return to the left heart increase. In order to maintain adequate peripheral perfusion, the left ventricular and aortic output increase with a concomitant decrease in the systemic vascular resistance. The increased output together with a large runoff into the main pulmonary artery account for the wide pulse pressure which is manifested clinically as bounding pulses.

Manifestations

The patient with a small ductus arteriosus is usually asymptomatic. The physical examination might show some widening of the pulse pressure. The palpable cardiac activity is usually normal. The first and second heart sounds are normal, and there is a continuous murmur audible in the left infraclavicular area, upper sternal border, and back (Fig. 7-2A). The murmur starts shortly after the first heart sound, peaks around the second sound, and extends into, but not necessarily throughout, diastole. The continuous murmur is a function of the continuous pressure gradient and, therefore, shunt between the aorta and pulmonary artery. The electrocardiogram and chest x-ray are usually within normal limits.

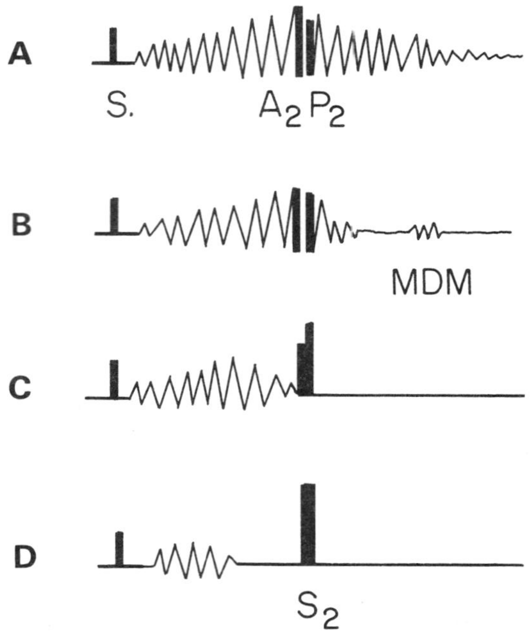

Figure 7–2 Schematic illustration of the progressive modification of the ductus murmur. (A) Patent ductus with normal pulmonary artery pressure. Continuous murmur heard at the left infraclavicular area. Note the peak around the second heart sound. (B) At the apex of the same patient, the continuous murmur is shorter, and there is a mid-diastolic rumble. (C) Large ductus with dynamic pulmonary hypertension. The second sound is now single with increase in the pulmonic component. The systolic murmur peaks in late systole. There is no diastolic component. (D) Pulmonary hypertension with increased resistance. The second sound is booming. There is a short systolic ejection murmur.

Moderate and Large Ductus with Normal Pulmonary Vascular Resistance (Fig. 7-3)

In the presence of a large PDA, the normal postnatal pulmonary vascular maturation may be delayed. When full maturation does occur, however, a large left-to-right shunt through the ductus is established with increased pulmonary blood flow, large volume overload on the left heart, and widening pulse pressure. This commonly occurs at 6-12 weeks of age, depending upon the rate of fall of pulmonary vascular resistance. The development of cardiac failure in these infants is related to the ability of the left ventricle to handle the increased volume load.

The hemodynamic disturbances and the influence on the pulmonary vasculature are similar to those encountered in VSD. In the presence of a large shunt, the pulmonary artery pressure increases to approximate systemic level, a situation known as dynamic or hyperkinetic pulmonary hypertension. When dynamic pulmonary hypertension persists unchecked, progressive pulmonary vascular changes may develop and lead to irreversible pulmonary hypertension.

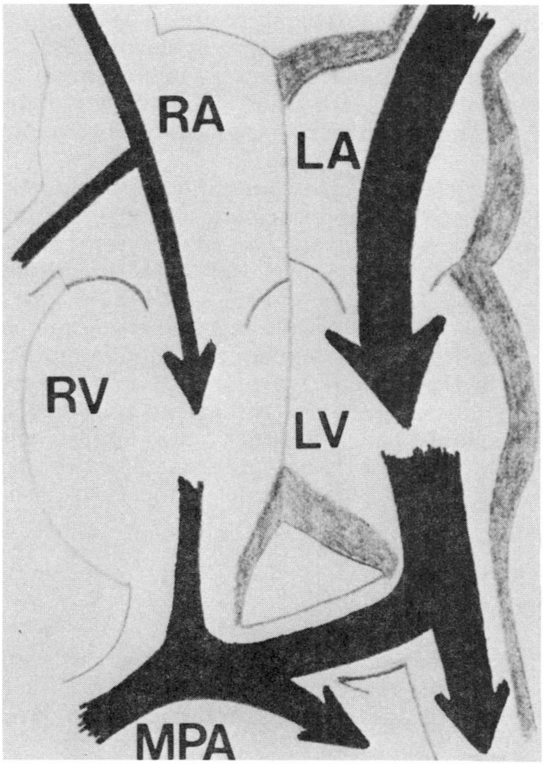

Figure 7-3 Schematic representation of a heart with moderate PDA. There is a large left-to-right shunt at the ductal level, resulting in increased return to the left atrium and ventricle. There is evidence of left atrial and left ventricular hypertrophy.

Manifestations

The infant may appear well or may be reported to have tachypnea. At approximately 6-8 weeks of age, he begins feeding poorly, tires easily, and perspires excessively, especially during feeding. He becomes more tachypneic and often is treated for one or two episodes of upper respiratory infection or "pneumonia" without improvement. On physical examination, he is small for age with signs of congestive heart failure. The pulses are bounding with a large pulse pressure. Chest deformity is often present and related to the enlarged heart. The precordium is hyperdynamic to palpation with evidence of an enlarged left ventricle. The first heart sound is accentuated, and the second heart sound is often masked by the loud continuous murmur (Fig. 7-2A). The murmur starts shortly after the first heart sound, peaks at the second sound, and ends late in diastole. It is heard best at the upper left sternal border and back. A diastolic flow rumble is audible at the apex (Fig. 7-2B). This low-frequency diastolic murmur is related to a large volume returning from the lungs into the left atrium and crossing the mitral valve (see Figs. 7-1, 7-3). Scattered rales may be heard, and hepatomegaly of variable degree is present.

The electrocardiogram shows left ventricular hypertrophy, and possibly left atrial enlargement (Fig. 7-4A). The chest x-ray reveals cardiomegaly, left ventricular, left atrial, and main pulmonary artery enlargement (Fig. 7-5). The ascending aorta is also enlarged. Pulmonary blood flow is increased, often with evidence of pulmonary venous congestion manifested by Kerley B lines and wet fissures.

When the ductus arteriosus is large, the clinical presentation is similar, but more exaggerated than that of a moderate ductus. Physical examination shows a small-for-age, scrawny, tachypneic, tachycardiac infant with suprasternal and subcostal retractions who is sweating profusely. The pulses are bounding, and the precordium is hyperactive. The second heart sound is accentuated; an ejection systolic murmur that peaks in late systole is audible at the upper left sternal border (see Fig. 7-2C). The diastolic component may be completely absent or represented as an extension of the systolic murmur into early diastole. A diastolic flow rumble is present at the apex. Evidence of cardiac failure is usually present. The electrocardiogram invariably shows biventricular hypertrophy and left atrial enlargement (see Fig. 7-4B). The radiological manifestations are similar to those described with moderate-size ductus with possible association of pulmonary edema (Fig. 7-6).

Large Ductus with Increased
Pulmonary Vascular Resistance

Large ductus with increased pulmonary vascular resistance is the end-stage of longstanding large left-to-right shunt. Increased pulmonary vascular resistance develops secondary to anatomic vascular changes with a decrease in the

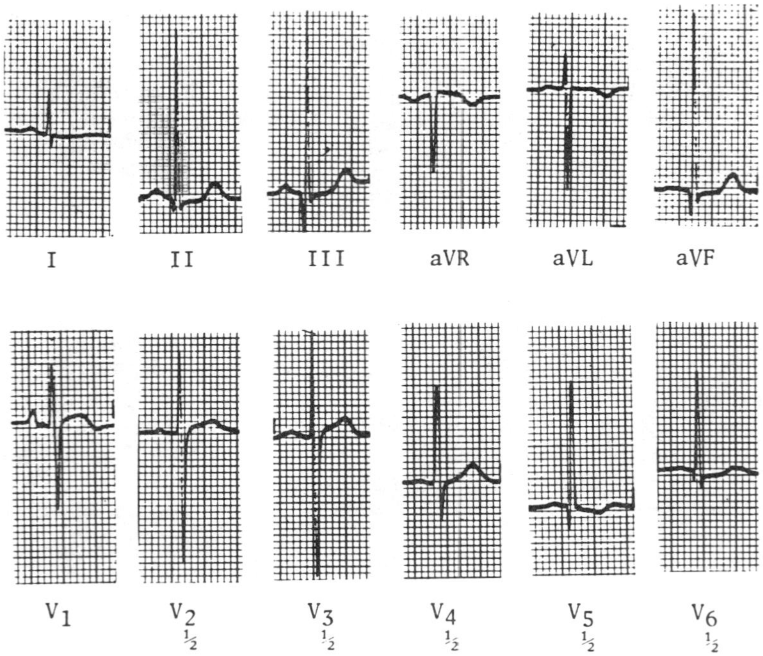

Figure 7-4A EKG of a 4-year-old with moderate PDA. Note the left ventricular hypertrophy manifested by large inferior and left precordial forces (see also B and C).

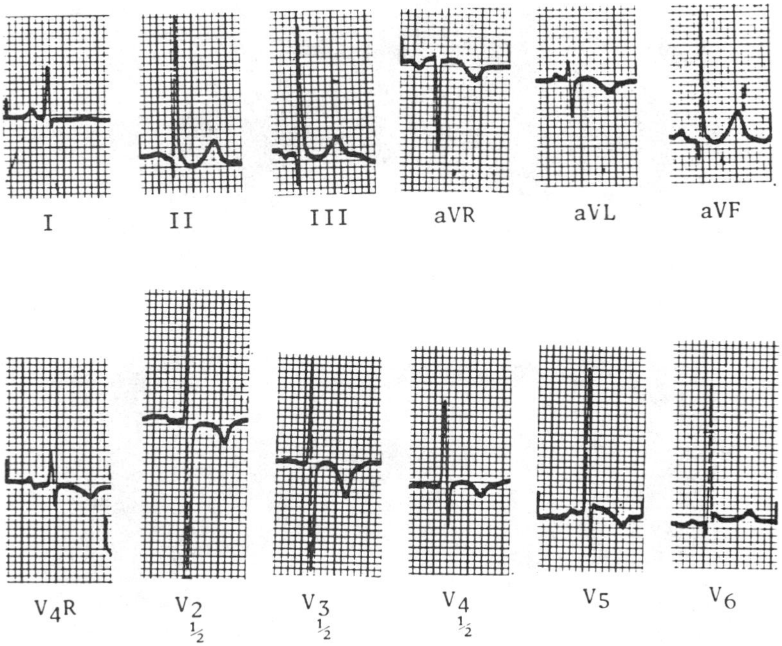

Figure 7–4B A 3-year-old with large PDA and dynamic pulmonary hypertension. There is evidence of biventricular hypertrophy (see also A and C).

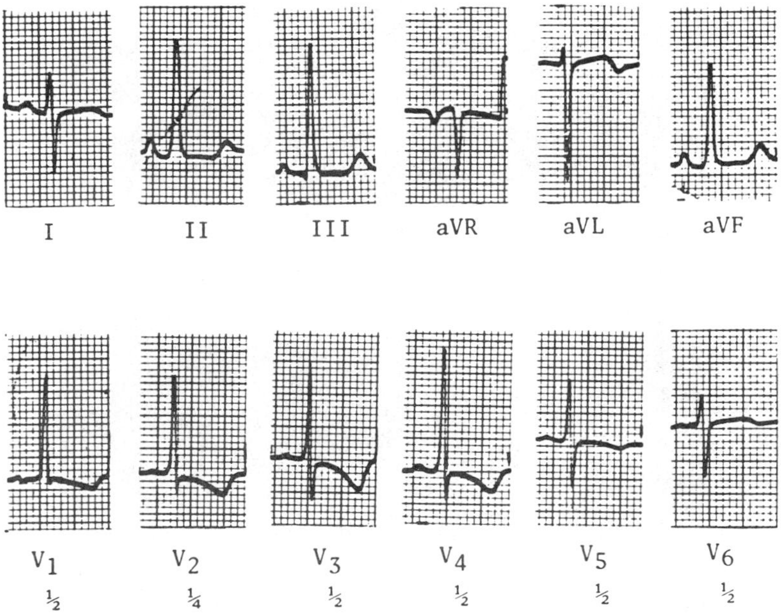

Figure 7–4C A 6-year-old with PDA, pulmonary hypertension, and increased pulmonary vascular resistance. Right axis deviation and right ventricular hypertrophy predominate (see also A and B).

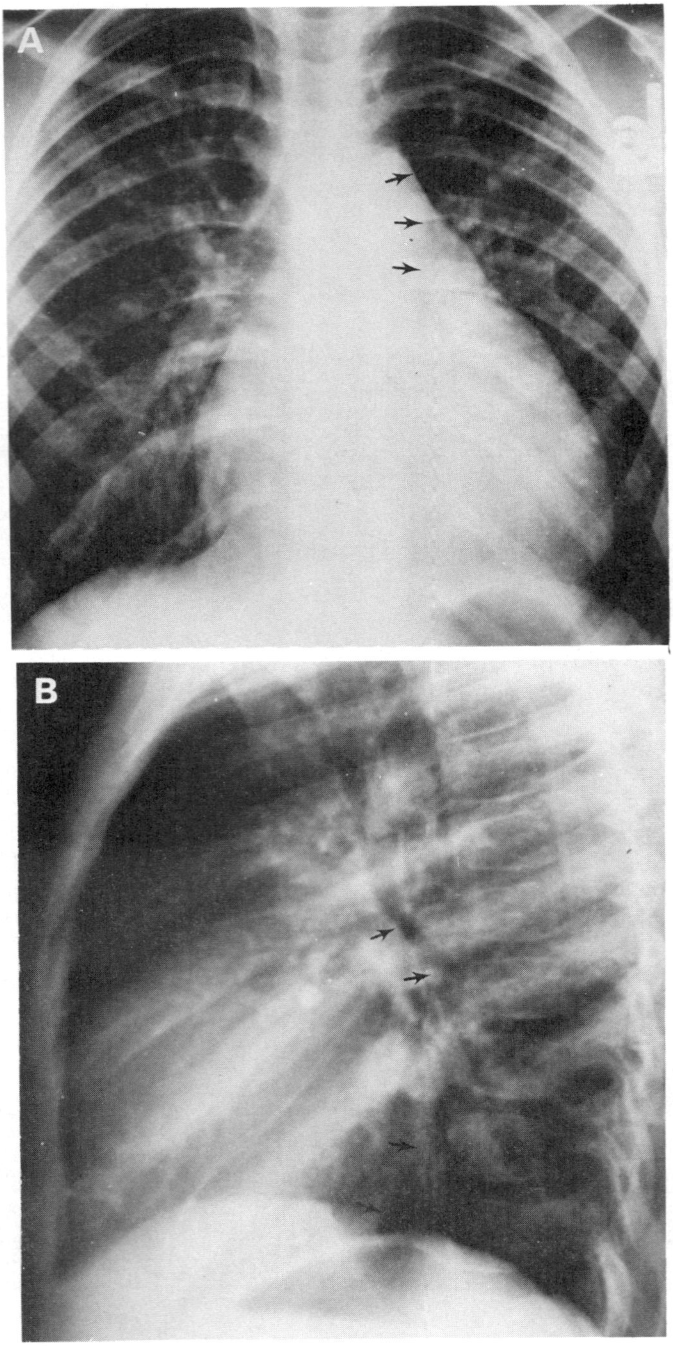

Figure 7–5 A 3-year-old with moderate-size patent ductus arteriosus and normal pulmonary artery pressure. (A) Note cardiomegaly with elongated cardiac apex. The descending aorta is enlarged (arrows). There is also increased pulmonary vascularity. (B) The lateral projection reveals left atrial (upper arrows) and left ventricular (lower arrows) enlargement.

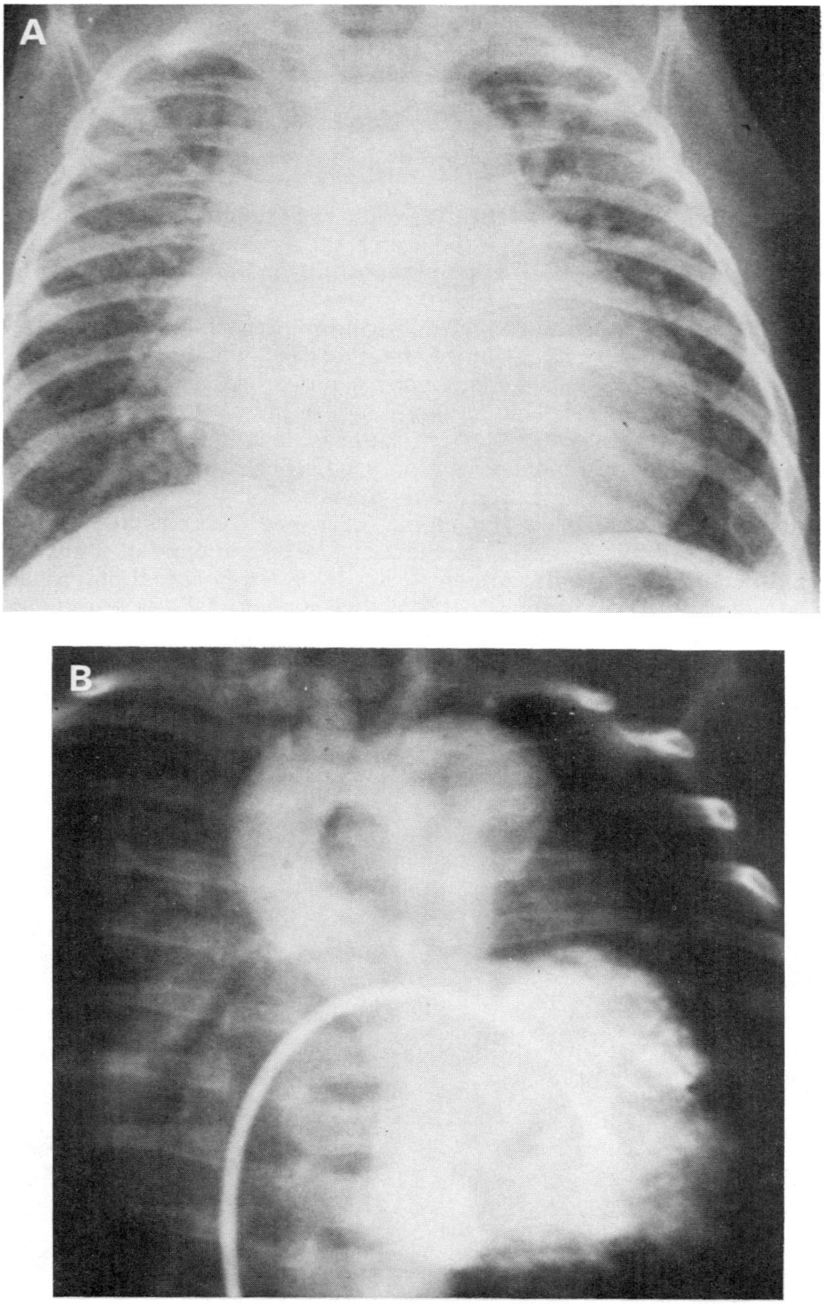

Figure 7–6 A 3-month-old with a large ductus and dynamic pulmonary hypertension in congestive heart failure. (A) Note the marked cardiomegaly, enlarged main pulmonary artery, increased pulmonary vascularity, and pulmonary edema. (B) Left ventricular angiogram of the same patient. The left ventricle is dilated and thick-walled. The descending aorta is enlarged. There is opacification of a markedly dilated pulmonary artery via the patent ductus.

cross-sectional diameter of the pulmonary tree and concomitant decrease in the left-to-right shunt. When the pulmonary vascular changes are severe enough to elevate the pulmonary vascular resistance to systemic levels, a right-to-left shunt develops (the evolution of these changes are discussed in detail in Chap. 4).

Manifestations

Patients with increased pulmonary vascular resistance are often asymptomatic. When pulmonary resistance is increased above the systemic level, a right-to-left shunt is established, and the patients become tachypneic with exertional dyspnea and cyanosis. Clubbing may or may not be present depending upon the severity and duration of hypoxemia. Associated with longstanding pulmonary hypertension is often growth retardation. Inspection of the chest reveals precordial bulge and a right ventricular impulse. The second heart sound is usually palpable. On auscultation the second heart sound is single and loud. Since the resistance is equal in both systemic and pulmonary circulation, there is no shunt and, therefore, no murmur or only a short ejection murmur at the upper left sternal border (see Fig. 7-2D).

The electrocardiogram shows right axis deviation, right ventricular hypertrophy and, occasionally, right atrial enlargement (Fig. 7-4C). The radiologic examination shows a normal or mildly increased cardiac size with evidence of right ventricular and main pulmonary artery enlargement (Fig. 7-7). The central pulmonary vessels are large with sudden pruning manifested as discrepancy in size between the central and peripheral vessels. Peripheral pulmonary blood flow appears normal to decreased.

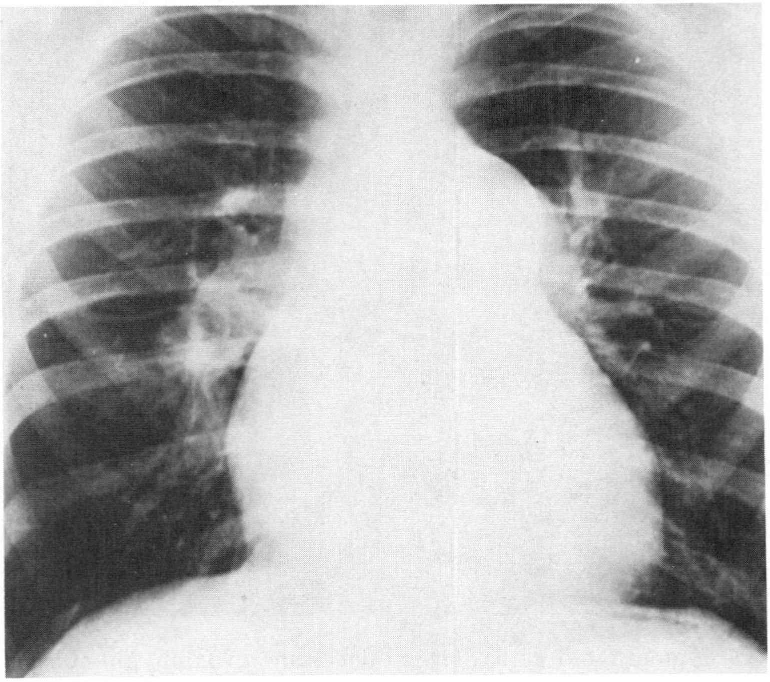

Figure 7-7A A 7-year-old with patent ductus arteriosus and pulmonary hypertension associated with increased resistance. The heart size is normal. Markedly dilated main pulmonary artery is noted as well as both main branches. There is pruning of the right and left branch. Peripheral pulmonary vascularity is decreased.

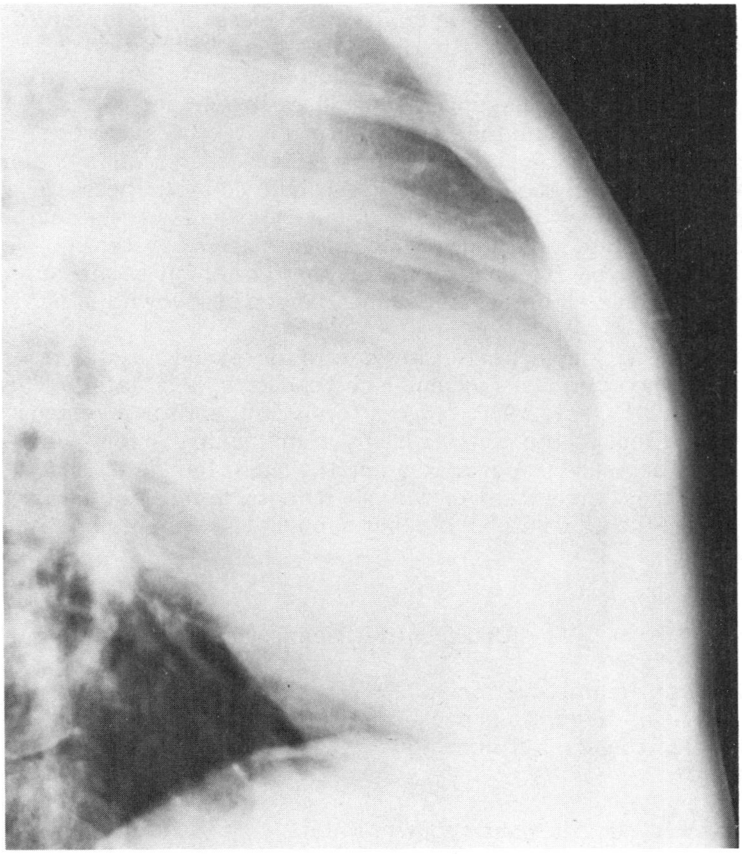

Figure 7-7B A 7-year-old with patent ductus arteriosus and pulmonary hypertension associated with increased resistance. Lateral projection of the same shows a dilated right ventricle with loss of the normal retrosternal clear space.

Echocardiographic Findings

The echocardiographic manifestations of patent ductus arteriosus, utilizing the M-mode technique, are identical to ventricular septal defect (q.v.). The study is thus not diagnostic of patent ductus, but reflects of the volume of the left-to-right shunt (see p. 218). Direct imaging of the patent ductus has been achieved in selected cases with two-dimensional techniques.

Cardiac Catheterization

The venous catheter manipulated into the pulmonary artery can almost invariably pass via the patent ductus into the ascending aorta. This catheter passage is typical in the uncomplicated ductus, and no angiogram is necessary. Left-to-right shunt is demonstrated by increased oxygen saturation at the main pulmonary artery level. The magnitude of the stepup is proportional to the magnitude of the shunt. If an angiogram is performed, however, there is prompt opacification of the pulmonary artery from the aorta via the ductus (Fig. 7-6B). In the small ductus, the pressures in the cardiac chambers and both great vessels are normal except for possibly a mild increase in the aortic pulse pressure. In the moderate-size ductus, the right-sided, left atrial and left ventricular end-diastolic pressure may be mildly to moderately elevated. The aortic pulse pressure is increased. In large defects, the right ventricular and main pulmonary arterial pressures approach systemic systolic pressure. The aortic diastolic pressure is decreased and, in the presence of severe congestive failure, the left ventricular end-diastolic pressure may be elevated. In large defects with increased pulmonary vascular resistance, the right ventricular and main pulmonary arterial pressures are at systemic levels. However, there is little or no evidence of a left-to-right shunt as measured by oximetry. There may be a right-to-left shunt (oxygen stepdown at the descending aorta).

When pulmonary artery hypertension due to increased resistance is suspected, the reactivity of the pulmonary vascular bed should be evaluated. This can be done by having the patient inhale 100% oxygen for 10 min and then remeasuring pressure and oxygen saturations in the vena cava, main pulmonary artery, and aorta. If either pulmonary pressure has decreased or the shunt has increased, it is indicative of reversible changes, the extent of which will determine the operability. This can also be done by injecting an alpha-blocker such as tolazoline directly into the main pulmonary artery.

Differential Diagnosis

Since the salient manifestations of PDA are bounding pulses and continuous murmur, differential diagnosis is presented for both. The diagnosis is usually apparent on clinical grounds, but occasionally cannot be made prior to cardiac catheterization.

A. Entities associated with continuous murmur.
   1. Venous hum: Is heard best in the sitting position. Diastole is accentuated and disappears upon compression of the ipsilateral jugular vein.
   2. Aorticopulmonary communication: May be clinically indistinguishable from PDA. The diagnosis is established at cardiac catheterization.
   3. Coronary arteriovenous fistula: A continuous superficial murmur heard within the cardiac borders. The diastolic component is often louder.
   4. Pulmonary AV fistula: The murmur may be located anywhere over the lung fields. If of sufficient magnitude, the AV malformation can be seen radiographically within the lung parenchyma. Cyanosis and clubbing may be apparent.
   5. Peripheral pulmonic stenosis: May give rise to continuous murmur all over the chest. This is unassociated with bounding pulses.

B. Entities associated with bounding pulses.
   1. Aorticopulmonary communication (window, surgical shunt).
   2. Aortic insufficiency with ventricular septal defect.
   3. Systemic AV fistula.
   4. Truncus arteriosus with insufficient truncal valve and/or increased pulmonary blood flow.

Careful examination of the chest x-ray, EKG, and physical examination will often point to the correct diagnosis.

Treatment, Course, and Prognosis

The patient with a small defect is asymptomatic and requires no medical management except for antibiotic prophylaxis during periods of potential bacteremia such as dental procedures, tonsillectomy, and so forth. Since the risk of surgery for this defect is equal to or smaller than the risk of bacterial endocarditis, it has been our practice to perform surgical ligation and division in all patients when diagnosed. This can be performed at any time.

Moderate and large PDA in failure should be treated with decongestive measures without delay. Digitalis and diuretics are administered, followed by surgery as soon as the patient's functional status has improved. There is no advantage in delaying surgical closure in this group since the failure may not be adequately controlled, and growth may be retarded.

Increased pulmonary vascular resistance generally develops beyond 2 years of age; however, occasionally isolated patients with reactive pulmonary vascular bed may develop it earlier without previous manifestation of congestive heart failure. Patients who develop vascular changes may progress to irreversible pulmonary hypertension. Surgical correction is not advisable in this group. The closure of the ductus removes the only alternative outlet available to the pulmonary circulation. This may result in an acute increase in a right-sided pressure, right heart failure, inability to maintain systemic circulation, and subsequent death. This complication should not be encountered if adequate and thoughtful management of this lesion is afforded in infancy and childhood.

Patent Ductus Arteriosus of Prematurity

Patent ductus arteriosus is encountered in approximately 60% of prematures with birth weights under 1750 g. This phenomenon is thought to be related to the increased sensitivity of the ductal smooth muscle to endogenously produced prostaglandins. These prostaglandins inhibit the vessel's ability to contract in response to oxygen. It appears that PDA is more frequent in infants with respiratory distress syndrome than in the unaffected infant.

The incidence of this problem has increased significantly in the last several years. This may be related to improved respiratory care and, therefore, improved survival of these infants and also to the increased intravenous fluids administered. For those infants who recover from the respiratory difficulty and congestive failure, the ductus arteriosus obliterates spontaneously within the first 3 months of life.

Clinical Manifestations in the Premature Infant

The most frequent mode of presentation is that of a 1500–1750-g baby who is initially stable or improving from respiratory distress syndrome, but starts to deteriorate at 6–7 days of age. A murmur is usually audible at the left upper sternal border. The murmur is initially a short systolic ejection one and increases in intensity and duration. This is associated with tachypnea, tachycardia, hyperdynamic precordium, bounding pulses, and fluid retention. Almost invariably, the development of a significant ductal shunt is associated with increased episodes of apnea and evidence of CO_2 retention.

Infants under 1000 g usually present with significant respiratory distress syndrome and seem to exhibit signs of a significant ductal shunting somewhat earlier than those above 1500 g. A possible explanation for the absence of a large left-to-right shunt immediately at birth might be related to the respiratory distress and subsequent increased pulmonary vascular resistance. When ventilatory function improves, pulmonary resistance declines with the appearance of a left-to-right shunt.

The electrocardiogram is generally normal, but chest roentgenograms often show a progressive cardiac enlargement (Fig. 7-8A), increased pulmonary arterial flow, and venous congestion.

The diagnosis of a hemodynamically significant left-to-right shunt in prematures may be difficult. There is usually no difficulty in patients exhibiting classical physical findings and symptoms. It has been shown, however, that patients with a significant documented left-to-right shunt might not have a murmur. The electrocardiogram is not helpful, and the chest x-ray may be misleading; therefore, a more sensitive tool, independent of the physical and other laboratory findings, was needed in order to better evaluate the magnitude of the left-to-right shunt.

Recently, the noninvasive echocardiographic technique has been utilized to assess the magnitude of the shunt. The left atrium and aortic dimensions can easily be measured and expressed as a ratio. The left atrial dimension is related to the large pulmonary blood flow and, in this case, to a large PDA. The normal left atrial-to-aortic (LA/Ao) ratio is 0.7-0.9, but in the presence of a large left-to-right shunt and a large left atrium the ratio is over 1.0 (Fig. 7-9). This concept has been widely applied to the diagnosis and followup of these patients. Return to normal of this ratio can be demonstrated immediately after surgical closure of the ductus.

Cardiac catheterization is usually avoided in these patients because of transport problems and the size of the vessels. The shunt through the ductus can be angiographically confirmed by positioning of the umbilical arterial catheter at the level of the ductus; contrast material can be injected through the catheter and a one-frame portable radiograph taken at the appropriate time. In the presence of a large shunt, the dye opacifies the aorta and main pulmonary artery. Similarly, this can be done by injecting saline in the same location while recording a simultaneous echocardiogram from the suprasternal position. In the presence of a PDA, microbubbles of the injectate appear in the aorta and subsequently in the right pulmonary artery, whereas if the ductus is closed, the microbubbles appear only in the aorta.

Treatment

Infants with congestive heart failure generally respond well to fluid restriction, diuretics, and maintenance of the hematocrit above 40%. Digitalis has been shown to be of little value in most infants since the primary problem is one of the effect of a large flow and pulmonary hypertension on pulmonary ventilatory characteristics rather than being related to depressed myocardial function. A small subset of infants will show myocardial failure, and in these patients digitalization is indicated. Ventricular performance can be assessed from the echocardiogram. Many infants require some form of respiratory assistance. With the advent of improved ventilatory care, it has become feasible to institute continuous positive airway pressure which causes significant improvement and enables the physician to reduce the infant's inspired oxygen concentration.

In spite of ventilatory assistance, a few continue to deteriorate, manifesting elevated arterial pCO_2. These few infants ultimately require surgical division of the ductus (see Fig. 7-8B). This can be easily performed in the neonatal intensive care unit, avoiding the risks of transport.

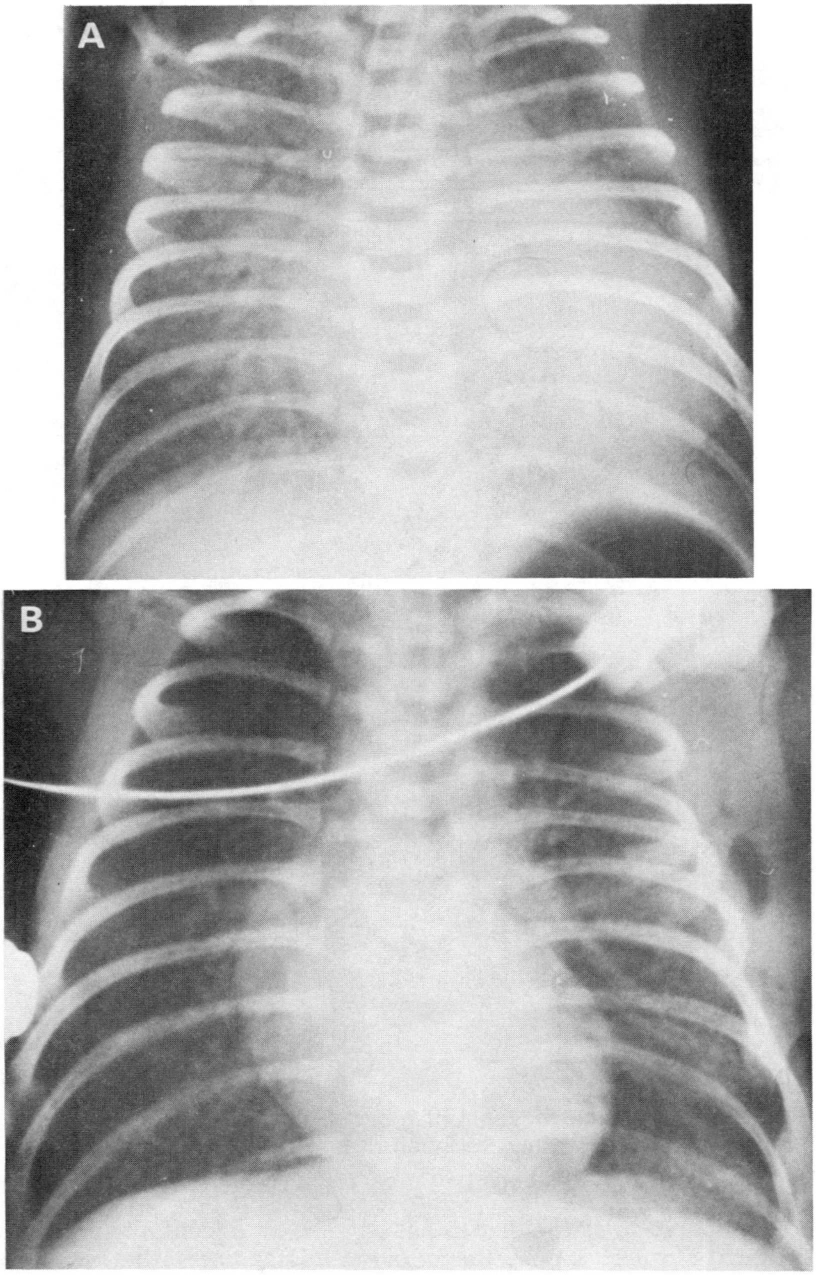

Figure 7-8 A 20-day-old premature with clinical findings of large patent ductus arteriosus and congestive failure necessitating respiratory assistance. (A) There is cardiomegaly with left ventricular and left atrial enlargement. The pulmonary arterial flow is markedly increased with evidence of pulmonary edema. (B) The same patient shortly after surgical ligation of the ductus. There is still air in the subcutaneous tissue at the site of thoracotomy. Note the marked diminution in cardiac size and pulmonary vascularity.

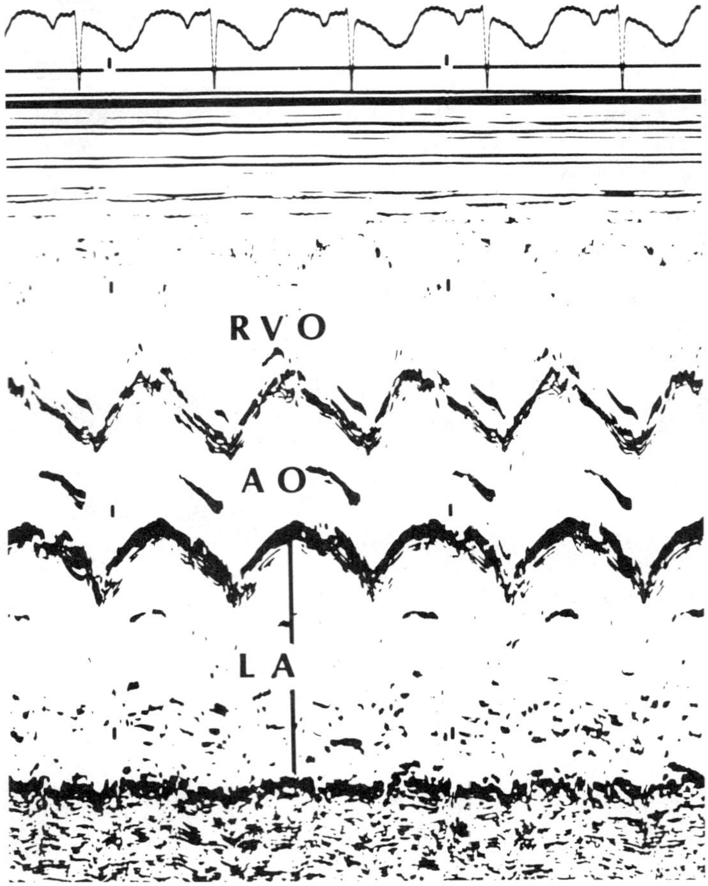

Figure 7-9 M-mode echocardiogram of a premature infant with a large PDA. Left atrium (LA) is large with markedly abnormal LA/Ao ratio.

Medical manipulation of the ductus has become an acceptable effective alternative to surgical closure. Indomethacin (a prostaglandin synthetase inhibitor) has been shown to induce PDA closure. Enteral administration of three 0.2-mg/kg doses at 8-hr intervals appears to induce ductal closure in approximately 80% of the patients. There is a marked age-dependent difference in ductal smooth muscle response to prostaglandin. Likewise, indomethacin proved to be more effective in producing contraction at the more immature vessel. The side-effects that should be watched for are transient impaired renal function and mild gastrointestinal bleeding.

Bibliography

Clyman RI, Mauray F, Rudolph AM, Heyman MA: Age dependent sensitivity of the lamb ductus arteriosus to indomethacin and prostaglandins. J Pediatr 96:94, 1980.

Krovetz LJ, Warden HE: Patent ductus arteriosus. An analysis of 515 surgically proved cases. Dis Chest 42:46, 1962.

McMurphy DM, Heyman MA, Rudolph AM, Melmon KL: Developmental changes in constriction of the ductus arteriosus response to oxygen and vasoactive substances in the isolated ductus arteriosus of the fetal lamb. Pediatr Res 6:231, 1972.

Neal WA, Bessinger FB, Hunt CE, Lucas RV: Patent ductus arteriosus complicating respiratory distress syndrome. J Pediatr 86:127, 1975.

Rowe RD, Lowe JB: Auscultation in the diagnosis of persistent ductus arteriosus in infancy. New Zea Med J 63:195, 1964.

Rudolph AM, Heyman MA: Medical treatment of the ductus arteriosus. Hosp Prac p. 57, February, 1977.

Rudolph AM, Mayer FE, Nadas AS, Gross RE: Patent ductus arteriosus. A clinical and hemodynamic study of 23 patients in the first year of life. Pediatrics 22:892, 1958.

Silverman NH, Lewis AB, Heyman MA, Rudolph AM: Echocardiographic assessment of ductus arteriosus shunt in premature infants. Circulation 50:821, 1974.

Chapter 8

ENDOCARDIAL CUSHION DEFECT

Endocardial cushion defects constitute a spectrum of anomalies that result from an abnormal development of the endocardial cushions. These defects are conveniently divided into the partial form or ostium primum defect and the complete form or common atrioventricular canal.

Anatomical and Embryologic Considerations

The endocardial cushions are located in the primitive atrioventricular canal. The two main cushions, the anterior and posterior, grow toward each other to divide the common atrioventricular canal into two separate openings, the ultimate mitral and tricuspid orifices (Fig. 8-1). The endocardial cushions also contribute to the membranous part of the ventricular septum, the anterior leaflet of the mitral valve, the medial leaflet of the tricuspid valve, and to the closure of the atrial septum or ostium primum (Figs. 8-2A,B). Therefore, any maldevelopment of these structures may induce a variety of defects (Figs. 8-2C,D, 8-3).

The most common variety of the partial endocardial cushion defect is the ostium primum defect. In this anomaly there is almost complete fusion of the endocardial cushions so that the annuli of the tricuspid and mitral valves are well formed. Incomplete fusion of the left portion of the anterior and posterior endocardial cushions accounts for the cleft in the anterior mitral valve leaflet. Associated is the defect in the septum primum located immediately above the annulus of the mitral and tricuspid valves (Figs. 8-2C, 8-3, 8-4, and see Fig. 5-2, p. 178).

Complete endocardial cushion defect is attributed to absence of fusion of the anterior and posterior endocardial cushions, resulting in a common atrioventricular valve orifice (Figs. 8-2C, 8-3, 8-5). As the name implies, there is failure of development of separate mitral and tricuspid rings. There is also a defect in the lower portion of the interatrial septum and upper portion of the interventricular septum. In essence, all four chambers communicate through this atrioventricular canal.

Partial Endocardial Cushion Defect (Ostium Primum Defect)

Partial endocardial cushion defect is one-fourth as common as secundum atrial septal defect (ASD).

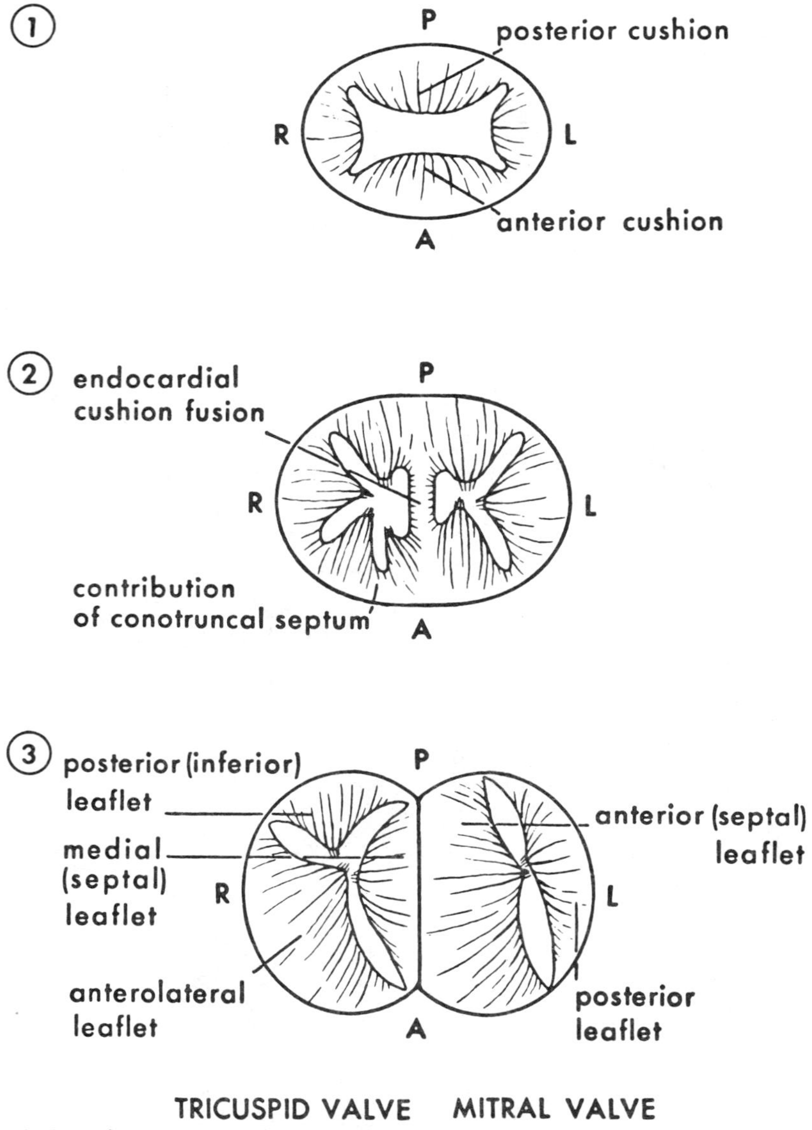

Figure 8-1 Diagram showing the primitive atrioventricular canal and the stages of development of the tricuspid and mitral valves from the primitive endocardial cushions. (From Rudolph AM, Congenital Diseases of the Heart, 1974, by permission of Year Book Medical Puslishers, Inc., Chicago.)

Hemodynamic Considerations

The hemodynamic abnormality which exists in a simple secundum ASD is reproduced in this anomaly; consequently, there is a large left-to-right shunt in the atrial level. In addition, because of the cleft mitral valve (Figs. 8-2A, 8-4), there may be a variable degree of mitral regurgitation resulting in an additional left ventricular overwork. The severity of the regurgitation depends upon the size of the cleft and the degree of tissue deficiency of the mitral valve. The anatomy is such that the regurgitant blood streams from the left ventricle through the cleft and the interatrial defect into the right atrium, thereby producing an obligatory left-ventricular-to-right-atrial shunt.

Manifestations

The lesion may be discovered in infancy because of the prominent murmur of mitral insufficiency. The symptoms and signs are similar to those described for ostium secundum atrial septal defects. They are related to the magnitude of the left-to-right shunt at the atrial level and the magnitude of mitral regurgitation or left-ventricular-to-right-atrial shunt. The children usually develop normally, but some may be slightly underweight.

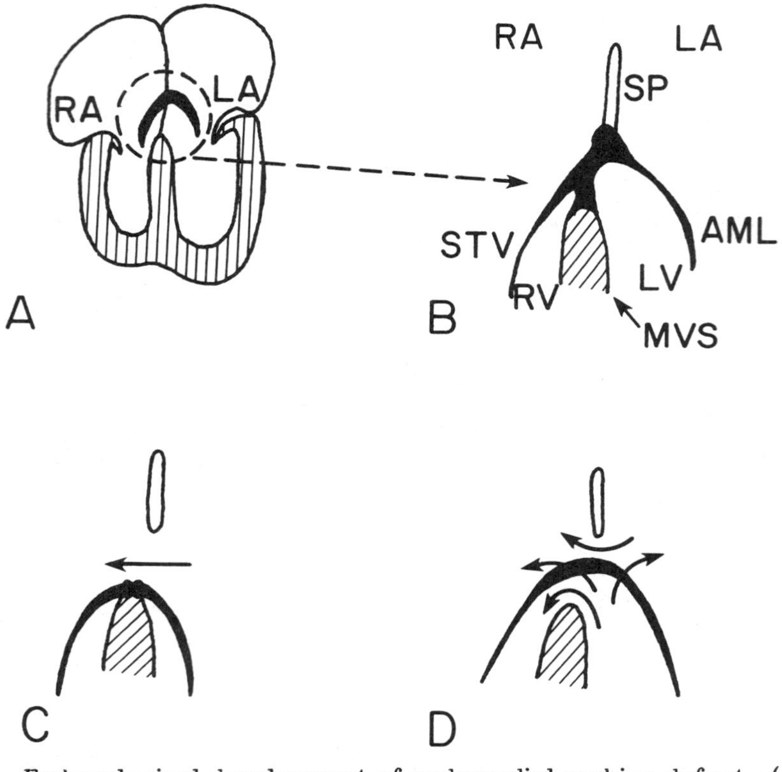

Figure 8–2 Embryological development of endocardial cushion defect. (A) Frontal section of a normal heart; the circle delineates the structures derived from the endocardial cushions. (B) Closeup of this area. The blackened structures are derived from the endocardial cushions; namely, the membranous ventricular septum on the top of the muscular septum (MVS), septal leaflet of the tricuspid valve (STV), anterior leaflet of the mitral valve (AMV), and the lower portion of the septum primum (SP). (C) Partial endocardial cushion defect. There is a defect in the septum with resultant left-to-right shunt. Note the abnormal insertion of the mitral and tricuspid leaflet at the crest of the muscular ventricular septum. (D) Complete endocardial cushion defect. There is an atrial septal defect, ventricular septal defect, and a common atrioventricular valve. (Adapted from Baron MG: Endocardial Cushion Defects, Ped Clin North Am. 4:343, December 1968.)

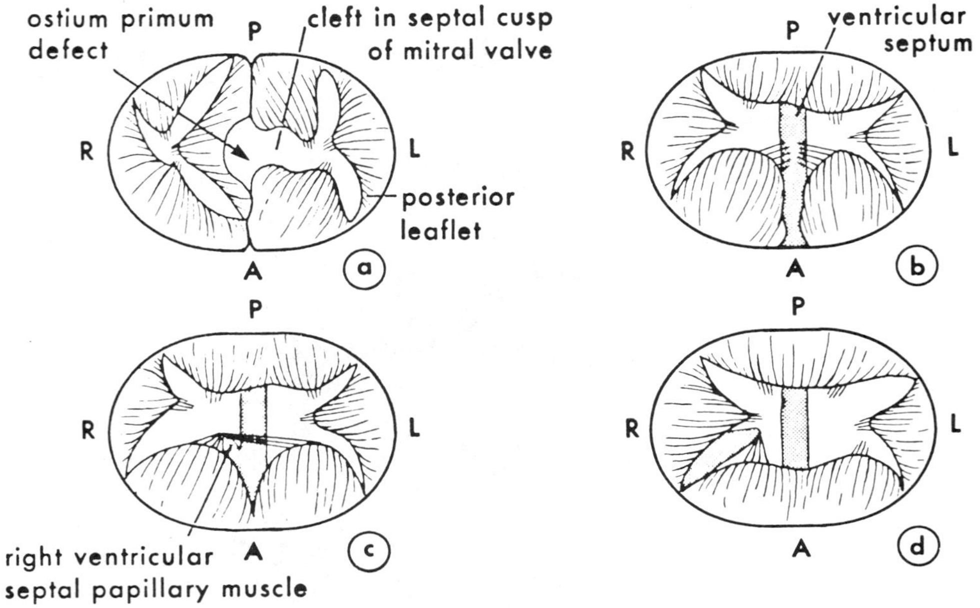

Figure 8-3 Defects of the atrioventricular valves in different types of endocardial cushion defects. (A) Ostium primum defect with cleft anterior leaflet of the mitral valve. (B) Complete endocardial cushion defect; the chordae from the anterior divided leaflet insert at the crest of the ventricular septum. (C) Complete endocardial cushion defect; partial separation of the anterior leaflet. Chordae from the mitral portion of this leaflet cross the ventricular septal defect to the right-sided papillary muscle. (D) Complete endocardial cushion defect; undivided anterior leaflet. (From Rudolph AM: Congenital Diseases of the Heart, 1974, by permission of Year Book Medical Publishers, Inc., Chicago.)

Physical Examination

The precordium is hyperactive with a prominent right ventricular impulse. The first heart sound is normal, and the second heart sound is widely split without respiratory variation. There is usually an ejection systolic murmur heard at the upper left sternal border radiating toward both lung fields. A murmur of mitral insufficiency may or may not be heard. There is often a low-frequency early diastolic rumble at the lower left sternal border. This murmur is related to a large flow through the tricuspid valve (see Fig. 5-4, p. 180).

Electrocardiogram

Characteristically, there is left axis deviation (Fig. 8-6). The mean frontal axis may be -20° to -90°. The vector loop rotates counterclockwise in the frontal plane.

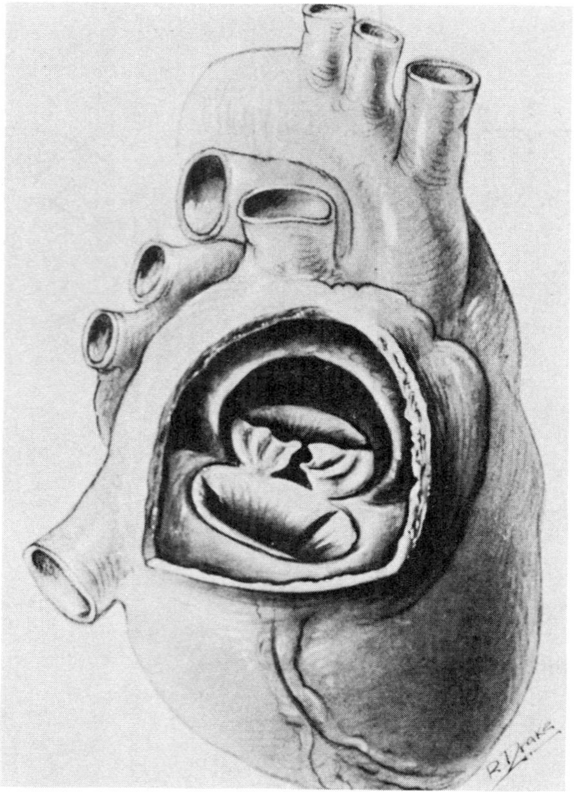

Figure 8-4 Ostium primum defect. The right atrial free wall is removed. The cleft mitral leaflet can be seen through the ostium primum defect. (From Moss AJ, Adams FH: Heart Disease in Infants, Children and Adolescents, p. 302, 1968, by permission of the Williams and Wilkins Co., Baltimore.)

Frequently, there is prolongation of the atrioventricular conduction manifested as a prolonged PR interval. Delayed right ventricular depolarization is invariably present and is indicative of right ventricular hypertrophy. In the presence of severe mitral regurgitation, left ventricular overload may be present as well.

Radiologic Evaluation

The appearance of the heart on chest radiograph may be indistinguishable from that of ASD 2° defect. A varying degree of cardiomegaly is present, depending on the size of the left-to-right shunt. There is invariable right ventricular, right atrial, and main pulmonary artery enlargement. In the presence of significant mitral regurgitation, left ventricular enlargement may also be present (Fig. 8-7).

Echocardiographic Findings

Dilatation of the right ventricle and paradoxical motion of the interventricular septum as manifestations of right ventricular volume overload due to the left-to-right shunt at the atrial level are the usual M-mode findings. Depending upon the

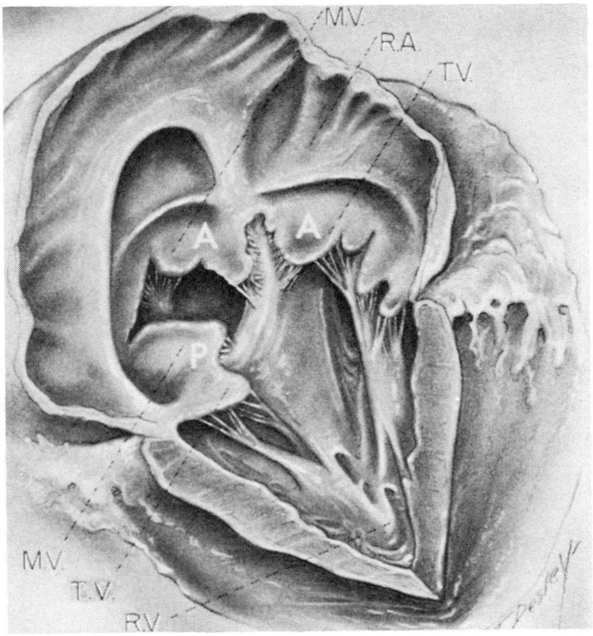

Figure 8-5 Complete endocardial cushion defect. The right atrium (RA) and right ventricular (RV) free wall are removed. The ventricular septal defect, atrial septal defect, and single AV valve were seen. A - anterior, P - posterior, MV - mitral valve, TV - tricuspid valve. (From Moss AJ, Adams FH: Heart Disease in Infants, Children and Adolescents, p. 202, 1968, by permission of the Williams and Wilkins Co., Baltimore.)

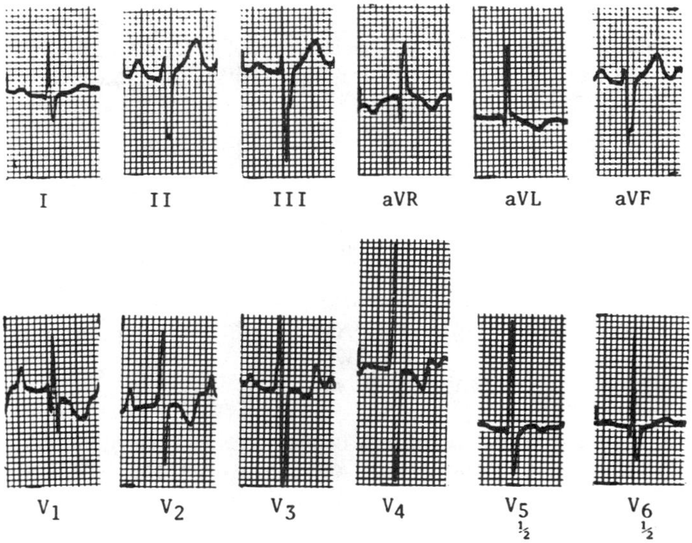

Figure 8-6 Electrocardiogram of a 5-year-old with ostium primum defect and significant mitral regurgitation. Note the superior left axis deviation in the frontal plane (-70°), 1° AV block, right atrial and biventricular enlargement.

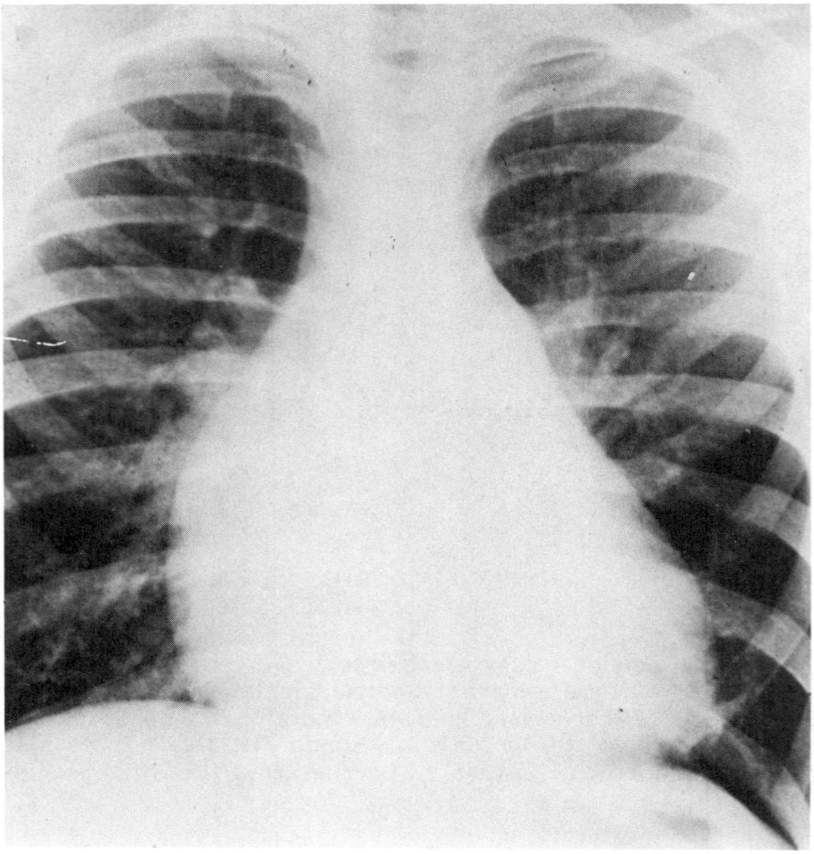

Figure 8–7 A 6-year-old with ostium primum defect. The cardiac silhouette is enlarged with prominent right atrium, left ventricle, and main pulmonary artery segment. Arterial pulmonary vascularity is increased.

degree of abnormality of the mitral valve, there may be prolonged diastolic approximation between the anterior mitral leaflet and the interventricular septum and also difficulty in imaging both the mitral valve and the posterior ventricular wall simultaneously. Notice, however, a good deal of variation in this lesion. Two-dimensional techniques may allow clearer delineation of the type of atrial septal defect and will often visualize the mitral valve more clearly.

Cardiac Catheterization and Angiography

A large left-to-right shunt can be demonstrated at the atrial level by comparing right atrial and superior vena caval oxygen saturations. The left-to-right shunt can also be demonstrated angiographically by an injection of contrast material into the main pulmonary artery or left atrium. If the patient is positioned in the left anterior oblique projection with the head and thorax elevated 45° (hepatoclavicular projection), the interatrial septum is placed in profile, and the location of the atrial septal defect clearly defined. The left ventricular angiogram demonstrates a typical gooseneck deformity of the outflow tract resulting from a deficient membranous ventricular septum and, consequently, an abnormal insertion of the anterior mitral valve leaflet on the crest of the muscular septum (Figs. 8-8B, C, 8-9). The cleft in the mitral valve is seen best during ventricular systole (Fig. 8-8B).

The catheter passage across the atrial septal defect is characteristic. Since the defect in the atrial septum is low, the catheter passage into the left ventricle is quite low as compared to a similar passage through an ostium secundum defect (Fig. 8-10).

Course and Prognosis

Congestive heart failure is more common in this anomaly than in secundum atrial septal defect. The failure is usually apparent before 5 years of age and is associated with poor prognosis. Pulmonary vascular disease rarely develops before adolescence, and the course is similar to that of secundum atrial septal defect. Bacterial endocarditis is more commonly seen with this anomaly as compared with ASD secundum. This is related to the mitral valve malformation.

Treatment

Surgical repair of this anomaly is more complicated than closure of a secundum atrial septal defect. The difficulty is related to the extent of mitral valve involvement. The mitral valve is not only cleft but deficient in tissue. If the cleft is surgically closed, the valve may become foreshortened, and severe regurgitation or stenosis result. It is now customary to ignore the mitral valve cleft if the mitral valve is competent. If significant insufficiency is present, the cleft should be

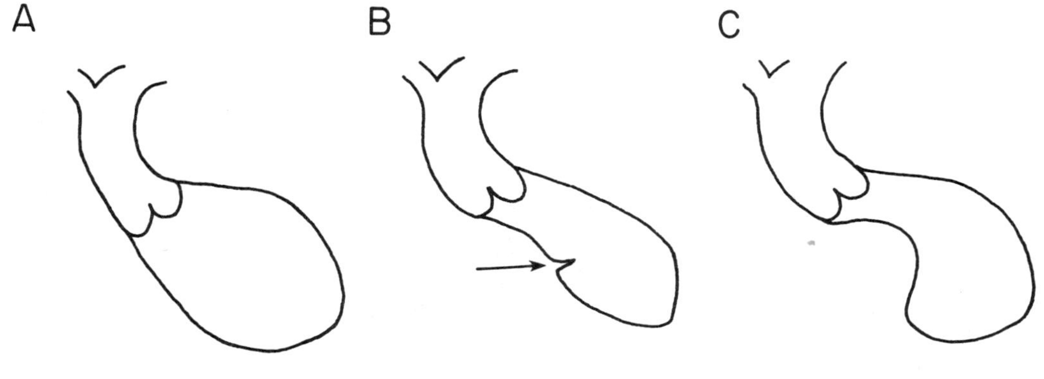

Figure 8-8 Angiographic appearance of the left ventricle in: (A) Normal heart where smooth wide-open outflow tract is seen. (B) Endocardial cushion defect, systole. Note the gooseneck deformity of the outflow tract which is related to abnormal attachment of the anterior leaflet of the mitral valve. The mitral valve cleft is well demonstrated (arrow). (C) Endocardial cushion defect, diastole. The gooseneck deformity or scooped-out outflow tract is accentuated during diastole. The cleft is not seen.

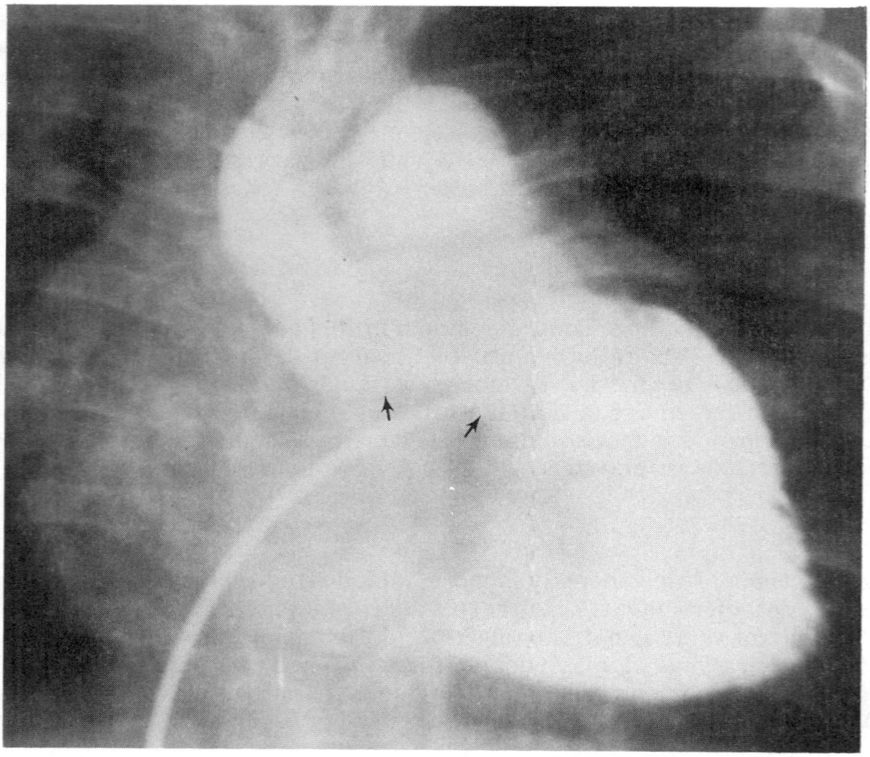

Figure 8–9 Endocardial cushion defect. Left ventricular angiogram, diastolic phase showing the typical gooseneck deformity of the outflow tract (arrows).

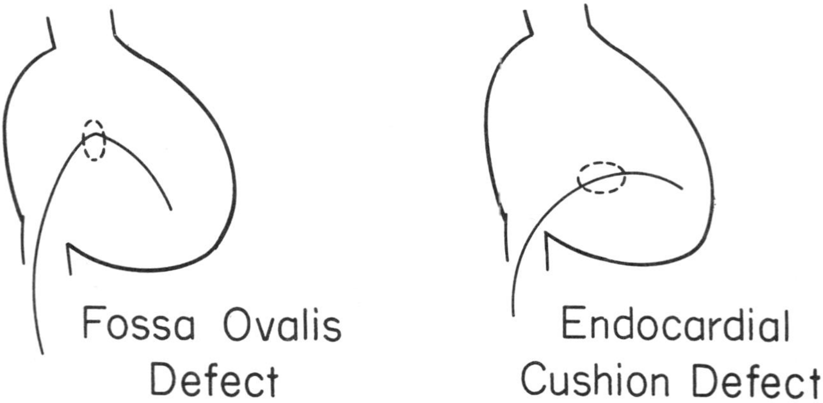

Figure 8–10 Comparison of the catheter passage in fossa ovalis (ostium secundum) defect and endocardial cushion defect. In fossa ovalis defect, the catheter crosses the defect in a more cranialward location and makes an acute bend to enter the left ventricle. In an endocardial cushion defect the defect is low and the course of the catheter into the left ventricle is low and flat.

repaired taking precaution not to shorten the valve; occasionally this is not possible, and mitral valve replacement is necessary. Surgery for asymptomatic children is recommended at 5-7 years of age.

Differential Diagnosis

Ostium secundum defect and partial anomalous pulmonary venous return should always be considered. The clinical presentation, physical examination, and symptomatology may be similar. The electrocardiogram with its superior left axis in the frontal plane and 1° AV block are helpful in distinguishing endocardial cushion defect from the other entities. Rarely, the electrocardiogram may not exhibit these features.

Complete Endocardial Cushion Defect

Incidence and Associated Anomalies

The lesion of complete endocardial cushion defect occurs in approximately 2% of all patients with congenital heart disease. It may occur as an isolated lesion in otherwise normal individuals. These defects are, however, encountered often in association with other anomalies. It is the most common congenital heart defect among patients with Down syndrome and has been frequently seen with the asplenia and polysplenia syndromes. There are other cardiac lesions associated with endocardial cushion defect such as pulmonic stenosis and patent ductus arteriosus.

Anatomy

The lesion consists of a common tricuspid and mitral orifice and a defect in the interatrial septum as well as the upper interventricular septum (Figs. 8-2D, 8-3, 8-5).

Hemodynamic Considerations

Shunting through the atrial septal defect and ventricular septal defect is dependent upon factors discussed in the respective sections, namely, the pressure relationship between the two ventricles and the outflow resistances. When pulmonary vascular resistance (PVR) is lower than systemic resistance, such as occurs postnatally, the direction of shunting is left to right. In most infants with this anomaly, the pulmonary vascular resistance falls significantly in the first 6-8 weeks, a large left-to-right shunt is then established, and cardiac failure commonly occurs.

The degree of competence of the atrioventricular valve is crucial in determining the physiological disturbances. The clinical status is definitely worsened by the presence of atrioventricular valve incompetence or obligatory shunt. In the latter, the left-to-right shunt occurs from a high pressure to low pressure chamber, namely, from the left ventricle via the common atrioventricular valve directly into the right atrium. This shunt is called an obligatory shunt since it does not depend upon changes in pulmonary vascular resistance. It also hastens the development of pulmonary vascular disease.

Manifestations

Symptoms usually occur early in infancy. The clinical presentation is diverse, depending upon the relative size of the atrial septal defect, ventricular septal defect, and the competency of the atrioventricular valve.

Physical Examination

In general, the children are small and undernourished with hyperactive precordium. Usually, both left and right ventricular impulses can be felt. The first heart sound may be accentuated, and the second sound is loud. The presence or absence of a widely split second sound depends upon the size of the atrial septal defect. A rough, loud holosystolic murmur is usually audible at the lower left sternal border with or without a palpable thrill. A low-frequency mid-diastolic rumble is audible at the apex and left sternal border. These physical signs are often indistinguishable from those of a large ventricular septal defect. When significant AV valve dysfunction is present, symptoms occur early in infancy and progress rapidly to severe heart failure. With increased pulmonary vascular resistance, there is cyanosis first on exertion and then at rest, progressing to right heart failure. Right ventricular impulse is prominent as well as a palpable second heart sound. The murmur is almost inaudible, accompanied by a loud booming single second sound.

Electrocardiogram

As with partial endocardial cushion defect, there is prolongation of the AV conduction and abnormality of the frontal plane axis (Fig. 8-11). Characteristically, the frontal plane QRS axis ranges from -40° to -150° with evidence of biventricular hypertrophy. Right ventricular hypertrophy is usually seen in patients with pulmonary hypertension and increased vascular resistance.

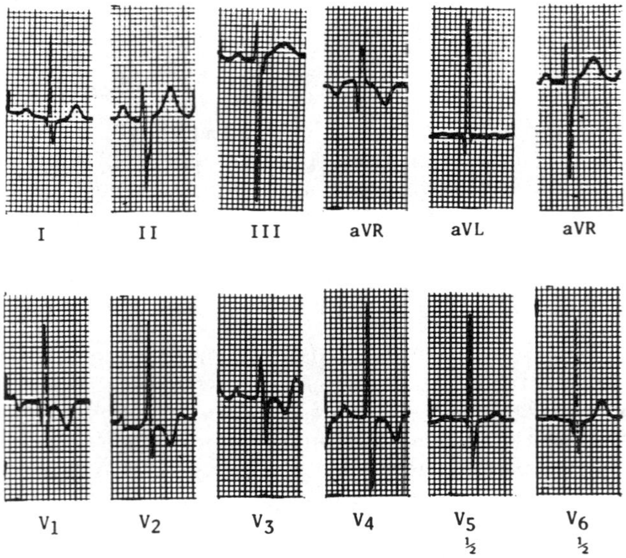

Figure 8-11 Electrocardiogram of a 5-year-old with complete endocardial cushion defect. The frontal plane axis is -60° with counterclockwise rotation, and there is a 1° AV block, suggestion of left atrial enlargement, and biventricular hypertrophy.

Radiological Features

The heart is always large; its contour is suggestive of enlargement of all four chambers (Fig. 8-12). Right atrial enlargement is common. The main pulmonary artery is prominent with large pulmonary blood flow. There is nothing specific on the chest radiograph to distinguish it from a large VSD except the presence of right atrial enlargement. The characteristic lumbar vertebrae configuration associated with Down syndrome (cephalocaudad dimension greater than anteroposterior dimension) seen on the latter chest film would suggest the diagnosis of an endocardial cushion defect (Fig. 8-12B).

Echocardiographic Findings

M-mode findings will reflect right ventricular volume overload as is true with the partial endocardial cushion defect. If there is a large left-to-right shunt at the ventricular level or significant atrioventricular valve incompetence, left ventricular dilatation may be present as well. Findings indicative of pulmonary hypertension may be seen. Perhaps the most useful finding is that which is related to the common atrioventricular valve. The opening motion of the anterior mitral leaflet appears to cross the plane of the interventricular septum with continuity between mitral and tricuspid valves (see Fig. 2-78). The relationship of this finding to the anatomy is fairly straightforward. The common AV valve is typically well imaged with two-dimensional techniques, and both atrial and ventricular septal defects may be identified although such imaging defines only anatomy. The

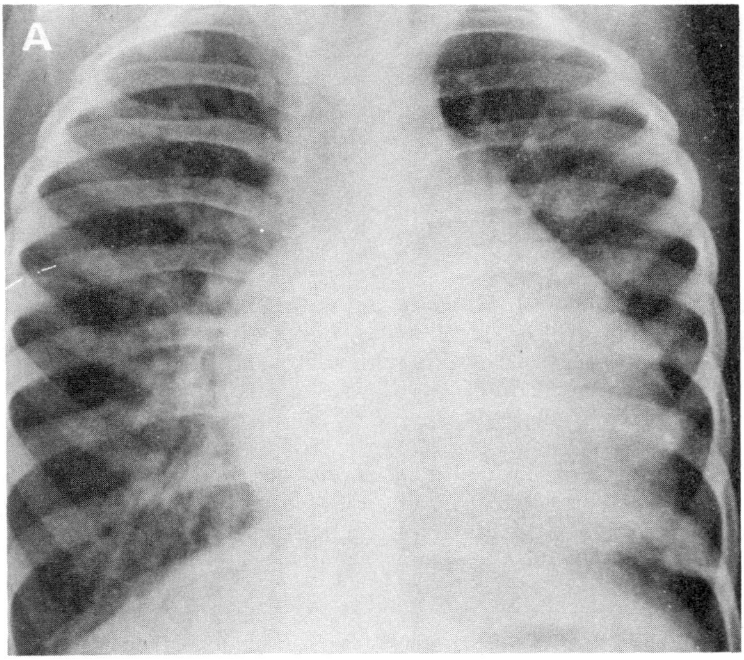

Figure 8-12A Chest x-ray of a 6-year-old with Down syndrome and endocardial cushion defect. Posteroanterior projection shows cardiomegaly involving all four chambers with prominent main pulmonary artery segment and increased pulmonary vascularity.

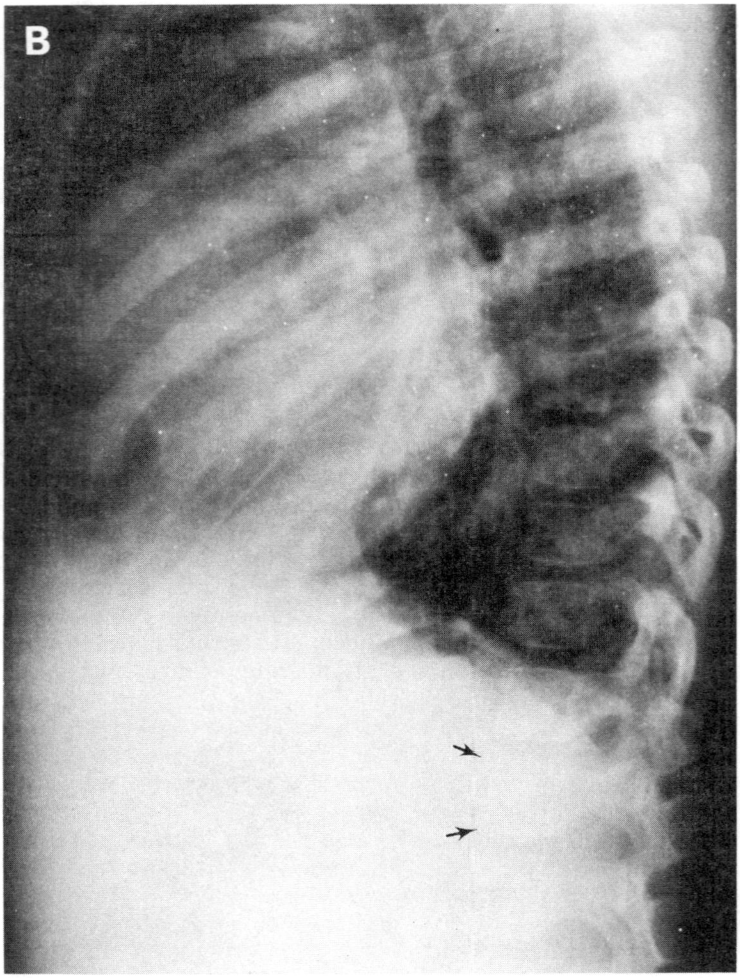

Figure 8-12B Chest x-ray of a 6-year-old with Down syndrome and endocardial cushion defect. The lateral projection shows left atrial, left ventricular, and right ventricular enlargement. Note the lumbar vertebrae; they are taller than wide, characteristic of Down syndrome.

The degree to which the structural components are functionally important can be inferred only indirectly in terms of ventricular overload. This is clearly a situation where careful cardiac catheterization is mandatory.

Cardiac Catheterization

The venous catheter entering the right atrium can be freely manipulated into all four chambers and usually into both pulmonary artery and aorta (via the VSD). The catheter passage into the left ventricle is characteristic (see Fig. 8-10). There is increased oxygen saturation in both right atrium and ventricle, indicative of a large left-to-right shunt. In the presence of an incompetent AV valve, there is free shunting of blood between all four chambers.

The right ventricular pressure is often at systemic levels with evidence of increased pulmonary blood flow. In the presence of pulmonary hypertension related to pulmonary vascular disease, there may be no appreciable left-to-right shunt, and there could be a net right-to-left shunt. The left ventricular angiogram, apart from showing a left-to-right shunt and possibly incompetent AV valve, has a characteristic appearance or gooseneck deformity relating to the abnormal insertion of the mitral valve (Figs. 8-8, 8-9). The cleft mitral valve can often be seen (Fig. 8-8).

Differential Diagnosis

Endocardial cushion defect must be considered in any infant with a large left-to-right shunt, congestive heart failure, and Down syndrome. This may, however, occur in patients who are otherwise normal. Lesions such as ventricular septal defect, truncus arteriosus, single ventricle and tricuspid atresia with a large VSD may present similar features. The most helpful tool in the differential diagnosis is the electrocardiogram with superior left axis deviation in the frontal plane. Left axis deviation is usually present in tricuspid atresia; however, the latter does not exhibit right ventricular hypertrophy.

Most untreated patients die within the first year of life; the cause of death is heart failure and/or pneumonia. If the patient survives infancy and childhood, progressive pulmonary vascular disease occurs and appears to develop sooner than in patients with uncomplicated ventricular septal defect.

Treatment

Conventional medical treatment is instituted when heart failure is diagnosed. If the cardiac failure is not controlled, surgery should be undertaken. Complete correction of the defect is feasible; however, this is a complicated procedure which is associated with a relatively surgical mortality, particularly in infancy.

Banding of the main pulmonary artery could be performed as a palliative procedure in some patients. This procedure, however, is not recommended in the presence of an incompetent atrioventricular valve. Banding affords symptomatic relief which is usually proportional to the reduction in pulmonary blood flow if the major shunt is at the ventricular level. Definitive surgery can then be done at a later date when reconstruction and/or replacement of the atrioventricular valves may be more feasible.

Bibliography

Baron MG: Endocardial cushion defects. Rad Clin North Am 6:343, 1968.

Greenwood RD, Nadas AS: The clinical course of cardiac disease in Down syndrome. Pediatrics 58:893, 1976.

McCabe JC, Engle ME, Gay WA, Ebert PA: Surgical treatment of endocardial cushion defects. Am J Cardiol 39:72, 1977.

Rabinowitz JG, Moseley JE: The lateral lumbar spine in Down syndrome — a new Roentgen feature. Radiology 83:74-79, 1964.

Somerville J: Atrioventricular defects. Mod Concepts Cardiovasc Dis 40:33, 1971.

Somerville J: Ostium primum defect: factors causing deterioration in the natural history. Brit Heart J 27:413, 1965.

Tenchoff L, Stamm SJ: An analysis of 35 cases of the complete form of persistent common atrioventricular canal. Circulation 48:416, 1973.

Van Mierop LHS, Alley RD, Kausel HW, Stranahan A: The anatomy and embryology of endocardial cushion defect. J Thorac Cardiovasc Surg 43:71, 1962.

Weyn AS, Bartle SH, Nolan TB, Dammann JF: Atrial septal defect, primum type. Circulation 32:III-13, December 1965.

Chapter 9

PULMONIC STENOSIS

Pulmonic stenosis implies anatomic obstruction to right ventricular outflow with a systolic pressure gradient between the right ventricle and pulmonary artery. Anatomic obstruction may be subvalvular (infundibular), valvular, or result from segmental narrowing of the pulmonary trunk or its branches (Fig. 9-1). Occasionally obstructing anomalous muscle bundles in the right ventricular cavity may be found. More than one site of obstruction may occur in some patients. Although the lesion occurs commonly in association with other cardiac defects, only isolated pulmonic stenosis will be considered in detail here.

Incidence

Valvular pulmonic stenosis with intact ventricular septum accounts for approximately 10% of congenital cardiac anomalies and ranks fourth or fifth in frequency in the experience of most large centers. In association with other cardiac malformations, some form of pulmonic stenosis is present in another 10–15% of cases.

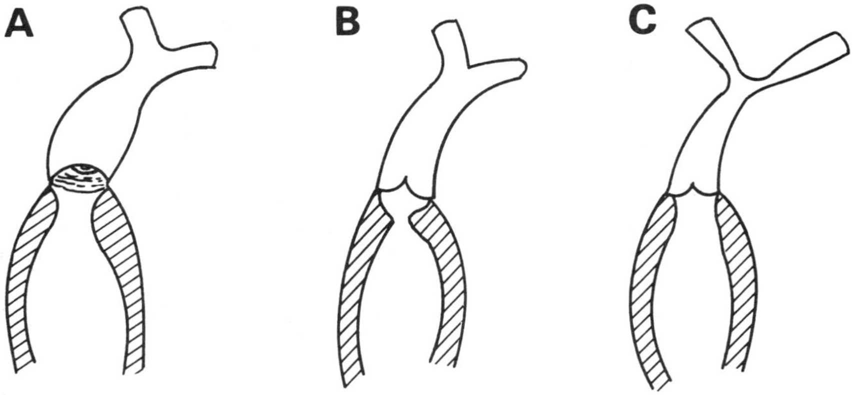

Figure 9–1 Types of pulmonic obstruction. (A) Pulmonic valvular stenosis. The valve is domed with small central orifice. Poststenotic dilatation of the pulmonary trunk is present. Secondary infundibular hypertrophy mildly encroaches on the subvalvular region. (B) Primary infundibular obstruction. Poststenotic dilatation of the pulmonary trunk is not present. (C) Stenosis of the pulmonary branches at their origin.

Embryology and Anatomy

Valvular pulmonic stenosis results from a developmental abnormality of the valve cusps or faulty commissural formation with commissural fusion. Although the embryological insult resulting in this abnormality is not usually known, the role of maternal infection with rubella virus in some cases has been clearly documented.

By far the most common site of stenosis is the pulmonic valve. Infundibular narrowing due to muscular hypertrophy is a common accompanying finding, but is not often of hemodynamic significance. Spontaneous regression usually follows surgical relief of the stenotic valve. Although rare, isolated infundibular stenosis may occur. The valve typically is thickened with commissural fusion, resulting in a small central orifice which may vary from 1 cm in mild stenosis to 2-3 mm in severe stenosis. A variable degree of hypoplasia of the pulmonic annulus may be present, particularly when pulmonic stenosis is part of more complex defects (e.g., tetralogy of Fallot). In the Noonan syndrome a particularly fibrotic, dysplastic, and thickened valve may be present.

Peripheral pulmonic stenosis or distal pulmonary artery stenosis may involve the main branches or, diffusely, the small peripheral arteries. This anomaly, in association with patent ductus arteriosus, is the most frequent cardiovascular anomaly associated with the rubella syndrome.

Hemodynamics

Increased resistance to right ventricular ejection is the major hemodynamic abnormality. This results in increased right ventricular pressure work and right ventricular hypertrophy, proportional to the severity of obstruction. The presence of an intact ventricular septum (and competent tricuspid valve) permits only one pathway of flow from the right ventricle (i.e., across the stenotic valve). Consequently, the pressure required to overcome resistance imposed by the stenosis may be considerable and well in excess of left ventricular pressure.

Although mild stenosis usually does not progress significantly, severe obstruction may increase in absolute or relative terms as the patient grows. Right ventricular output in response to demands of growth or stress may thus be limited and, eventually, ventricular dilatation and manifestations of congestive heart failure may appear. In absence of right-to-left shunting or right ventricular failure, pulmonary blood flow is normal, and cyanosis is absent. In severe cases, abnormal right ventricular compliance may elevate right atrial pressure above that of the left atrium, resulting in right-to-left shunting across a patent foramen ovale (central cyanosis). With the onset of congestive failure, peripheral cyanosis due to increased oxygen extraction by the tissues also may occur.

Manifestations

Development of symptomatology is related primarily to the severity of obstruction. Patients with mild-to-moderate stenosis remain asymptomatic. Severe stenosis may result in symptoms ranging from mild exertional fatigue and dyspnea to variable cyanosis and congestive heart failure.

In the neonate severe stenosis may result in the early appearance of congestive heart failure and cyanosis. The latter is due to left-to-right shunting across the foramen ovale which is almost invariably present at this age, especially if the right ventricular end-diastolic pressure is elevated. Hypoxemia commonly dominates the clinical features and may be complicated by severe congestive failure by 2-3 weeks of age. The examination reveals an exaggerated right ventricular parasternal impulse. A systolic thrill may be felt at the pulmonic area. A loud, harsh systolic ejection murmur is heard at the mid and upper left sternum with precordial radiation. At times, an additional harsh, long systolic murmur representing tricuspid regurgitation may be present along the lower left sternum and right sternal edge. In the presence of severe failure, the stenotic murmur may be atypical or absent.

The pulmonic component of the second sound is diminished or inaudible and the aortic component somewhat obscured by the murmur. A pulmonary ejection click, characteristic of valvular pulmonic stenosis in the older patient, may be absent in the neonate. Large jugular venous A waves, often difficult to detect in the newborn, may be coincident with a presystolic pulsation of an enlarged liver.

Marked cardiomegaly (cardiothoracic ratio exceeding 0.6) and pulmonary hypovascularity are characteristic radiographic features of the neonate with severe pulmonic stenosis and congestive failure. Poststenotic dilatation of the pulmonary trunk is usually not visible at this age.

The electrocardiogram demonstrates marked right axis deviation and right ventricular hypertrophy characterized by abnormally tall, pure R waves or a qR pattern in the right precordium. Deep S waves are present over the left precordium. However, in some infants, depending on the degree of development of the right ventricle, an unusually leftward axis may be seen associated with left or, less often, combined ventricular hypertrophy. The latter changes are more often seen when the right ventricle is somewhat hypoplastic and right-to-left shunting across the foramen ovale is present. In approximately one-half of cases, right atrial enlargement (tall, peaked P waves in II, III, and right precordial leads) is present.

Beyond the neonatal period pulmonic stenosis usually presents features distinctive enough to permit accurate clinical diagnosis. Patients with mild-to-moderate stenosis are usually asymptomatic, and the presence of the defect is identified by the characteristic pulmonic ejection murmur.

Severe pulmonic stenosis usually is symptomatic. Mild exertional fatigue and dyspnea are common, and strenuous effort may result in cyanosis, dizziness, or syncope. Except in infancy, severe pulmonic stenosis infrequently results in congestive heart failure until the second or third decades. Once present, failure may progress rapidly and respond poorly to medical therapy.

On physical examination the presence of mild stenosis is suggested only by a systolic ejection murmur at the pulmonic area usually preceded by an early ejection click. More severe stenosis results in a prominent right ventricular parasternal systolic impulse. A systolic thrill is almost invariably present at the upper left sternal border, frequently extending into the suprasternal notch and neck. Auscultation reveals a normal first heart sound. The second heart sound is widely split and relatively fixed in severe obstruction. Slight respiratory variation without expiratory fusion may be present in less severe stenosis. Except in very severe stenosis with immobile valve, a systolic ejection click is almost always heard. The murmur is typically harsh, crescendo-decrescendo, maximum at the third left interspace, and radiates up the left sternal border toward the infraclavicular region. Extension into the neck is not unusual.

Stenosis of increasing severity results in a murmur of longer duration and later peak intensity, a diminished intensity of both the ejection click and pulmonic closure, and an increased width of splitting of the second sound. Pulmonic closure may be somewhat obscured, however, by the murmur. A prominent fourth sound, if present, also suggests severe obstruction.

The electrocardiogram in mild stenosis may be normal. More significant disease results in right axis deviation and right ventricular hypertrophy. In general, the worse the obstruction, the greater the degree of both axis deviation and hypertrophy. A qR pattern in right precordial leads in this lesion suggests severe stenosis as does an R wave exceeding 20 mm in lead V_1 (Fig. 9-2).

On chest roentgenogram the heart usually is not enlarged in the transverse diameter, but a rounded, uplifted apex, characteristic of right ventricular prominence, is seen. In the left lateral view, encroachment on the retrosternal space may be noted (Fig. 9-3). The pulmonary artery segment, left branch, and occasionally right branch may show poststenotic dilatation. The peripheral vasculature is normal; however, vessels frequently appear of relatively small caliber even in the presence of normal pulmonary blood flow.

Echocardiogram

Echocardiographic evaluation of the pulmonic valve may suggest stenosis by the presence of premature opening of the cusps. This phenomenon, an exaggeration of normal presystolic motion of the valve leaflet following atrial systole, is due to the more forceful atrial contraction occasioned by abnormal ventricular compliance (see Fig. 2-77, p. 112). Thickening of the anterior right ventricular wall may be a secondary finding.

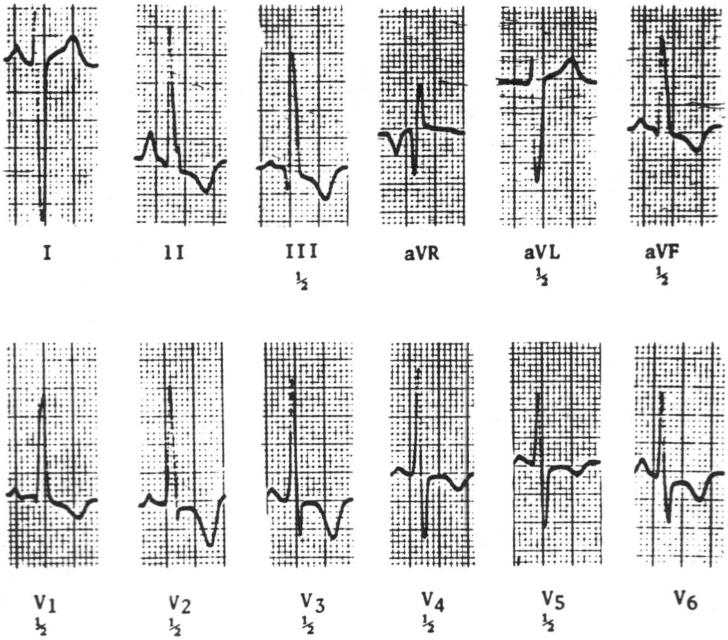

Figure 9-2 Electrocardiogram in extremely severe valvular pulmonic stenosis showing right axis deviation, severe right ventricular hypertrophy, and right atrial enlargement. Note qR pattern in V_1, $\frac{1}{2}$ standardization in V_1-V_5, and inverted T waves across the precordium. Right ventricular systolic pressure is 230 mmHg.

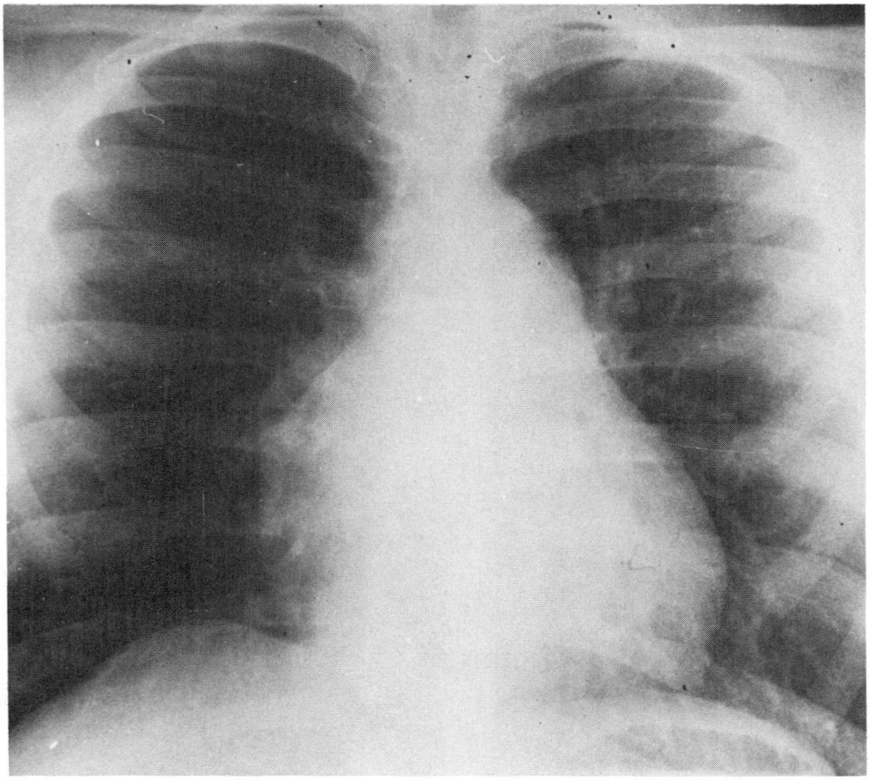

Figure 9–3A Chest roentgenogram of patient with valvular pulmonic stenosis. Frontal view. The apex is rounded and uplifted and the pulmonary trunk dilated (poststenotic).

Cardiac Catheterization

Cardiac catheterization is indicated in any symptomatic patient suspected to have pulmonic stenosis and in any patient with clinical features suggesting significant obstruction. The cyanotic infant and those with signs of congestive failure, in particular, require prompt evaluation. Catheterization permits precise definition of the anatomy including possible associated defects, site and severity of stenosis, and site of right-to-left shunting if present. Saturation studies demonstrate no evidence of left-to-right shunting, but variable right-to-left shunting across the foramen ovale may be found.

In mild-to-moderate stenosis, right atrial mean pressure is normal, but slightly prominent A waves may be seen. Mean atrial pressure may be considerably elevated in severe stenosis. Right ventricular systolic pressure at rest is elevated in proportion to the severity of stenosis, but always exceeds 30–35 mmHg with a pressure gradient across the stenotic valve exceeding 10 mmHg. Empirically, mild stenosis is indicated by a right ventricular systolic pressure less than 50 mmHg, moderate stenosis by a pressure exceeding 50 mmHg, but less than systemic and severe stenosis by right ventricular pressure in excess of systemic (Fig. 9–4).

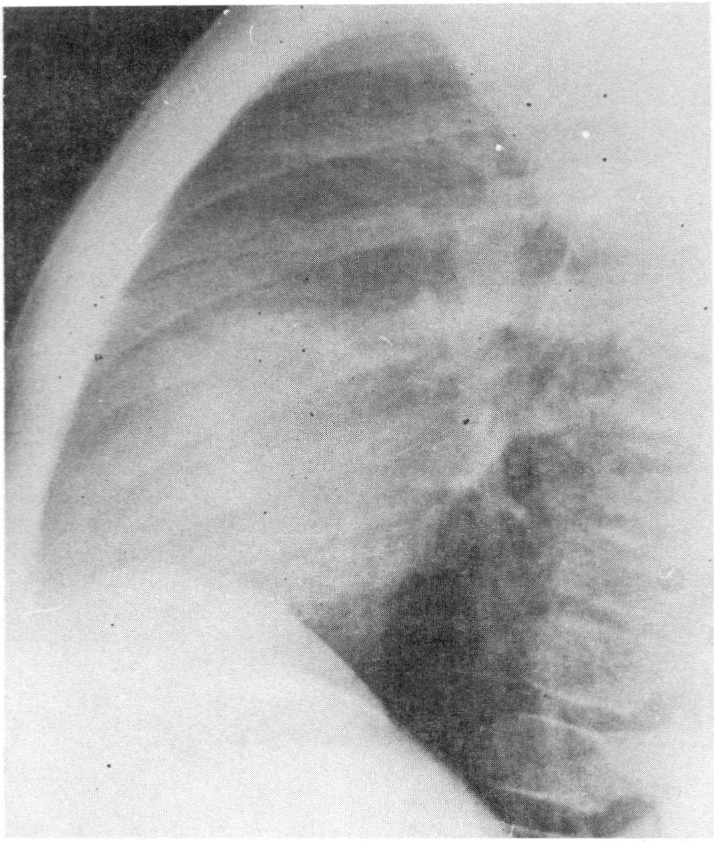

Figure 9-3B Chest roentgenogram of patient with valvular pulmonic stenosis. Left lateral view. Right ventricular enlargement encroaches on the retrosternal space.

Right ventricular pressures exceeding 250 mmHg occasionally are seen. Except in severe stenosis, the pulmonary artery is usually entered and pressures are normal. With severe stenosis, mean pulmonary pressure is reduced with marked damping of the phasic curve and, occasionally, the Venturi effect results in recording of a negative pressure in the high-velocity stream near the site of obstruction. Passage of the catheter across a severely stenotic orifice may cause nearly complete occlusion, resulting in an acute decline in cardiac output. Catheter withdrawal from the pulmonary artery will define the pressure gradient across the obstructive site and, in patients with associated infundibular stenosis, may identify two levels of pressure change.

Angiocardiography in the right ventricle reveals a heavily trabeculated and possibly dilated right ventricle. In the lateral view, the valve appears domed and thickened with a jet of contrast streaming through the small orifice. The pulmonary artery usually is dilated considerably, but the degree of dilatation does not correlate with the severity of stenosis. Dilatation of the left and occasionally both pulmonary branches also may be noted. Narrowing of the hypertrophied infundibulum may be seen in systole (Fig. 9-5).

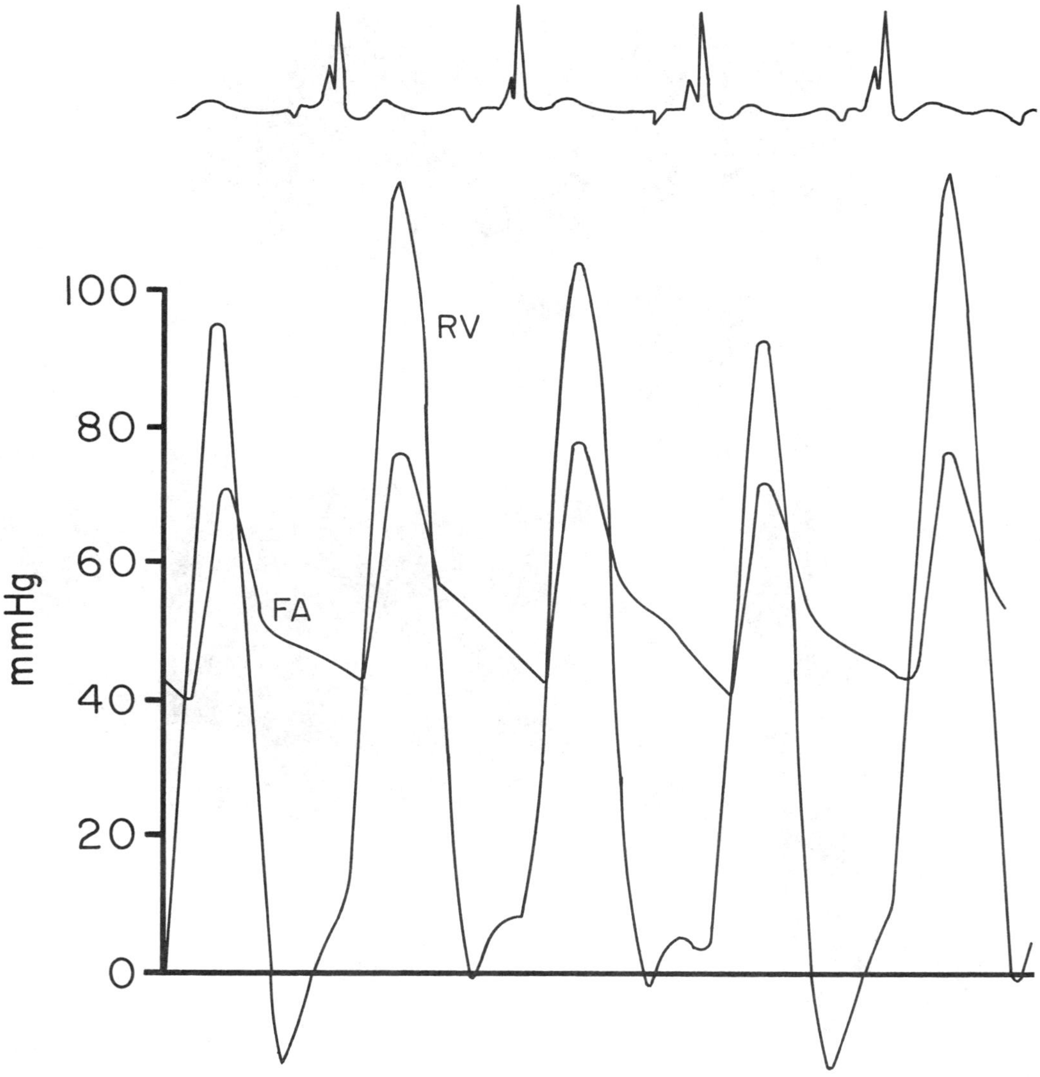

Figure 9-4 Suprasystemic pressure in the right ventricle (RV), simultaneously recorded with femoral artery pressure (FA), in a young infant with severe pulmonic valvular stenosis.

Course and Prognosis

In the absence of severe obstruction, the course of patients with pulmonic stenosis is generally favorable. Moderate stenosis remains stable in the majority of patients, but serial followup may reveal signs of worsening in some cases, as evidenced by progressive electrocardiographic changes and/or development of symptoms. Surgery may therefore become necessary in some individuals in this category. Symptoms are usually present in patients with severe stenosis and, without surgery,

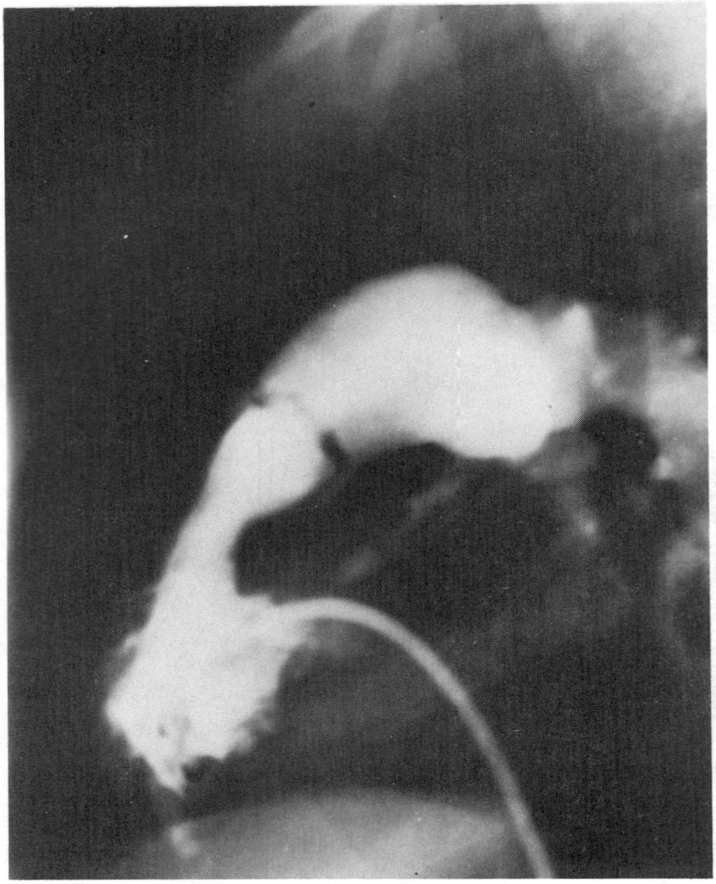

Figure 9–5 Lateral view of right ventricular angiocardiogram of patient with severe valvular pulmonic stenosis. The pulmonic valve is thickened and domed in systole. There is poststenotic dilatation of the pulmonary trunk and moderate infundibular narrowing.

eventual deterioration may be anticipated. Congestive heart failure is a particularly ominous development resulting in considerable mortality, even with surgery.

Patients presenting beyond infancy with mild stenosis rarely show significant progression of their lesion. However, the course of infants under 1 year of age with initially mild stenosis appears to be less predictable and may in some instances progress to severe obstruction in later childhood. Periodic clinical evaluation, therefore, is especially important for those presenting at this age.

Treatment

Regardless of symptoms, all patients with right ventricular systolic pressure at rest equal to or exceeding systemic pressure should have surgical relief of their obstruction. Valvulotomy under direct vision utilizing cardiopulmonary bypass is the preferred approach. Associated obstructive infundibular hypertrophy may warrant infundibulectomy. Patients with mild stenosis require no surgical therapy but should receive routine bacterial endocarditis prophylaxis, as indicated.

The decision regarding surgery in asymptomatic patients with moderately severe pulmonic stenosis is less well defined. Some regard a resting right ventricular pressure exceeding 75 mmHg as an indication for elective pulmonary valvulotomy. Factors other than pressure alone often require consideration in these patients including age, cardiac output, and hemodynamic response to stress.

Postoperatively there is usually prompt relief of symptoms and more gradual improvement of electrocardiographic changes. Residual mild obstruction indicates that small postoperative pressure gradients may be present. Mild pulmonic regurgitation may be produced as a result of the valvulotomy. Neither of these is usually of hemodynamic significance. Bacterial endocarditis, although uncommon, is a potential risk both pre- and postoperative, and appropriate prophylactic measures should be followed in all patients.

Differential Diagnosis

Clinical features are usually sufficiently distinctive to permit accurate clinical diagnosis. Severe pulmonic stenosis in the neonate may mimic other cyanotic lesions seen at this age such as transposition of the great arteries, tetralogy of Fallot, and pulmonic atresia with intact ventricular septum. Mild pulmonic stenosis primarily may suggest secundum atrial septal defect or functional pulmonary ejection murmur.

Bibliography

Campbell M: The natural history of congenital pulmonary stenosis. Brit Heart J 31:394, 1969.

Ellison RC, Freedom RM, Keane JF, Nugent EW, Rowe RD, Miettinen OS: Indirect assessment of pulmonary stenosis. Circulation 56 (Supp. I):14, 1977.

Engle MA, Ito T, Goldberg HP: The fate of patients with pulmonic stenosis. Circulation 30:554, 1964.

Gersony WM, Bernhard WF, Nadas AS, Gross RE: Diagnosis and surgical treatment of infants with critical pulmonary outflow obstruction. Circulation 35:765, 1967.

Mody MR: The natural history of uncomplicated pulmonic stenosis. Am Heart J 90:317-321, 1975.

Moller JH, Adams P, Jr.: The natural history of pulmonary valvular stenosis. Serial cardiac catheterizations in 21 children. Am J Cardiol 16:654, 1965.

Mustard WT, Jain SC, Trusler GA: Pulmonary stenosis in the first year of life. Brit Heart J 30:255, 1968.

Nugent EW, Freedom RM, Nora JJ, Ellison RC, Rowe RD, Nadas AS: Clinical course in pulmonary stenosis. Circulation 56 (Suppl. I)I:38, 1977.

Vogelpoel L, Schrire V: Auscultatory and phonocardiographic assessment of Fallot's tetralogy. Circulation 22:73, 1960.

Vogelpoel L, Schrire V: Auscultatory and phonocardiographic assessment of pulmonary stenosis with intact ventricular septum. Circulation 22:55, 1960.

Chapter 10

AORTIC STENOSIS

Aortic stenosis implies the presence of obstruction to left ventricular ejection with a systolic pressure gradient between the left ventricle and aorta. Left ventricular outflow obstruction occurs in several anatomic sites: supravalvular, valvular, and subvalvular (Fig. 10-1). The latter may exist as a discrete subvalvular lesion or as a more diffusely obstructive cardiomyopathy (idiopathic hypertrophic subaortic stenosis). Only aortic valvular stenosis, the most common form, is considered here in detail.

Incidence

Although not a common cause of morbidity and mortality in young infants, aortic stenosis occurs with a frequency of approximately 3-6% among patients with congenital heart disease. It has been suggested that the incidence is considerably higher and that many adults with "acquired" aortic valve stenosis, in fact, may represent progressive degenerative changes in a congenitally abnormal (bicuspid) valve. A distinct male sex predominance (4:1) has been noted.

Embryology and Anatomy

As is true for most congenital cardiac malformations, the embrylogic alteration resulting in the various forms of aortic stenosis is not entirely clear. Intrauterine endocarditis, endocardial fibroelastosis, and abnormal fetal flow patterns have been suggested as possible factors. Idiopathic hypertrophic subaortic stenosis in some instances has demonstrated a familial occurrence, while supravalvular aortic stenosis has been related to abnormal vitamin D metabolism in the mother and/or fetus.

In the vast majority of cases (75%) aortic stenosis is valvular and, most often, the valve is bicuspid. Isolated congenitally bicuspid aortic valve appears to be an extremely common malformation, and has been suggested to be perhaps the most frequent of all cardiac malformations. It is the most common lesion found in association with coarctation of the aorta with an observed incidence as high as 75%. A bicuspid aortic valve usually is of no hemodynamic significance in early life, but may account for significant obstruction in later years, due to progressive degenerative changes and calcification.

A B C D

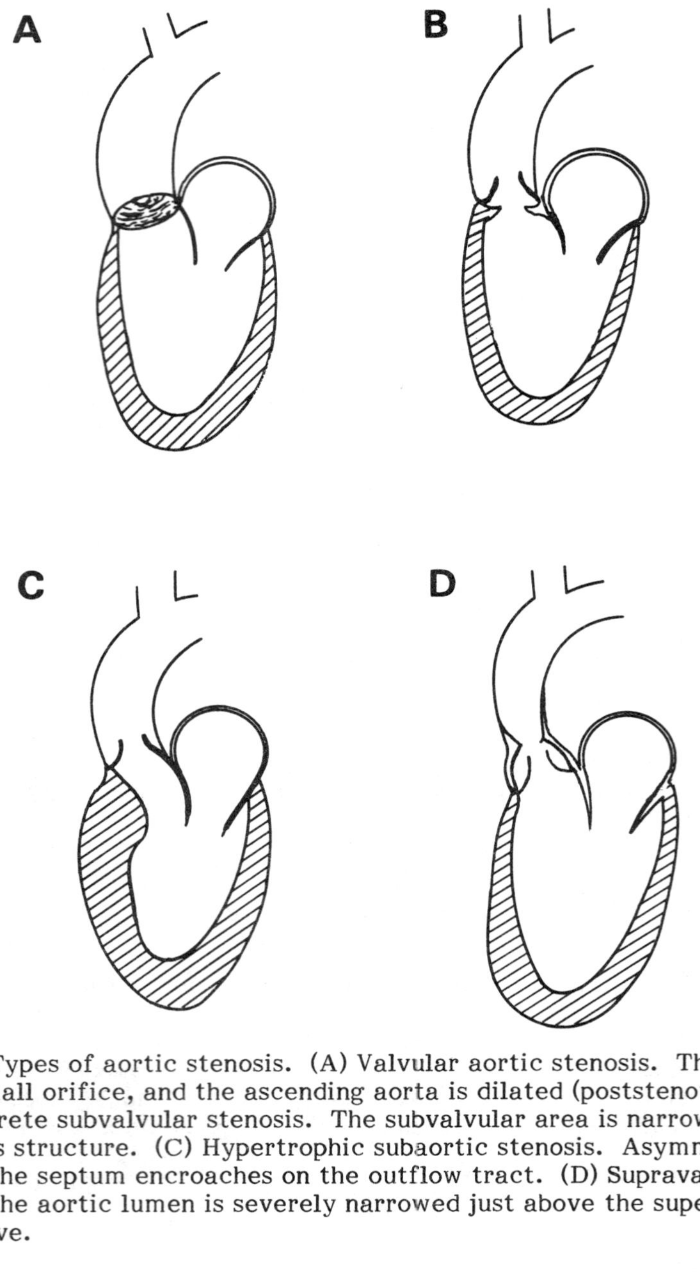

Figure 10-1 Types of aortic stenosis. (A) Valvular aortic stenosis. The valve is domed with small orifice, and the ascending aorta is dilated (poststenotic dilatation). (B) Discrete subvalvular stenosis. The subvalvular area is narrowed by a ringlike fibrous structure. (C) Hypertrophic subaortic stenosis. Asymmetrical thickening of the septum encroaches on the outflow tract. (D) Supravalvular aortic stenosis. The aortic lumen is severely narrowed just above the superior margins of the valve.

Less commonly, the stenotic valve is tricuspid with variable commissural fusion and leaflet thickening. Rarely, in the more severe lesions, the valve is unicuspid. Typically, the valve has a domed configuration with eccentric orifice. Usually, the annulus is of normal size, but hypoplasia of variable degree may be seen. A characteristic feature is poststenotic dilatation of the ascending aorta, particularly the anterior aspect. Presumably this is related to the chronic effects of high-velocity turbulence impinging on the vessel wall in this area.

Discrete subaortic stenosis occurs as a localized membranous diaphragm with small orifice or as a fibrous ring encircling the outflow tract, usually within 2 cm of the aortic annulus. The aortic valve may be entirely normal, although thickening of the leaflets may be present. The fibrous ring at times extends to the ventricular surface of the anterior mitral leaflet and, occasionally, a component of localized muscular obstruction is also present.

Idiopathic hypertrophic subaortic stenosis creates obstruction by disproportionate thickening of septal muscle in the region of the outflow tract. Encroachment on the left ventricular outflow tract by abnormal anterior systolic movement of the septal mitral leaflet is also a feature. This lesion is considered a form of cardiomyopathy and is discussed in Chap. 24.

Supravalvular aortic stenosis most often occurs as a feature of a syndrome characterized in part by typically abnormal facies, dental abnormalities, mental retardation, and in many instances peripheral pulmonary arterial stenosis. The site of aortic obstruction is usually localized at the upper margins of the sinuses of Valsalva above the attachment of the aortic cusps. A discrete fibrous ring or diaphragm may be present, but an "hourglass" deformity or more diffuse narrowing of the ascending aorta and proximal arch may also occur.

Hemodynamics

Regardless of the site of obstruction, aortic stenosis exaggerates left ventricular pressure work by imposing abnormal resistance to ejection. The increase in pressure work is related to the severity of obstruction. An otherwise healthy myocardium will respond to increasing obstruction by generation of higher pressure in order to maintain adequate flow and pressure in the systemic circuit. Myocardial hypertrophy results in an effective compensatory mechanism until a critical degree of obstruction is present, generally considered to be a valve cross-sectional area in the range of 0.5-0.7 cm^2/m^2. Below this critical valve area, more severe alterations consisting of left ventricular dilatation and elevated left ventricular end-diastolic volume may occur. Left ventricular isovolumic contraction time, ejection time, and total systole are prolonged. Initially, mean left atrial pressure and left ventricular end-diastolic pressure may be normal except in more severe obstruction. Progressive left ventricular hypertrophy and/or impaired myocardial function may lead to loss of ventricular compliance, requiring more forceful atrial contraction. The usual dominant V wave of the left atrial phasic pressure curve is replaced by a prominent A wave, and mean left atrial pressure and left ventricular end-diastolic pressure rise accordingly. These compensatory mechanisms may permit normal resting cardiac output and stroke volume. However, critical obstruction limits the ability of the left ventricle to increase output with stress. With the onset of left ventricular failure, cardiac output declines even at rest, and left ventricular end-diastolic pressure and mean left atrial pressure may rise considerably. These changes are reflected in elevation of pulmonary venous pressure and the appearance of pulmonary edema.

Progressive left ventricular hypertrophy results in increasing myocardial oxygen demands. The ability of the coronary circulation to meet these demands may be compromised by abnormally high intramural pressures and shortening of diastole (when major coronary flow occurs) as well as other factors.

Manifestations

Aortic Stenosis in the Infant

Isolated aortic valvular stenosis is an uncommon cause of cardiac symptomatology in early infancy. Although the lesion more often presents in the second month of life, it is occasionally responsible for critical illness in the newborn period. Severe congestive heart failure is usually the major manifestation. Tachypnea, dyspnea, irritability, and diaphoresis are common. The dusky pallor of poor perfusion may be present, and diffuse rales may be heard. Infants in profound failure may have little or no murmur. In others it may be atypical, frequently more prominent at the lower left sternal edge or apex than at the aortic area. Improved myocardial contractility following medical therapy may result in an intensified and more typical stenotic murmur. More often than not, an aortic ejection click is heard in these infants, but like the murmur, may be absent when severe congestive heart failure is present. Pulses may be generally weak, a feature which may suggest the hypoplastic left heart complex in the newborn.

Abnormal left ventricular forces, occasionally with strain pattern, may be present in the electrocardiogram of the newborn with severe aortic stenosis (Fig. 10-2). However, combined or right ventricular hypertrophy and right atrial enlargement may be seen as a result of pulmonary hypertension secondary to elevated left atrial and left ventricular diastolic pressures.

Chest roentgenogram may be normal, but in the presence of congestive failure, left ventricular and left atrial enlargement, pulmonary venous engorgement and secondary right ventricular enlargement may occur. In contrast to older patients, the ascending aorta is usually not dilated (Fig. 10-3).

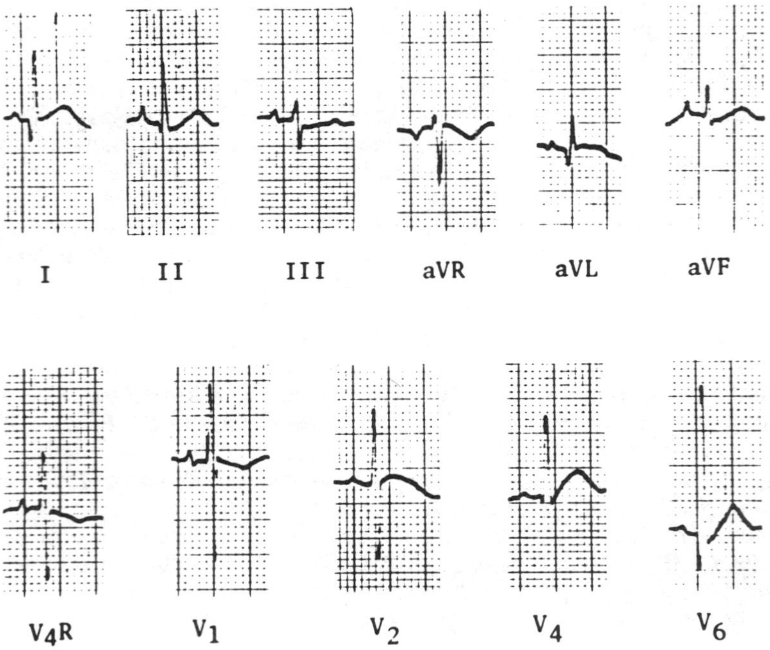

Figure 10-2 Electrocardiogram of neonate with severe valvular aortic stenosis and congestive heart failure. The frontal plane QRS axis is leftward for a neonate. Note prominent leftward forces and Q waves in left precordial leads.

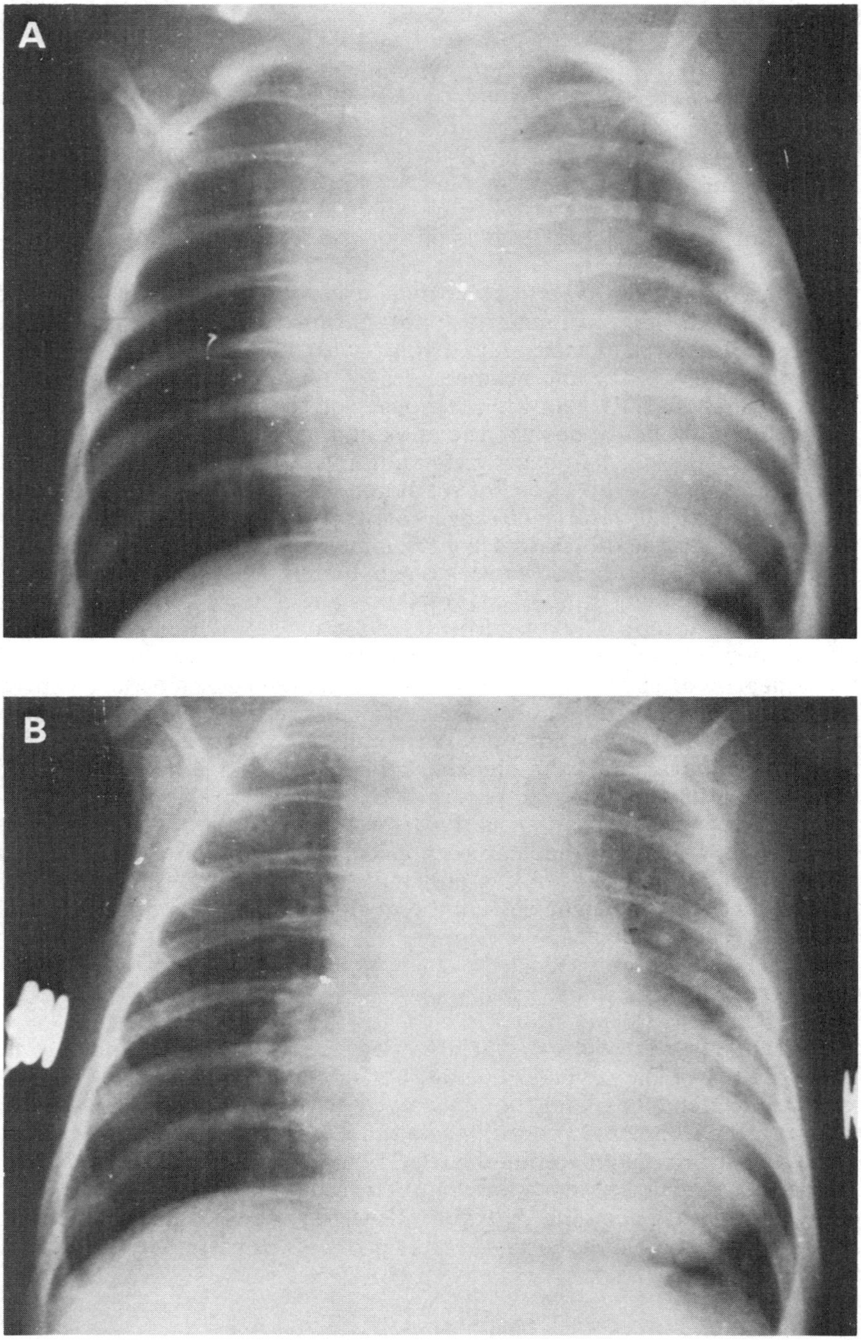

Figure 10-3 Critical aortic stenosis in a neonate. (A) The heart is greatly enlarged, and there is pulmonary venous congestion. A transaortic valve systolic pressure gradient of 45 mmHg was measured at cardiac catheterization. Aortic valvulotomy was performed. (B) Postoperative film 4 days later shows significant reduction in cardiac size.

Aortic Stenosis in Childhood

Beyond infancy, patients with aortic valvular stenosis may be relatively asymptomatic, even with severe obstruction. Growth and development are usually unimpaired. Symptomatic patients may complain of exertional fatigue and dyspnea. As a rule, symptoms suggest obstruction of at least moderate severity. Severe stenosis may result in anginal chest pain and occasionally syncope, both considered ominous manifestations. However, absence of symptoms does not imply hemodynamically unimportant disease, a fact that is one of the pitfalls in clinical assessment of this lesion.

On physical examination, aortic stenosis is usually suggested by the presence of a typical stenotic ejection murmur of variable intensity. The murmur peaks in mid-to-late systole and is of maximum intensity at the upper right sternal edge, less often at the midleft sternum or apex. Radiation into the neck, especially the right side, is a usual feature. Marking the onset of the murmur in most cases is a constant ejection click heard best at the apex and aortic areas. Usually a systolic thrill is palpable at the cardiac base, extending into the suprasternal notch and carotids. The presence of a precordial thrill generally implies a systolic pressure gradient of at least 20-30 mmHg. Severe aortic obstruction is usually characterized by a very forceful sustained left ventricular systolic impulse at the apex which may be displaced laterally and downward. A palpable presystolic impulse related to altered left ventricular filling characteristics and a more forceful left atrial contraction may be noted. The auscultatory counterpart of this is a prominent fourth heart sound. As severity increases, the stenotic murmur peaks later in systole, and the degree of splitting of the second sound decreases as left ventricular ejection is prolonged. Extreme delay of aortic closure may lead to paradoxical splitting. Progressive impairment of valve mobility results in decreasing intensity and eventual disappearance of the ejection click. In perhaps one-fourth of patients, an early diastolic murmur of aortic regurgitation may be present.

Although the blood pressure is usually within normal range, the pulse pressure may be diminished, a feature that can be appreciated by palpation of the arterial pulses. Because of normal physiologic augmentation of the distal arterial pulse pressure, the character of pulsations can be evaluated best by palpation of the more centrally located carotid pulses.

Electrocardiogram

Left ventricular hypertrophy of variable degree is the usual electrocardiographic finding (Fig. 10-4). The severity of obstruction, however, does not consistently correlate with EKG changes, and the older patient with severe aortic stenosis may have a normal or near-normal recording. In most instances, the presence of severe left ventricular hypertrophy combined with ST-segment depression and T-wave inversion in the left precordial leads (strain pattern) indicates severe stenosis, provided the patient is not receiving digitalis. However, approximately 25% of patients with severe stenosis show only voltage criteria of left ventricular hypertrophy with normal T waves.

Radiologic Features

The heart size, in the absence of failure, may be normal or minimally enlarged with a straight left border and downward-directed apex in the frontal view. Posterior prominence of the left ventricle may be seen in the lateral projection. Left atrial enlargement, a feature suggesting severe obstruction, may be present in both

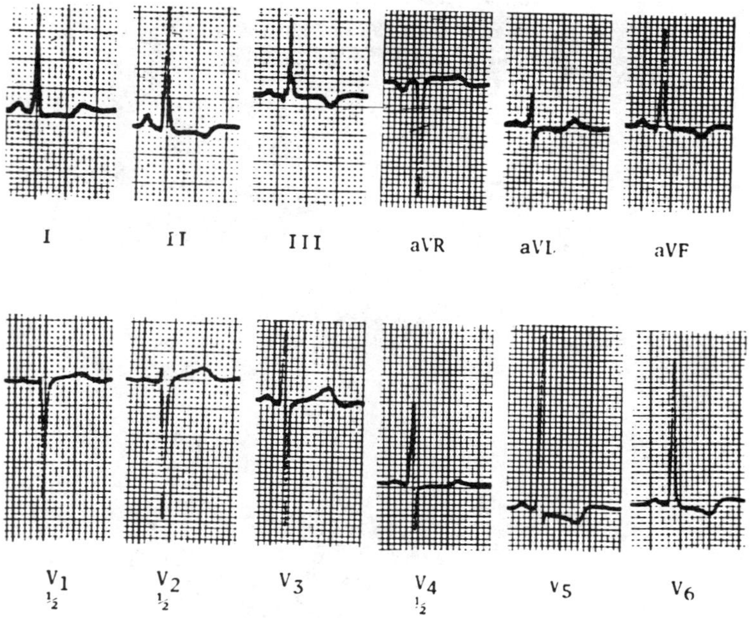

Figure 10–4 Electrocardiogram of a 12-year-old child with severe valvular aortic stenosis. Left ventricular hypertrophy and strain pattern. ST-segment depression and T-wave inversion in left precordial leads are present.

views. Poststenotic dilatation of the ascending aorta is a characteristic radiographic feature of this lesion. Pulmonary venous hypertension manifested by distended lymphatics (Kerly B lines) usually indicates severe obstruction and impending pulmonary edema.

Echocardiography

Echocardiographic recording of the stenotic aortic valve characteristically demonstrates multiple echoes from the thickened leaflets, particularly in diastole. Eccentricity of the diastolic closure line is a common but inconsistent feature of bicuspid aortic valve. Restricted opening of the stenotic valve also can be recorded in some cases. Secondary echocardiographic features include thickening of the septum and left ventricular posterior wall. Attempts have been made to correlate various echocardiographic measurements of left ventricular function with the severity of hemodynamic obstruction. Left ventricular ejection time, preejection period, and mean velocity of circumferential fiber shortening have shown inconsistent correlation. Measurement of the shortening fraction of the left ventricle in children with aortic stenosis has suggested that values greater than 40% correlate with an aortic valve systolic pressure gradient greater than 45 mmHg. This determination may be of value in identifying those patients with more severe obstruction. An echocardiographic formula employing the ratio of systolic left ventricular dimension and systolic posterior wall thickness multiplied by 225 was found to be a reliable prediction of peak left ventricular pressure in preoperative patients (Fig. 10-5). Hopefully, continued correlative studies eventually will permit reliable noninvasive evaluation of the severity of this lesion.

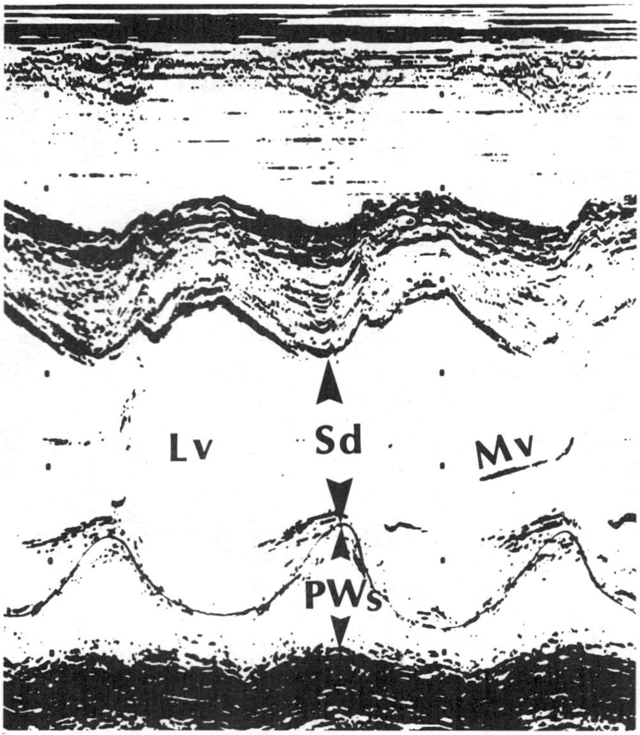

Figure 10–5 Left ventricular echocardiogram indicating site used for end-systolic measurement. PW_S - posterior wall (systole), Sd - systolic dimension, MV - mitral valve, LV - left ventricle. LV systolic pressure, PW_S/Sd x 225. In this patient the LV pressure was estimated to be 174 mmHg.

Cardiac Catheterization

Cardiac catheterization is essential in the assessment of symptomatic patients with aortic stenosis and those with clinical features suggesting severe obstruction. Presently, this procedure is the only satisfactory means for accurately determining the severity of obstruction. Accurate evaluation of the hemodynamic severity of obstruction requires measurement of both cardiac output and systolic pressure gradient across the stenotic site. When cardiac output is normal, a peak systolic pressure gradient exceeding 75 mmHg at rest or a calculated valve area less than 0.7 cm^2/m^2 body surface area generally indicates critical obstruction (Fig. 10–6).

Left ventricular angiography demonstrates the thickened aortic valve, with domed configuration during systole and an eccentric jet impinging on the wall of the dilated ascending aorta (Fig. 10–7). The left ventricular wall usually appears thickened while the cavity is of near-normal size. If aortic regurgitation is present, aortography is indicated to estimate its severity. In the event that the left ventricle cannot be entered retrograde from the aorta, pulmonary cineangiography also may provide helpful information regarding valve mobility and orifice size.

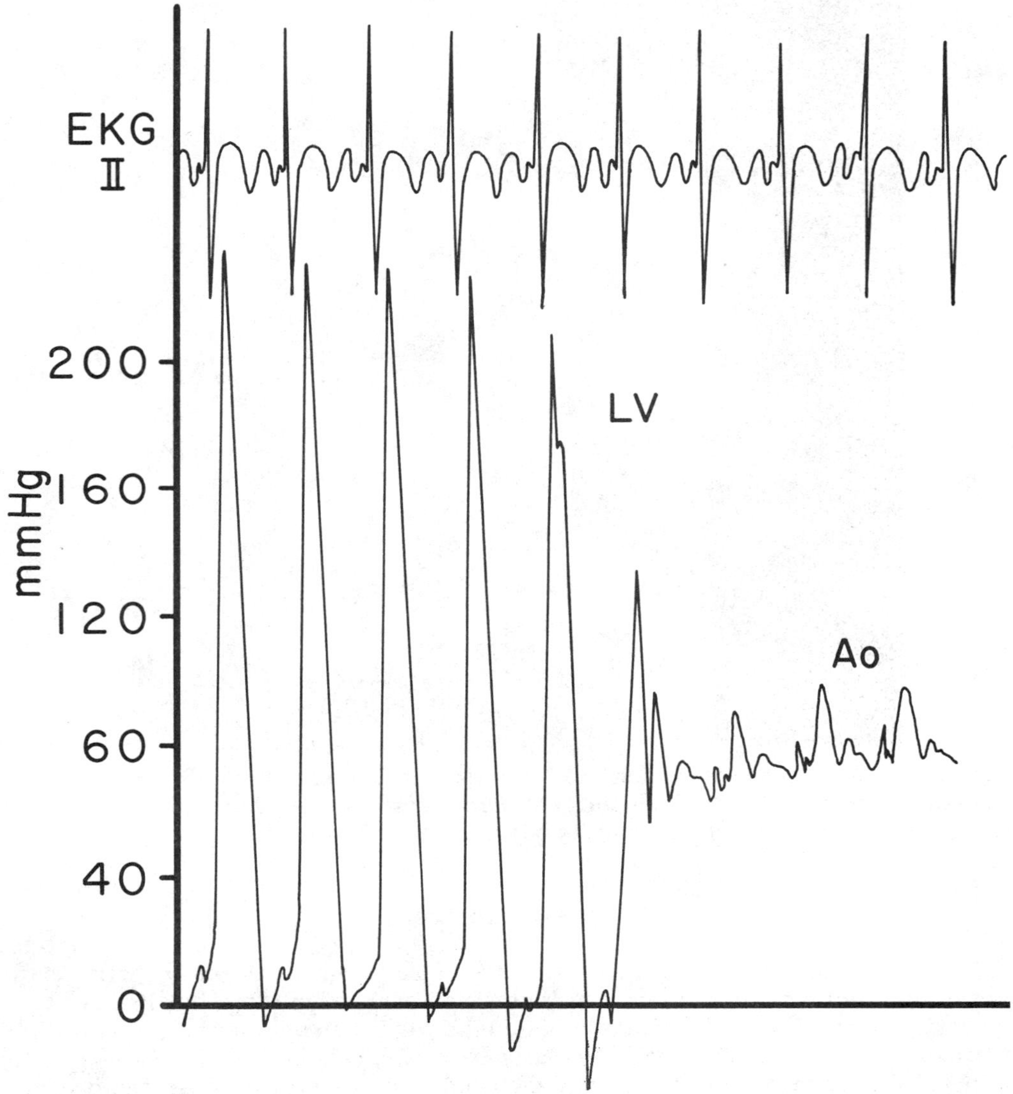

Figure 10–6 Withdrawal pressure curve recording from left ventricle to aorta. Note severe elevation of left ventricular systolic pressure and abrupt fall in systolic pressure as the catheter crosses the aortic valve to the ascending aorta.

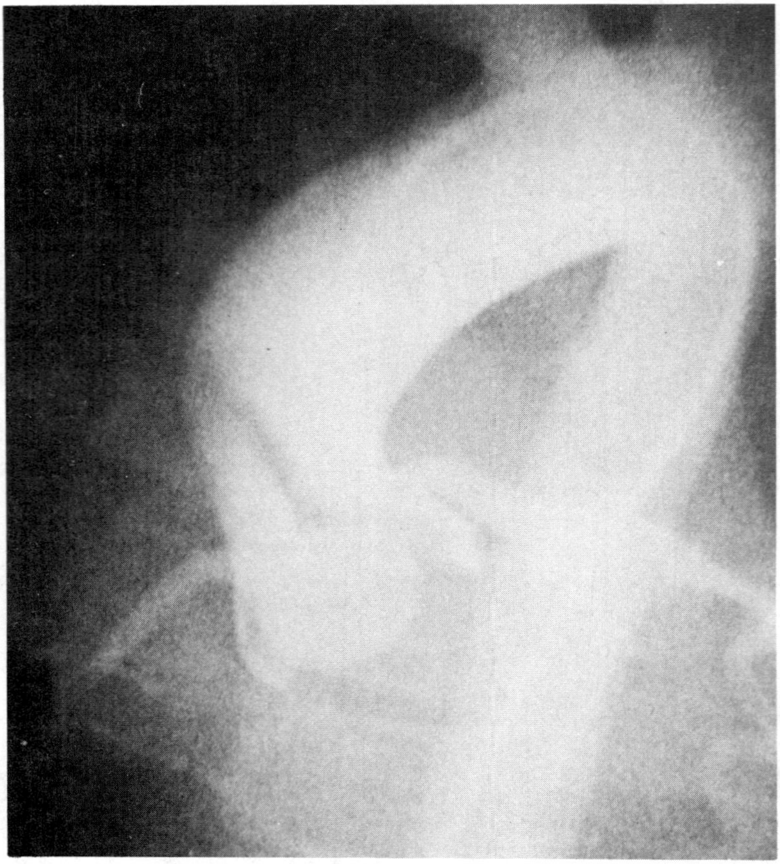

Figure 10–7 Aortogram in patient with severe aortic stenosis. Note the thickened, domed aortic valve. A jet of unopacified blood from the left ventricle impinges on the anterior aortic wall which exhibits poststenotic dilatation.

Course and Prognosis

The course and prognosis of this lesion are closely related to the severity of the obstruction. Mild valvular stenosis may cause no early symptoms, but in later years progressive sclerosis and calcification may lead to significant and symptomatic obstruction. In children, demands for increased cardiac output occasioned by growth and increasing activity may result in hemodynamic deterioration when the orifice size does not proportionately increase with growth or diminishes due to sclerotic change. Because of these features in the natural history of this lesion, participation in competitive sports is not recommended, in general, and specific restriction of strenuous activity is suggested for those with more severe obstruction.

Sudden death, presumably due to myocardial ischemia and dysrhythmia, is a potential hazard with a reported incidence up to 7.5%. In most such instances, significant prior symptoms have been present. Regular clinical reevaluation is indicated to detect early manifestations of deterioration, and periodic reassessment of hemodynamics by cardiac catheterization will be indicated in most patients. As in other cardiac malformations, current recommendations regarding bacterial endocarditis prophylaxis should be strictly followed in every patient.

Treatment

Patients with severe aortic valvular stenosis should undergo surgical treatment. For most, the initial procedure involves valve commissurotomy under direct vision during cardiopulmonary bypass. This can provide satisfactory relief of obstruction unless severe hypoplasia of the valve annulus coexists. Invariably, some degree of aortic regurgitation is present following this procedure. Obviously, all such patients have a residual valvular abnormality which may undergo progressive degenerative changes at a variable rate. Hemodynamic reassessment by cardiac catheterization at one year postoperatively and at 5-year intervals thereafter has been suggested. Most will eventually require reoperation, frequently necessitating prosthetic valve replacement.

When severe hypoplasia of the annulus is present, surgical therapy is more difficult. Procedures for expansion of the annulus have met with variable success.

Discrete Subvalvular Aortic Stenosis

Discrete subaortic stenosis, while less frequent than valvular obstruction, similarly exhibits a male sex predominance (2:1). Consistent differentiation between valvular and subvalvular obstruction on a clinical basis is not possible. Certain differences in their clinical features do exist but are by no means diagnostic. In the symptomatic infant with findings suggesting aortic stenosis, discrete subaortic obstruction would be only a remote consideration. While the ejection murmur is similar in both lesions, an ejection click is rarely present in subaortic stenosis. Aortic regurgitation, however, is more frequent, apparently resulting from cusp trauma by the high-velocity subvalvular jet. Dilatation of the ascending aorta may occur with both lesions but is less apparent with subaortic stenosis. Electrocardiographic features are similar. Echocardiography in subaortic stenosis may show transient early systolic closure of the aortic cusps, a helpful but nondiagnostic feature. In some instances, the two-dimensional echocardiogram is most useful in detecting a discrete constant subaortic thickening encroaching on the outflow tract.

Clear differentiation is possible only with cardiac catheterization and angiocardiography. Catheter withdrawal from the left ventricle to aorta may clearly identify the subvalvular location of the obstruction. Left ventricular angiography usually outlines a ringlike obstruction a short distance below the aortic root. Some degree of valve thickening is not unusual. Aortogram confirms valvular regurgitation when present. Treatment of this lesion is surgical excision employing cardiopulmonary bypass. Surgical results are usually quite good, although residual or recurrent obstruction has been noted occasionally.

Supravalvular Aortic Stenosis

Supravalvular aortic stenosis most often occurs as a component of a specific clinical picture, featuring a peculiar characteristic elfin facies, mental retardation, dental abnormalities, and stenosis of both pulmonary and systemic peripheral arteries. The lesion has been related to the syndrome of idiopathic infantile hypercalcemia, a condition of deranged vitamin D metabolism in the fetus and/or mother.

Experimentally, the lesion has been seen in the offspring of pregnant rabbits given excesses of vitamin D. When the metabolic, cardiac, and distinctive phenotypic features coexist, the term supravalvular aortic stenosis syndrome or the Williams syndrome has been applied.

Occasionally, the aortic lesion and pulmonary arterial stenosis are seen as sporadic or familial occurrences without other features of the syndrome. Autosomal dominant transmission with variable expressivity has been noted in some familial cases.

Three major anatomic variants of supravalvular obstruction are seen. An annular constriction at the superior margin of the sinuses of Valsalva, producing an hourglass deformity, is the most common form. Associated thickening of the aortic cusps and adherence of their free margin to the stenotic ridge may be noted. A fibrous or fibromuscular supravalvular diaphragm with small orifice characterizes the membranous type. Least common is diffuse hypoplasia of the entire ascending aorta. Since the obstruction in this lesion is above the origin of the coronary vessels, they are subjected to the same high pressure as the left ventricle. Consequently, the coronary arteries are unusually large, thick-walled, and tortuous, and premature arteriosclerotic changes may be present even in children.

Clinical recognition of this lesion is facilitated in most instances by the typical phenotypic features. The facial resemblance of one to another is striking. Features include prominent forehead, flat nasal bridge with broad nares, epicanthal folds, malformed teeth, and small mandible. Strabismus, prominent upper lip, and some degree of mental retardation are also common. The typical murmur of aortic stenosis is present, but the aortic closure may be unusually prominent, due to the high pressure in the aortic root. In some cases a significantly higher blood pressure is present in the right arm than in the left.

The electrocardiogram usually shows left ventricular hypertrophy, but biventricular or right ventricular hypertrophy may occur when significant stenosis of the pulmonary arterial branches is also present.

Roentgenographic features are nonspecific. Dilatation of the ascending aorta is almost never present. Withdrawal pressure recording from left ventricle to ascending aorta, during cardiac catheterization, demonstrates a systolic pressure gradient just above the aortic valve, and permits evaluation of its hemodynamic severity. The extent and location of the obstruction is further clarified by angiocardiography (Fig. 10-8). Since pulmonary branch stenosis is common, catheterization and angiography of the right heart also should be included.

Surgical therapy is indicated when warranted by the severity of obstruction. Hemodynamic criteria for surgery are similar to those for aortic valvular stenosis. However, surgical relief of this obstruction is technically more difficult, particularly when the ascending aorta is diffusely hypoplastic. Therefore, more careful patient selection is indicated, and surgery may be deferred in asymptomatic patients with less severe degrees of obstruction.

Differential Diagnosis

In the older infants and children, the features of aortic stenosis are usually sufficiently typical to permit clinical diagnosis without difficulty, although the type and severity of outflow obstruction cannot always be certain. Occasionally, the murmur of mild pulmonic stenosis or small ventricular septal defect may mimic that of aortic stenosis. The major problem of differential diagnosis exists in the young infant with critical aortic stenosis in congestive heart failure. Typical clinical findings are often absent in this situation. Weak pulses, absent or atypical murmur, and similar electrocardiographic and roentgenographic features may be seen in infants with aortic atresia, or other variants of the hypoplastic left heart syndrome, primary myocardial disease, and coarctation of the aorta. The hypoplastic left heart can now be excluded with the aid of the echocardiogram, particularly the two-dimensional. Cardiac catheterization and angiography are frequently necessary to clearly define the nature of the problem.

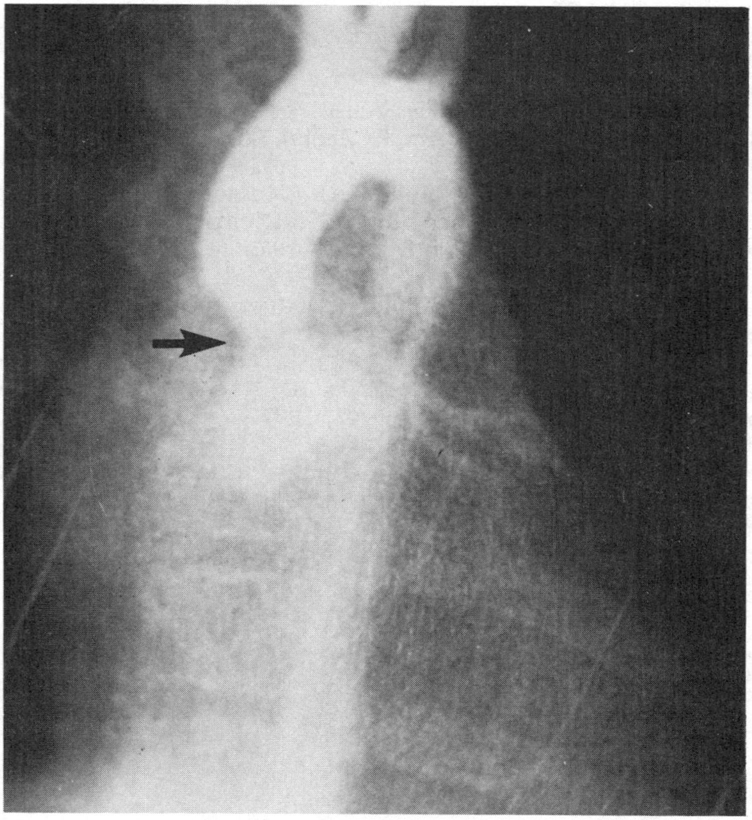

Figure 10–8 Aortogram of patient with supravalvular aortic stenosis. Note the site of obstruction (arrow) just above the aortic valve.

Bibliography

Beuren AJ, Schulze C, Eberle P, Harmjanz Apitz J: Syndrome of supravalvular aortic stenosis, peripheral pulmonary stenosis, mental retardation and similar facial appearance. Am J Cardiol 13:471, 1964.

Campbell M: The natural history of congenital aortic stenosis. Brit Heart J 30: 514, 1968.

Cohen LS, Friedman WF, Braunwald E: Natural history of mild congenital aortic stenosis elucidated by serial hemodynamic studies. Am J Cardiol 30:1, 1972.

Edmunds LH, Wagner HR, Heyman MA: Aortic valvulotomy in neonates. Circulation 61:421, 1980.

El-Said G, Galioto FM Jr, Mullins CE, McNamara DG: Natural hemodynamic history of congenital aortic stenosis in childhood. Am J Cardiol 30:6, 1972.

Friedman WF, Roberts WC: Vitamin D and the supravalvular aortic stenosis syndrome. The transplancental effects of vitamin D on the aorta of the rabbit. Circulation 34:77, 1966.

Jack WD II, Kelly DT: Long-term follow-up of valvulotomy for congenital aortic stenosis. Am J Cardiol 38:231, 1976.

Newfeld EA, Muster AJ, Paul MH, Idriss FS, Riker WL: Discrete subaortic stenosis in childhood. Study of 51 patients. Am J Cardiol 38:53, 1976.

Reis RL, Peterson LM, Mason DT, Simon AL, Morrow AG: Congenital fixed subvalvular aortic stenosis: an anatomical classification and correlations with operative results. Circulation 43 (Suppl. I):I-II, 1970.

Roberts WC: The congenitally bicuspid aortic valve. A study of 85 autopsy cases. Am J Cardiol 26:72, 1970.

Wagner HR, Ellison RC, Keane JF, Humphries JO, Nadas AS: Clinical course in aortic stenosis. Circulation 56 (Suppl. I):I-47, 1977.

Wagner HR, Weidman WH, Ellison RC, Miettinen OS: Indirect assessment of severity in aortic stenosis. Circulation 56 (Suppl. I):I-20, 1977.

Williams JCP, Barrett-Boyes BG, Lowe JB: Supravalvular aortic stenosis. Circulation 24:1311, 1961.

Chapter 11

COARCTATION OF THE AORTA

A localized congenital narrowing of the aortic lumen usually located near the site of the ligamentum arteriosus is referred to as coarctation of the aorta (Fig. 11-1).

Incidence

The defect is common, being noted in about 8% of all congenital cardiovascular malformations. Males are affected predominantly (2:1). It is the most common cardiovascular lesion seen in the Turner syndrome, where it occurs with an incidence of approximately 35%.

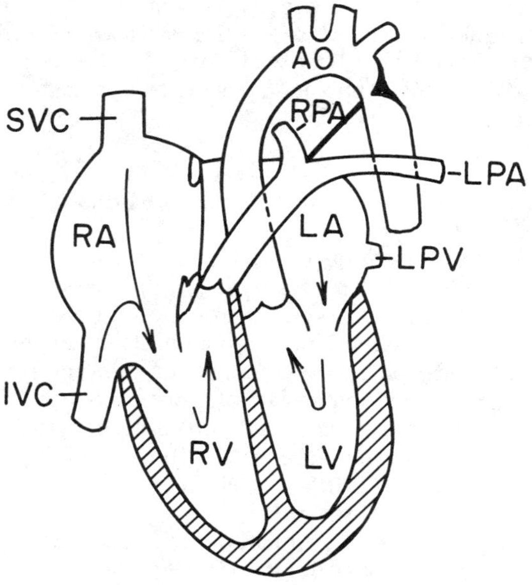

Figure 11-1 Coarctation of the aorta. A discrete intraluminal narrowing of the aorta beyond the origin of the left subclavian artery is present. Intracardiac circulation is normal. SVC - superior vena cava, IVC - inferior vena cava, RA - right atrium, LA - left atrium, RV - right ventricle, LV - left ventricle, AO - aorta, LPA - left pulmonary artery, RPA - right pulmonary artery.

Embryologic and Anatomical Considerations

Various theories to explain this developmental abnormality include constricting fibrosis around the aortic wall related to fibrotic obliteration of the ductus arteriosus, or developmental abnormality of the complex fetal arch system. The precise explanation remains unclear, but recently the concept has been suggested that altered fetal blood flow pathways, resulting from intracardiac malformations, secondarily produce developmental abnormality of various portions of the aortic arch.

Pathologically, the lesion is characterized by thickening of the media of the aortic wall, usually opposite the insertion of the ductus arteriosus, with protrusion into the aortic lumen in a shelflike fashion. Intimal thickening and sclerosis may contribute further to the degree of obstruction which may vary from minimal to near-total occlusion. The external appearance may give no clue as to the severity of internal obstruction. When total occlusion of the involved segment is present, the condition has been referred to as interruption of the aortic arch and has been considered a separate entity by some.

Although usually juxtaductal, the site of obstruction is variable and may occur between the left carotid and left subclavian arteries (rarely more proximally) or in the descending aorta (abdominal coarctation). When juxtaductal, the obstruction is likely to be localized, and associated defects are less common. When the obstruction is complete (interruption of the aortic arch) or characterized by diffuse hypoplasia of the segment between the left subclavian artery and ductus arteriosus (aortic isthmus), major, often complex, cardiovascular anomalies are frequently present. These include large ventricular septal defect, various forms of transposition of the great arteries, double-outlet right ventricle, and endocardial cushion defects. The most frequently associated lesion is bicuspid aortic valve, present in at least 50% of cases. Atrial septal defect, mitral valve anomalies, and other vascular abnormalities such as stenosis, atresia, or aberrancy of the subclavian arteries have been noted.

Hemodynamic Considerations

Coarctation results in resistance to aortic blood flow to the segment distal to the obstruction. Major adaptive mechanisms may be required to maintain adequate perfusion of the lower half of the body. These include elevation of blood pressure in the aortic compartment proximal to the obstruction, bypassing of the obstruction by development of collateral pathways of flow, and arteriolar vasoconstriction to maintain adequate mean perfusion pressure (approximately 55 mmHg) below the coarctation. Collateral pathways include transverse cervical, transverse scapular, intercostal, and internal mammary arteries. Dilatation of intercostal vessels may eventually result in erosion of the inferior rib margins (rib notching), a radiographically important feature in older patients.

The cause of the hypertension associated with coarctation of the aorta has been controversial and not completely understood. The role of both mechanical obstruction imposed by the coarcted segment and humoral features related to reduced pulsatile renal arterial flow have been considered. Multiple factors, both mechanical and humoral, may be involved.

Clinical Manifestations

Clinical features depend on severity of the obstruction, development of compensatory mechanisms, and presence of associated defects.

Coarctation in Childhood

In most instances coarctation produces no symptoms in the young infant, and the lesion is recognized incidentally during a routine childhood physical examination. A cardiac murmur or systolic hypertension in the upper extremities is the usual presenting feature. Occasionally, a history of headaches, leg muscle cramps, epistaxis, or exertional fatigue may be noted.

Normal growth and development are usually present. Cardiac examination reveals minimal or no left chest prominence, but the left ventricular apical impulse may be forceful, particularly if hypertension is present. A precordial thrill is usually absent, but a thrill in the suprasternal notch is common. On auscultation, the first heart sound may be accentuated if hypertension is present. Occasionally, a systolic ejection click at the apex and mildleft sternal border may suggest associated aortic valve abnormality.

A murmur is almost always audible but of variable character and intensity. A harsh systolic murmur peaking rather late in systole, representing flow across the stenotic site, may be heard maximally in the left upper back. Infrequently, a continuous murmur may occur at the coarcted site if the lumen is extremely small, but continuous bruits related to flow in collateral arterial vessels around the left shoulder and chest wall are not unusual. Systolic murmurs related to mitral regurgitation or aortic stenosis are not infrequent and, at times, auscultation may be dominated by the murmurs of other associated intracardiac lesions, such as ventricular septal defect.

The most characteristic feature of the examination is the discrepancy in blood pressures and pulses between the upper and lower extremities. Simple palpation, *simultaneously* of brachial and femoral pulses, may give an immediate clue to the presence of coarctation. Femoral pulses typically are delayed, weak, or absent; rarely are they normal. Comparison of both brachial pulses likewise may reveal a discrepancy suggesting subclavian artery stenosis or aberrant origin below the coarctation.

Blood pressure measurement in upper and lower extremities, using cuffs of appropriate dimensions, reveals higher systolic pressure in the arms, but diastolic pressures may be approximately equal. Significantly, not all patients, particularly younger ones, have true hypertension in the upper compartment. It is the disparity — the presence of relative hypertension in the upper compartment — that is important. However, true hypertension is seen with increasing frequency after 5 years of age, is present almost always after 10 years of age and, in some cases, may be severe.

Electrocardiogram

Electrocardiographic changes vary with severity of the lesion and associated malformations, and may be normal in uncomplicated cases without significant hypertension. Left ventricular hypertrophy of variable degree is the most common abnormality. Severe hypertrophy with left ventricular strain pattern should suggest a complicating problem, such as aortic stenosis.

Radiologic Features

Radiologic examination of the chest may be unremarkable, but older children are likely to show left ventricular prominence. Pulmonary vascularity is normal in the absence of complicating problems. The ascending aorta and aortic knob may appear dilated, and an indentation of the aorta just below the knob (coarcted site) with poststenotic dilatation of the descending aorta ("figure 3") may sometimes be seen along the left border of the spine (Fig. 11-2). The reverse of this configuration ("figure E") can be visualized as impressions on the barium-filled esophagus. Tortuous, dilated collateral intercostal arteries may produce erosion of the inferior rib margins (see Fig. 2-67, p. 98). This notching is characteristic, but not pathognomic of coarctation of the aorta. It is usually asymmetrical and confined to the posterior middle one-third of the fourth through the eighth ribs. The finding is not consistently present and is infrequently seen under 8 years of age.

Echocardiographic Findings

In the face of severe obstruction with significant upper body hypertension, the M-mode echocardiogram may reveal concentric left ventricular hypertrophy. A frequently associated bicuspid aortic valve may be identified by both M-mode and two-dimensional techniques (Fig. 2-76B). Utilizing the latter technique, the aortic arch and its branches may be imaged by placing the transducer in the suprasternal notch and directing it caudally and slightly posteriorly. It may be possible to image the coarctation of the aorta directly in this manner.

Cardiac Catheterization

Although coarctation of the aorta can be diagnosed clinically with confidence, the great frequency of associated malformations suggest that cardiac catheterization should be performed in every case. Opinion differs regarding this point,

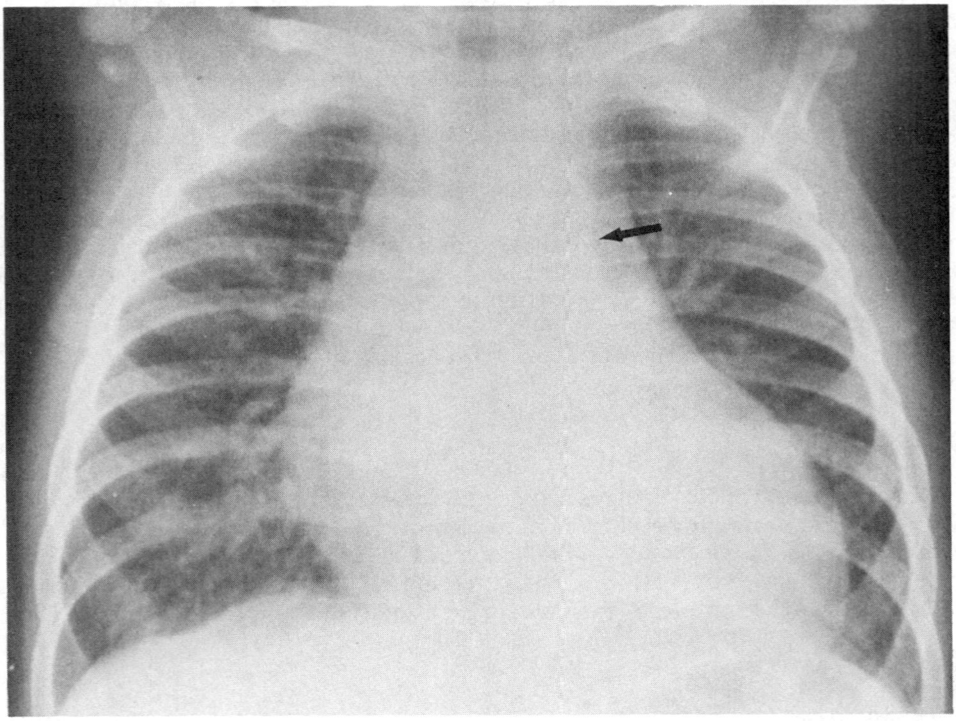

Figure 11-2 Chest roentgenogram of older infant with coarctation of the aorta. Cardiomegaly with left ventricular contour is present. Note indentation of aorta (arrow) suggesting figure 3 sign.

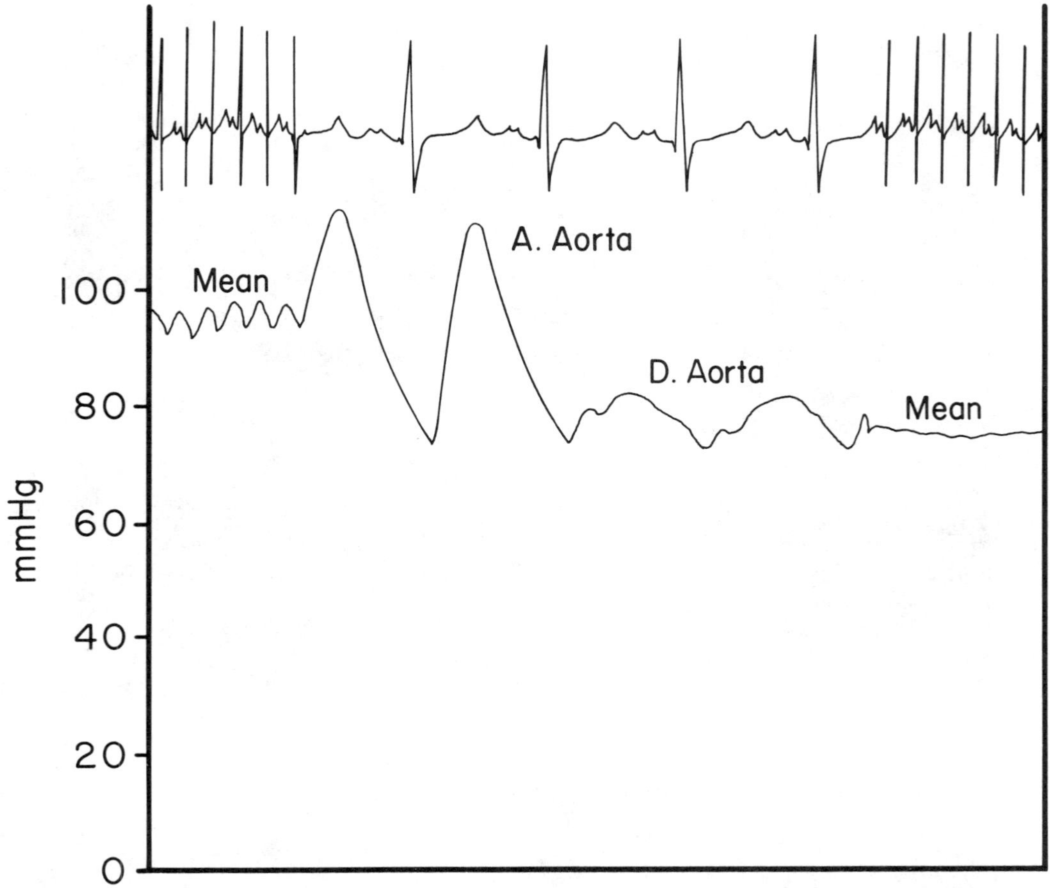

Figure 11-3 Pressure curve in ascending aorta (A. Aorta) and descending aorta (D. Aorta) above and below coarctation. Note rounded slow-rising curve below the obstruction with very narrow pulse pressure primarily due to damping of systolic pressure. Diastolic pressures above and below are equal.

however, except in the symptomatic young infant where complicating lesions are almost always present. In isolated coarctation, right heart catheterization usually reveals no abnormalities, but mild elevation of pulmonary arterial pressure and wedge pressure may be seen. Left heart catheterization may be achieved in some instances via a patent foramen ovale, but often requires the retrograde approach through the brachial or femoral artery. Systolic pressure in the left ventricle and ascending aorta are equal, and exceed that in the aorta distal to the coarcted segment. Diastolic pressures, however, are approximately equal. Proximal to the obstruction, the pulse pressure is wide, while distally the pressure curve exhibits a slow rise to a low, rounded peak resulting in a narrow pulse pressure of "sawtooth" configuration. It is this damped pulse pressure that is responsible for the weak or absent arterial pulses in the lower extremities (Fig. 11-3).

Angiographic visualization of the coarcted area by left ventricular or aortic root injection permits assessment of the site and extent of the obstruction as well as the adequacy of collateral arterial pathways (Fig. 11-4). The latter is a particularly important consideration in surgical correction of some patients.

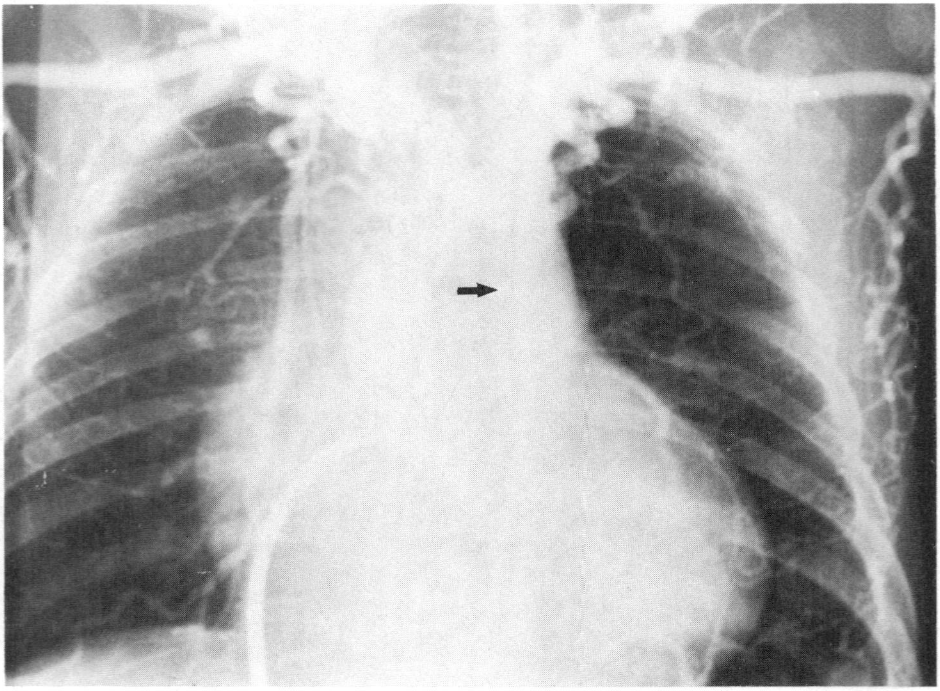

Figure 11-4 Angiogram of patient with severe aortic coarctation. The catheter advanced to the left ventricle by way of the foramen ovale. A discrete coarctation is seen (arrow). Note the extensive tortuous collateral arterial vessels.

Course and Prognosis

Most patients with simple coarctation are asymptomatic in the first two decades. Hypertension appears to progress through puberty, and related complications — cerebrovascular accidents, hypertensive encephalopathy, cerebral or aortic aneurysms — increase with age. Early operation may obviate many of these complications. However, persistent abnormal resistance in the vascular compartment, proximal to the coarctation, has been demonstrated in patients operated on as young as 5 years of age, suggesting that vascular damage in this lesion may be initiated at a very early age. The average age of survival without surgery is about 35 years. Death usually results from complications of hypertensive cardiovascular disease, intracranial bleed, or from bacterial endocarditis.

Treatment

Treatment of this lesion is surgical excision of the coarcted segment. Closure of a patent ductus, if present, is achieved at the same time. In most instances, anastomosis of the proximal and distal aortic segments can be accomplished, but if this is not feasible, insertion of an aortic graft may be necessary.

Recently, a repair employing a subclavian artery flap turned down to form the new anterior wall of the aorta at the site of the coarctation has been performed with great success (Fig. 11-5). The advantage of this procedure is that the posterior wall of the aorta remains intact supposedly allowing for better growth.

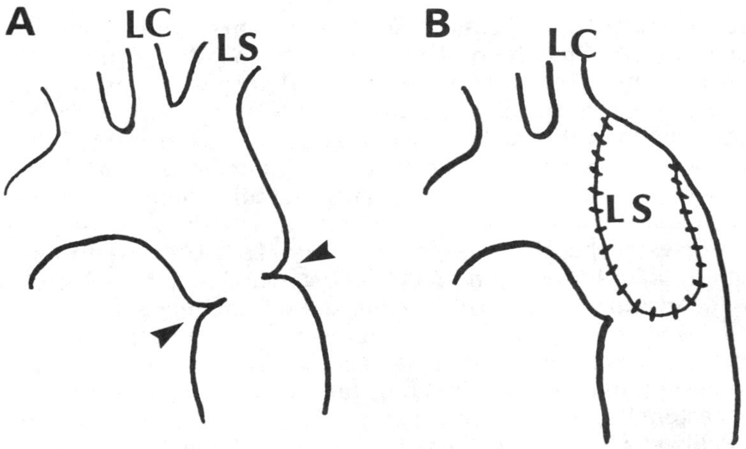

Figure 11–5 (A) Coarctation of the aorta (arrow heads). (B) The same aorta following repair with the subclavian flap. The subclavian artery is isolated, resected distally, opened longitudinally with an incision that continues down along the anterior wall of the aorta through the coarctation. The open subclavian artery is then turned down and sewn in place. LC - left carotid, LS - left subclavian.

Although opinions vary, the optimal age for elective repair is considered by many to be around 3-5 years. Circumstances may dictate earlier or somewhat later correction. Fatal cardiovascular complications appear to occur more frequently when hypertension has been longstanding and surgical correction delayed beyond 25 years of age.

Postoperative complications include hemorrhage, paradoxical hypertension, and necrotizing mesenteric arteritis. Postoperative hypertension of variable degree is seen in perhaps 50% of patients. This appears to be characterized by two phases. The first, occurring within 24 hr postoperatively, is apparently related to augmented sympathetic tone and is predominantly systolic in nature. The second phase occurs on the second to third day after surgery with more significant elevation of diastolic pressure, and appears to be a result of increased plasma renin-angiotensin activity. Both of these mechanisms may be active in the production of the postcoarctectomy syndrome which is seen in almost one-fifth of postoperative cases. This syndrome usually appears around the fourth day after surgery and is characterized by significant hypertension, abdominal pain, fever, vomiting, and leukocytosis. More severe cases may develop a necrotizing mesenteric arteritis. Most cases respond to conservative management with antihypertensive and bowel decompression. However, bowel infarction requiring surgical resection can occur, and occasional fatalities result.

Coarctation in Infancy

Isolated coarctation rarely presents in the neonate. Symptomatic coarctation at this age almost always is complicated by intracardiac anomalies, resulting in the early appearance of congestive heart failure. Except for the hypoplastic left heart complex in the first week, coarctation of the aorta is the most common cause of congestive heart failure in the first month of life. The usual manifestations of left ventricular failure in the infant — tachypnea, dyspnea, diaphoresis, tachycardia, feeding difficulty, and dusky pallor — are typical findings. Pulmonary rales and hepatomegaly may be present and, occasionally, peripheral edema may be noted. Cardiac auscultation may reveal a gallop rhythm, but murmurs are variable. A systolic regurgitant murmur along the left sternal border is commonly present, suggesting mitral insufficiency or associated ventricular septal defect. An ejection systolic murmur or a continuous murmur of associated patent ductus arteriosus may be present, and an apical mid-diastolic rumble is noted not infrequently. The second sound is usually narrowly split with an accentuated pulmonic component. Pulses in the upper extremities are often full. Right and left arm pulses are equal, unless the origin of the left subclavian artery is stenosed or the right subclavian originates aberrantly from the descending aorta. Femoral pulses and leg blood pressure in the neonate with coarctation may be variable, reflecting the status of the pulmonary vascular bed and patency of the ductus arteriosus. Typically, femoral pulses are weak and of late onset compared to the brachial pulse and, occasionally, may be impalpable. Systolic blood pressure in the upper extremities is always higher than that in the legs, although upper extremity blood pressure is not always significantly elevated above normal. Differences in systolic blood pressure in upper and lower extremities are more difficult to evaluate in the very young infant, since normally higher pressures in the upper extremities are present up to 9 months of age. Therefore, only values 20 mmHg or more above those obtained in the legs should be considered significant in this age group.

Electrocardiogram

The electrocardiogram of the young infant with simple coarctation is variable. Biventricular hypertrophy is common in infants in congestive heart failure, but isolated left ventricular hypertrophy is unusual at this age (Fig. 11-6). Right ventricular hypertrophy may be related to pulmonary congestion and secondary pulmonary hypertension, or to pulmonary hypertension secondary to communication of the pulmonary artery with the systemic circuit by way of a large ductus below the coarctation.

Radiologic Features

The chest roentgenogram usually reveals generalized cardiomegaly and pulmonary hypervascularity, due to pulmonary venous congestion and/or arterial engorgement if a left-to-right shunt coexists.

Echocardiographic Findings

Manifestations of associated lesions will dominate the echocardiographic picture in this group of patients. In the presence of an associated left-to-right shunt, one will generally see dilatation of the left heart. Left ventricular performance may be assessed as described previously in the M-mode recording. A bicuspid aortic valve may be identified, and occasionally in the newborn direct visualization of the coarctation via the suprasternal notch approach may be feasible.

Cardiac Catheterization

Cardiac catheterization findings are similar to those noted in older patients. Pulmonary artery and right ventricular pressures are normal or modestly elevated, unless a large left-to-right shunt is present. Complicating lesions are common and may be clinically silent. Therefore, evaluation of left heart structures is important in symptomatic infants, particularly if early surgical intervention is anticipated.

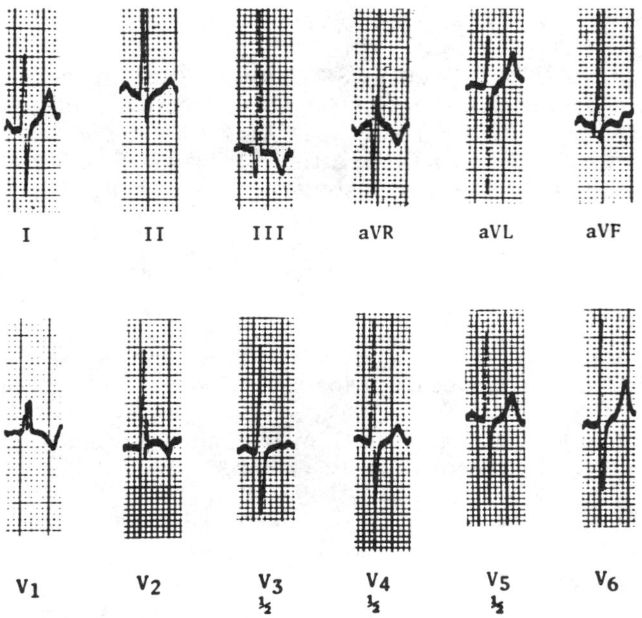

Figure 11-6 Electrocardiogram of an 8-month-old infant with severe uncomplicated coarctation of the aorta. Voltage changes suggest biventricular hypertrophy.

Treatment

Symptomatic neonates and young infants with coarctation initially should receive intensive medical management. The small minority having only solitary coarctation is likely to show satisfactory improvement, while those with major complicating lesions often respond poorly to medical management alone. Those infants not responding to vigorous medical therapy within a few days should undergo surgical correction of the coarctation. Associated malformations may require additional corrective or palliative procedures. Survival of 60-75% of these infants can be expected, but past experience suggests 25%, or perhaps more, will eventually require reoperation for recurrent obstruction. Newer operative techniques may reduce this figure significantly, however.

Differential Diagnosis

The differential diagnosis of coarctation of the aorta should present no problem if assessment of pulses and blood pressure in upper and lower extremities is a consistent part of every pediatric physical examination.

In the very young infant presenting with congestive heart failure, accurate assessment of pulses and blood pressure initially can be difficult, and other conditions, such as severe aortic stenosis, primary myocardial disease, or hypoplastic left heart complex, may enter into consideration. Reevaluation after anticongestive therapy is, therefore, important. At times, associated malformations, such as ventricular septal defect or more complex malformations (transposition of the great arteries) may dominate the clinical picture.

Bibliography

Connors JP, Hartmann AF Jr, Weldon CS: Considerations in the surgical management of infantile coarctation of the aorta. Am J Cardiol 36:489, 1975.

Maron BJ, Humphries JO, Rowe RD, Mellitis ED: Prognosis of surgically corrected coarctation of the arota: A 20-year postoperative appraisal. Circulation 47:119, 1973.

Nanton MA, Olley PM: Residual hypertension after coarctectomy in children. Am J Cardol 37:769, 1976.

Rocchini AP, Rosenthal A, Barger AC, Castaneda AR, Nadas AS: Pathogenesis of parodoxical hypertension after coarctation resection. Circulation 54:382, 1976.

Rudolph AM, Heyman MA, Spitznas U: Hemodynamic considerations in the development of narrowing of the aorta. Am J Cardiol 30:514, 1972.

Samanek M, Goetzova J, Fiserova J, Skovranek J: Differences in muscle blood flow in upper and lower extremities of patients after correction of coarctation of the aorta. Circulation 54:377, 1976.

Shinebourne EA, Elseed AM: Relation between fetal blood flow patterns, coarctation of the aorta and pulmonary blood flow. Brit Heart J 36:492, 1974.

Sinha SN, Kardatzke ML, Cole RB, Muster AJ, Wessel HU, Paul MH: Coarctation of the aorta in infancy. Circulation 40:385, 1969.

Chapter 12

TETRALOGY OF FALLOT

Tetralogy of Fallot is a cyanotic congenital cardiac abnormality classically encompassing four components (Fig. 12-1).

1. Large ventricular septal defect
2. Severe pulmonic stenosis
3. Aortic override of the ventricular septum
4. Right ventricular hypertrophy

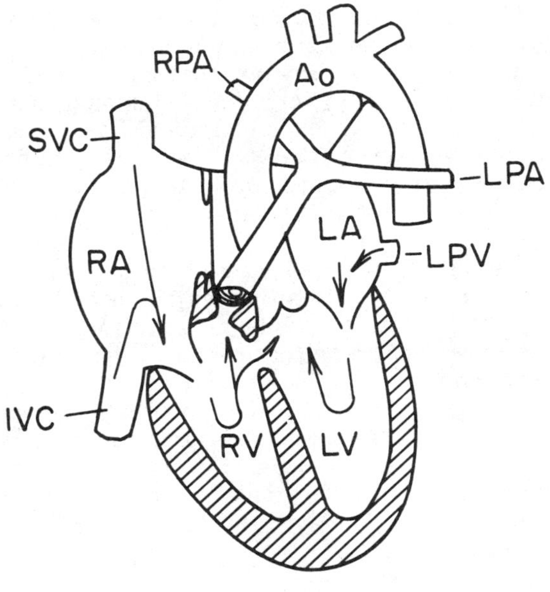

Figure 12-1 Circulation in tetralogy of Fallot. Infundibular and valvular pulmonic stenosis result in right-to-left shunting across the large ventricular septal defect. SVC - superior vena cava, IVC - inferior vena cava, RA - right atrium, LA - left atrium, RV - right ventricle, LV - left ventricle, Ao - aorta, RPA - right pulmonary artery, LPA - left pulmonary artery, LPV - left pulmonary vein.

Incidence

Tetralogy of Fallot is one of the most common cyanotic congenital heart defects. In most large patient series, tetralogy ranks fourth or fifth among all congenital cardiac malformations with an incidence of 10%. It is the most frequent cyanotic cardiac anomaly found in patients surviving infancy. In cyanotic neonates, tetralogy of Fallot is encountered less often than in transposition of the great arteries and, when seen at this age, is commonly associated with severe pulmonic stenosis or atresia.

Embryology and Anatomy

The embryological development of this defect is still not completely understood. The earlier concept that unequal septation of the truncus arteriosus by the developing spiral septum results in a large aortic and a small pulmonary component has been disputed. A more recent hypothesis relates the abnormality to diffuse underdevelopment of the subpulmonic conus with abnormal orientation and hypertrophy of the crista supraventricularis (infundibular stenosis). Faulty alignment of the crista (pariental band) to the ventricular septum and septal band prevents closure of the interventricular foramen (VSD). According to this concept, underdevelopment of the pulmonary artery, enlargement of the aorta, right ventricular hypertrophy, and a ductus arteriosus of somewhat reduced size are the secondary results of altered hemodynamics.

Infundibular obstruction is almost invariably present with or without additional obstruction at the pulmonic valve or beyond (stenotic or hypoplastic pulmonary artery and/or pulmonary branches). The obstruction typically is severe, and in extreme cases, atresia of the pulmonic valve and pulmonary arterial trunk exists. Uncommonly, there is congenital absence of the pulmonic valve, resulting in severe pulmonic regurgitation and aneurysmal dilatation of the pulmonary arteries. Segmental stenosis of one or both pulmonary branches, at their origin, may occur; and rarely is congenital absence of the left branch seen.

The ventricular septal defect is typically large, subcristal in location, and somewhat more anterior than usual. In size it approximates that of the aortic orifice, and offers free communication between the ventricles and between the right ventricle and aortic root. The aortic root is large, anteriorly displaced, and overrides the septal plane by as much as 75%, a feature not of great hemodynamic importance. A right aortic arch is present in approximately one-fourth of cases, and in some patients, atrial septal defect coexists (pentalogy of Fallot). Of surgical importance is the occasional presence of a major coronary branch crossing the right ventricular outflow tract at the usual site of ventriculotomy for surgical repair. The right ventricle is heavily trabeculated and hypertrophied, a result of increased pressure work.

Hemodynamics

Although four components are classically ascribed to tetralogy of Fallot, the hemodynamic alterations are basically dominated by the severity of right ventricular outflow obstruction. Usually of less relative importance are the size of the septal defect, the level of systemic vascular resistance, and phasic differences in pressure changes in the two ventricles.

The obstruction to right ventricular outflow results in a systolic pressure gradient between right ventricle and pulmonary artery, with right ventricular systolic hypertension and normal or low pulmonary artery pressures. Typically, the pulmonic stenosis is of sufficient severity that resistance to flow into the pulmonary artery exceeds resistance to flow into the aorta, via the large VSD. As a result, the right ventricle is required to generate abnormally high pressure, the level of which is limited by aortic outflow resistance. Systolic pressures in the right ventricle, left ventricle, and aorta are, therefore, essentially equal. This limitation of pressure workload on the right ventricle in tetralogy is one reason for the rare incidence of congestive heart failure. In contrast, the right ventricular pressure burden resulting from comparably severe pulmonic stenosis with intact ventricular septum might induce right ventricular pressure considerably in excess of systemic, and congestive failure is not uncommon.

The volume and direction of ventricular shunting in tetralogy, basically, is a function of the severity of the pulmonic stenosis. Less severe stenosis may allow primarily left-to-right shunting with a small right-to-left component and minimal systemic arterial unsaturation (precyanotic or pink tetralogy), while more severe stenosis produces predominent right-to-left shunting with severe unsaturation. The pulmonic stenosis represents essentially fixed obstruction which may increase relatively, or absolutely, in severity. In either case, the result is limitation of pulmonary blood flow in response to growth or exertion. Eventually, some patients may develop extensive bronchial arterial collateral flow which may achieve levels up to 2.0 $L/min/m^2$.

As pulmonary blood flow (and pulmonary venous return) is reduced by increasing severity of pulmonic stenosis, the magnitude of right-to-left shunt is increased. Since systemic arterial saturation is a function of the relative proportions of unsaturated (right-to-left shunt) and saturated (pulmonary venous) blood ejected into the aorta (mixing site) by the right and left ventricles, respectively, the severity of pulmonic stenosis plays a major role in the intensity of arterial unsaturation and clinical manifestations and hypoxia.

Manifestations

Approximately one-third of neonates with tetralogy are intensely cyanotic at birth or shortly thereafter, but a lesser degree of cyanosis is apparent at birth in about one-half of cases. Cyanosis at birth usually indicates the most severe form of the defect (pulmonic atresia or severe stenosis) with a closed or constricted ductus of insufficient size to maintain an adequate pulmonary blood flow. A murmur in such cases may be absent, of soft, nonspecific, pulmonary ejection quality, or continuous (suggesting patency of the ductus). In some infants, closure of the ductus may result in rapidly progressive cyanosis and hypoxia. Cyanosis developing more slowly with age may reflect increasing severity of outflow obstruction. Occasionally, cyanosis may be inapparent until 6 months of age or later.

Early manifestations of hypoxia include mild resting tachypnea, followed by fatigue, dyspnea, and hyperpnea with exertion. Cyanosis may intensify with activity and with crying or straining. More severe hypoxia may result in apparent delay of motor development. In the child who has begun to walk, squatting following exertion may become a prominent clinical feature. This posture is an acquired phenomenon in which physiologic changes leading to increased arterial oxygen saturation have been clearly demonstrated. Basically, the squatting posture imposes mechanical vascular impedance, resulting in increased systemic arterial resistance and reduced venous return from the lower extremities. The net effect is transient reduction of right-to-left shunting and increased pulmonary blood flow leading to improved systemic arterial saturation. Although common in younger children, squatting is usually abandoned by older children because of social pressures. Acute attacks of intense cyanosis and hyperpnea are a more serious hypoxic manifestation in tetralogy of Fallot, but are not limited to this specific cyanotic defect (see Chap. 4 for further discussion of hyperpneic spells).

Infants with milder forms of the defect may exhibit minimal or absent cyanosis in the early months after birth. Cyanosis, and accompanying symptoms of effort dyspnea and hyperpnea, appear near the end of the first year and progress with age. Paroxysmal hyperpneic spells are less common and less severe, but squatting with exertion is frequent after the age of walking. Impairment of physical activity varies from mild to severe.

Physical examination typically reveals a cyanotic patient with mild-to-moderate hyperpnea at rest. Patients with less severe arterial unsaturation may lack truly cyanotic coloration, but may demonstrate a reddish, plethoric appearance of the terminal digits, cheeks, ear lobes, and other sites of high-capillary density. Although uncommon in young infants, clubbing of the digits is characteristic in older infants and children. Clubbing is characterized by convex deformation of the nails with elevation of the base of the nail and broadening of the terminal portion of the digits. Early changes, best seen in the thumbs, consist of loss of fine wrinkling of the skin overlying the base of the nail.

Cardiac examination reveals a relatively quiet precordium with little or no precordial prominence. The dominant impulse is represented by the right ventricle at the lower left sternal border or xiphoid area. A systolic thrill, usually not intense, may be palpable along the midleft sternal border. A stenotic systolic murmur at the pulmonic area is almost always present, but is lacking in neonates with pulmonary atresia. The intensity varies inversely with the severity of outflow obstruction. The character of this murmur differs from that of pulmonic stenosis with intact ventricular septum by its earlier systolic peaking and more uniform intensity during systole.

Significant variation in the intensity of the murmur may occur during alterations in the patient's physiologic state. A usually loud stenotic murmur may diminish or even disappear during an acute hyperpneic spell when flow across the obstructive outflow tract is greatly decreased. The first heart sound is often prominent, and the second sound single represented only the aortic component. If audible, the pulmonic component is muffled and late. Typically, S_2 is louder with more severe degrees of infundibular hypoplasia (stenosis) because of the greater degree of aortic overriding that is present. Occasionally, a systolic ejection click related to the dilated ascending aorta is present. Pulses are normal or slightly prominent.

Electrocardiogram

Electrocardiography reveals right axis deviation and right ventricular hypertrophy of variable severity (Fig. 12-2). In those with milder degrees of pulmonic stenosis and predominent left-to-right shunt, biventricular hypertrophy is occasionally seen.

Echocardiography

Echocardiographic features of tetralogy of Fallot are somewhat similar to those seen in truncus arteriosus and include apparent breakup of septal continuity with the

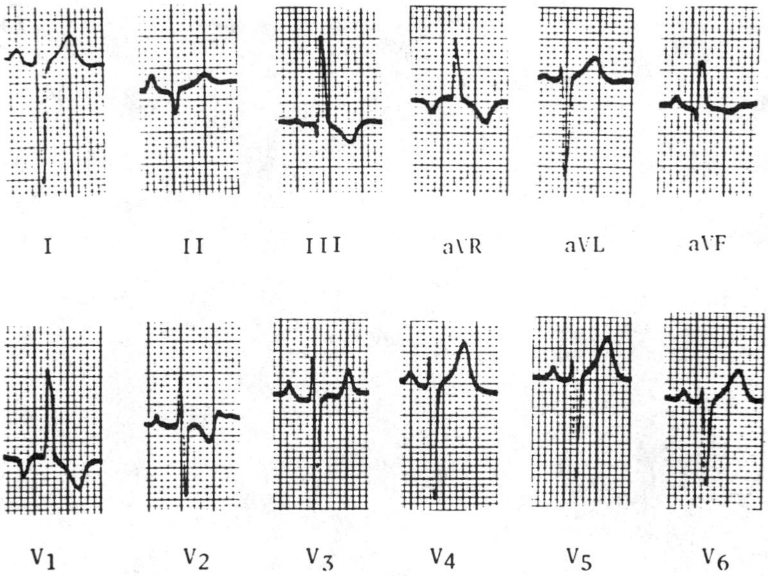

Figure 12–2 Electrocardiogram of child with tetralogy of Fallot showing right axis deviation and right ventricular hypertrophy characteristic of this defect.

anterior aortic wall in conjunction with anterior displacement of a dilated aortic root (overriding) but with maintenance of mitral-aortic continuity. Usually, however, the aorta is much larger in truncus and left atrial enlargement more likely. Unless atretic, the pulmonic valve can usually be demonstrated in tetralogy but not in truncus, a major distinguishing feature.

Radiologic Features

Chest roentgenogram demonstrates a normal cardiac size with rounded, uplifted apex suggesting a right ventricular contour. The left upper cardiac border is concave, with deficiency of the main pulmonary artery segment. Hilar vessels are relatively small, and peripheral vasculature is diminished. A somewhat reticular vascular pattern may be seen in those with bronchial collateral circulation. The ascending aorta and aortic knob may appear prominent, and in approximately 25% the aortic arch is on the right (Fig. 12-3).

Cardiac Catheterization

Cardiac catheterization and angiocardiography are essential for complete evaluation of the patient with tetralogy of Fallot, in anticipation of surgical intervention. Of particular importance are the anatomy of the obstructive outflow tract, adequacy of the pulmonary arteries, size of the ventricular chambers, presence of unusual muscle bundles of the right ventricle, and possible abnormal coronary artery distribution over the infundibulum.

Mean right atrial pressure is usually within normal range, although prominent A waves may be present in the phasic curve. Right ventricular systolic pressure is equal to that in the left ventricle and aorta. The pressure curve contour is nearly identical to that of the left ventricle, in contrast to isolated pulmonic stenosis in

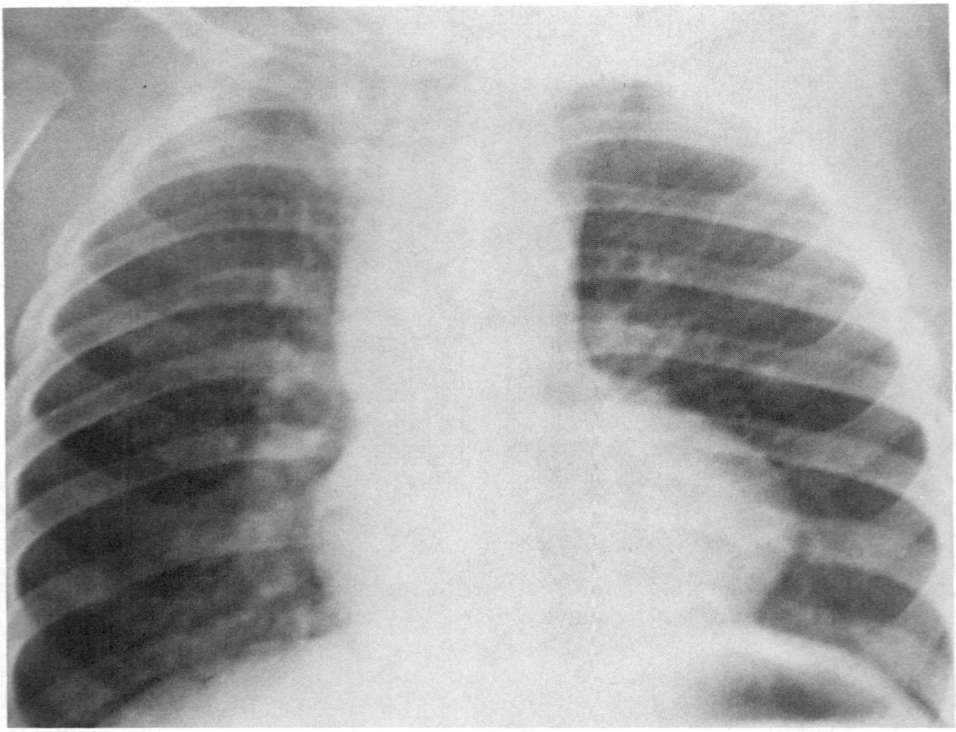

Figure 12–3 Roentgenogram of infant with tetralogy of Fallot. The heart is small, apex uplifted with right ventricular contour, and a concavity at the site of the pulmonary artery is seen. Pulmonary vessels are peripherally reduced. Note prominent aorta.

which the upstroke is slightly delayed, the curve is more triangular, and the peak may exceed systemic pressures. Pulmonary artery pressure is usually low, the pulse pressure narrow, and withdrawal from pulmonary artery to right ventricle demonstrates a systolic gradient often at both valvular and infundibular sites.

Frequently, the catheter passes from right ventricle into the ascending aorta via the ventricular septal defect, permitting selective aortography to evaluate coronary distribution and anatomy of the vessels arising from the arch. In infants, particularly, the foramen ovale may be transversed, allowing evaluation of left heart pressures, saturations, and selective left ventricular angiography.

Left atrial saturation is normal in the absence of right-to-left shunting across the atrial septum. Left ventricular saturation is usually similar to that of the left atrium since the right-to-left ventricular shunt is directed predominantly into the aorta. Aortic saturation represents a mixture of output from both ventricles. Consequently, the actual level of saturation is influenced by total pulmonary blood flow and the volume of right-to-left shunt, and may range from 90–30% or less. Aortic saturation generally is greater than that in the right ventricle but less than that in the left ventricle. Typically, mixed systemic venous saturation is low with no evidence of left-to-right shunt. A mild respiratory alkalosis related to persistent hyperventilation is not uncommon.

Patients with less severe pulmonary stenosis may demonstrate near-normal mixed systemic venous saturation with evidence of variable left-to-right shunt into the right ventricle. Pulmonary blood flow is correspondingly greater, and less severe arterial unsaturation is present.

Angiographic studies with contrast injection into the right ventricle typically reveal a heavily trabeculated chamber which is slightly dilated. Almost simultaneously, both aorta and pulmonary artery opacify. The size and location of the ventricular septal defect usually is well defined by the right-to-left shunt which frequently opacifies the left ventricle, as well. The infundibulum usually appears narrow along its entire length, but an infundibular chamber may be present in some cases. Often, the infundibulum appears dynamic with almost total systolic obliteration. The pulmonic annulus varies from normal size to severe hypoplasia, and the pulmonic valve is thickened and stenotic. The pulmonary trunk and branches also may appear locally stenotic or diffusely hypoplastic (Fig. 12-4). The newer angled or axial projections have contributed greatly to the preoperative evaluation of the anatomy of tetralogy. The right ventricular outflow tract is best seen in the elongated right anterior oblique view, which is a 30° right anterior oblique projection combined with a 30° cephalocaudad angulation (Fig. 12-5). The VSD is evaluated following right ventricular injection of contrast medium in the long axis (60° LAO - 30° craniocaudad) or hepatoclavicular (45° LAO - 30° craniocaudad) projections. Finally, the structure of the pulmonary arteries can be clearly demonstrated by injection of contrast into the right ventricular outflow tract or main pulmonary artery in the PA projection with 45° cephalocaudad angulation. If not demonstrated otherwise, aortography may be necessary to assess the coronary arterial distribution and vessels arising from the arch.

Course and Prognosis

Infants with tetralogy of Fallot follow a variable course depending on severity of the lesion. Those with pulmonary atresia or severe stenosis may succumb early from profound hypoxia unless subjected to surgical intervention. Rarely do they survive the first year of life. The occasional such infant surviving into the second year may develop extensive bronchial collateral circulation, sufficient to maintain a severely compromised existence for several years. Intense cyanosis, severe polycythemia, and exercise intolerance are charactersitic, and survival beyond the second decade is unusual.

Less severely affected infants are more typical of the lesion, with cyanosis appearing later, during the first year of life. In some, hypoxic spells appear after the first few months, while others remain relatively symptom-free until the age of walking, when exertional dyspnea, fatigue, and squatting appear. Cyanosis and polycythemia are present in variable severity, and survival may extend into the third decade. Those with mildest affliction, so-called pink tetralogy, may remain acyanotic until mid-childhood or later. Symptoms with exertion are minimal, and survival into the third or fourth decades may occur.

Complications associated with tetralogy of Fallot are those that may potentially occur with any cyanotic defect with right-to-left shunting. These include severe polycythemia, brain abscess, bacterial endocarditis, thrombotic episodes, and hemorrhagic disorders.

Treatment

Management of the patient with tetralogy of Fallot is influenced by age, severity of the lesion, and clinical course, and includes both medical and surgical

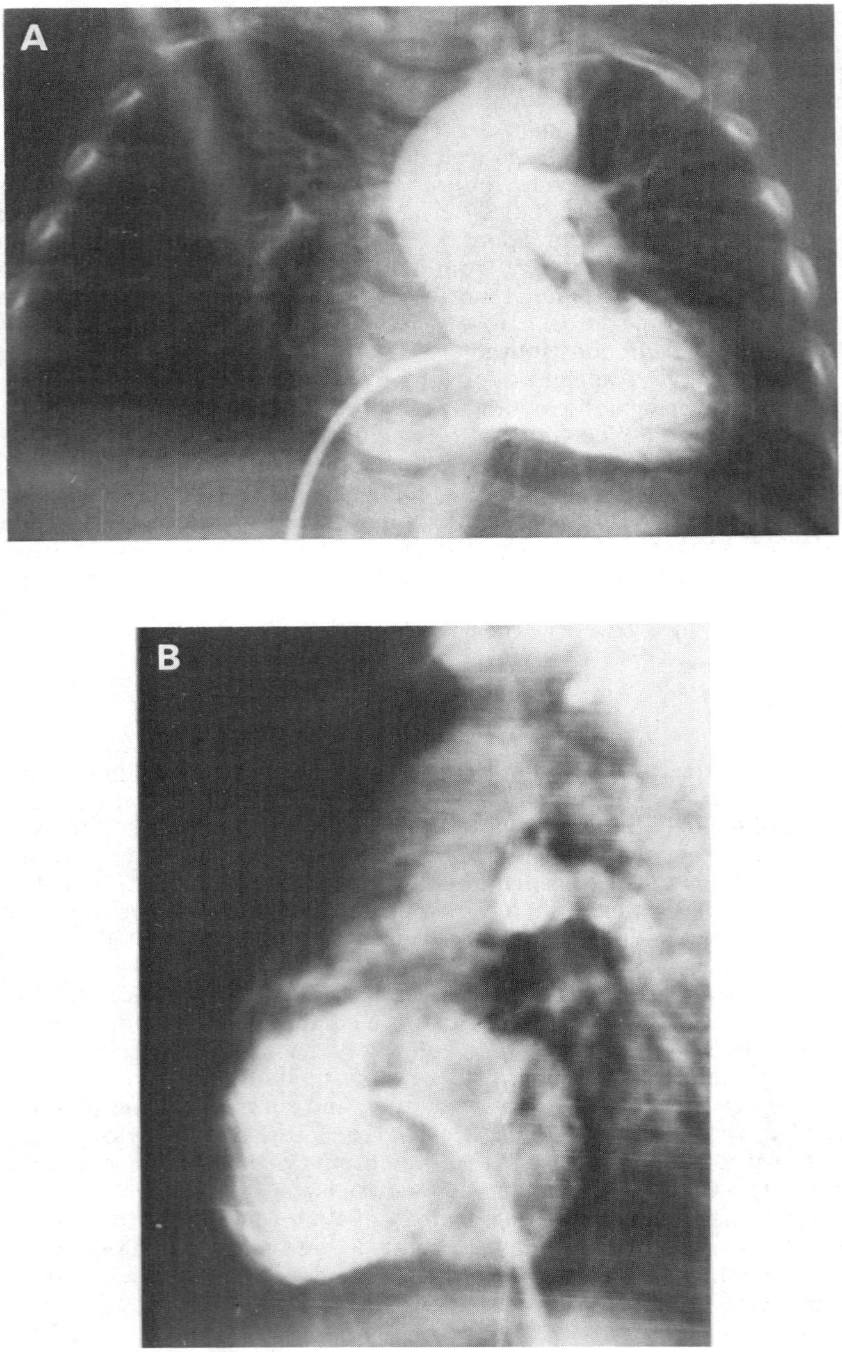

Figure 12–4 Tetralogy of Fallot, right ventricular angiogram. (A) In the frontal view both ventricles and both great arteries opacify almost simultaneously. The aorta is considerably enlarged. The pulmonary trunk is small, and severe infundibular and valvular stenosis is present. Pulmonary vessels opacify poorly. (B) Lateral view. Both ventricles are opacified from the right ventricular injection, and the large aorta overrides the ventricular septum.

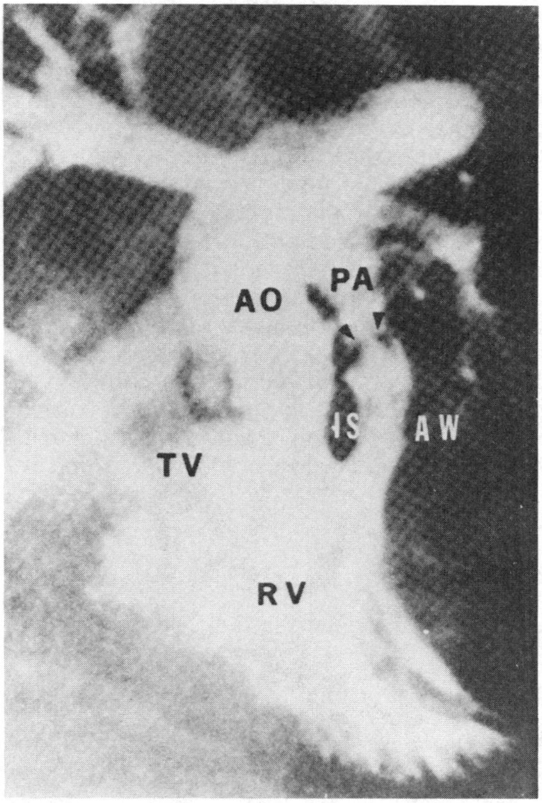

Figure 12-5 Right ventricular injection, elongated right anterior oblique view in tetralogy of Fallot. In this projection the stenotic pulmonic valve (arrows) as well as the diffuse infundibular narrowing immediately beneath the valve are well demonstrated. Right-to-left shunting through the ventricular septal defect with opacification of the aorta is also seen. Ao - ascending aorta, TV - tricuspid valve, RV - right ventricle, IS - infundibular septum, AW - right ventricular anterior wall, PA - main pulmonary artery. (Reproduced from Soto et al.: Tetralogy of Fallot: An angiographic-pathologic correlative study. Circulation, Volume 64, September, 1981, by permission of the American Heart Association, Inc.)

considerations. Pertinent aspects of medical management include treatment of acute hypoxic spells, close observation for evidence of increasing hypoxia, maintenance of an optimum hemoglobin level (Chap. 4), and bacterial endocarditis prophylaxis.

Antibiotics for the prophylaxis of bacterial endocarditis should be administered in accordance with current recommendations (Chap. 26). Even following surgical repair, patients should continue to receive prophylaxis, since residual operative anatomic abnormality is almost invariably present.

Severely hypoxic newborns with critical pulmonic stenosis or atresia may achieve effective short-term palliation following the infusion of prostaglandin E_1 into the descending aorta (at the upstream end of the ductus arteriosus) or even intravenously. If the ductus has not closed completely, it may be dilated by this drug, allowing marked improvement in pulmonary blood flow and arterial oxygenation. This allows for less hurried surgical intervention in a nonacidotic infant who is, therefore, a much better surgical risk.

Very young infants, particularly cyanotic neonates, usually undergo a palliative shunt procedure to increase pulmonary blood flow. The choice of shunt often depends on anatomical considerations and the surgeon's experience and preference. The Blalock-Taussig anastomosis in which the divided subclavian artery (preferably on the side of the innominate artery) is anastomosed end-to-side to the pulmonary artery is the procedure of choice. An equally acceptable alternative is a shunt between the ascenting aorta and main pulmonary artery utilizing a short prosthetic conduit. Direct aorticopulmonary anastomoses (Waterstons or Potts shunts) have significant complications and are used only rarely (Fig. 12-6).

Currently, in many centers, total correction has been achieved successfully in very young infants. Undoubtedly, this approach will become more generally employed as further experience and refinements of technique permit. Total correction basically consists of patch closure of the ventricular septal defect (via right ventriculotomy) and adequate relief of pulmonic stenosis at all existing sites. Invariably, this requires resection of infundibular musculature and, usually, pulmonary valvotomy. Enlargement of the outflow tract and pulmonary arteries by insertion of a patch may be necessary in some cases. Physiologic correction of pulmonary

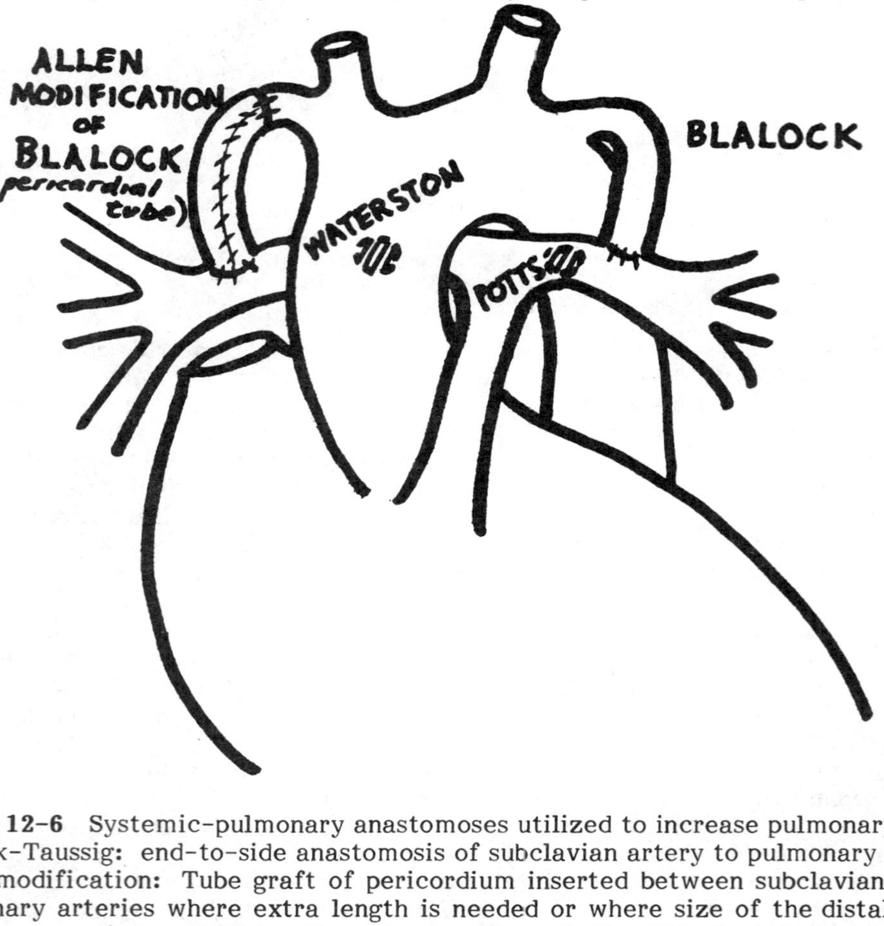

Figure 12-6 Systemic-pulmonary anastomoses utilized to increase pulmonary flow. Blalock-Taussig: end-to-side anastomosis of subclavian artery to pulmonary artery. Allen modification: Tube graft of pericordium inserted between subclavian and pulmonary arteries where extra length is needed or where size of the distal subclavian artery is too small to allow adequate flow. Potts: Side-to-side anastomosis of left pulmonary artery and descending aorta. Waterston: Side-to-side anastomosis of the right pulmonary artery and the ascending aorta.

atresia, the most extreme form of tetralogy, may be successful in selected cases by insertion of an external valved conduit between the right ventricle and pulmonary artery.

Postoperatively, almost all patients who have undergone total correction of tetralogy have residual murmurs of pulmonic stenosis and occasionally regurgitation. We feel that all patients should undergo elective cardiac catheterization a year or so following surgery. The repair is considered satisfactory if the VSD is completely closed and there is little (less than 20 torr) or no gradient across the right ventricular outflow tract. Such patients are usually asymptomatic and lead active lives, although the ultimate long-term prognosis remains to be demonstrated. Ventricular ectopy is encountered in approximately 10% of postop patients, usually in the context of persistently elevated right ventricular pressure. This is a major concern as there is a small, but definite, incidence of late sudden death following repair of tetralogy of Fallot which is felt to be arrhythmia-related. It is becoming the practice in most centers to obtain periodic 24-hr ambulatory EKG monitoring (Holter monitoring) and exercise EKGs to evaluate the presence or absence of post-repair ventricular ectopy. Frequent or multiform PVCs or those occurring in couplets, triplets, or runs should probably be treated although this issue is not yet completely clarified.

Differential Diagnosis

Most lesions presenting with cyanosis in the newborn period must be considered. The more common ones include tricuspid atresia, transposition of the great arteries, severe pulmonic stenosis, or atresia with intact ventricular septum and truncus arteriosus.

Bibliography

Bonchek LI, Starr A, Sunderland CO, Menashe VD: Natural history of tetralogy of Fallot in infancy: clinical classification and therapeutic implications. Circulation 48:392, 1973.

Goldman BS, Mustard WT, Trusler GS: Total correction of tetralogy of Fallot: review of ten years exerience. Brit Heart J 30:463, 1968.

Guntheroth WG, Morgan BC, Mullins GL: Physiologic studies of paroxysmal hyperpnea in cyanotic congenital heart disease. Circulation 31:70, 1965.

Kirklin JW, Karp RB: The Tetralogy of Fallot from Surgical Viewpoint. W. B. Saunders Co., Philadelphia, 1970.

Levin AR, Boineau JP, Spach MS, Canent RV, Capp MP, Anderson PA: Ventricular pressure flow dynamics in tetralogy of Fallot. Circulation 34:4, 1966.

Shinebourne EA, Anderson RH, Bower JJ: Variations in clinical presentation of Fallot's tetralogy in infancy. Angiographic and pathogenic implications. Brit Heart J 37:946, 1975.

Soto B, Pacifico AD, Ceballos R, Bargeron LB Jr: Tetralogy of Fallot. An angiographic-pathologic correlative study. Circulation 64:558, 1981.

Sunderland CO, Matarazzo RG, Lees MH, Menashe VD, Bonchek LI, Rosenberg JA, Starr A: Total correction of tetralogy of Fallot in infancy: postoperative hemodynamic evaluation. Circulation 43:398, 1973.

Van Praagh R, Van Praagh S, Nebesar RA, Muster AJ, Sinha SN, Paul MH: Tetralogy of Fallot: underdevelopment of the pulmonary infundibulum and its sequelae. Am J Cardiol 26:25, 1970.

Vogelpoel L, Schrire V: Auscultatory and phonocardiographic assessment of Fallot's tetralogy. Circulation 22:73, 1960.

Chapter 13

TRICUSPID ATRESIA

Tricuspid atresia implies complete failure of development of the tricuspid valve, resulting in lack of direct communication between the right atrium and right ventricle. Normal forward flow through the right heart obviously cannot occur, and all systemic venous return must flow across the atrial septum to the left heart both pre- and postnatally.

Incidence

The lesion is not common, accounting for about 3% of cardiac malformations. However, the defect should always be considered in the differential diagnosis of cyanotic infants and children.

Embryology and Anatomy

The embryologic cause of the anomaly is not fully understood. Various hypotheses include abnormal development of the AV canal resulting in malalignment of the ventricular septum with the atria causing obstruction of the tricuspid orifice, abnormal development of the right portion of the endocardial cushions, or early fusion of the tricuspid leaflets due possibly to *in utero* infection.

Several anatomic variants of this lesion are recognized as differing primarily in the relationships of the great arteries (normal or transposed), presence or absence of ventricular septal defect, and presence or absence of pulmonary stenosis or atresia. Over two-thirds of cases have normally related great arteries and, in the most common form, a ventricular septal defect and some degree of right ventricular outflow obstruction are present. To some extent, the right ventricle is usually hypoplastic, consisting of an infundibular portion of variable size. The left ventricle, left atrium, and mitral orifice are enlarged. Infrequently, pulmonary atresia is present, the ventricular septum is intact, and the right ventricle is absent or slitlike. Pulmonary blood flow is then dependent on patency of the ductus arteriosus and bronchial collateral circulation. When transposition of the great arteries is present, the ventricular septal defect is most often large and the pulmonary artery unobstructed.

Hemodynamics

Hemodynamics depend on the underlying associated abnormalities, but certain common features are present. In all cases, systemic venous blood must enter the left atrium and ventricle, where mixing occurs with pulmonary circulations by various pathways, depending on the associated abnormalities (Fig. 13-1). Systemic arterial unsaturation is always present, but the degree is influenced by total pulmonary blood flow. When anatomic arrangements permit large pulmonary flow, arterial saturation is relatively high and cyanosis minimal. Conversely, low-volume pulmonary flow may result in extreme cyanosis and hypoxia.

Since the left atrium and ventricle must handle the combined systemic and pulmonary venous return pre- and postnatally, these chambers, as well as the mitral orifice, are usually enlarged. When pulmonary flow is increased, volume overload of the left heart may result in congestive failure.

The interatrial communication in most cases consists of a patent foramen ovale. Not uncommonly, this communication is, or becomes, obstructive, resulting in inadequate decompression of the right atrium and progressive signs of systemic venous congestion.

Clinical Manifestations

The clinical manifestations of tricuspid atresia present considerable variation determined by the underlying anatomy. The great majority of affected infants have normally related great arteries, diminished pulmonary blood flow, and present

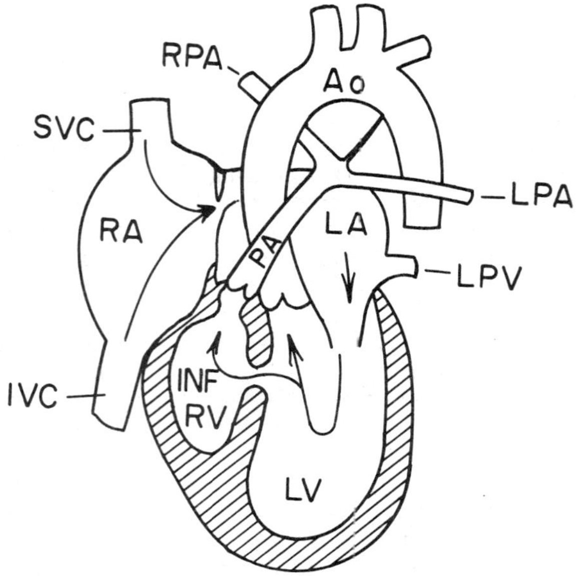

Figure 13-1 The circulation in tricuspid atresia. Systemic venous return shunts across the foramen ovale to the left side. The small right ventricle communicates with the left ventricle by way of a ventricular septal defect, and infundibular obstruction is present. SVC - superior vena cava, IVC - inferior vena cava, RA - right atrium, LA - left atrium, INF. RV - infundibulum, right ventricle, LV - left ventricle, Ao - aorta, RPA - right pulmonary artery, LPA - left pulmonary artery, PA - pulmonary artery.

early in infancy with moderate-to-severe cyanosis. Although occasionally delayed by late closure of the ductus arteriosus, cyanosis is usually apparent within the first week or two of life, and often progresses rapidly. Tachypnea and dyspnea usually are noted, and acute hypoxic spells may occur in early infancy. Such spells signify critical impairment of pulmonary blood flow and an urgent need for surgical therapy.

Physical examination reveals a relatively quiet precordium with minimal or no cardiomegaly. In about one-third of patients, a systolic thrill is palpable along the mid and upper left sternal edge. The first heart sound is normal, and the second sound single, or a soft pulmonic component noted. A harsh systolic murmur of moderate intensity is present at the mid and upper left sternal border in about one-half of cases. This murmur may be related to the ventricular septal defect and/or pulmonic stenosis.

Liver size is variable depending on the presence of heart failure and the degree of patency of the interatrial septum. Significant obstruction to interatrial communication or congestive failure may result in considerable hepatomegaly with a definite presystolic hepatic pulsation coincident with large A waves in the neck vein pulsations. These latter findings may be difficult to evaluate, however, in the young infant.

In tricuspid atresia associated with transposition of the great arteries, the relatively hypoplastic right ventricle gives rise to the aorta, while the left ventricle perfuses the pulmonary trunk. Pulmonary blood flow typically is increased. Congestive heart failure is the usual presenting manifestation, and cyanosis is less intense. Dyspnea, tachypnea, pulsatile hepatomegaly, and edema are prominent features. Cardiomegaly with hyperdynamic precordium is characteristic, and a significant systolic murmur at the midleft sternal border is nearly always present. A systolic thrill parasternally and an apical diastolic filling rumble may be noted.

Electrocardiogram

The electrocardiogram is always abnormal and usually provides information of diagnostic importance, even in the newborn. Characteristic features include prominent left axis deviation, left ventricular hypertrophy, and insignificant right ventricular forces (Fig. 13-2). In 80-90% of cases, left axis deviation, most often between +15° and -60°, is present even in the neonate. The infrequent occurrence of normal or right axis is usually associated with the less common anatomic variants with transposition, or pulmonary atresia with nontransposed arteries.

Left ventricular hypertrophy is almost always present, although changes suggesting isolated right ventricular hypertrophy occasionally are seen. The neonate may show dominant left ventricular forces with diminished rightward forces, a mature pattern of left ventricular hypertrophy for age. Right atrial enlargement is present in about one-half of patients. Left atrial enlargement also may be present, particularly in older infants with increased pulmonary blood flow.

Echocardiographic Features

When pulmonary blood flow is markedly diminished, the right ventricle and pulmonary valve may be extremely difficult or impossible to image. The tricuspid valve of course cannot be detected. A larger right ventricle may be encountered in the presence of a moderate-to-large ventricular septal defect. This anatomy is best demonstrated by two-dimensional techniques which allow clear delineation of

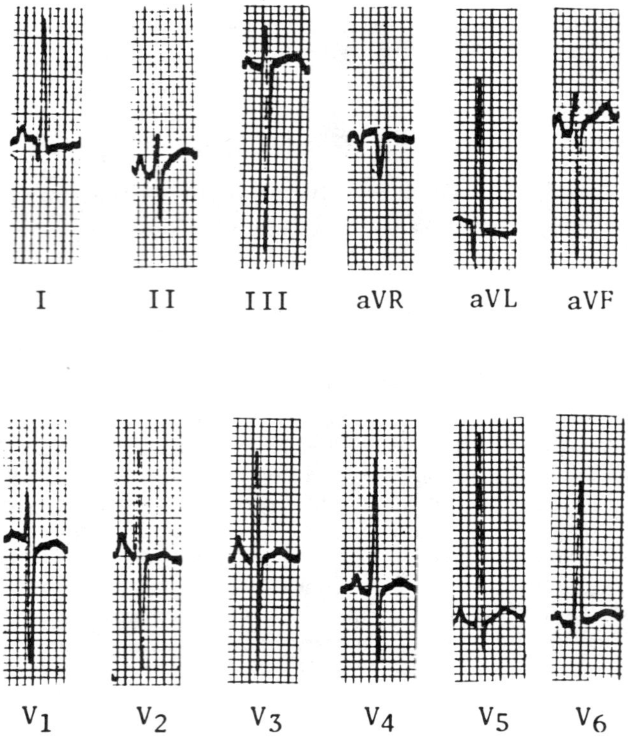

Figure 13–2 Electrocardiogram of 4-day-old infant with tricuspid atresia showing left superior axis deviation and dominant left ventricular forces suggesting left ventricular hypertrophy in a neonate.

the size of the right ventricle, as well as the relationship of the great arteries and the presence of an interatrial communication.

Radiologic Features

Infants with tricuspid atresia and obstruction to pulmonary blood flow have normal cardiac size and diminished pulmonary vascularity on chest roentgenogram (Fig. 13-3). Various cardiac contours have been described, but about one-half of patients have a prominent left heart border and rounded apex. The right atrium may appear prominent, but often is rather straight, close to or overlying the vertebral column. Associated transposition of the great vessels results in a narrow cardiac base and "egg-on-side" contour characteristic of other transposition malformations. If the underlying anatomy favors increased pulmonary blood flow, the heart appears significantly enlarged and pulmonary vasculature quite prominent. The diminutive right ventricle may be suspected on the basis of oblique views.

Cardiac Catheterization

Cardiac catheterization reveals a right-to-left shunt at the atrial level. The atrial septum is readily crossed with the catheter, but the right ventricle cannot be entered from the right atrium. Nearly identical saturation is found in the left

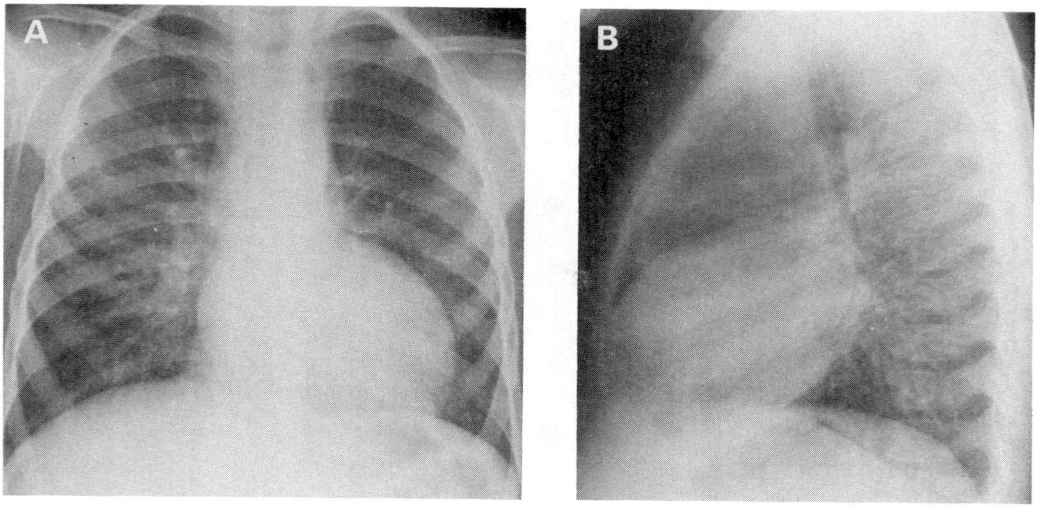

Figure 13-3 Chest roentgenogram of patient with tricuspid atresia and moderate obstruction to pulmonary blood flow. (A) Frontal view shows normal transverse cardiac diameter but sharply convex left border with concave pulmonary artery segment. The right heart border is rather straight. Pulmonary vasculature is slightly prominent. (B) Lateral view. Note unusually clear retrosternal space suggesting small right ventricle.

atrium and left ventricle, due to almost complete admixture of pulmonary and systemic venous blood. Systemic arterial unsaturation, which is always present, is inversely proportional to pulmonary blood flow.

Mean right atrial pressure is always increased and exceeds or equals mean left atrial pressure. Left atrial pressure is determined both by left ventricular end-diastolic pressure and the volume of pulmonary venous return. When pulmonary flow is large or left ventricular end-diastolic pressure elevated, as in congestive failure, left atrial pressure is increased. Left ventricular systolic pressure and aortic pressures are usually normal.

Although the foramen ovale usually is of adequate size, functional obstruction may result from elevation of left atrial pressure, a finding likely to occur when pulmonary blood flow is increased. In some instances this results in considerable elevation of right atrial pressure to maintain the necessary right-to-left shunt and promotes signs of systemic venous congestion.

Because of anatomical factors, determination of right ventricular and pulmonary arterial pressures is difficult. Usually, they are variable, depending on the size of the ventricular septal defect and associated pulmonary stenosis. Right ventricular pressure may equal that in the left ventricle, but usually is somewhat less. Right ventricular outflow obstruction — valvular, subvalvular, or combined — may be present and is best defined by angiocardiography.

Contrast injection into the right atrium reveals lack of direct inflow into the right ventricle (Fig. 13-4). In typical sequence, contrast opacifies the right atrium, left atrium, left ventricle, aorta, and pulmonary artery. In the frontal view a characteristic filling defect may be seen at the usual right ventricular inflow area. Left heart chambers, as well as the right atrium, are enlarged. Evaluation of the ventricular septal defect, right ventricle, and the great arteries — features of surgical importance — usually can be achieved best by left ventricular injection.

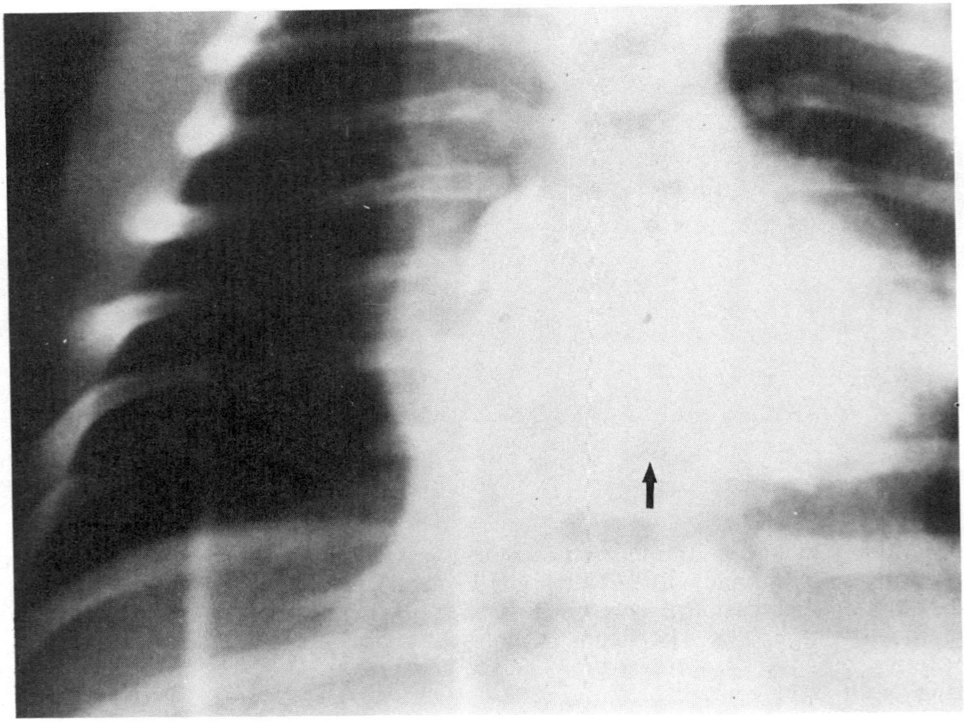

Figure 13-4 Right atrial angiogram. The contrast medium has passed to the left atrium and ventricle. There is reflex into the inferior vena cava and hepatic veins. A triangular filling defect (arrow) is present at the usual site of the right ventricle.

Course and Prognosis

The course and prognosis of infants with tricuspid atresia vary with the underlying anatomy, but in general the prognosis is guarded at best. Without surgical treatment, approximately two-thirds of affected infants succumb within the first year of life, most within the first 6 months. Those with restrictive VSD or severe pulmonic stenosis have the worst outlook, and deterioration may occur following increasing pulmonic stenosis or spontaneous closure of the VSD. Infants with severely increased pulmonary blood flow likewise do poorly, while those with moderately increased pulmonary flow appear to have the best outlook. Death is usually related to severe hypoxia, congestive heart failure, or other complicating factors. Palliative surgery has clearly improved the early prognosis, and the development of physiologically corrective techniques is a promising step toward increased long-term survival.

Treatment

Treatment is, for the most part, surgical. Anticongestive therapy and supportive measures may provide only transient benefit in symptomatic patients. Since the foramen ovale has the potential to be obstructive, an adequate interatrial communication should be assured in each case. Usually this can be accomplished in the infant by balloon atrial septostomy (Rashkind procedure) at the time of original cardiac catheterization. This procedure often is not feasible in older patients, however, and surgical atrial septectomy may be necessary (Blalock-Hanlon procedure). Newborns with critical pulmonic stenosis or atresia and ductus-dependent pulmonary blood flow may be temporarily palliated by infusion of prostaglandin E_1. This will dilate the ductus arteriosus, increasing pulmonary blood flow and decreasing hypoxemia.

Both palliative and physiologically corrective surgical procedures are available for this lesion. Cyanotic infants with restricted pulmonary blood flow require a shunt to increase flow to the lungs. Any one of several types of shunt procedures can be utilized, including ascending aorta to right pulmonary artery (Waterston), descending aorta to left pulmonary artery (Potts), subclavian artery to pulmonary artery (Blalock-Taussig), and superior vena cava to the right pulmonary artery (Glenn). All have their advantages and disadvantages, but none is consistently satisfactory. The Blalock-Taussig shunt provides a more controlled pulmonary blood flow usually without pulmonary hypertension, but carries a greater mortality in the very young infant and is less likely to maintain adequate flow as the child grows, requiring reoperation. Excessive pulmonary blood flow and pulmonary hypertension are more frequent complications of the Waterston or Potts shunts; the former may produce kinking of the pulmonary artery restricting flow to the ipsilateral lung. The Glenn anastomosis will provide good long-term palliation with low pulmonary artery pressure but carries an unacceptable mortality under 1 year of age. The choice usually depends on the infant's age, size of the vessels to be utilized, individual anatomy, and the surgeon's personal experience and preference.

When excessive pulmonary blood flow exists, congestive heart failure is often present. If failure is medically uncontrollable, the reduction in pulmonary blood flow achieved by surgical banding of the pulmonary artery may be beneficial.

In selected cases, physiologic correction may be achieved by the insertion of a prosthetic conduit, with or without a procine valve, between the right atrium and the right ventricle or pulmonary artery or by direct anastomosis of the right atrium to the right ventricle. At the same time, the atrial and ventricular septal defects are closed, thereby establishing physiologically normal circulatory pathways. Early success with this technique, or variations thereof, have been encouraging. Prerequisite conditions for this operation, (known as the Fontan procedure) include normal pulmonary artery pressure and resistance, age over 3 years, adequate distal pulmonary arteries, normal sinus rhythm, and normal left ventricular function.

Differential Diagnosis

Tricuspid atresia is the primary consideration in the cyanotic infant with pronounced electrocardiographic left axis deviation and dominant left ventricular forces. Usually, these features permit clinical diagnosis of the most common type of tricuspid atresia, but the presentation of more complicated variants is less typical.

Other lesions associated with left axis deviation and left ventricular hypertrophy include endocardial cushion defects, single ventricle, and truncus arteriosus. Infants with pulmonary atresia with intact ventricular septum occasionally may present a relative left axis for age, but usually not superiorly oriented. Cardiac catheterization and angiographic studies are essential for precise differentiation.

Bibliography

Dick M, Fyler DC, Nadas AS: Tricuspid atresia: clinical course in 101 patients. Am J Cardiol 36:327, 1975.

Fontan F, Baudet E: Surgical repair of tricuspid atresia. Thorax 26:240, 1971.

Gamboz R, Gersony WM, Nadas AS: The electrocardiogram in tricuspid atresia and pulmonary atresia with intact ventricular septum. Circulation 34:24, 1966.

Glenn WWL, Ordway NK, Talner NS, Call EP Jr: Circulatory bypass of the right side of the heart. IV. Shunt between superior vena cava and distal right pulmonary artery: report of clinical application in thirty-eight cases. Circulation 31:172, 1965.

Rao PS: Natural history of the ventricular septal defect in tricuspid atresia and its surgical implications. Brit Heart J 39:276, 1977.

Stanton RE, Lurie PR, Lindasmith GG, Meyer BW: The Fontan procedure for tricuspid atresia. Circulation 64 (Suppl II):140, 1981.

Tandon R, Edwards JE: Tricuspid atresia: a re-evaluation and classification. J Thoracic Cardiovasc Surg 67:530, 1974.

Williams WG, Rubis L, Fowler RS, Rao MK, Trusler GA, Mustard WT: Tricuspid atresia: results of treatment in 160 children. Am J Cardiol 38:235, 1976.

Chapter 14

PULMONARY ATRESIA WITH INTACT VENTRICULAR SEPTUM

Atresia of the pulmonary valve may occur with intact ventricular septum or with ventricular septal defect. The latter is generally considered a severe form of tetralogy of Fallot and is discussed in Chap. 12.

Incidence

Pulmonary atresia with intact ventricular septum is an uncommon defect. In autopsy studies it accounts for approximately 3% of congenital cardiac malformations, but in newborn infants dying with congenital heart disease, pulmonary atresia with intact ventricular septum ranks second to transposition of the great arteries.

Embryology and Anatomy

The malformation is characterized by complete failure of development of the pulmonary valve, resulting in no communication between right ventricle and pulmonary artery. Usually a membranous diaphragm with rudimentary raphe can be identified (80%), but occasionally infundibular atresia and, less commonly, atresia of the main pulmonary artery are present. The lesion is usually classified into two types.

Type I: With small tricuspid orifice and small right ventricle
Type II: With tricuspid insufficiency and large right ventricle

The tricuspid valve in type-I pulmonary atresia with intact ventricular septum is small and somewhat stenotic, but not greatly deformed. In type II the tricuspid valve may exhibit abnormalities resembling those seen in Ebstein malformation. When severe right ventricular hypoplasia is present, prominent intramyocardial sinusoids may communicate with the coronary arteries. In the presence of significant tricuspid insufficiency, the right ventricular cavity tends to be normal or enlarged. In either case, right atrial enlargement is present, and the atrial septum patent, usually via the foramen ovale. The right ventricular wall commonly is quite thick, and in those with a small cavity considerable fibrosis of the endocardium may be present. Pulmonary blood flow is dependent on patency of the ductus arteriosus, which undergoes closure at a variable time, usually within a few weeks after birth. Although usually underdeveloped, the pulmonary trunk tends to be larger than in infants with pulmonary atresia and ventricular septal defect. The left atrium, mitral valve, and left ventricle are enlarged, and the left ventricular wall hypertrophied. The aorta is normally related.

Hemodynamics

Blood entering the right ventricle may flow in small quantities via myocardial sinusoids to the coronary vessels and aorta, but most regurgitates into the right atrium across a variably incompetent tricuspid valve. Since normal forward flow through the right ventricle is not possible, blood entering the right atrium must flow predominantly across the atrial septum to the left heart chambers. Ductal left-to-right shunting is essential for survival of the affected newborn, and the volume of such flow directly influences the severity of cyanosis (Fig. 14-1).

Manifestations

Most infants with pulmonary atresia and intact ventricular septum present with obvious cyanosis in early postnatal life. Cyanosis usually progresses in the neonatal period, often becoming intense with manifestations of hypoxemia. The early appearance of congestive heart failure with associated dyspnea and hepatomegaly occurs in about one-half of infants.

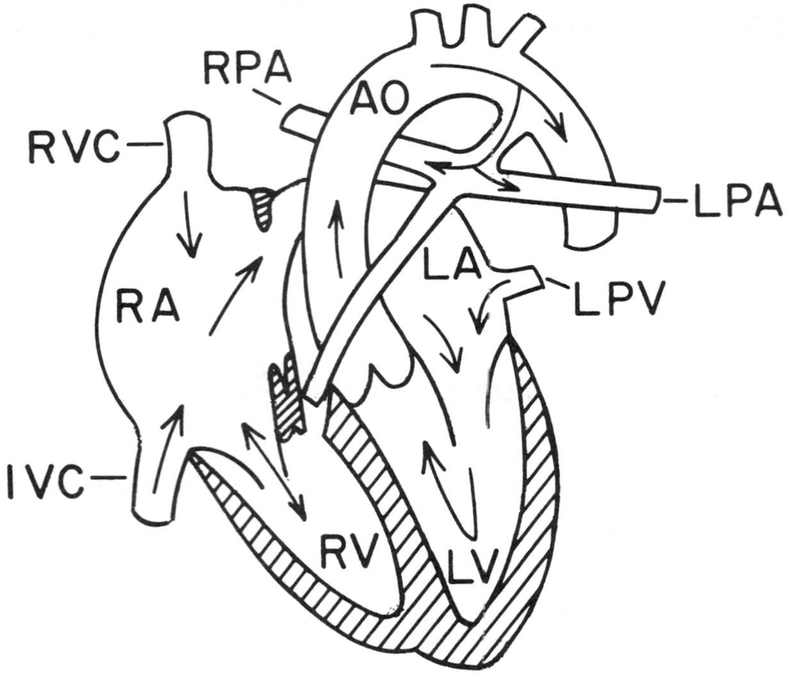

Figure 14-1 Circulation in pulmonary atresia with intact ventricular septum. Pulmonary arterial blood flow is by way of the patent ductus arteriosus. The only pathway of exit from the right heart is across the foramen ovale (or by way of myocardial sinusoids).

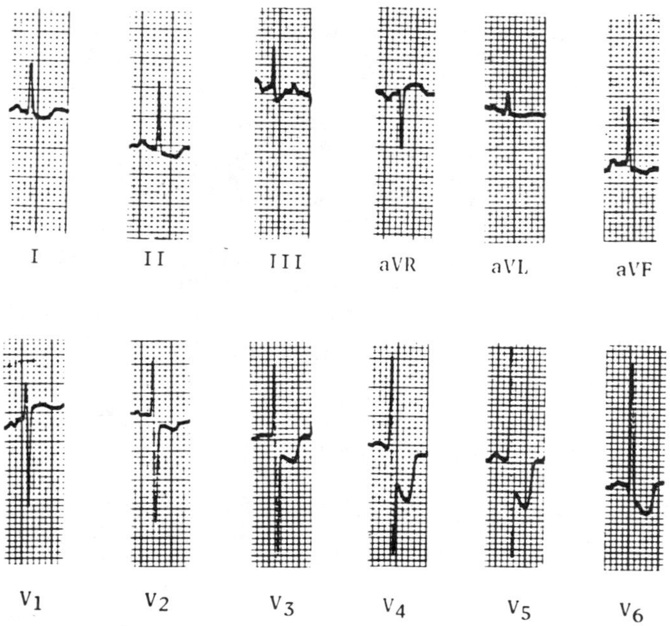

Figure 14–2 Electrocardiogram of a 3-week-old infant with pulmonary atresia and intact ventricular septum. A relative left axis deviation for age is present. Dominant left ventricular forces are present in the precordial leads with abnormal T waves.

Cardiac examination may reveal prominent jugular A waves coincident with presystolic hepatic pulsations. Heart size is variable, but often a xiphoid or left parasternal impulse is present. Auscultation reveals a loud single second sound. Murmurs are not striking and may be nonspecific or absent. An early systolic murmur at the lower left sternal edge related to tricuspid regurgitation or a continuous murmur related to ductal shunting may be heard. Disappearance of the latter may coincide with increasing cyanosis and clinical deterioration.

Electrocardiogram

The electrocardiogram usually shows a positive frontal plane QRS axis which may vary widely from -10° - $+120^\circ$. This is an important feature differentiating this lesion from tricuspid atresia, which typically shows a marked left superior axis.

Right atrial enlargement is usual, and biatrial enlargement may be present. Left ventricular dominance or hypertrophy is characteristic, especially of those with small right ventricle (Fig. 14-2). When the right ventricle is of near-normal size, precordial evidence of right ventricular hypertrophy or occasionally biventricular hypertrophy may be seen.

Echocardiographic Features

Typical echocardiographic findings are those of an extremely hypoplastic right ventricle with inability to visualize the pulmonic valve. The tricuspid valve is usually imaged, but its excursion is much reduced. In the presence of significant tricuspid regurgitation, the right ventricle may be of normal size or even dilated, however. An atrial septal defect may be imaged by two-dimensional techniques, and the left ventricle is usually dilated.

Radiologic Features

Chest roentgenogram may initially appear normal in the neonate. Cardiomegaly is usually apparent within a few days after birth and pulmonary vascular markings reduced. The right atrium appears prominent, as does the aortic knob. The pulmonary artery segment may appear normal, but a straight or concave segment is often present (Fig. 14-3).

Cardiac Catheterization

Cardiac catheterization reveals elevated right atrial pressure with large A waves. Right ventricular pressure is abnormally high and commonly exceeds systemic pressure. The pulmonary artery cannot be entered from the right ventricle. The left heart is usually entered by way of the atrial septum and normal pressures

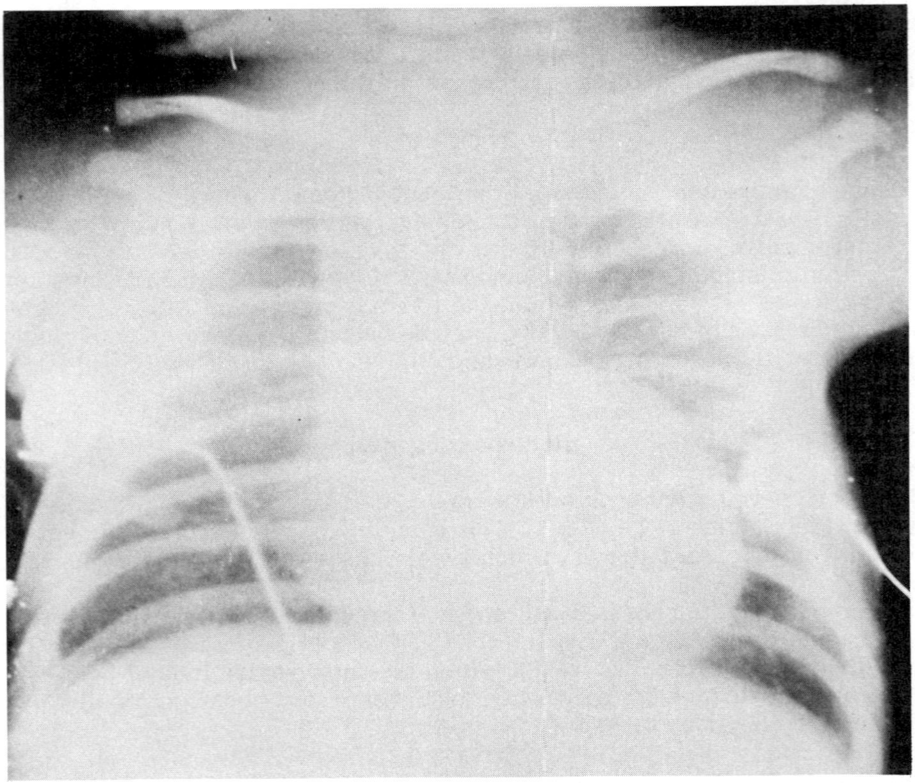

Figure 14-3 Chest roentgenogram of infant with pulmonary atresia and intact ventricular septum. The pulmonary artery segment is ill-defined, and peripheral pulmonary vasculature is reduced.

recorded. Saturations in the left atrium, ventricle, and aorta are reduced, usually markedly so.

Diagnosis rests on angiocardiographic studies which demonstrates no filling of the pulmonary artery from right ventricular injection. The infundibulum is small and ends blindly. The right ventricular cavity may be small and irregular with poor contractility and prominent sinusoids which may drain in retrograde fashion through the coronary circulation to the aorta (Fig. 14-4). Variable tricuspid regurgitation is usually present, and contrast clears the right ventricle very slowly. The left atrium and ventricle appear somewhat enlarged, and the ventricular septum is intact. Opacification of the pulmonary branches by way of the patent ductus is usually demonstrated, often filling the main pulmonary artery retrograde to its root.

Course and Prognosis

Survival is dependent on patency of the ductus arteriosus as a source of pulmonary blood flow. Without surgery the lesion is invariably fatal. Most infants die within 2 weeks after birth, and survival beyond 2 months is unusual.

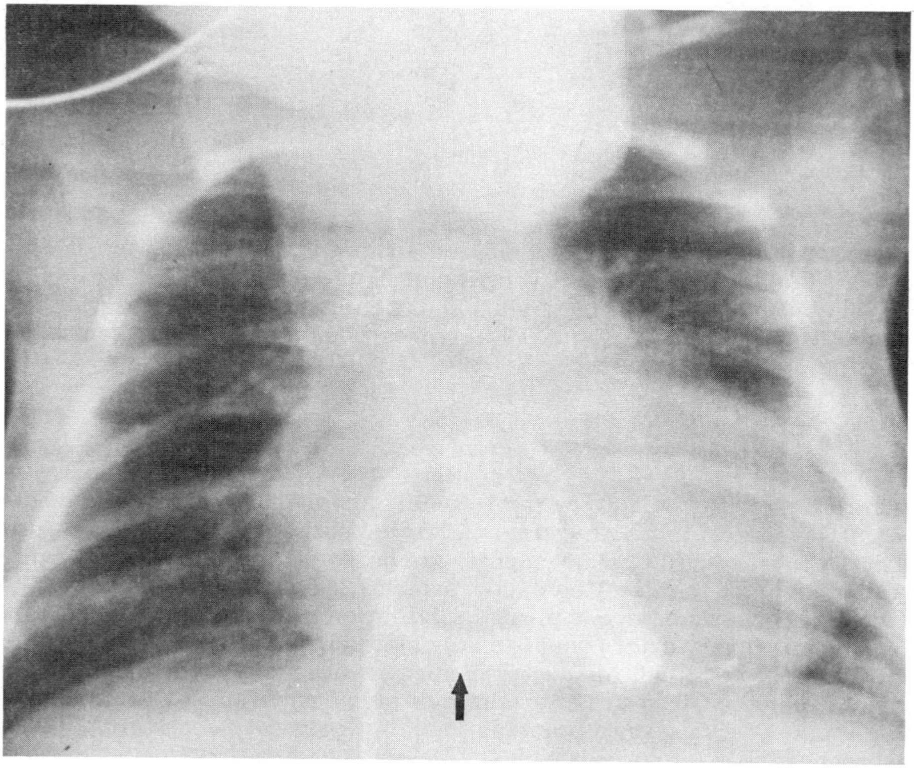

Figure 14-4A Right ventricular angiogram of infant with pulmonary atresia and intact ventricular septum. Frontal view shows diminutive ventricular cavity, prominent intramyocardial sinusoids with communication with the coronary circulation (arrow).

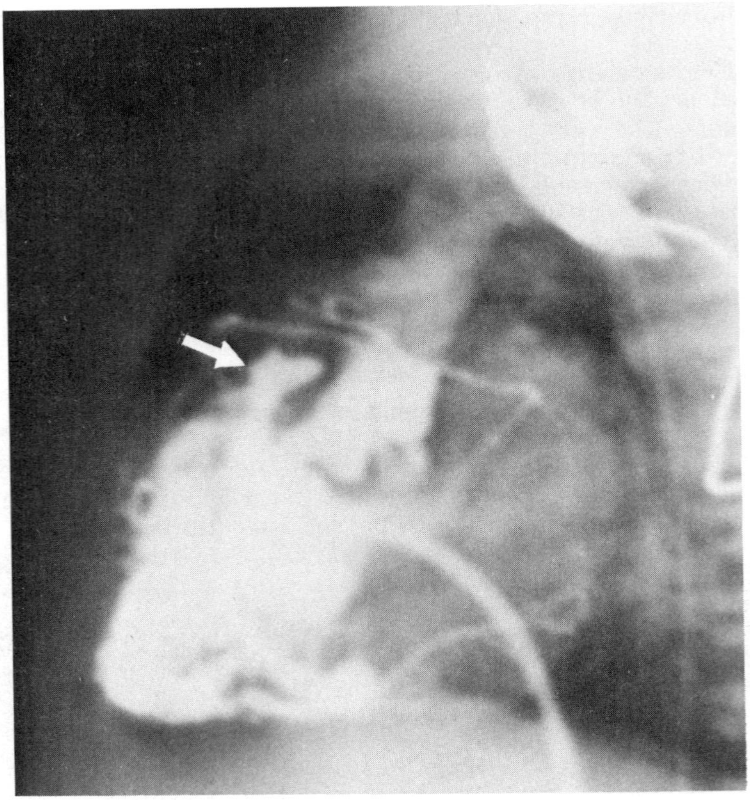

Figure 14–4B Right ventricular angiogram of infant with pulmonary atresia and intact ventricular septum. Right ventricular cavity better defined in the left lateral view. Hypoplastic infundibulum ends blindly (arrow) just anterior to the aortic root which is opacified by way of retrograde coronary flow from intramyocardial sinusoidal connections.

Treatment

Facilitation of the obligatory right-to-left atrial shunt can be achieved by balloon atrial septostomy at the time of cardiac catheterization, thus assuring unobstructed interatrial flow. Temporary improvement results from the infusion of prostaglandin E_1 to dilate the ductus arteriosus and improve pulmonary blood flow until surgery can be accomplished. Palliation can be achieved by establishing a systemic-pulmonary artery shunt to augment pulmonary blood flow. This should be considered even though the ductus is open because of the capricious and unreliable nature of this structure as a source of pulmonary flow. This procedure alone permits immediate survival of many infants, but does not necessarily improve long-range prognosis.

Recently, an arterial shunt operation has been combined with pulmonary valvotomy, hopefully to promote some measure of forward right ventricle-to-pulmonary artery flow. This approach has resulted in growth of the right ventricular cavity in some patients. For those infants with pulmonary vessels and right ventricle of adequate size, physiologic correction can be achieved by use of a valved external conduit between the right ventricle and pulmonary artery. Results of this approach in selected cases have been encouraging.

Differential Diagnosis

Because of the left ventricular predominance on EKG, tricuspid atresia is the lesion most resembling pulmonic atresia; the former generally shows a superior plane axis. Other lesions with pulmonary hypoperfusion would include tetralogy of Fallot, transposition with pulmonic stenosis and VSD, single ventricle, or other admixture lesions with severe pulmonic stenosis or atresia. Critical pulmonic stenosis with right heart failure and a right-to-left shunt at the atrial level may resemble pulmonary atresia closely; however, the degree of hypoxemia is generally less severe, and a stenotic murmur is present in most cases.

Bibliography

Bharati S, McAllister HA Jr, Chiemmongkoltip P, Lev M: Congenital pulmonary atresia with tricuspid insufficiency: morphologic study. Am J Cardiol 40:70, 1977.

Cole RB, Muster AJ, Lev M: Pulmonary atresia with intact ventricular septum. Am J Cardiol 21:23, 1968.

Dhanavaravibul S, Nora JJ, McNamara DG: Pulmonary valvular atresia with intact ventricular septum: problems in diagnosis and results of treatment. J Pediatr 77: 1010, 1970.

Luckstead EF, Mattioli L, Crosby IK, Reed WA, Diehl AM: Two-stage palliative surgical approach for pulmonary atresia with intact ventricular septum (type I). Am J Cardiol 29:490, 1972.

Shams A, Fowler RS, Trusler GA, et al.: Pulmonary atresia with intact ventricular septum. Report of 50 cases. Pediatrics 43:370, 1971.

Chapter 15

TRANSPOSITION OF THE GREAT ARTERIES

Although the term transposition of the great arteries includes a number of anatomically diverse, and often complicated, abnormalities, it is most commonly used to refer to lesions where there is ventriculoarterial discordance (i.e., where the arteries come off the wrong ventricles). The most commonly encountered entity, complete D-transposition, is characterized by the aorta originating anteriorly from the right ventricle and the pulmonary artery posteriorly from the left ventricle (Fig. 15-1). As a result, unoxygenated systemic venous blood is ejected into the aorta while oxygenated pulmonary venous blood is recirculated through the lungs. The two major circulations are, therefore, separate and parallel, instead of in normal series.

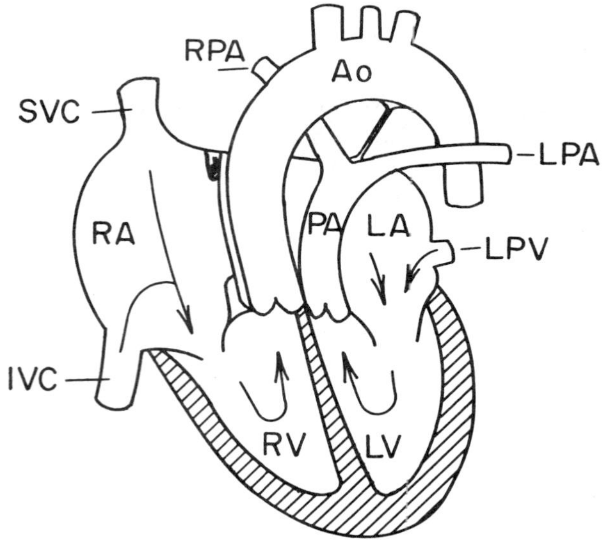

Figure 15-1 Circulation in D-transposition without associated defect. The aorta arising from the right ventricle receives systemic venous blood, while pulmonary venous blood without access to the systemic circuit is recirculated through the lungs. SVC - superior vena cava, IVC - inferior vena cava, RA - right atrium, LA - left atrium, RV - right ventricle, LV - left ventricle, Ao - aorta, PA - pulmonary artery, RPA - right pulmonary artery, LPA - left pulmonary artery, LPV - left pulmonary vein.

Although there are numerous anatomic variations, only D-transposition will be discussed in detail. A brief description is also given of an infrequent variant, corrected transposition of the great arteries (L-transposition). For more complete discussion of the transposition complexes, the reader is referred to the bibliography.

Incidence

Transposition of the great arteries is a common cyanotic defect which has been said to account for most deaths from congenital heart disease in the first 2 months of life. Among infants born with congenital heart malformations, transposition is found in approximately 8% of cases, but ranks first among neonates presenting with cyanosis. There is a dominant male sex incidence at birth (70%). In the past, 90% of affected infants did not survive the first year of life, most succumbing in the early weeks after birth.

Embryology and Anatomy

The older concept of straight-line septation of the truncus arteriosus has been disputed by the differential conal growth hypothesis. According to this widely accepted theory, the primitive conotruncus undergoes straight-line division with the aorta anterior to the pulmonary artery. Normally, the developing cardiac tube loops to the right (D-loop) as a result of differential tissue growth, causing the great arteries to lie in a side-by-side relationship with the aorta to the right of the pulmonary artery. At this stage, distal conal tissue is thought to be present beneath both great vessels. Subsequent expansion and growth of the subpulmonic conal tissue, with regression of subaortic conus, leads to rotation of the vessels with the aorta moving posteriorly in relation to the right ventricle. Absence of subaortic conus results in direct fibrous continuity between the posterior aortic annulus and anterior (septal) leaflet of the mitral valve. Subpulmonic conal tissue (infundibulum) prevents continuity of the pulmonary annulus with either atrioventricular (AV) valve.

Transposition is thought to result when the subpulmonic conus regresses while expansion and growth of the subaortic conus occurs. This results in anterior migration of the pulmonary artery above the left ventricle; with rare exception aortic-mitral fibrous continuity is lacking. This concept, therefore, attributes transposition to developmental abnormality of the distal conus, the hallmark of which is origin of the aorta above the morphological right ventricle and origin of the pulmonary artery above the morphological left ventricle, typically with discontinuity between aortic and mitral valves. Not infrequently, transposition is complicated by associated malformations, including ventricular septal defect, pulmonic stenosis, patent ductus arteriosus, and coarctation of the aorta.

Hemodynamics

Complete transposition of the great arteries results in loss of the normal sequential relationship between pulmonary and systemic circulations. In the absence of communication between the two circuits, oxygenated blood has no access to the systemic circulation, and body tissues, including myocardium, as perfused with systemic venous blood of low-oxygen content (Fig. 15-2).

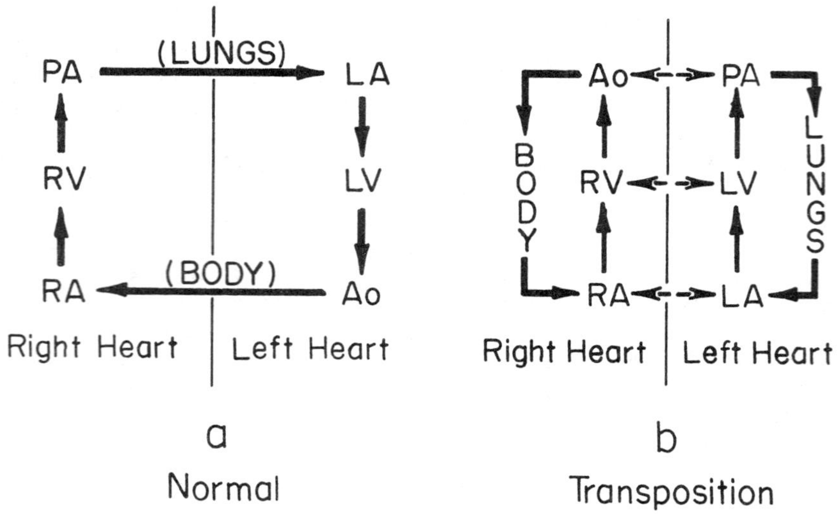

Figure 15-2 Normal in-series circulating pathway contrasted to parallel circulation in transposition of the great arteries. Intercirculatory shunting (broken arrows) necessary for survival in transposition may occur between the atria (foramen ovale or atrial septal defect), the ventricles (ventricular septal defect), the great arteries (ductus arteriosus), or combinations of these. SVC - superior vena cava, IVC - inferior vena cava, RA - right atrium, LA - left atrium, RV - right ventricle, LV - left ventricle, Ao - aorta, PA - pulmonary artery, RPA - right pulmonary artery, LPA - left pulmonary artery, LPV - left pulmonary vein.

In the fetus, shunts at the foramen ovale and ductus arteriosus minimize the effects of this lesion. However, postnatal closure of fetal pathways results in severe impairment of oxygen delivery into the systemic circuit, leading to hypoxia. Survival beyond the neonatal period is dependent, therefore, on sufficient intercirculatory mixing by any of several pathways: atrial septal defect or foramen ovale, ventricular septal defect, patent ductus arteriosus, or bronchopulmonary collaterals. Closure of the ductus arteriosus occurs at a variable time after birth, a factor which may clearly influence the clinical course. While favoring mixing between the two circuits, persistent patency of the ductus often is associated with early onset of pulmonary vascular disease.

The right ventricle in each case is required to generate pressure sufficient to perfuse the systemic circuit, while left ventricular pressure is governed by pulmonary vascular resistance or the resistance imposed by pulmonic stenosis.

The same pressure-resistance-flow relationships that govern shunts in other defects apply also to transposition, although the shunting mechanisms involved in this lesion are more complex. The physiologic consequences differ, however, because of the parallel nature of the two circuits. Left ventricle (or atrium) to right ventricle (or atrium) shunting augments systemic saturation and blood flow, while right-to-left shunting augments pulmonary blood flow but reduces pulmonary arterial saturation. It is also apparent that unidirectional shunts cannot exist in this lesion or else one circuit would drain entirely into the other. Bidirectional shunting of equal net magnitude must, therefore, be present. In the presence of two shunts (e.g., ASD-VSD or ASD-PDA). Shunting is typically predominantly in one direction at one level and in the opposite direction at the second level. Thus, if both atrial and ventricular septal defects are present without severe pulmonic stenosis, the shunts go mainly from left atrium to right atrium and from right ventricle to left ventricle.

As in other cyanotic malformations, the degree of hypoxia is dependent on the volume of pulmonary blood flow and the adequacy of mixing between systemic and pulmonary circuits. Patients with inadequate mixing or with obstruction to pulmonary blood flow have greater cyanosis, while those with high-volume pulmonary flow and good mixing reflect minimal cyanosis. In the presence of a large ventricular septal defect without pulmonic stenosis, excessive pulmonary flow and left ventricular volume overload may occur as pulmonary vascular resistance declines postnatally. The appearance of cardiomegaly and congestive failure in this situation is dependent on the changing postnatal relationships of pulmonary and systemic vascular resistances, characteristic of a large ventricular septal defect in general, and may be delayed for several weeks after birth.

Pulmonic stenosis, usually fibrous subpulmonic obstruction, is often present with ventricular septal defect, or can develop and progress postnatally. Although variable, it is typically severe, compromising pulmonary blood flow and contributing to the severity of cyanosis. More recently a dynamic type of subpulmonic resembling hypertrophic subaortic stenosis has been recognized. This usually occurs in the absence of a ventricular septal defect and may have significant adverse effects on venoarterial mixing and pulmonary blood flow.

The most desirable associated lesion in transposition of the great arteries is a large atrial septal defect which allows free bidirectional shunting with good mixing but without transmission of high-pressure pulsatile flow into the pulmonary bed. Although left ventricular volume work is increased, pressure remains low, and congestive failure is not usually seen.

Regardless of the type of shunt lesion present, the incidence of early development of pulmonary vascular disease is usually high in transposition of the great arteries. The reasons for this are multifactorial and incompletely understood. A possible relationship to bronchial arterial collateral flow has been suggested.

Manifestations

The clinical features of transposition are influenced considerably by the presence of associated defects, but the major manifestations are hypoxemia with or without congestive heart failure. Typically, the newborn infant with transposition is a male of above average birth weight. Not uncommonly, there is a maternal history of diabetes mellitus. When intercirculatory mixing is inadequate, cyanosis is usually present at birth, but may be delayed for several hours. Symptoms initially are absent and the physical examination may reveal nothing unusual. Murmurs are usually absent, but a nonspecific grade 2-3/6 systolic ejection murmur may be heard at the midleft sternal border. The electrocardiogram shows the normal right ventricular dominance of the neonate. The chest roentgenogram frequently reveals cardiac size, contour, and pulmonary vasculature to be unremarkable. However, typical radiographic features are often apparent in the first week of life. Characteristically, the thymic shadow is small or absent, the cardiac contour has an "egg-on-side" appearance, and the mediastinal supracardiac shadow is narrow in the frontal view. The latter is related to the malpositioned great vessels which lie in a more direct anteroposterior relationship, and are more centrally placed than normal. Widening of the superior mediastinal shadow may be apparent on the lateral view due to these vessel relationships. The pulmonary artery segment cannot be clearly identified, but vasculature may appear somewhat accentuated (Fig. 15-3). The combination of increased pulmonary vascular markings and

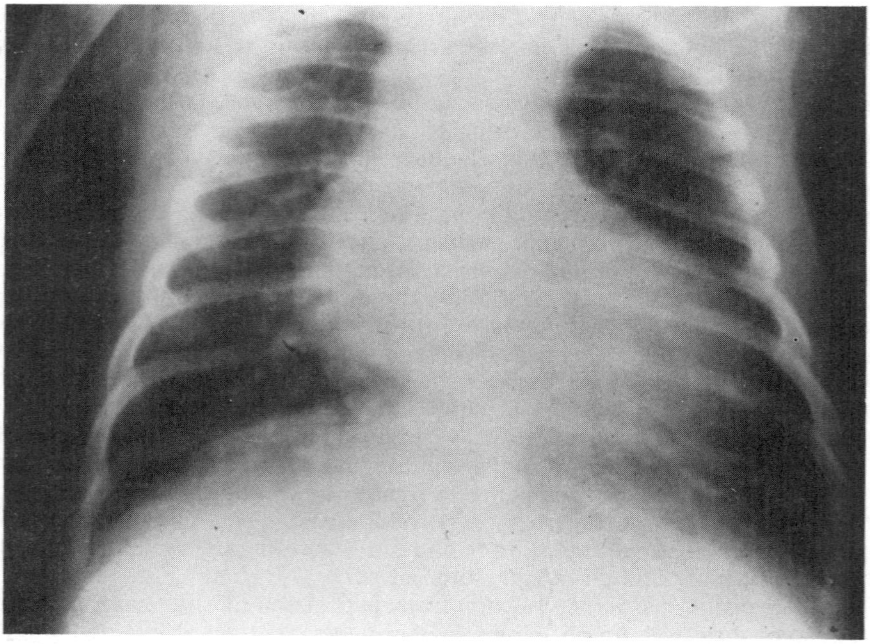

Figure 15-3 Newborn with D-TGA and intact ventricular septum. Classic "egg-on-side" cardiac contour is seen with narrow mediastinum. Pulmonary arterial markings are prominent.

severe hypoxemia is highly suggestive, if not pathognomonic, of transposition with inadequate mixing (i.e., intact ventricular septum).

Arterial blood gas determinations initially may reveal normal pH and pCO_2 and a low pO_2 (30-40 torr or less) which does not significantly improve with oxygen administration. As pO_2 declines, manifestations of hypoxia develop. Tachypnea and hyperpnea result in lowering of pCO_2, while metabolic acidosis induced by tissue hypoxia leads to falling pH. The latter usually marks the onset of clinical deterioration which may progress rapidly.

When a large ventricular septal defect is present, symptoms may be delayed as pulmonary vascular resistance follows the usual postnatal decline. The time of appearance of symptoms varies but may be as early as 2-4 weeks. Manifestations are predominantly those of large left-to-right shunt with pulmonary plethora, left ventricular volume overload, and congestive failure. Resting tachypnea, followed by dyspnea, irritability, diaphoresis, and fatigue resulting from the effort of feeding are common. Cyanosis may be unimpressive, often manifested as a dusky pallor. Cardiac examination may reveal prominent impulses, both parasternally and at the apex, but a thrill is not often felt. A harsh systolic murmur of grade 3/6 intensity may develop along the lower left sternal border. Often this murmur is slightly less than holosystolic, and does not exhibit the typical rightward radiation of the usual ventricular septal defect, since the turbulent stream is directed posteriorly toward the left ventricle. The mid-diastolic apical rumble of exaggerated left ventricular filling may be present. Both S_1 and S_2 are prominent with narrow splitting of S_2.

In most such infants, electrocardiographic and roentgenographic abnormalities appear with increasing frequency after the second week of life. Right ventricular hypertrophy is almost invariably present, and combined hypertrophy is quite common. Evidence for right and left atrial enlargement may also be noted (Fig. 15-4). Roentgenographic findings include the characteristic narrow supracardiac mediastinal shadow and egg-on-side contour with definite, and often pronounced, generalized cardiomegaly. Pulmonary hypervascularity of both arterial and venous patterns may be seen (Fig. 15-5).

When pulmonary stenosis exists with ventricular septal defect, the clinical features resemble those of tetralogy of Fallot. The clinical presentation is influenced greatly by the severity of pulmonic stenosis. Initially after birth, such infants, although often cyanotic, may exhibit no distress until closure of the ductus arteriosus results in accentuation of cyanosis and symptoms of hypoxia. Physical findings are not greatly different from those already described, with the exception of a systolic murmur of stenotic quality at the midleft sternal border. This murmur is related to the pulmonic stenosis, but differs from the usual in that it radiates most prominently toward the upper right sternal edge (mimicking aortic stenosis) along the course of the malpositioned pulmonary artery.

Significant pulmonic stenosis may be reflected in the electrocardiogram by relatively prominent left posterior forces. The x-ray features do not differ significantly from those already described except that pulmonary vascularity may be reduced when stenosis is severe. Poststenotic dilatation of the pulmonary trunk cannot be visualized.

Echocardiography

With the M-mode technique, altered anteroposterior relationships of the great arteries may permit simultaneous recording of both semilunar valves, a suggestive but nondiagnostic feature. In some patients it may be possible to define the anterior semilunar valve as being located to the right of the posterior valve. Two-

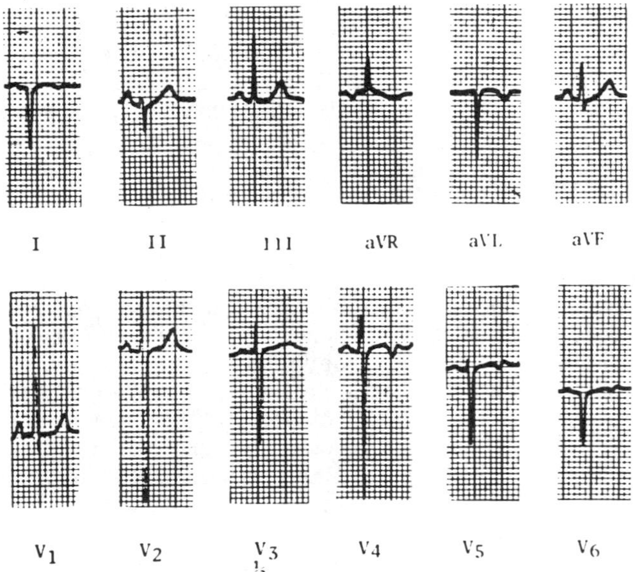

Figure 15-4 Electrocardiogram of infant with D-transposition of the great arteries and ventricular septal defect. Right axis deviation and right ventricular hypertrophy are present.

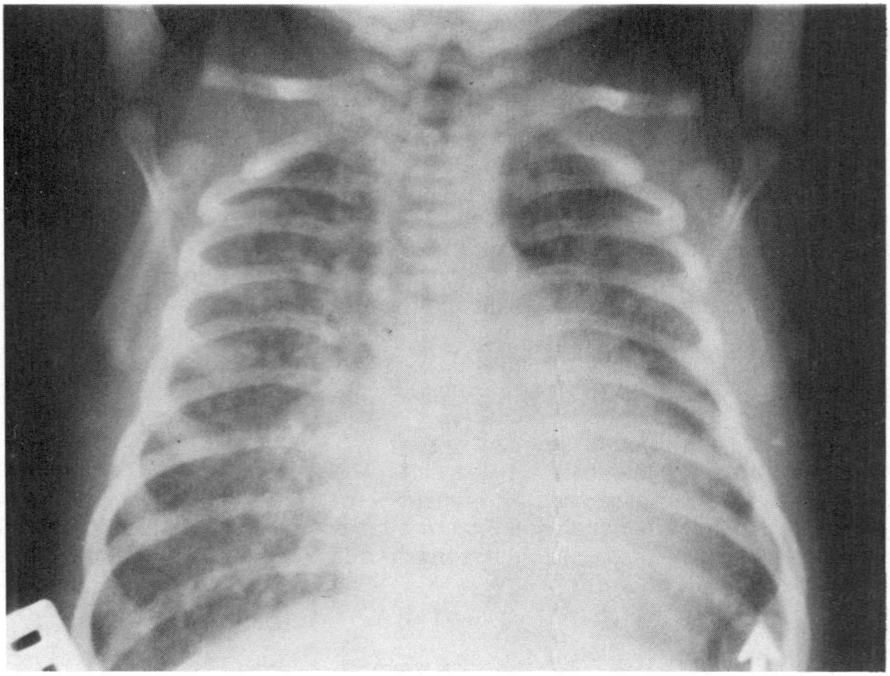

Figure 15–5 Chest roentgenogram of infant with D-transposition of the great arteries and ventricular septal defect. The thymus is absent or small, the heart enlarged, the cardiac base narrow, and neither great artery is clearly visible. Pulmonary arterial and venous congestion is present.

dimensional techniques allow for better delineation of the spacial relationship of the semilunar valves and the course of the great arteries as well as permitting evaluation of the status of the left ventricular outflow tract and septal defects.

Cardiac Catheterization

Cardiac catheterization is an essential aspect of the early management of the infant with transposition of the great arteries. Neonates and young infants with this lesion are often critically ill and in precarious hemodynamic and acid-base balance. Rapid deterioration may occur, particularly when severe hypoxemia exists. It is desirable, however, to achieve, as nearly as possible, optimal stability of these infants prior to and during the catheterization procedure. This requires maintenance of body temperature, correction and maintenance of blood glucose levels, administration of oxygen, and close monitoring of arterial blood gases to avoid progressive metabolic acidosis. Correction of hypocalcemia and other electrolyte imbalance may be indicated. Anticongestive therapy should be instituted promptly if heart failure is present. If these measures improve the infant's condition, the urgency of catheterization is diminished but should not be long delayed, since any improvement is not usually sustained. Failure of improvement only increases the need for prompt diagnostic studies and balloon septostomy.

Oxygen saturation studies may reveal extremely low levels in the right atrium, right ventricle, and aorta in infants with inadequate intercirculatory mixing. Occasionally, evidence of small left-to-right shunt at the atrial level may be seen. In most infants, the atrial septum is easily traversed via the foramen ovale, and pulmonary venous, left atrial, and left ventricular saturations are found to be normal.

Mean left atrial pressure is usually slightly elevated with a dominant V wave in the phasic curve. Left atrial pressure may exceed right atrial pressure when the interatrial communication is small. However, the presence of equal right and left atrial pressures does not necessarily indicate free communication between these chambers, since other factors influence these pressure relationships.

Right ventricular and aortic pressures are at expected systemic levels. Left ventricular and pulmonary artery pressures are more variable, and direct measurement of pulmonary arterial pressure is of utmost importance. Because of its location, catheterization of the pulmonary artery may be difficult but can usually be accomplished utilizing a balloon-tip flow-directed catheter or by various techniques using a guidewire to direct the catheter tip toward the pulmonary valve once the mitral valve has been crossed. If the ductus is widely patent or a large ventricular septal defect is present, left ventricular and pulmonary arterial systolic pressures usually are near systemic levels. The presence of severe pulmonic stenosis with large ventricular septal defect results in equal ventricular pressures but normal pulmonary artery pressure. With intact ventricular septum and closed ductus arteriosus, left ventricular and pulmonary artery pressures may be near normal; however, in the immediate newborn period persistence of increased pulmonary vascular resistance aggravated by hypoxemia may result in markedly elevated left heart pressures.

Careful cineangiocardiographic evaluation is essential to complete understanding of the spectrum of abnormalities present. Injections should be made in both ventricles with biplane filming to delineate the ventriculoarterial relationships, positioning of the atrioventricular valves, ventricular function, presence of ventricular septal defect or patent ductus arteriosus, and anatomy of the left ventricular outflow tract. In the traditional posteroanterior and lateral projections, the aorta can be seen to arise from the right ventricle, to the right and anterior of the pulmonary artery (Fig. 15-6). The latter may actually be almost directly posterior to the aorta. The interventricular septum can be evaluated more precisely in the long axis or hepatoclavicular views (see Chap. 12). These projections also lend themselves better to the assessment of the AV valves and left ventricular outflow tract (i.e., the presence or absence of pulmonic stenosis). Aortography may be necessary to demonstrate the ductus arteriosus and/or bronchial collateral vessels.

Treatment

One of the most important aspects of medical management of the infant with transposition is in preparation for cardiac catheterization and balloon septostomy, as previously discussed. Medical management is otherwise rather limited to supportive care, pending definitive surgical therapy. Balloon atrial septostomy as a palliative therapeutic technique is now considered an integral part of the catheterization procedure in this lesion. This procedure, promoted by Rashkind and Miller, requires passage of a special balloon-tipped catheter across the foramen ovale into the left atrium where the balloon is inflated with dilute contrast solution under fluoroscopic monitoring. The inflated balloon is jerked rapidly across

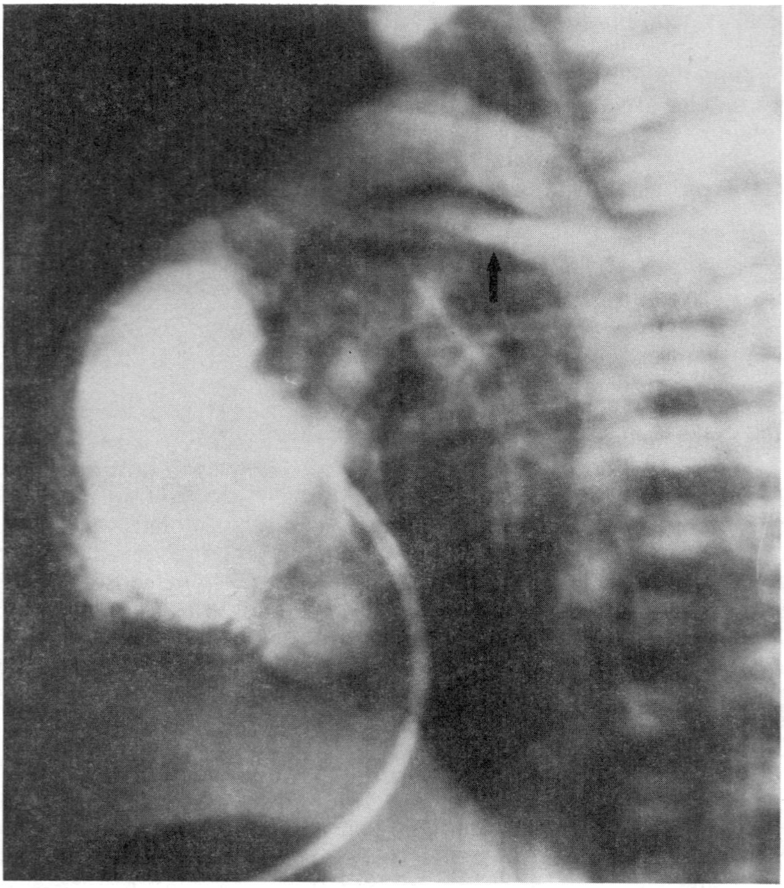

Figure 15–6 Right ventricular angiogram, lateral view. The aorta arises anteriorly from the right ventricle, with the pulmonary artery posteriorly above the left ventricle which is incompletely opacified by way of a ventricular septal defect. A patent ductus arteriosus is also present (arrow).

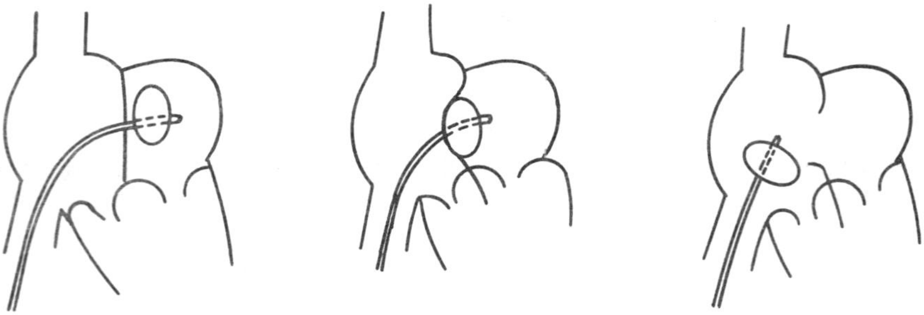

Figure 15–7 Diagrammatic illustration of balloon atrial septostomy. The balloon-tipped catheter, uninflated, is passed across the foramen ovale to the left atrium; the balloon is inflated with diluted contrast media and jerked sharply across the septum creating a tear in the thin foramen ovale tissue.

the atrial septum, creating a tear in the thin foramen tissue (Fig. 15-7). Usually, this is repeated several times to ensure an adequate opening, and the inflated balloon may be used to estimate the final size of the opening produced. When successful, this effectively creates a large atrial septal defect allowing reduction of left atrial pressure and effective mixing between the two circulations. This procedure usually is beneficial and should be attempted in all cases, regardless of associated cardiac defects. Results are often immediate and dramatic. Close observation is advisable for several days after this procedure, however, since improvement is sometimes only temporary. The reasons for this are not always clear, but may be related to inadequate tearing or only stretching of the foramen ovale.

If arterial pO_2 remains in the range of 26-30 torr or higher with no evidence of decreasing pH, decreasing pCO_2, or increasing negative base excess, and if there is no evidence of distress, observation may be continued to include evaluation of the weight gain and stability of the cardiac size. Decline in the pO_2 below these levels or signs of impending acidosis are indications that further intervention is necessary. Repeat balloon atrial septostomy may succeed in tearing the valve of the foramen ovale which was only stretched previously. An alternative approach is the use of a newly designed catheter which employs the knife blade to actually cut the septum; we have not personally evaluated this technique although it appears promising. Surgical excision of the interatrial septum (Blalock-Hanlon procedure) is only infrequently necessary. Should systemic arterial oxygenation remain inadequate following creation of an ASD, a trial infusion of prostaglandin E_1 (PGE_1) may be of benefit. Given either intraarterially at the aortic end of the ductus or intravenously, this drug may act to dilate the ductus and/or reduce pulmonary vascular resistance. Both effects would lead to increased pulmonary blood flow and improve venoarterial mixing at the atrial level as a result of the increase in pulmonary venous return.

Should improvement result, PGE_1 should be tapered and discontinued within a few days; in some cases the improvement has been sustained, allowing further intervention to be delayed. If secondary deterioration occurs or if there was no response to PGE_1, surgical intervention is mandatory. The current procedure of choice is physiologic correction by means of intraatrial rerouting of the venous return directing systemic venous blood to the left ventricle and pulmonary artery and pulmonary venous blood to the aorta. There are several procedural variations (Mustard, Senning, or Shumaker techniques), and the choice among them is beyond the scope of this text.

If the initial palliative approach proves satisfactory, surgery may be deferred, although the optimal age for physiologic correction is not clear. A major factor in the ultimate outcome is the development of pulmonary vascular disease with increased resistance. In patients with intact ventricular septum, such changes are uncommon before 2 years of age, but may occur earlier leading some centers to undertake physiologic correction between 6 and 12 months of age; other groups prefer to wait until about 2 years because of greater technical ease which can be achieved. Unfortunately, surgery does not always prevent the pulmonary vascular changes for reasons that are not clear. Another definitive surgical approach that remains to be evaluated is the Jatene procedure in which the great arteries are divided above the sinuses of Valsalva and reattached to the appropriate ventricles; the coronary arteries must be disconnected from the former aortic sinuses and implanted into the proximal portion of the old pulmonary artery (new aorta). The success of this approach has been limited by the fact that left ventricular myocardial mass in patients with intact ventricular septum is less than normal left ventricular mass by 3-4 months of age, and the left ventricle may not be able to handle the abrupt increase in pressure work that arterial switching may impose.

Options to overcome this problem would include performance of this operation prior to 4 months of age or doing a two-stage repair with the first stage consisting of pulmonary arterial banding to increase the left ventricular mass.

Transposition with large ventricular septal defect is usually complicated by congestive failure for which the usual medical therapy is indicated. By reducing left atrial and pulmonary venous pressure, balloon septostomy may provide distinct improvement, but poor control of failure may require surgical intervention. Banding of the pulmonary artery may be appropriate for these infants. This procedure, however, is not without significant morbidity and mortality, and, in the experience of some centers, correction by Mustard or related techniques is preferred even in very young patients.

It is in the patients with VSD that the risk of rapidly progressive increase in pulmonary vascular disease is greatest, with most patients exhibiting high fixed resistance by 2 years of age. Pulmonary artery banding may protect against these vascular changes as well as relieve failure; but such protection is not uniform, and any infant with D-transposition of the great arteries and VSD should have repeat cardiac catheterization by no later than 6 months of age, regardless of whether or not pulmonary artery banding was carried out. If pulmonary artery pressure is significantly elevated, intraatrial repair and closure of the ventricular septal defect should be performed fairly rapidly. If banding has lowered the pulmonary artery pressure to near normal, the second-stage repair could be deferred until 1-2 years of age. Pulmonary vascular resistance elevation to levels which preclude surgery should be encountered only rarely with current management techniques. When such elevation has occurred, a palliative intraatrial repair (leaving the VSD open) may improve the patient symptomatically and retard the progression of the pulmonary vascular disease by reducing hypoxemia.

If severe pulmonic stenosis is an associated problem, the infant commonly suffers from inadequate pulmonary blood flow and, in addition to atrial septostomy, a systemic-pulmonary artery shunt is indicated. Choices include ascending aorta-right pulmonary artery (Waterston), descending aorta-left pulmonary artery (Potts), or subclavian artery-pulmonary artery (Blalock-Taussig). Where feasible, the subclavian artery-pulmonary artery anastomosis is generally preferred. Surgical correction of this complex is complicated, particularly by the presence of the pulmonic stenosis. Valvular obstruction can be relieved by commissurotomy through an incision in the artery above the valve, but the posterior location of the vessel complicates this technique. Furthermore, the stenosis is often subvalvular, alone or combined with valvular obstruction. The location and the risk of significant complications, including damage to the mitral apparatus and surgical heart block, have made this a formidable lesion to attack directly, and inadequate relief of the obstruction has been a major factor in the previously high surgical mortality. The outlook was approved markedly with the development by Rastelli of a technique of repair involving patch closure of the ventricular septal defect in such a way that the left ventricular output is directed to the aorta and placement of an external valve conduit between the right ventricle and previously transected pulmonary artery. Primarily because of limitations in the size of the conduit that can be inserted, this procedure is best performed between 2 and 5 years of age. The presence of dynamic muscular subpulmonic stenosis with resultant limitation of pulmonary flow is probably best handled by intraatrial repair in early infancy.

Course and Prognosis

The diagnosis of transposition of the great arteries at one time implied a dismal prognosis with almost certain demise before the end of the first year of life. Several factors have contributed to a remarkably improved outlook for these patients. Notable among these are improved understanding of the pathophysiology of this defect; more aggressive diagnostic, medical, surgical, and postoperative management; development of the balloon atrial septostomy technique in the early management of the critically ill infant; and new and refined techniques in palliation and physiologic correction of this lesion and its commonly associated malformation.

Even with palliation alone, the majority of affected infants now survive the critical early months of life and eventually become candidates for further surgical therapy. The intraatrial repair is currently the most successful approach with mortality of less than 10% in cases of uncomplicated transposition. The age at which to perform this operation clearly must be individualized, but the present trend is toward as early correction as feasible; success has been achieved in infants less than 6 months in many centers. Early surgical correction obviates one of the major potential complications of this disease in older patients (i.e., development of pulmonary vascular obstructive disease). Irreversible vascular changes have been clearly demonstrated in patients, beginning in the second year of life.

The long-range outlook for infants having intraatrial repair at an early age is not yet defined. Earlier problems of serious postoperative arrhythmias have been reduced but not eliminated by carefully avoiding damage both to the sinus node and, insofar as possible, to the internodal conduction pathways during placement of the baffle. The early enthusiasm for this procedure as a "curative" operation, however, has been tempered by the late occurrence of various other complications, such as venae caval obstruction, pulmonary venous obstruction, leakage of the baffle, inadequate residual right atrial volume, and tricuspid insufficiency. How growth may affect the function of this baffle, when inserted in the small heart of a young infant, is not yet determined; neither is the long-range performance of the right ventricle as a systemic chamber. Although much has been achieved, overall results are still suboptimal. A recent study has shown that approximately 50% of appropriately treated children with D-transposition will survive to 5 years of age with no complications, and another 20% will be alive but with residual defects.

Differential Diagnosis

Transposition of the great arteries must be differentiated from other lesions presenting with cyanosis and/or congestive heart failure in early infancy. Transposition with inadequate intercirculatory mixing presents with cyanosis and hypoxia without significant murmur. Such findings are also seen in other cyanotic heart defects, such as pulmonary atresia with intact ventricular septum, tricuspid atresia, severe tetralogy of Fallot, and double-outlet right ventricle. Pulmonary vascularity on chest roentgenogram charactersitically is reduced in these lesions, and heart size is small in contrast to the normal or prominent vascularity and increased heart size with narrow base seen in transposition. However, when complex transposition is associated with significant pulmonic stenosis and reduced pulmonary blood flow, clinical differentiation from other cyanotic defects with reduced pulmonary flow may not be possible.

When a large ventricular septal defect without pulmonic stenosis coexists with transposed great arteries, congestive heart failure usually dominates the clinical picture with less prominent, often mild cyanosis.

Isolated large ventricular septal defect, truncus arteriosus, tricuspid atresia with large pulmonary flow single ventricle, or double-outlet right ventricle without pulmonic stenosis must be considered. Although the typical clinical picture of transposition of the great arteries may be readily recognized, precise diagnosis must often depend on cardiac catheterization and angiocardiographic studies.

Corrected Transposition of the Great Arteries

In the less common variant of transposition of the great arteries, corrected transposition or L-transposition, the primitive cardiac tube loops to the left. This results in morphologic inversion of the developing ventricular chambers, that is, the morphologic right ventricle (with its tricuspid atrioventricular valve) is left-sided and the morphologic left ventricle (with its bicuspid atrioventricular valve) is right-sided (bulboventricular inversion).

In the developing conotruncus, the aorta lies to the left of the pulmonary artery. Growth of the subaortic conus results in anterior rotation of this vessel above the left-sided (morphologic right) ventricle, while the pulmonary trunk is posteriorly oriented above the right-sided (morphologic left) ventricle. The leftward ventricle (morphologic right ventricle with a tricuspid AV valve) receives oxygenated blood from the left atrium and ejects into the displaced aorta. The rightward ventricle (morphologic left ventricle with bicuspid AV valve) receives venous blood from the right atrium and ejects into the pulmonary artery. As a result, the pathway of blood flow is physiologically correct, hence the term corrected transposition. Of surgical importance is abnormal distribution of major coronary vessels. An inherent feature of ventricular inversion is reversal of the bundle branches of the conduction system, resulting in the anatomic left bundle branch lying on the right side of the septum and the right bundle on the left side. This results in reversal of the direction of initial forces (septal) of ventricular depolarization. Characteristically, this produces initial Q waves in left precordial leads, a diagnostically important electrocardiographic feature of this lesion.

The majority of cases have significant associated anomalies, including ventricular septal defect, pulmonic stenosis, single ventricle, and an Ebsteinlike malformation of the left-sided tricuspid AV valve. This form of transposition also is frequently associated with congenital absence of the spleen or polysplenia. Corrected transposition is a very uncommon lesion accounting for less than 1% of clinical cases of congenital heart disease. Approximately two-thirds of cases are males.

In the absence of associated defects, patients with L-transposition may be entirely asymptomatic and may pass unrecognized. Clinical features are usually those of the associated malformations which characteristically lead to symptoms early in life. Symptoms may be as diverse as congestive heart failure, cyanosis, or debiliating arrhythmias which not infrequently occur (paroxysmal tachycardia, Wolff-Parkinson-White syndrome, or complete heart block), even when there are no additional defects.

When associated malformations are absent, physical examination may be unremarkable. However, the leftward, anteriorly malplaced aorta may produce an unusually loud, single second sound at the midleft sternal border. Splitting of S_2 may be better heard at the right sternal border. Murmurs of associated pulmonic stenosis or incompetence of the left AV valve may be somewhat atypical in location because of the abnormal anatomic relationships.

Electrocardiographic features may suggest the diagnosis of this lesion. Typical changes are reversal of the precordial Q wave pattern, atrioventricular conduction abnormalities (preexcitation or varying degrees of atrioventricular block), and various supraventricular arrhythmias. Evidence of chamber hypertrophy is dependent on the hemodynamics of associated defects (Fig. 15-8).

Specific roentgenographic findings likewise are influenced by associated malformations, but suggestive features may be noted. Most typical is a shoulderlike prominence of the left midcardiac border corresponding to the malpositioned ascending aorta. the pulmonary artery segment may not be visible, but, in some, the right pulmonary hilar vessels are unusually prominent, particularly if a left-to-right shunt exists (Fig. 15-9). Without associated malformations, the chest roentgenogram may be unremarkable.

Diagnosis in most cases depends on angiocardiographic information which demonstrates the abnormal great artery relationships and the morphologic anatomy of the inverted ventricles. Two-dimensional echocardiography may demonstrate the abnormal arterial relationships.

Surgical treatment, when indicated by the severity of coexisting lesions, is complicated by abnormal anatomical relationships. Of major surgical concern are the abnormal coronary artery distribution which complicates ventriculotomy and the malpositioned conduction system which increases the risk of surgical heart block.

The course and prognosis of this lesion is primarily governed by the associated cardiac abnormalities. Supraventricular arrhythmias occur in about 15% of patients

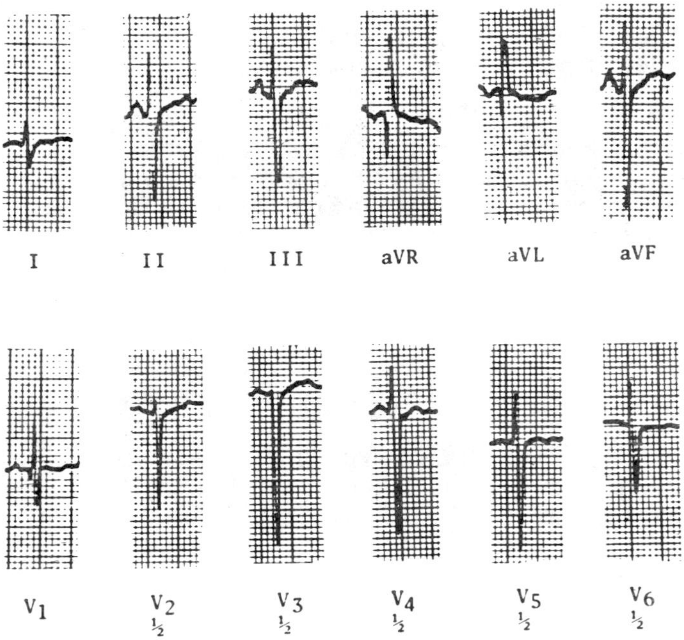

Figure 15-8 Electrocardiogram of infant with L-transposition and complex associated cardiac anomalies. Note the left superior axis, Q wave in V_1 and absence of Q waves in left precordial leads.

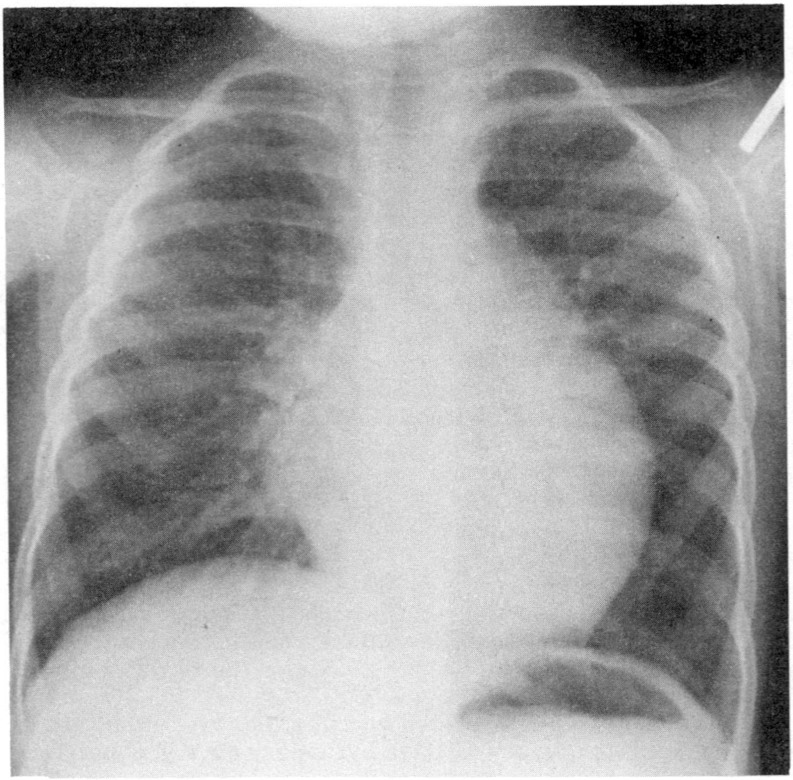

Figure 15-9 Chest roentgenogram of child with L-transposition. Note the long convexity to the left upper cardiac border due to the malplaced ascending aorta.

and complete AV block in another 10-15%; such dysrhythmias may dominate the clinical picture, especially when no associated defects are present. Death in complicated cases usually occurs in infants and mostly in the first 6 months. Survival into the eighth decade has been reported when no other intracardiac anomalies exist. The ability of the morphologic right ventricle to function as the systemic ventricle over a long period of time has been the subject of some concern, but the degree to which this complicates the clinical course is not clear.

Bibliography

Aziz KU, Paul MH, Rowe RD: Bronchopulmonary circulation in D-transposition of the great arteries: possible role in genesis of accelerated pulmonary vascular disease. Am J Cardiol 39:432, 1973.

Gutgessell HP, Garson A, McNamara DF: Prognosis for newborns with transposition of the great arteries. Am J Cardiol 44:96, 1979.

Lang P, Freed MD, Bierman FZ, Norwood WI Jr, Nadas AS: Use of prostaglandin E_1 in infants with D-transposition of the great arteries and intact ventricular septum. Am J Cardiol 44:76, 1979.

Mair DD, Danielson GK, Wallace RB, McGoon DC: Long-term follow-up of Mustard operation survivors. Circulation 49 and 50 (Suppl II):II-46, 1973.

Mair DD, Ritter DG, Danielson GK, Wallace RB, McGoon DC: The palliative Mustard operation: rationale and results. Am J Cardiol 37:762, 1976.

Mustard WT: Successful two-stage correction of transposition of the great vessels. Surgery 55:469, 1964.

Neufeld EA, Paul MH, Muster AJ, Idriss FS: Pulmonary vascular disease in complete transposition of the great arteries: a study of 200 patients. Am J Cardiol 34:75, 1974.

Rashkind WJ, Miller WW: Creation of an atrial septal defect without thoracotomy; a palliative approach to complete transposition of the great arteries. JAMA 196: 991, 1966.

Van Praagh R, Perez-Trevino C, Lopex-Cuellar M, Baker FW, Zuberbuhler JR, Quero V, Perez VM, Moreno F, Van Praagh S: Transposition of the great arteries with posterior aorta, anterior pulmonary artery, subpulmonary conus and fibrous continuity between aortic and atrioventricular valves. Am J Cardiol 28:621, 1971.

Van Praagh R, Van Praagh S: Isolated ventricular inversion. A consideration of the morphogenesis, definition and diagnosis of non-transposed and transposed great arteries. Am J Cardiol 17:395, 1966.

Chapter 16

TRUNCUS ARTERIOSUS

Persistent truncus arteriosus is an uncommon malformation characterized by the presence of a single arterial trunk arising from the heart, providing systemic, pulmonary, and coronary circulations (Fig. 16–1).

Incidence

The lesion accounts for approximately 3% of cardiac malformations. Clinical recognition of this defect is important, however, since current surgical techniques permit palliation or physiologic correction.

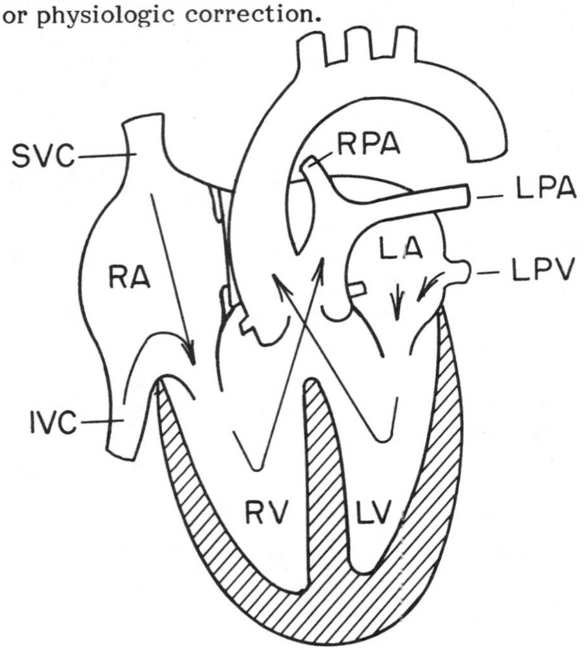

Figure 16–1 Truncus arteriosus. The ventricular septal defect underlying the truncal root permits both ventricles to eject into the common vessel which supplies systemic, pulmonary, and coronary circulation. SVC - superior vena cava, IVC - inferior vena cava, RA - right atrium, LA - left atrium, RV - right ventricle, LV - left ventricle, RPA - right pulmonary artery, LPA - left pulmonary artery, LPV - left pulmonary vein.

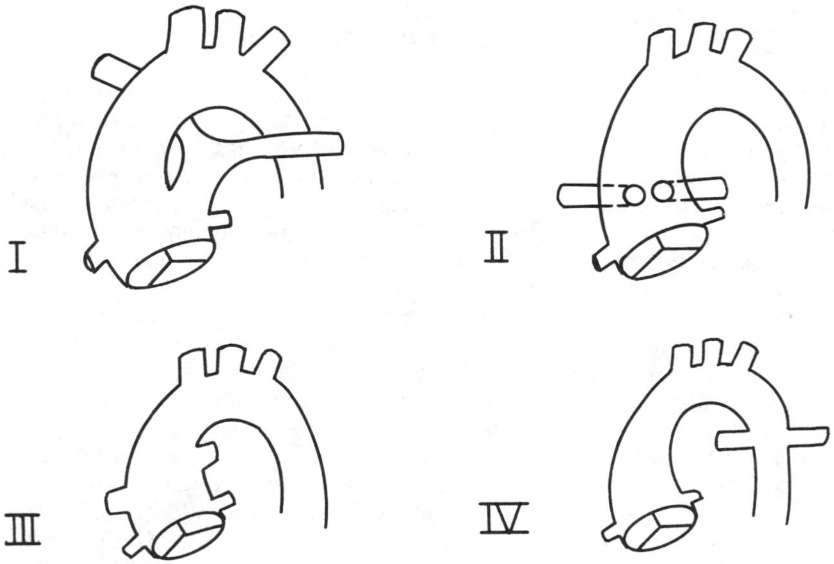

Figure 16–2 Four types of truncus arteriosus (see text for explanation).

Embryology and Anatomy

The embryologic origin of this malformation remains controversial. The classic embryological concept attributes this malformation to failure of division of the conotruncus, while others consider that the defect results from total atresia of the subpulmonic infundibulum with partial or complete absence of pulmonic leaflets and partial or complete absence of the aorticopulmonary septum. A large ventricular septal defect is almost invariably a component of the complex, and allows communication of both ventricles with the common trunk. The etiology of abnormal embryologic formation resulting in this defect is not known, but the role of abnormal blood flow patterns in early fetal development has been suggested. Although variable, the truncal valve most often consists of three cusps. Several anatomic classifications have been proposed. The one which has been most widely accepted is that of Collett and Edwards (Fig. 16–2).

Type I: A single pulmonary trunk arises near the base of the truncus and divides into right and left branches.
Type II: The right and left pulmonary arteries arise separately, but close together, usually from the posterior aspect of the ascending truncus.
Type III: The pulmonary arteries arise independently and more laterally from either side of the truncus.
Type IV: Absence of true pulmonary arteries with pulmonary supply via large bronchial arteries.

Inclusion of type IV as a true variant is somewhat controversial since it does not fulfill the basic definition of the lesion. Less commonly, asymmetrical or more complex origins of the pulmonary arteries may occur. The most common associated anomaly is right aortic arch, present in approximately 30% of cases. Truncal valve insufficiency is present in about 20% of patients and stenosis in 11%. Less commonly, arch anomalies such as coarctation, hypoplasia, or interruption may occur.

Hemodynamics

Blood from both ventricles is ejected directly into the common trunk where more or less complete mixing occurs. This admixture is distributed to the pulmonary, systemic, and coronary circuits. Essentially equal systolic pressures exist in the truncus and both ventricles. The hemodynamics are determined, therefore, by the relative resistances to flow into the systemic and pulmonary vascular beds. Pulmonary blood flow is influenced both by pulmonary arteriolar resistance and the size of the pulmonary arteries. Consequently, small or stenotic pulmonary arteries may be important features of some cases.

Since intercirculatory mixing exists, systemic arterial saturation is always reduced. As in other admixture lesions, the level of saturation is influenced greatly by the volume of pulmonary blood flow. In the neonate with large pulmonary vessels, pulmonary blood flow is limited by the usual high pulmonary vascular resistance, but may soon become excessive as pulmonary resistance declines postnatally. In some cases this decline is unusually rapid, and cardiac failure due to large pulmonary flow and left ventricular volume overload may occur within the first week of life. More typically, pulmonary resistance falls more slowly over a 2-3 week period, and symptoms may appear about this time. Because the pulmonary circuit may be exposed to high pressure and flow, obstructive pulmonary vascular disease is a major potential complication which can appear as early as the first year of life.

Stenotic or diffusely small pulmonary arteries may limit the volume of pulmonary flow after birth. In these infants, congestive heart failure is not likely, but the degree of arterial unsaturation may be greater and may progress in the face of increased oxygen needs associated with growth. Such restriction of flow, however, does impart protection against the development of pulmonary hypertension. When pulmonary blood flow is totally by way of systemic collaterals, the lungs are typically hypoperfused with significant hypoxemia. Less frequently, collaterals may be large and flow normal or increased; in this situation, the hemodynamic picture may resemble that seen when large pulmonary arteries are present.

Clinical Manifestations

Clinical features are determined primarily by the status of the pulmonary arteries and pulmonary vascular bed. Infants with pulmonary stenosis or high pulmonary vascular resistance are usually cyanotic in the neonatal period and may present symptoms of hypoxemia, features which are particularly characteristic of type IV truncus. When large pulmonary arteries are present, cyanosis is initially minimal, occasionally unrecognized, and may actually decrease as pulmonary vascular resistance declines. Such infants may develop congestive failure as early as the first week, but usually signs of failure are delayed until the second or third week.

Precordial palpation reveals a prominent left parasternal or substernal impulse and a systolic thrill may be felt at the second or third left interspace. In over two-thirds a heart murmur is present within the first month of life. This murmur may be a harsh holosystolic murmur at the left sternal edge, suggesting a ventricular septal defect, or only a soft systolic ejection murmur at the base. Occasionally, an ejection murmur at the upper right sternal edge mimics aortic stenosis. Stenotic pulmonary arteries may be suggested by a continuous murmur at the pulmonic area, often extending over both sides of the upper chest. Excessive pulmonary blood flow may result in an apical diastolic rumble due to augmented mitral flow. Two other auscutatory features of diagnostic value are the presence of a prominent systolic ejection click heard both at the base and apex, and a high-pitched decrescendo diastolic murmur along the left sternal border due to insufficiency of the truncal valve. The first sound is normal, but the second sound is typically loud and single, although narrow splitting may be suggested at times. Pulmonary rales and hepatomegaly may be noted when congestive failure is present. Although blood pressure is usually within normal range, a wide pulse pressure with brisk pulses is common when pulmonary flow is high.

Electrocardiogram

The most frequent electrocardiographic feature is combined ventricular hypertrophy, although uncommonly isolated right or left ventricular hypertrophy may be seen. The electrical axis is usually within normal range for age, or slightly rightward (Fig. 16-3). A normal electrocardiogram may be present in infants under 2 weeks of age.

Radiologic Features

Radiographic features may be nonspecific although significant cardiomegaly and pulmonary hypervascularity are present in most. The apparent ascending aorta and knob are sometimes unusually prominent, and in approximately 30% of cases the arch is on the right. The main pulmonary artery typically appears small or ill-defined, but the left pulmonary branch may appear to exit from the hilum at an unusually high level. Left atrial enlargement is frequently present if pulmonary flow is increased (Fig. 16-4).

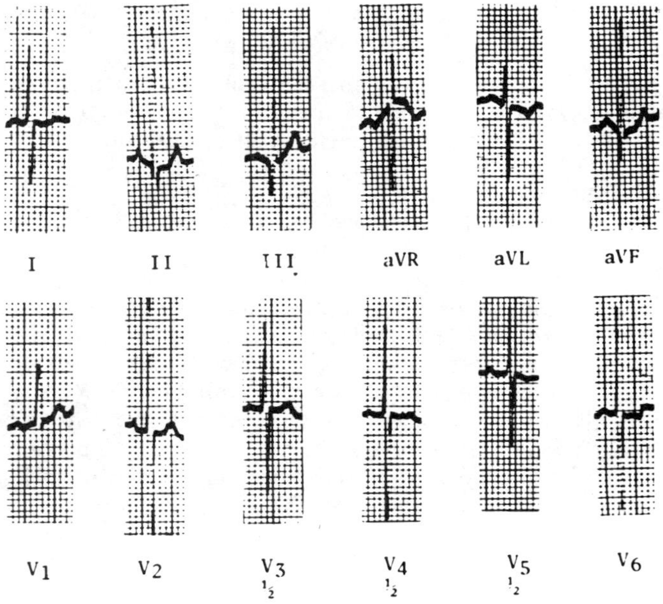

Figure 16-3 Electrocardiogram of infant with truncus arteriosus, type I, demonstrating characteristic biventricular hypertrophy.

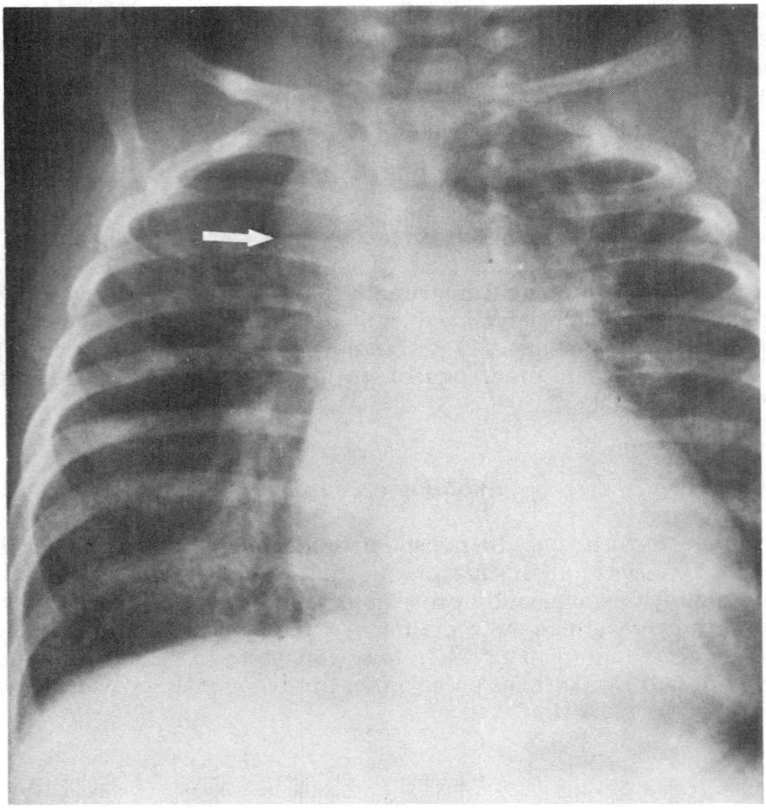

Figure 16-4 Chest roentgenogram of infant with type I truncus. Cardiomegaly, pulmonary hypervascularity, and a right aortic arch (arrow) are present. Note the superior position of the left pulmonary branch in the hilum.

Echocardiographic Findings

As is true in the case of tetralogy, the primary echocardiographic feature is aortic (truncal) overriding of the interventricular septum (i.e., discontinuity between the anterior aortic wall and the septum). The truncal root is dilated, but normal continuity with the mitral valve is preserved. Both ventricles may show dilatation and hypertrophy, more so with high pulmonary flow in which case left atrial dilatation is also present. Right ventricular outflow tract and pulmonic valve are not seen. Abnormalities of the truncal valve may be recognized. The ventricular septal defect and origin of the pulmonary arteries may be easily demonstrated by two-dimensional techniques.

Cardiac Catheterization

Usually the catheter readily enters the truncus from the right ventricle, but passage into the pulmonary arteries may be difficult, depending on their origin from the trunk. Saturation studies consistently reveal systemic arterial unsaturation of variable degree. Evidence of left-to-right shunting in the right ventricular outflow tract may be seen, but saturations in the aorta and pulmonary artery are essentially equal, due to admixture in the common trunk. However, occasionally saturation in the pulmonary artery is slightly less than systemic. This more often occurs in type I anatomy and is due to preferential streaming. Systolic pressures are essentially equal in the ventricles, the truncus, and (in the absence of stenosis) the pulmonary arteries.

Angiocardiography is essential to the diagnosis of this lesion. Injection into the proximal portion of the truncus best defines the abnormal origin of the pulmonary vessels, particularly when both anteroposterior and lateral views are obtained. Delineation of the anatomy of the pulmonary arteries is especially important for surgical considerations (Fig. 16-5) as is accurate assessment of any abnormality of the truncal valve.

Course and Prognosis

Although the clinical course of this lesion is variable, the prognosis is generally poor without surgical intervention. The majority of infants fail to survive the first year of life. Most deaths occur within the first 6 months, with many of these within the first 6 weeks of life. Death in infancy usually results from congestive heart failure or, less often, from complications of severe hypoxemia. Patients surviving infancy with unobstructed pulmonary flow may eventually succumb to progressive obstructive pulmonary vascular disease.

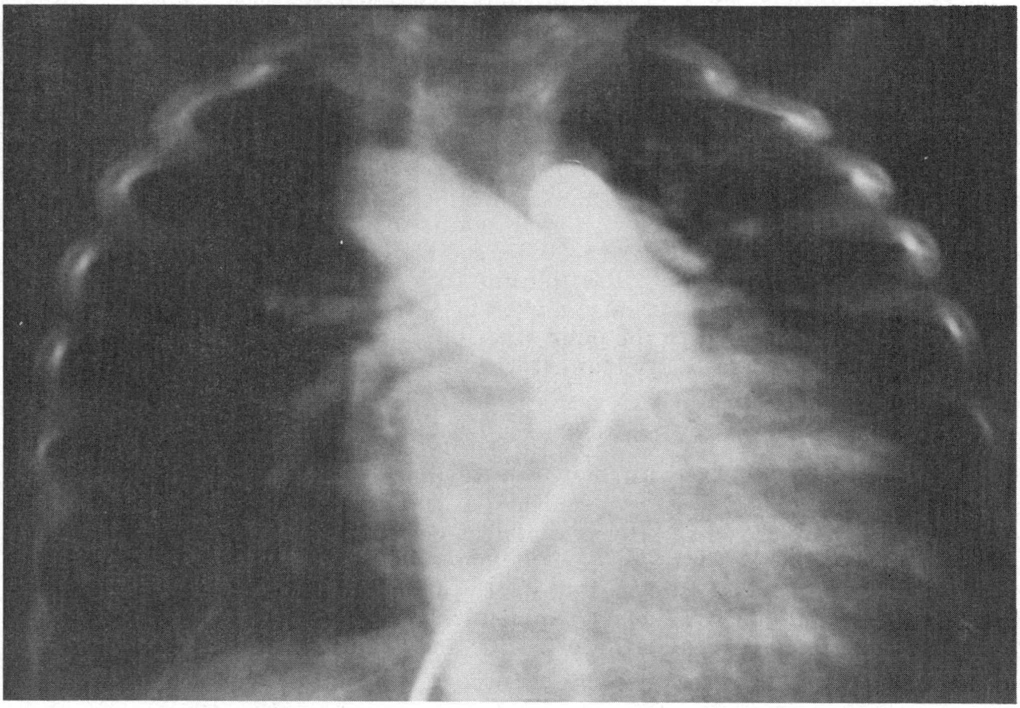

Figure 16-5 Angiogram, truncus arteriosus, type I (same patient). The catheter tip is in the ascending portion of the truncus. The large common pulmonary trunk arises from the left posterior aspect of the truncus. The arch and descending aorta are on the right. Note the high origin of the left pulmonary branch.

In some individuals, pulmonary blood flow and pressures are effectively balanced by an appropriate degree of pulmonary stenosis and, in these, survival into the third or fourth decade is possible. Surgical advances have significantly improved the immediate prognosis for many patients with this malformation, but long-term results of physiologic correction are not yet clearly defined.

Treatment

Manifestations of congestive failure should be vigorously treated with digitalis and, if indicated, diuretics. Every effort should be made in providing adequate nutrition, a goal which may be difficult to achieve as these infants are often too ill to feed properly. Medical management is usually unsuccessful as there is no way to reduce the excessive and often torrential pulmonary blood flow and attendant pulmonary hypertension. Thus, the treatment of this lesion is primarily surgical. Two approaches are available: palliation and physiological correction.

Palliation can be achieved in those patients having excessive pulmonary blood flow by banding the common pulmonary segment (type I) or right and left branches, individually (types II, III). In the latter instance both branches, if large, must be banded, otherwise increased flow to the unbanded side may lead to the development of pulmonary vascular disease. Banding has met generally with only moderate success. Technical problems and late complications have dampened earlier enthusiasm for this procedure. In young infants with pulmonary stenosis and inadequate pulmonary blood flow, some type of systemic-pulmonary artery shunt can be performed with expected alleviation of cyanosis and hypoxemia.

Patients with appropriate pulmonary artery anatomy without prohibitive pulmonary vascular disease may be candidates for reconstructive physiological correction. This consists of dividing the pulmonary arteries from the truncus and closure of the ventricular septal defect to incorporate the truncal root into the left ventricle. Communication between the right ventricle and pulmonary circuit is accomplished by means of an external valved conduit. Although the best candidate for this approach would appear to be over 2 years of age with controlled congestive failure and normal pulmonary vascular resistance, such patients are rare, and surgical intervention is usually mandatory within the first 12-18 months of life. Recent experience with open heart surgery in even very small infants in the first months of life is very encouraging to the point where pulmonary arterial banding has no place in the management of truncus arteriosus. Definitive repair is clearly the proper approach at any age.

Differential Diagnosis

This lesion may present features which suggest numerous other malformations, both cyanotic and acyanotic. Large ventricular septal defect with pulmonary hypertension, tetralogy of Fallot, patent ductus arteriosus, and transposition of the great arteries are among the more common lesions to be considered. Diagnosis, however, depends on careful catheterization and angiographic studies.

Bibliography

Calder L, Van Praagh R, Van Praagh S, Sears WP, Corwin R, Levy A, Keith JD, Paul MH: Truncus arteriosus communis. Clinical, angiocardiographic and pathologic findings in 100 patients. Am Heart J 92:23, 1976.

Collett RW, Edwards JE: Persistent truncus arteriosus; a classification according to anatomic types. Surg Clin North Am 29:1245, 1949.

Edwards JE, McGoon DC: Absence of anatomic origin from the heart of pulmonary arterial supply. Circulation 47:393, 1974.

Mair DD, Ritter DG, Davis GD, Wallace RB, Danielson DK, McGoon DC: Selection of patients with truncus arteriosus for surgical correction: anatomic and hemodynamic considerations. Circulation 49:144, 1974.

Marcelletti C, McGoon DC, Danielson GK, Wallace RB, Mair TD: Early and late results of surgical repair of truncus arteriosus. Circulation 55:636, 1977.

Stark J, Gandi D, deLeval M, McCartney F, Taylor JFN: Surgical treatment of persistent truncus arteriosus in the first year of life. Brit Heart J 40:1280, 1978.

Sullivan H, Sulayman R, Replogle R, Arcilla RA: Surgical correction of truncus arteriosus in infancy. Am J Cardiol 38:113, 1976.

Thiene G, Bortolotti U, Gallucci V, Terribile V, Pellegrino PA: Anatomical study of truncus arteriosus communis with embryological and surgical considerations. Brit Heart J 38:1109, 1976.

Van Praagh R, Van Praagh S: The anatomy of common aorticopulmonary trunk (truncus arteriosus communis) and its embryologic implications. A study of 57 necropsy cases. Am J Cardiol 16:406, 1965.

Chapter 17

TOTAL ANOMALOUS PULMONARY VENOUS DRAINAGE

Total anomalous pulmonary venous drainage (TAPVD) is characterized by abnormal connection of all pulmonary veins to the systemic venous circuit instead of to the left atrium. Several anatomic variants have been recognized, forming the basis for a generally accepted classification (Fig. 17-1).

1. *Supracardiac:* A confluence of the four pulmonary veins behind the left atrium joins a persistent vertical vein (persistent left superior vena cava) which ascends to the left innominate and then to the right superior vena cava. In some instances, the common pulmonary vein directly enters the right superior vena cava posteriorly at its junction with the right atrium.
2. *Cardiac:* Drainage of the four pulmonary veins into the coronary sinus or connection of the veins directly into the right atrium.
3. *Infracardiac:* A confluent single venous trunk courses downward behind the left atrium, traversing the diaphragm anterior to the esophagus to connect with a systemic vein: portal (most common), ductus venosus, hepatic, or inferior vena cava.
4. *Mixed:* Combinations of 1, 2, and 3.

In each type the anomalous pathway may be obstructed to a variable degree, although obstruction is most frequent with infracardiac connections.

Incidence

The lesion is not common, accounting for less than 2% of clinical congenital cardiac malformation. In newborn autopsy series the defect has been reported in up to 4% of cases. The sex incidence is equal except for male predominance in TAPVD to the portal vein.

Embryology and Anatomy

The developmental disturbance resulting in this malformation is still undefined. The pulmonary vascular bed, derived from the splanchnic plexus, in early development has no communication with the heart and is drained by primitive venous branches, the right and left cardinal veins, and umbilicovitelline veins. Communication is eventually established normally by development of an outgrowth, the

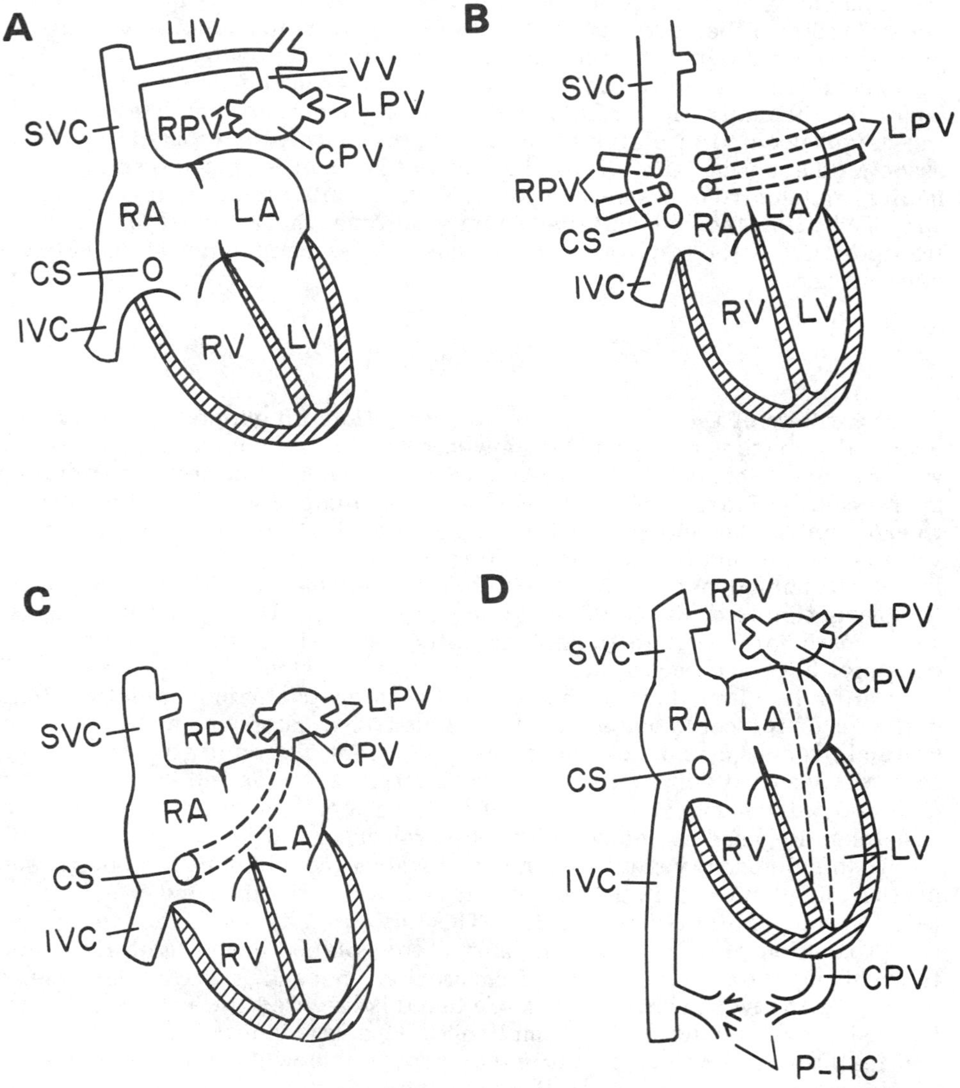

Figure 17–1 Types of total anomalous pulmonary venous drainage. (A) Supracardiac drainage to the superior vena cava. (B) Cardiac drainage directly into the right atrium. (C) Cardiac drainage by way of the coronary sinus. (D) Infradiaphragmatic connections into the portal-hepatic system. SVC - superior vena cava, IVC - inferior vena cava, RA - right atrium, LA - left atrium, CS - coronary sinus, RV - right ventricle, LV - left ventricle, LPV - left pulmonary vein, RPV - right pulmonary vein, CPV - common pulmonary vein, LIV - left innominate vein, VV - vertical vein, PHC - portal-hepatic connections, LPA - left pulmonary artery, RPA - right pulmonary artery.

common pulmonary venous trunk, from the area of the left atrium. This common trunk connects with the primitive pulmonary venous system and is eventually incorporated into the posterior wall of the left atrium in such a way that the four pulmonary veins enter this chamber directly and individually.

A developmental disturbance at various stages in this process is thought to account for the anatomic variants of this lesion encountered clinically. Most often, the defect occurs in isolated form, but approximately one-fourth of patients have associated abnormalities. These include patent ductus arteriosus, aortic arch anomalies, and ventricular septal defect. More complicated defects usually accompany TAPVD in the congenital asplenia syndrome where endocardial cushion defects, transposition of the great arteries, anomalous systemic veins, and single ventricle may be seen.

Hemodynamics

Regardless of the site of anatomic connection, all pulmonary venous return eventually reaches the right atrium where essentially complete admixture occurs with systemic venous return. Adequate communication with the systemic circuit is an essential feature of this lesion, since systemic flow must be maintained. Although ventricular and aortopulmonary communications may occur, in most cases the sole communication is a patent foramen ovale or atrial septal defect. The most important hemodynamic consideration in this anomaly is the presence or absence of obstruction to drainage of the pulmonary veins. Although obstruction is classically associated with infradiaphragmatic connections, similar obstruction hemodynamics have been noted in almost all forms. Obstruction may be related to several factors including inadequacy of the interatrial communication, length and diameter of the common pulmonary venous trunk, narrowing at the entrance to the systemic venous circuit, compression by adjacent anatomic structures (e.g., passage of a vertical vein of the supracardiac type between the left main stem bronchus and pulmonary artery) and, in the case of communication with the portal vein, resistance imposed by the portal-hepatic vascular bed.

When pulmonary venous return is not obstructed, pulmonary blood flow increases postnatally, due to declining pulmonary vascular resistance and changing compliance relationships of the two ventricles. This has two major effects. One is to increase the proportion of saturated pulmonary venous blood in the right atrial admixture, thus raising the absolute level of saturation. Second, there is increased volume loading of the right ventricle as more blood is directed toward the pathway of falling resistance and increasing compliance. Cyanosis is less prominent in such cases, and features of congestive failure may appear somewhat later. Pulmonary hypertension due to excessive blood flow and some element of increased pulmonary vascular resistance is commonly present.

When obstruction is present, pulmonary venous pressure rises as blood flow through the lungs increases after birth. If of sufficient magnitude, this may promote transudation of fluid into the alveoli (pulmonary edema) and the development of passive pulmonary arterial hypertension. The latter is frequently complemented by a component of pulmonary arteriolar vasoconstriction.

Manifestations

The clinical manifestations reflect primarily the degree of obstruction to the pulmonary veins and the presence or absence of significant pulmonary hypertension.

Pulmonary hypertension of significant degree is present in approximately two-thirds and is due to pulmonary venous obstruction in the vast majority (80%).

Infants without pulmonary venous obstruction or significant pulmonary hypertension fare better and may present clinical signs of heart disease at a somewhat later age. Cyanosis may be present at birth, only to improve as pulmonary vascular resistance subsequently falls and pulmonary blood flow increases. Augmented right heart volume work eventually may result in signs of congestive heart failure in the early weeks of life, but generally, symptoms of mild dyspnea, cyanosis, and fatigue are more common; symptoms may be entirely lacking, however. Growth and development may be somewhat impaired. Physical examination may reveal minimal cyanosis or a mildly plethoric appearance, and mild clubbing may be present in older patients. Slight tachypnea is present, but lungs are clear. The overactive cardiac impulse is predominantly right ventricular at the xiphold and lower left sternal areas. Auscultation reveals a loud first heart sound and a well-split and fixed second heart sound. The pulmonic component is of normal or mildly accentuated intensity. Frequently, third and fourth heart sounds are present, resulting in a gallop quality. A soft pulmonic systolic ejection murmur is usually heard, and a right ventricular diastolic filling rumble is typically present along the lower left sternal border. At times, flow through the anomalous pulmonary venous pathway may be audible as a soft continuous murmur.

Increased volume work of the right heart is reflected in the electrocardiographic changes of right axis deviation and right atrial and right ventricular hypertrophy (Fig. 17-2). A qR pattern is often seen in right precordial leads but is not specific for this lesion. Older children may demonstrate a less rightward axis and better developed left ventricular forces in the precordial leads.

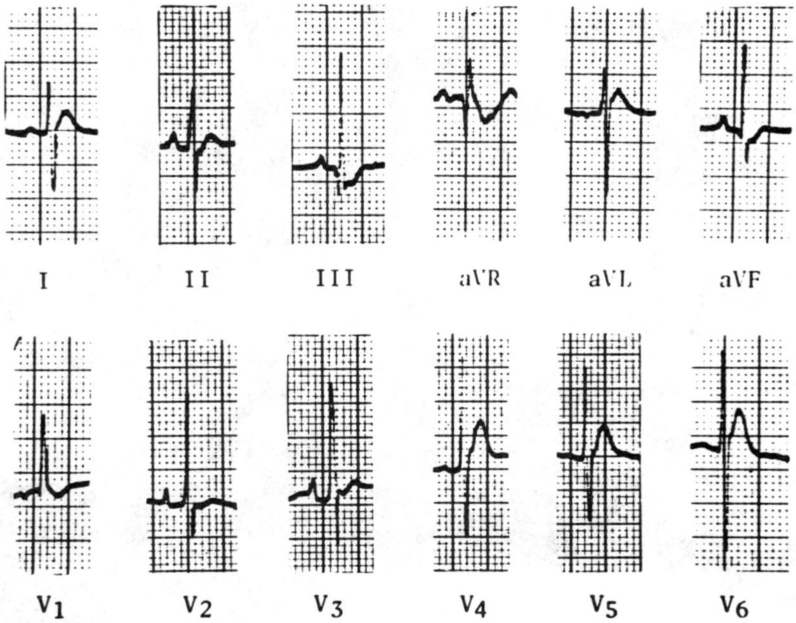

Figure 17-2 Electrocardiogram of infant with total anomalous pulmonary venous drainage. The QRS axis is directed to the right, and right ventricular hypertrophy is present. (Note qR pattern in V_1.)

The chest roentgenogram shows significant cardiomegaly, predominantly involving the right atrium and right ventricle. The pulmonary artery segment and its branches are dilated, and peripheral pulmonary vessels are engorged. Drainage by way of the persistent vertical vein and left innominate vein may result in the classical "snowman" or "figure-of-eight" configuration, a feature not usually identifiable before 4-6 months of age (Fig. 17-3). Drainage into the coronary sinus may be suggested by a low-lying double-density on the right heart border or in the lateral view by a posterior bulge adjacent to the left atrium. Anomalous veins entering the superior vena cava usually do so at its junction with the right atrium, producing an ill-defined vascular density at this site.

Infants with pulmonary venous obstruction usually exhibit some degree of cyanosis at birth, or shortly thereafter, often accompanied by tachypnea and dyspnea. With severe obstruction, these features are progressive, and the infant rapidly appears quite ill. Occasionally, when obstruction is less severe, symptoms may appear later in the first few weeks after birth with moderate cyanosis and congestive heart failure predominantly at this time.

The major manifestations in the infant with severe pulmonary venous obstruction are cyanosis and marked respiratory distress, usually appearing within the first few days of life. Respiratory rate and effort are increased, a result of pulmonary venous and lymphatic engorgement. Generalized diffuse fine inspiratory rales are audible. The precordium is not exceedingly overactive, and a dominant right ventricular impulse is present. Auscultation reveals a loud first heart sound. The second heart sound is narrowly split, and the pulmonic component is accentuated by pulmonary hypertension. Murmurs are frequently absent, but occasionally a soft nonspecific pulmonic ejection murmur is heard. In some infants a systolic murmur in the xiphoid area may suggest tricuspid regurgitation.

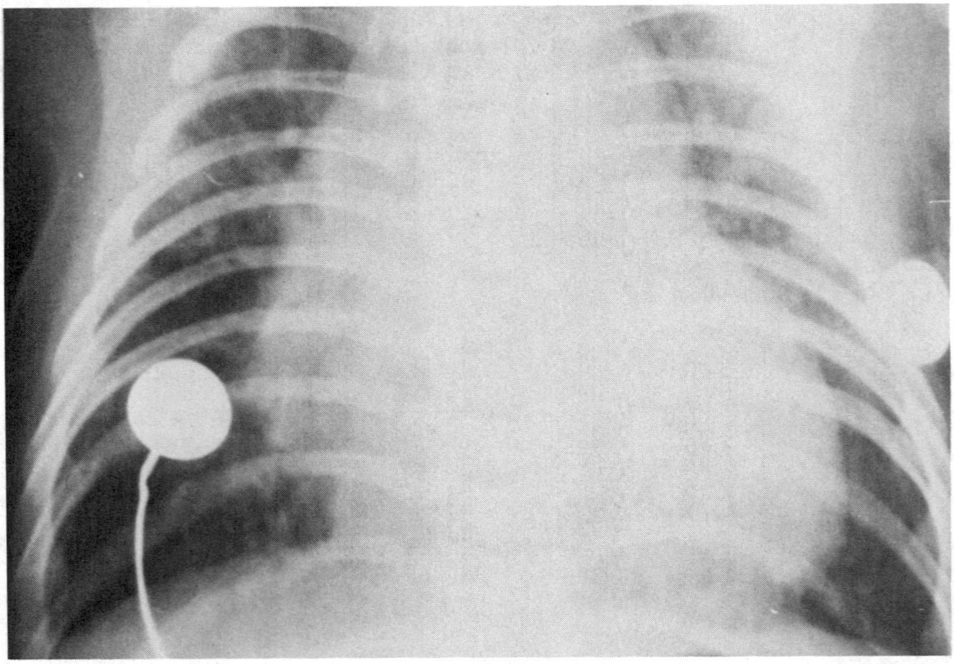

Figure 17-3 Chest roentgenogram of infant with TAPVD to the superior vena cava. Note the wide supracardiac mediastinal shadow characteristic of the snowman appearance.

Hepatomegaly is noted when right ventricular failure has developed. Systemic blood pressure and pulses may be normal initially, but often pulses generally feel diminished. Weak pulses are likely to be present when either obstruction to pulmonary veins is severe, or the interatrial communication is restrictive and the ductus arteriosus is closed.

The electrocardiogram, not remarkably different from those without obstruction, shows right axis deviation, right atrial enlargement, right ventricular hypertrophy, and minimal left ventricular forces.

When pulmonary venous obstruction is severe, the chest roentgenogram characteristically shows a normal or small heart size with diffuse pulmonary edema manifested by granular opacity of the lungs ("ground-glass" appearance). The heart borders and hilar structures may be difficult or impossible to identify (Fig. 17-4).

Echocardiographic Findings

Manifestations of this lesion have been variable. The right ventricle may appear large, the left atrium small or near normal size, and abnormal septal motion characteristic of right ventricular volume overload may be seen. In some instances, an echo-free space, posterior to the left atrial wall, has been seen on M-mode echocardiography correlating with the common pulmonary venous trunk. Two-dimensional techniques allow for better assessment of the common venous confluence as well as, often, the nature of the connection with the right atrium. Evaluation of cardiac chamber size is also better achieved by this approach.

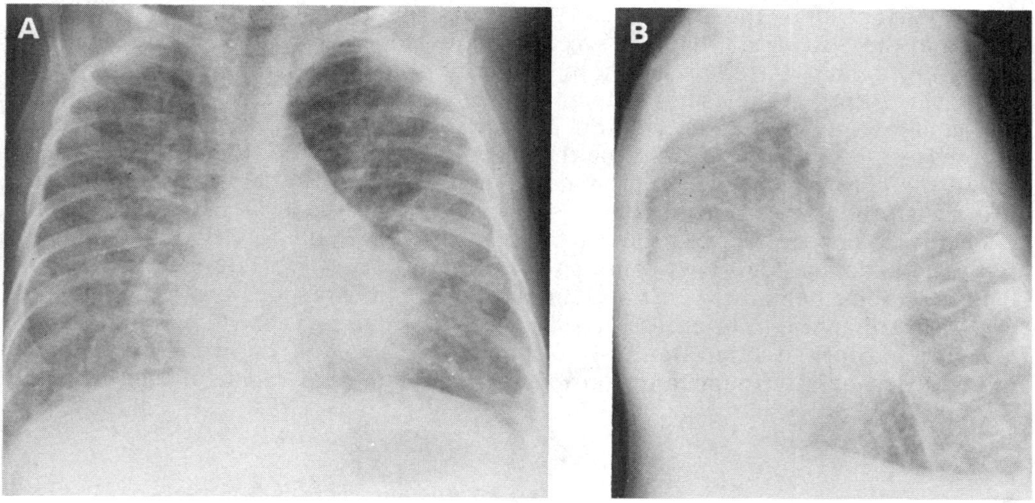

Figure 17-4 Chest roentgenogram of obstructive type of TAPVD. (A) The heart is not significantly enlarged. Diffuse pulmonary edema is present, partially obscuring the cardiac borders. (B) In the lateral view the cardiac borders are ill-defined, and there is fluid in the fissures.

Cardiac Catheterization

Thorough study is essential to establish the diagnosis, determine the site of drainage of all pulmonary veins, the site of venous obstruction, if present, and to assess the adequacy of the interatrial communication. Assessment of pulmonary vascular resistance also is essential, of course, particularly in older patients. Right atrial mean pressure usually exceeds left atrial mean pressure to a variable degree. The degree of elevation is influenced particularly by the size of the interatrial opening. The A wave is usually dominant in both atrial chambers, although of lesser magnitude in the left atrium.

Right ventricular and pulmonary arterial pressures are dependent on pulmonary vascular resistance and the severity of pulmonary venous obstruction, and may equal or exceed systemic levels. The majority have systolic pressures greater than 50% of systemic, although near-normal pulmonary artery pressure may be seen in the older patients who do not have venous obstruction. Right ventricular end-diastolic pressure usually is elevated when pulmonary venous obstruction or congestive failure is present. Pulmonary arterial wedge pressure is increased, often severely so, in those patients with obstructed pulmonary veins. Left ventricular and systemic arterial pressures are usually normal except when severe obstruction of the pulmonary veins or a restrictive foramen ovale impairs left ventricular output.

Since essentially complete admixture of pulmonary and systemic venous blood occurs in the right atrium, oxygen saturation values are nearly identical in all cardiac chambers and both great arteries. The actual level of saturation may vary considerably, however, depending on total pulmonary blood flow, and to some extent, the presence of preferential streaming. Systemic saturation values ranging from less than 30% to greater than 90% have been observed, the higher levels being seen in the absence of severe pulmonary hypertension. In most, however, significant unsaturation is present with variations less than 5% at all sites.

Selective angiocardiographic studies are essential to define the anatomy and site of connection of the anomalous veins, the site of venous obstruction (if present), and the left atrial chamber size. The anomalous veins and their connections usually are demonstrated by injection of contrast into the pulmonary artery, following through to the phase of pulmonary venous filling. Drainage to the superior vena cava by way of the left vertical and innominate veins presents a striking picture of the anatomy responsible for the snowman appearance (Fig. 17-5). Connection to the coronary sinus may produce an opacified density behind and communicating with the lower right atrium.

Subdiaphragmatic connections at times may be difficult to visualize because of high resistance and low flow, common to this pathway. Usually, however, the confluence of veins behind the left atrium and the common venous trunk descending through the diaphragm to enter the systemic veins can be seen (Fig. 17-6). Injection into the left atrium allows evaluation of left heart structures. Left atrial size is an especially important consideration for surgical repair of the critically ill infant.

Course and Prognosis

Prognosis for this lesion is generally related to the severity of pulmonary hypertension. Infants with severe pulmonary venous obstruction rarely survive more than a few weeks to months and often deteriorate rapidly within the first days of life. Those with hyperkinetic pulmonary hypertension may survive somewhat longer, but

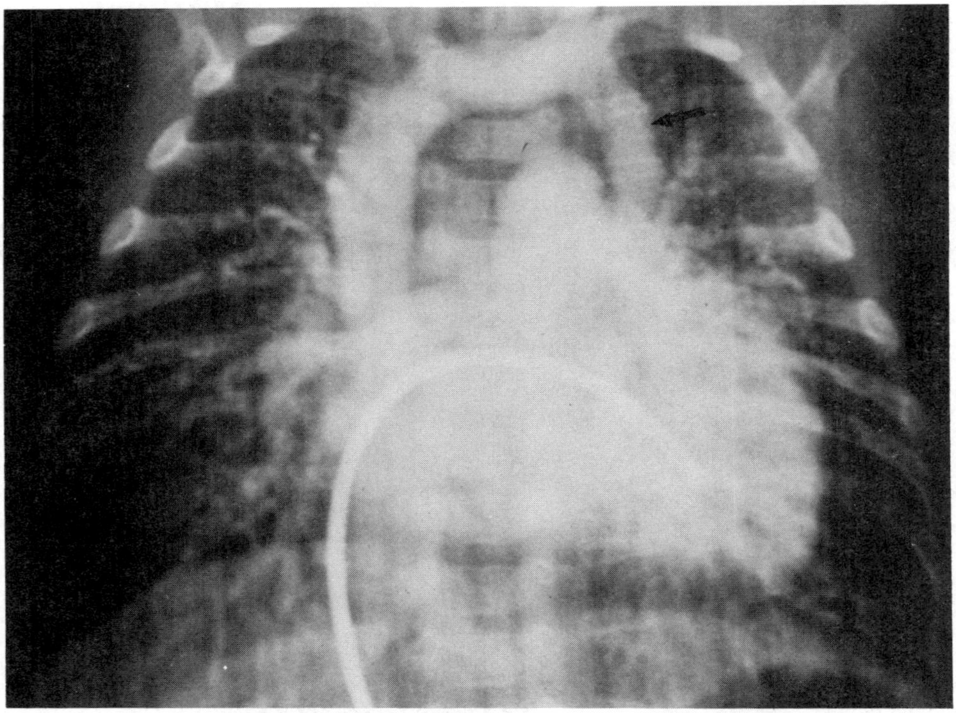

Figure 17–5A Right ventricular angiocardiogram of infant with TAPVD to the superior vena cava; pulmonary venous phase. The pulmonary veins communicate with the vertical vein (along left border of the spine, arrow) and innominate vein which crosses the right to enter the superior vena cava. Contrast medium is recirculating through the pulmonary artery.

are at risk to develop pulmonary vascular obstruction at an early age, even within the first year. The occasional patient without pulmonary hypertension clinically resembles secundum atrial septal defect and may survive into the second decade with few symptoms.

Treatment

Treatment of this lesion is primarily surgical. Manifestations of heart failure are treated with the usual anticongestive measures. The infant with pulmonary edema from pulmonary venous obstruction, however, may not show significant response since the problem is a mechanical one. Ventilatory assistance with continuous positive airway pressure (CPAP) may improve the pulmonary edema as well as pulmonary gaseous exchange.

Balloon atrial septostomy should be considered at the time of catheterization in all infants with this lesion to ensure unobstructed interatrial communication, particularly if right atrial pressure significantly exceeds left atrial pressure. The surgical approach varies somewhat with the underlying anatomy; but basically, utilizing cardiopulmonary bypass, the common pulmonary venous trunk is anastomosed to the left atrium by as large an opening as possible, and its anamalous connection is obliterated. Concurrently, the left atrial, and if necessary the right

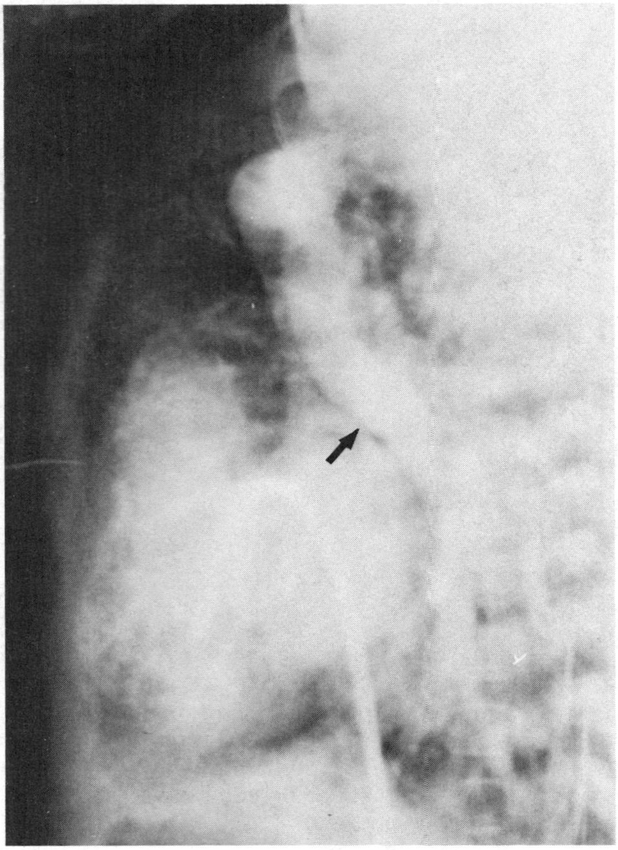

Figure 17–5B Right ventricular angiocardiogram of infant with TAPVD to the superior vena cava; pulmonary venous phase. Lateral view demonstrates the retrocardiac relations of the anomalous pulmonary venous channels.

atrial cavities, may be enlarged by various techniques and the interatrial communication closed. When the pulmonary veins connect directly to the right atrium or by way of the coronary sinus, flow is directed to the left atrium utilizing an interatrial baffle of pericardium. Mortality remains high in the young infant with pulmonary venous obstruction and heart failure, but is 10% or less in older patients with little pulmonary hypertension.

Differential Diagnosis

The presence of cyanosis and radiographic evidence of severe pulmonary venous congestion without cardiomegaly in the neonate would always direct consideration to the diagnosis of total anomalous venous return of the obstructive type, usually with infradiaphragmatic connections.

Other lesions associated with significant pulmonary venous hypertension include hypoplastic left heart syndrome, cor triatriatum, and atresia of the pulmonary veins, the last two of which are less common. In those without obstruction, increased pulmonary flow and congestive failure may lead one to suspect lesions such as transposition of the great arteries, single ventricle without pulmonic stenosis, and truncus arteriosus, among others. Differentiation from primary respiratory disorders in the neonate also can be difficult at times.

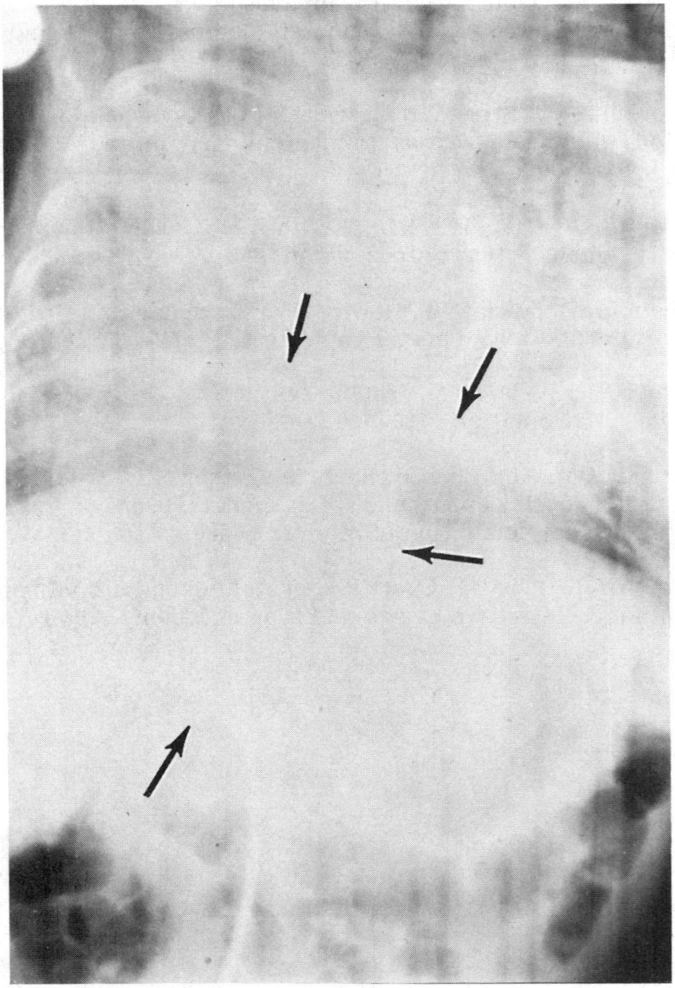

Figure 17-6 Pulmonary artery angiogram (pulmonary venous phase) showing confluence of pulmonary veins behind the heart (upper arrows). The common pulmonary vein (middle arrow) passes inferiorly to a large subdiaphragmatic pool (lower arrow) draining into the hepatic system.

Bibliography

Behrendt DM, Aberdeen E, Waterson DJ, Bonham-Carter RE: Total anomalous pulmonary venous drainage in infants. I. Clinical and hemodynamic findings, methods, and results of operation in 37 cases. Circulation 46:347, 1972.

Clark DR, Stark J, Deleval M, Pincott JR, Taylor JFN: Total anomalous pulmonary venous drainage in infancy. Brit Heart J 39:436, 1977.

Duff DF, Nihill MR, McNamara DG: Infradiaphragmatic total anomalous pulmonary venous return: review of clinical and pathological findings and results of operation in 28 cases. Brit Heart J 39:619, 1977.

Gersony WM, Bowman FO, Steeg CN, Hayes CJ, Jesse MJ, Malm JR: Management of total anomalous pulmonary venous drainage in early infancy. Circulation 43 and 44 (Suppl I):1-19, 1970.

Mathew R, Thilenius OG, Replogle RL, Arcilla RA: Cardiac function in total anomalous pulmonary venous return before and after surgery. Circulation 55:361, 1977.

Mortera C, Tyman M, Goodwin AW, Hunter S: Infradiaphragmatic total anomalous pulmonary venous connection to portal vein. Brit Heart J 39:685, 1977.

Paquet M, Gutgesell H: Echocardiographic features of total anomalous pulmonary venous connections. Circulation 51:599, 1975.

Silove ED, Behrendt DM, Aberdeen E, Bonham-Carter RE: Total anomalous pulmonary venous drainage. II. Spontaneous functional closure of interatrial communication after surgical correction in infancy. Circulation 46:357, 1972.

Turley K, Tucker WY, Ullyot DJ, Ebert PA: Total anomalous pulmonary venous connection in infancy: influence of age and type of lesion. Am J Cardiol 45:92, 1980.

Chapter 18

DOUBLE-OUTLET RIGHT VENTRICLE

Origin of both great arteries from the right ventricle (double-outlet right ventricle) is a relatively rare congenital cardiac malformation. Clinically, the lesion probably accounts for less than 1% of congenital cardiac malformations but is seen in up to 3% of infants dying from heart disease in the first months of life.

Embryology and Anatomy

Basically, the defect consists of a malposition of the great arteries such that both vessels arise solely or predominantly from the right ventricle (Fig. 18-1). The only outlet from the left ventricle is a ventricular septal defect, supracristal (subpulmonic) or infracristal (subaortic) in location. Infrequently the septal defect is uncommitted. Those cases with subpulmonic ventricular septal defect are often referred to as the Taussig-Bing malformation. Various classifications have been proposed, based on the location of the ventricular septal defect. The great arteries may be in normal relationship, lying side by side with the aorta to the right of the pulmonary artery and, although externally their relationships may appear normal, the aortic valve is abnormally high, lying in the same plane as the pulmonic valve. Conal tissue commonly is present beneath both arteries (double conus), and usually neither the aortic nor pulmonic annulus is in fibrous continuity with the mitral valve. Pulmonic stenosis, usually subpulmonic, may be associated, and other malformations, including atrioventricular canal defect, mitral atresia or stenosis, and coarctation of the aorta, are present not infrequently.

Hemodynamics

The only outlet for the left ventricle is the ventricular septal defect. The size and location of this defect, the presence of pulmonic stenosis, and other associated malformations influence the hemodynamic alterations. Basically, the right ventricle ejects into both systemic and pulmonary circuits and must, therefore, always generate abnormally high pressure. The left ventricle must empty into the right ventricle by way of the ventricular septal defect, which, if obstructive, may augment left ventricular pressure work. Depending on the location of the septal defect, the left ventricle may preferentially eject into either the aorta or pulmonary artery, a feature which affects the degree of cyanosis. However, since admixture of saturated and unsaturated blood always occurs, systemic saturation is influenced predominantly by total pulmonary blood flow.

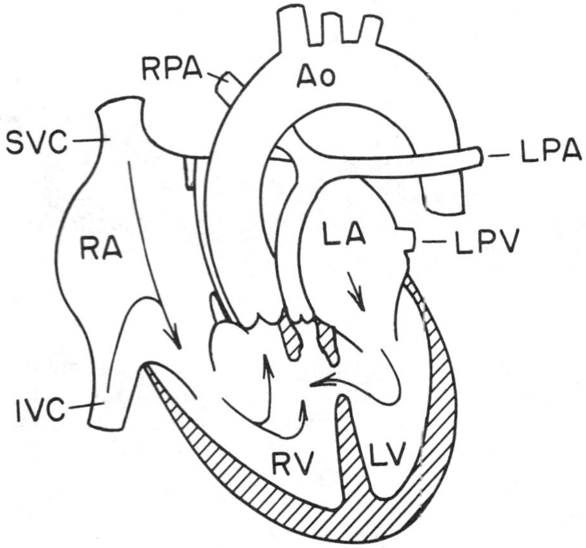

Figure 18–1 Circulatory pathways in double-outlet right ventricle with pulmonic stenosis. Both great vessels arise side by side from the right ventricle anterior to the ventricular septum with the semilunar valves at the same level. Subpulmonic obstruction is present, and the pulmonary artery is small. The left ventricle can eject only by way of the ventricular septal defect. SVC - superior vena cava, IVC - inferior vena cava, RA - right atrium, LA - left atrium, RV - right ventricle, LV - left ventricle, Ao - aorta, RPA - right pulmonary artery, LPA - left pulmonary artery, LPV - left pulmonary vein.

Manifestations

This group of malformations presents a spectrum of clinical manifestations related to the underlying anatomic variations. Commonly, the ventricular septal defect is subaortic, pulmonic stenosis is present, and the clinical features resemble those of tetralogy of Fallot. Those with subpulmonic ventricular septal defect without pulmonic stenosis clinically may resemble transposition of the great arteries, while other variants without pulmonic stenosis may suggest ventricular septal defect with pulmonary hypertension.

The majority of patients are recognized early to have heart disease: frequently, noncardiac congenital malformations are also present. Those with pulmonic stenosis commonly present with cyanosis in early infancy, and manifestations of hypoxemia dominate the clinical picture. Cyanosis, clubbing, and moderate cardiomegaly are present with a stenotic systolic murmur at the left sternal border, terminated by a loud single second sound. The electrocardiogram in these infants reveals right axis deviation and right ventricular hypertrophy. A pattern of right bundle branch block and prolonged AV conduction is often present. Roentgenographic features are similar to those of tetralogy of Fallot with right ventricular contour and hypovascular lungs.

Without pulmonic stenosis, pulmonary blood flow generally is excessive, cyanosis is less apparent, and congestive heart failure often appears within the first 2 months of life. Features of the physical examination are those of large ventricular septal defect, cardiomegaly, hyperdynamic precordium, lower left parasternal thrill, and holosystolic murmur. The pulmonic component of the second sound is always accentuated, reflecting the raised pulmonary arterial pressure. The electrocardiogram may suggest right or combined hypertrophy (Fig. 18-2).

The electrocardiogram in those with subaortic ventricular septal defect without pulmonic stenosis typically shows marked left superior axis (-30 - -180°) with right ventricular hypertrophy, a helpful diagnostic clue. Roentgenographic features are nonspecific, resembling those of a large ventricular septal defect with pulmonary hypertension, that is, generalized cardiomegaly, hypervascularity, and dilated pulmonary trunk (Fig. 18-3).

Echocardiography

M-mode echocardiographic features are suggestive but not diagnostic. Typically, there is lack of continuity between the anterior mitral leaflet and posterior aortic wall, but other conditions may produce similar findings. Secondary changes include right ventricular hypertrophy, variable enlargement of the left atrium and left ventricle, and difficulty in simultaneously visualizing both anterior and posterior walls of the aortic root. Two-dimensional techniques allow better evaluation of the origin of the great arteries and may possibly identify the ventricular septal defec

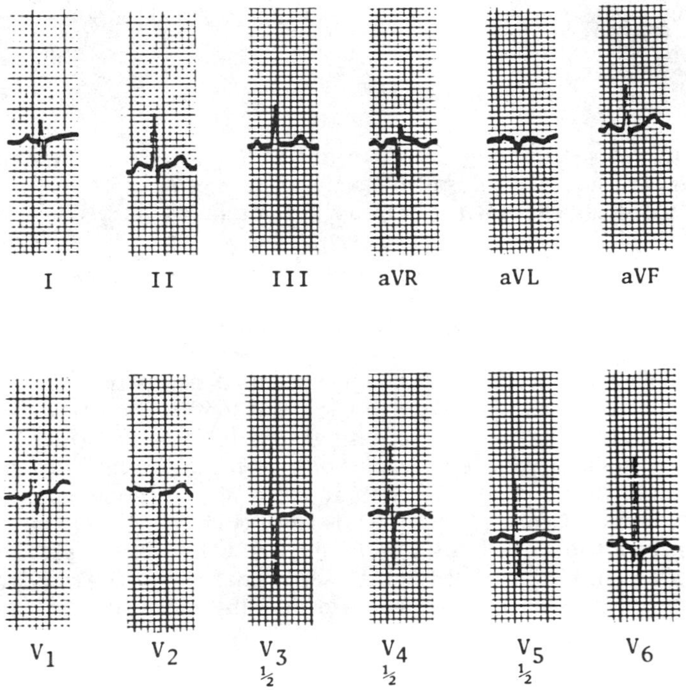

Figure 18-2 Electrocardiogram of 5-week-old infant with double-outlet right ventricle, subpulmonic ventricular septal defect (Taussig-Bing type) without pulmonic stenosis. Pulmonary hypertension was present. Midprecordial voltages are prominent and upright T waves in right precordial leads suggest right ventricular hypertrophy.

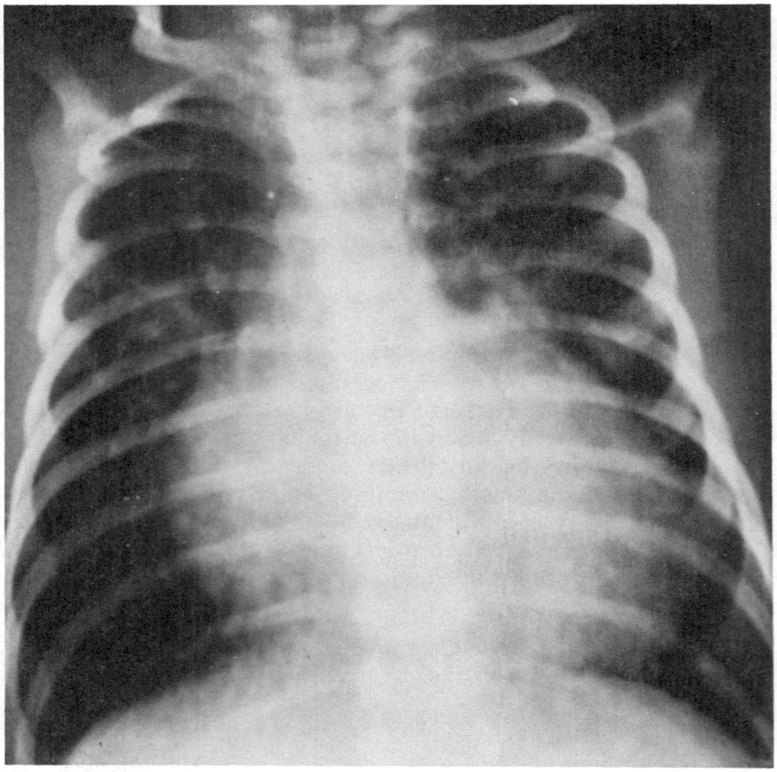

Figure 18-3 Chest roentgenogram of infant with double-outlet right ventricle and subpulmonic ventricular septal defect without pulmonic stenosis. The heart is enlarged and pulmonary vasculature increased. The pulmonary trunk is not well defined, however.

Cardiac Catheterization

Diagnosis of this anomaly and its variations is based primarily on angiocardiographic studies. Contrast injected into the right ventricle reveals simultaneous opacification of both great arteries, arising clearly from the right ventricle; the aortic valve in abnormally high position; both semilunar valves at the same level, with superimposition of the root of both arteries above the right ventricle in the lateral view and conal tissue present bilaterally (Fig. 18-4). On retrograde passage, the catheter enters the right ventricle from the aorta. Left ventriculography may reveal the relationship of the ventricular septal defect to the crista, and often shows a characteristic tunnellike channel extending from the septal defect to the aortic root.

Course and Prognosis

The course and prognosis depend on the basic anatomy and associated cardiac malformations. A significant number succumb to congestive heart failure or hypoxemia in early infancy. Those surviving with excessive pulmonary flow later may

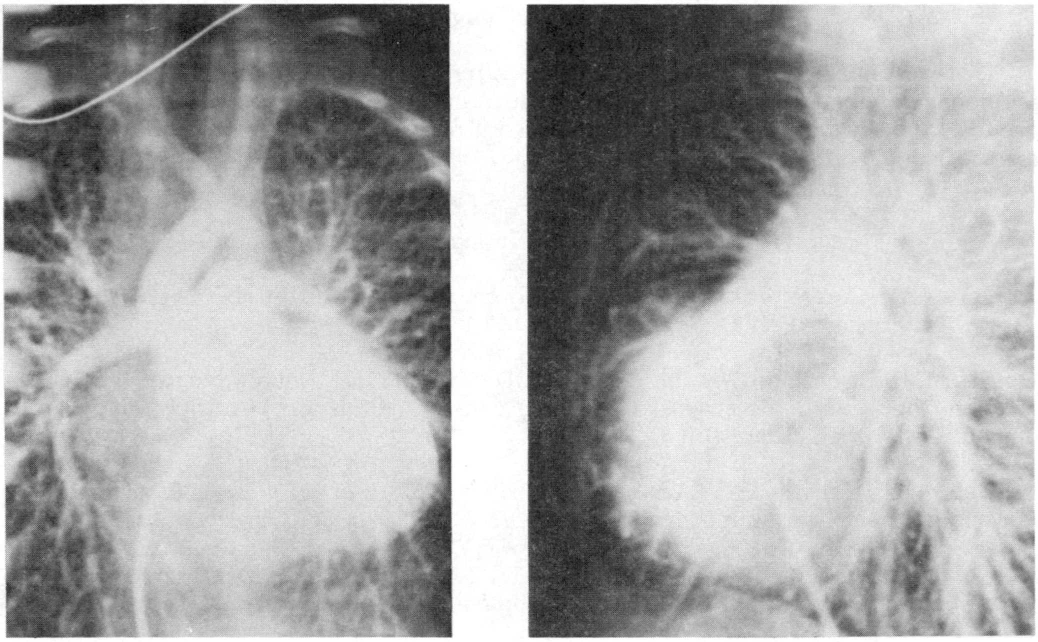

Figure 18–4 Angiocardiogram of child with double-outlet right ventricle without pulmonic stenosis, right ventricular injection. (A) Frontal view shows simultaneous opacification of both great arteries which lie side by side. (B) Lateral view. The origin of both arteries is superimposed and lies anterior to the ventricular septum.

develop pulmonary vascular disease. Complicating anomalies, both cardiac and noncardiac, often contribute to early demise.

Treatment

Congestive heart failure is, of course, managed as usual. Surgical therapy is both palliative and corrective. Infants with inadequate pulmonary blood flow can be symptomatically improved by a systemic-pulmonary artery shunt. If pulmonary blood flow is excessive, banding of the pulmonary artery may be beneficial but is not without risk. Surgical correction can be achieved, but is technically difficult and often complicated by associated cardiac lesions. Closure of the ventricular septal defect in the usual manner results in catastrophe, since a blind left ventricle results. Preoperative recognition of the presence of double-outlet right ventricle, therefore, is essential. When feasible, the left ventricular outflow may be directed into the aorta by means of a patch baffle extending from the ventricular septal defect to the aortic root. In some cases a more complicated approach has been used with closure of the ventricular septal defect, insertion of an external valved conduit between the left ventricle and pulmonary artery (creating in essence, transposition of the great arteries), followed by a Mustard procedure to reroute the venous inflows. Results have been satisfactory in selected cases.

Differential Diagnosis

Differential diagnosis primarily includes large ventricular septal defect with pulmonary hypertension, tetralogy of Fallot, and complete transposition of the great arteries. Clinical differentiation is not possible, and one must depend on angiocardiographic analysis.

Bibliography

Cameron AH, Acerete F, Quero M, Castro MC: Double outlet right ventricle. Study of 27 cases. Brit Heart J 38:1124, 1976.

Gomes MMR, Weidman WH, McGoon DC, Danielson GK: Double outlet right ventricle without pulmonic stenosis: surgical considerations and results of operation. Circulation 43, 44 (Suppl I):I-31, 1970.

Neufeld HN, Dushane JW, Edwards JE: Origin of both great vessels from the right ventricle. II. With pulmonary stenosis. Circulation 23:603, 1961.

Neufeld HN, DuShane JW, Wood EH, Kirklin JW, Edwards JE: Origin of both great vessels from the right ventricle. I. Without pulmonary stenosis. Circulation 23:399, 1961.

Sondheimer HM, Freedom RM, Olley PM: Double outlet right ventricle: clinical spectrum and prognosis. Am J Cardiol 39:709, 1977.

Sridaromont S, Feldt RH, Ritter DG, Davis GD, Edwards JE: Double outlet right ventricle: hemodynamic and anatomic correlations. Am J Cardiol 38:85, 1976.

Van Praagh R: What is the Taussig-Bing malformation? Circulation 38:445, 1968.

Zamora R, Moller JH, Edwards JE: Double outlet right ventricle — anatomic types and associated anomalies. Chest 68:672, 1975.

Chapter 19

HYPOPLASTIC LEFT HEART SYNDROME

Representing the hypoplastic left heart syndrome is a group of left-sided obstructive malformations associated with more or less severe hypoplasia of the left ventricle. Lesions most commonly encountered in this complex include atresia or severe hypoplasia and stenosis of the aortic and/or mitral valves and atresia or hypoplasia of the aortic arch. Coexistence of more than one anomaly is quite common.

Incidence

The complex is by no means rare and accounts for most cases of congestive heart failure in the first week of life. Among infants dying in the neonatal period from congenital cardiovascular malformation, hypoplastic left heart syndrome accounts for approximately 15-20% of cases. A slight male dominance (3:2) is seen.

Embryology and Anatomy

The etiology of this lesion is not known. Premature closure of the foramen ovale, resulting in abnormal fetal blood flow pathways, has been suggested but is not consistently found.

The most common and severe form of this complex is aortic valve atresia, the general features of which are representative of other lesions in this group. The aortic valve is represented by only a diaphragm extending across a very hypoplastic annulus. The coronary arteries originate normally and are of near-normal size.

The left ventricle usually is thick walled with a tiny cavity of sometimes slit-like proportions. Endocardial fibroelastosis of this chamber is frequently present. In approximately 90% of cases the ventricular septum is intact. The mitral annulus and valve are diminutive, and mitral valve atresia may coexist (25%). The left atrium is always small with a prolapsed foramen ovale (15%) or a true atrial septal defect. The right atrium, right ventricle, and pulmonary artery are considerably enlarged, and the latter communicates with the aorta by way of a large ductus arteriosus.

Hemodynamics

Forward flow through the left heart is not possible, a feature resulting in major hemodynamic disturbance, both in the fetus and after birth. In the fetus, blood from the inferior vena cava can no longer flow to the left atrium, but instead must pass into the right ventricle with the superior vena caval stream. Blood ejected into the pulmonary artery is distributed, in small part, to the fetal lungs with the greater portion entering the aorta by way of the ductus arteriosus. The ascending aorta and its branches (cerebral and coronary) are perfused in retrograde fashion (Fig. 19-1).

In cases where the mitral valve is patent, blood entering the diminutive left ventricular chamber must reflux back into the left atrium. Occasionally, the left ventricular cavity communicates by way of large myocardial sinusoids with the coronary circulation.

Left atrial and pulmonary venous hypertension may be considerable, especially when left atrial egress is dependent on an obstructive foramen ovale, and results in the characteristic presence of pulmonary edema. Pulmonary arterial hypertension is always present. This is due to both pulmonary venous hypertension and to the fact that the pulmonary artery supplies both pulmonary and systemic blood flow. Blood entering the aorta is an admixture of systemic and pulmonary venous return. Consequently, cyanosis is invariably present, the severity of which is dependent on total pulmonary blood flow.

After birth, the right ventricle continues to perfuse both the pulmonary and systemic circulations. The relative proportions of blood flow distributed to the

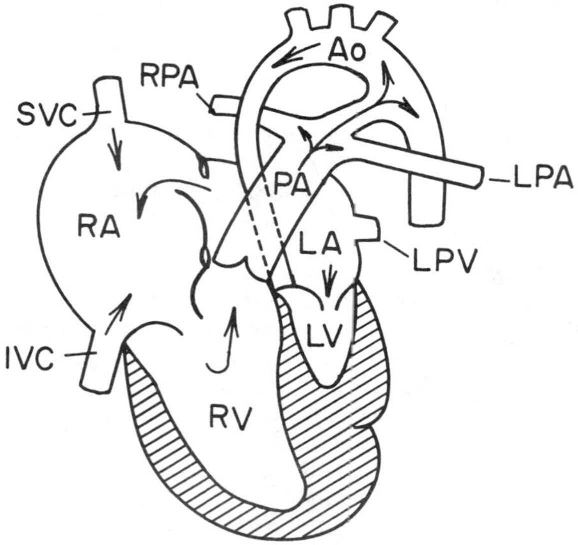

Figure 19-1 Circulatory pathways typical of hypoplastic left heart syndrome. The aortic valve is atretic, and the ascending aorta, left ventricle, mitral valve, and left atrium are hypoplastic. Blood exits from the left atrium across the foramen ovale. The aorta is supplied only by the ductus arteriosus with retrograde flow to the ascending aorta. SVC - superior vena cava, IVC - inferior vena cava, RA - right atrium, LA - left atrium, RV - right ventricle, LV - left ventricle, Ao - aorta, PA - pulmonary artery, LPA - left pulmonary artery, RPA - right pulmonary artery, LPV - left pulmonary vein.

lungs and to the systemic circuits depend on the ratio of total pulmonary resistance to systemic resistance. The former includes pulmonary vascular resistance and the resistance to outflow from the left atrium across the foramen ovale. The latter is a function of systemic vascular resistance and resistance to flow across the ductus arteriosis. Normal postnatal constriction of the ductus and/or declining pulmonary vascular resistance can lead to impairment of systemic perfusion, initiating the appearance of clinical symptomatology and progressive deterioration.

Manifestations

Surprisingly, infants born with this severe anomaly commonly appear normal at birth, although unrecognized tachypnea is frequently present. Characteristically, within 48-72 hr after delivery, the infant appears to acutely and rapidly deteriorate. Examination reveals dusky cyanosis, pallor, and signs of congestive failure: tachypnea, dyspnea, pulmonary rales, tachycardia, gallop rhythm, hepatomegaly, and a striking weakness or absence of all arterial pulses.

Electrocardiogram

The electrocardiogram commonly reveals right ventricular hypertrophy and right atrial enlargement, but occasionally may appear normal for age. A qR pattern in V_1 and absence of Q waves in left precordial leads are common (Fig. 19-2).

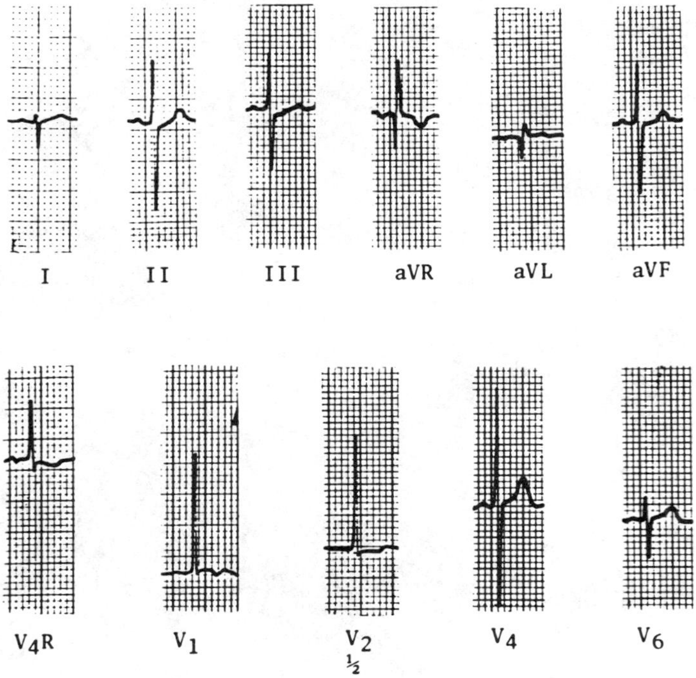

Figure 19-2 Electrocardiogram of neonate with hypoplastic left heart syndrome (aortic valve atresia). The frontal plane axis is directed rightward, and relative absence of left ventricular forces is noted in the precordial leads.

Radiologic Features

Chest roentgenogram reveals marked cardiomegaly of globular contour with prominent right atrium. Pulmonary venous engorgement and pulmonary edema are often pronounced (Fig. 19-3).

Echocardiography

Echocardiographic findings consist of abnormally large right ventricular cavity and tricuspid valve. If identified, the left ventricular cavity, mitral valve, aortic root, and left atrium are abnormally small. The echocardiographic demonstration of normal left heart anatomy clearly dictates against the diagnosis of hypoplastic left heart syndrome in the ill neonate.

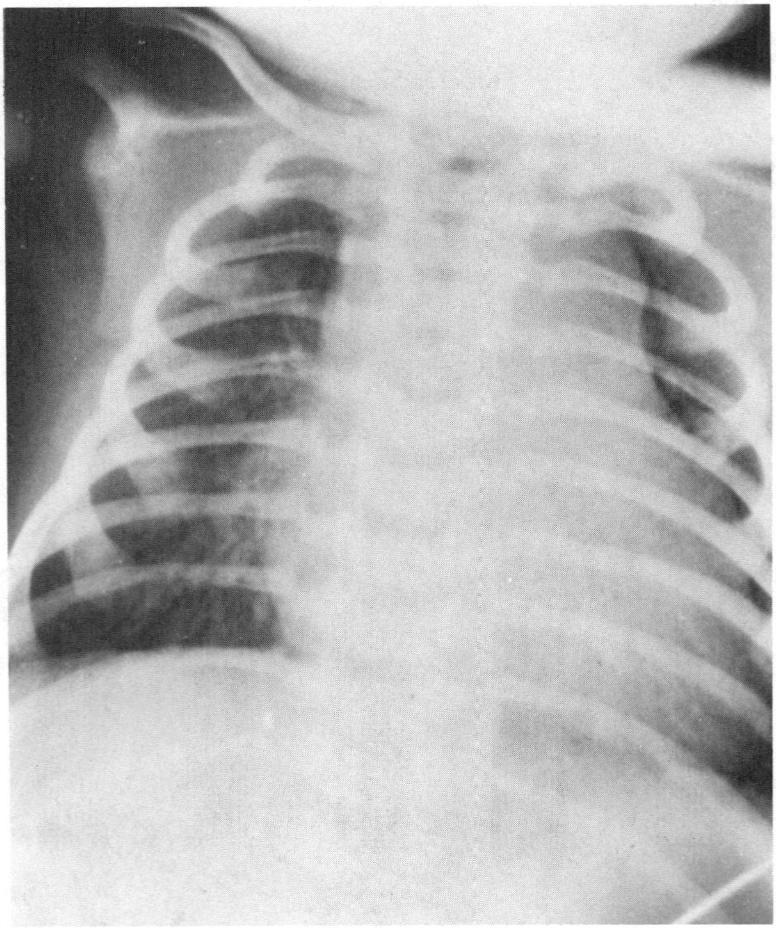

Figure 19-3 Chest roentgenogram of infant with aortic atresia. Severe cardiomegaly and pulmonary venous congestion are present.

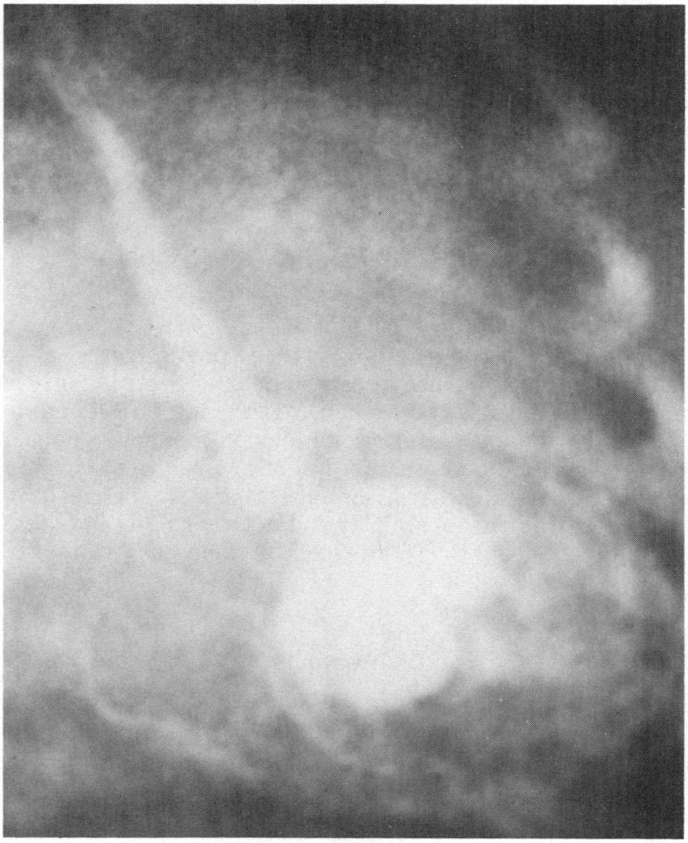

Figure 19-4 Angiocardiogram of infant with aortic atresia. The catheter was advanced across the atrial septum and through the mitral valve to the left ventricle. Note diminutive ventricular cavity. Opacification of the hypoplastic ascending aorta in this instance was by way of myocardial sinusoids and retrograde drainage through the coronary arteries.

Cardiac Catheterization

Cardiac catheterization reveals a left-to-right shunt at the atrial level. Oxygen saturation values of blood in the right ventricle, pulmonary artery, and aorta are similar. Left atrial pressure may be considerably elevated, always exceeding right atrial pressure. Right ventricular, pulmonary arterial, and aortic systolic pressures are essentially equal. Angiography with injection of contrast medium into the left atrium reveals a consistent flow pathway from left atrium to right atrium, right ventricle, pulmonary artery, and descending aorta; retrograde filling of the hypoplastic ascending aorta is commonly seen. The hypoplastic left ventricle occasionally can be entered if the mitral valve is not atretic (Fig. 19-4).

Treatment, Course, and Prognosis

Attempts at surgical palliation of this defect have not met with significant success. Trensient benefit may be achieved by balloon atrial septostomy to reduce left atrial and pulmonary venous pressure. Intensive medical therapy, likewise, usually provides only transient results. Most infants succumb within 48 hr after onset of symptomatology, and average age at death is approximately 5 days. Survival beyond 1 month of age is rare.

Differential Diagnosis

The sudden appearance of progressive, severe congestive heart failure in the first few days of life in an infant previously appearing well is quite characteristic for this syndrome. Other entities to be considered include critical aortic stenosis (without hypoplastic left heart), total anomalous pulmonary venous drainage, and complicated coarctation of the aorta. Fulminant sepsis with cardiovascular collapse may be suggested in some cases. Echocardiography is useful in evaluating left heart structures in this defect, but at times may reveal uncertain findings. Catheterization and angiographic studies may be necessary to identify other potentially salvageable conditions.

Bibliography

Deely WJ, Ehlers KH, Levin AR: Hypoplastic left heart syndrome. Anatomic, physiologic and therapeutic considerations. Am J Dis Child 121:168, 1971.

Krovetz LJ, Rowe RD, Scheibler GL: Hemodynamics of aortic valve atresia. Circulation 42:953, 1970.

Lundstrom NR: Ultrasound cardiographic studies of the mitral valve region in young infants with mitral atresia, mitral stenosis, hypoplasia of the left ventricle and cor triatriatum. Circulation 45:324, 1972.

Meyer RA, Kaplan S: Echocardiography in the diagnosis of hypoplasia of the left or right ventricles in the neonate. Circulation 46:55, 1972.

Noonan JA, Nadas AS: The hypoplastic left heart syndrome: an analysis of 101 cases. Pediatr Clin North Am 5:1029, 1958.

Roberts WC, Perry LC, Chandra RS, Meyers GE, Shapiro SR, Scott LP: Aortic valve atresia: a new classification based on necropsy study of 73 cases. Am J Cardiol 37:753, 1976.

Chapter 20

EBSTEIN ANOMALY OF THE TRICUSPID VALVE

Ebstein malformation is a deformity in which the tricuspid valve appears to attach not to the annulus fibrosus but to the right ventricular wall near the apex (Fig. 20-1). This downward or apical displacement of the attachment of the tricuspid valve involves primarily the posterior, and often the medial, leaflet, while the anterior leaflet is in a more or less normal position.

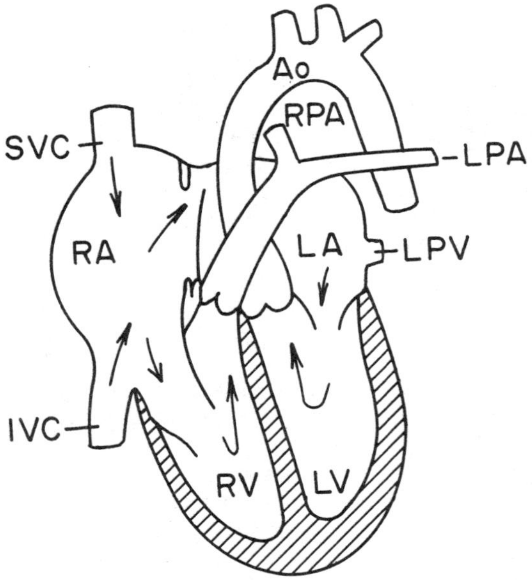

Figure 20-1 Ebstein anomaly of the tricuspid valve. Note the attachment of the tricuspid valve to the wall of the right ventricle resulting in incorporation of a portion of the ventricle into the atrium. SVC - superior vena cava, IVC - inferior vena cava, RA - right atrium, LA - left atrium, RV - right ventricle, LV - left ventricle, Ao - aorta, RPA - right pulmonary artery, LPA - left pulmonary artery, LPV - left pulmonary vein.

Incidence

Ebstein malformation is not a common defect and accounts for only 0.5-1.0% of congenital cardiac lesions. The lesions occur with equal frequency in both sexes, and familial cases have been observed.

Embryology and Anatomy

The embryologic explanation for this malformation is not entirely clear. A similar lesion of the left-sided AV valve may be seen in cases of corrected transposition (L-transposition) of the great arteries, where ventricular inversion is characteristically present. The valve abnormality ranges from mild and atypical to very severe, a fact accounting for the variable clinical expressivity. Because of the downwardly displaced attachments of the valve leaflets, that portion of the right ventricle above the valve is incorporated into the right atrium. As a result, the right atrium is large, and the right ventricular cavity is reduced in size. Infundibular obstruction may coexist. Associated cardiac defects occur in probably 50% of cases. Most commonly, these include atrial septal defect, ventricular septal defect, pulmonary stenosis, transposition of the great arteries, and patent ductus arteriosus.

Hemodynamics

Hemodynamic alterations range from minimal to severe, depending on the degree of malformation of the tricuspid valve, the size of the functioning right ventricular chamber, and the effects of associated cardiac lesions. Typically, the valve is variably incompetent, occasionally stenotic, and a right-to-left atrial shunt is commonly present. The right atrium and atrialized portion of the right ventricle are usually thin, and the latter, in particular, may exhibit poor contractility, often paradoxical to that of the true atrium.

Manifestations

Patients having mild variants of this anomaly are usually asymptomatic, with no more than minor EKG and roentgenographic findings, and may go unrecognized. Neonates with severe disease may exhibit intense cyanosis and profound heart failure, with death occurring in the neonatal period. Those less severely affected may be moderately cyanotic with cardiomegaly, prominent murmur, pulmonary hypovascularity, and failure to thrive during the first 2 or 3 months. Progressive improvement may occur as pulmonary resistance declines and right-to-left shunting diminishes. Exertional dyspnea, fatigue, and mild cyanosis may again become apparent at a later age.

More commonly, mild cyanosis and a murmur are the major features in the neonate, and patients remain asymptomatic in the early years. Episodes of supraventricular tachycardia may occur, however, especially in those exhibiting ventricular preexcitation conduction abnormality.

Physical examination reveals most patients to be acyanotic, or only minimally blue. Slight precordial prominence may be present. The precordium is not usually hyperdynamic, but a characteristic diffuse, rippling impulse across the precordium toward the apex is sometimes noted. Although slightly enlarged, the liver does not usually pulsate, and jugular venous pulses do not suggest tricuspid regurgitation. The most striking and characteristic feature at auscultation is the presence of a triple or quadruple rhythm composed of a late first sound, widely split second sound, and loud third and/or fourth sounds. Occasionally, a tricuspid opening sound is present. Usually heard is a systolic murmur of medium pitch and intensity, maximum at the lower left sternal edge or inside the apex. This murmur, representing tricuspid insufficiency, also may be associated with a soft pulmonic ejection murmur. Diastolic murmurs of a peculiar scratchy, superficial quality at the lower left sternal border sometimes combine with the tricuspid regurgitant murmur to produce a to-and-fro quality.

Electrocardiogram

The electrocardiogram is characterized by large P waves, right intraventricular conduction abnormality (RBBB), prolonged PR interval, and low-amplitude QRS complexes in the right precordium (Fig. 20-2). Wolff-Parkinson-White preexcitation conduction abnormality, type B, is present in approximately 9-30%. In lead V_1, P-wave amplitude may equal or exceed height of the R wave. Various arrhythmias may be seen, including premature beats, paroxysmal supraventricular tachycardia, atrial flutter and fibrillation, junctional rhythm, and atrioventricular dissociation.

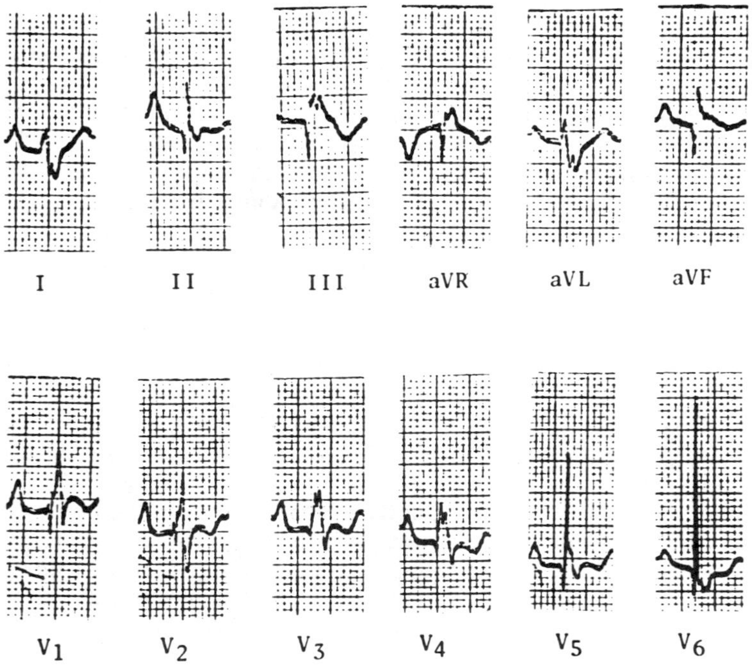

Figure 20-2 Electrocardiogram in Ebstein malformation showing first-degree atrioventricular block, right atrial enlargement, and splintered QRS complexes with terminal delay of rightward forces suggesting right bundle branch block.

Radiologic Features

Chest roentgenographic findings are variable. In most cases, cardiomegaly, sometimes severe, with marked right atrial enlargement, is present. A bulge along the upper left border producing a boxlike silhouette may sometimes be seen. In others the contour may suggest pericardial effusion. The pulmonary artery segment and pulmonary vasculature typically are diminished, but milder cases may show no definite abnormalities (Fig. 20-3).

Echocardiography

The major M-mode echocardiographic abnormality demonstrated in Ebstein malformation is significantly delayed tricuspid valve closure (more than 0.05 sec), with respect to mitral valve closure. This appears to be a feature specific for this lesion. Additional findings include abnormal septal motion, the ability to record the tricuspid valve in a more leftward position than normal, and increased amplitude of tricuspid valve motion. The abnormal position of the valve is better seen on two-dimensional studies.

Cardiac Catheterization

Although the risk of cardiac catheterization in this anomaly may be somewhat higher than average, it is no longer considered an extremely hazardous procedure. Paroxysmal dysrhythmia is a troublesome complication of catheterization, especially prone to occur in the presence of gross cardiomegaly. Catheterization usually reveals an atrial septal defect with right-to-left or bidirectional shunting. Systemic arterial saturation is less than normal in approximately 50% of cases. Elevated right atrial pressure is noted in the majority with a dominant V wave. Unless complicated by pulmonic stenosis, right ventricular and pulmonary artery systolic pressures are normal, but right ventricular end-diastolic pressure may be elevated. Coiling of the catheter in the large right atrium is not unusual, and passage to the pulmonary artery may be technically difficult.

Intracardiac electrocardiography has proven useful in the diagnosis of this lesion. Withdrawal of the electrode catheter through the right heart, while simultaneously recording pressure, demonstrates a right ventricular electrocardiographic pattern synchronous with a right atrial pressure curve, as the catheter crosses the displaced tricuspid valve to the atrialized portion of the ventricle. On further withdrawal, as the true tricuspid annulus is crossed, the expected right atrial pressure and right atrial electrocardiographic pattern coincide. Both false-positive and false-negative results have been noted.

Right ventricular angiography usually reveals the displacement of the tricuspid valve toward the right ventricular apex, well leftward of its normal position. Tricuspid regurgitation, with slow disappearance of contrast from the right heart, may be noted. Two distinct notches in the inferior border of the right atrial chamber may be seen in the frontal view, one representing the true tricuspid annulus, the other the site of displaced attachment.

Cineangiographic studies may reveal paradoxical or asynchronous motion of the ventricular and atrial components of the right atrial chamber. Visualization of the right coronary artery in the atrioventricular groove is a useful landmark identifying the site of the true tricuspid annulus.

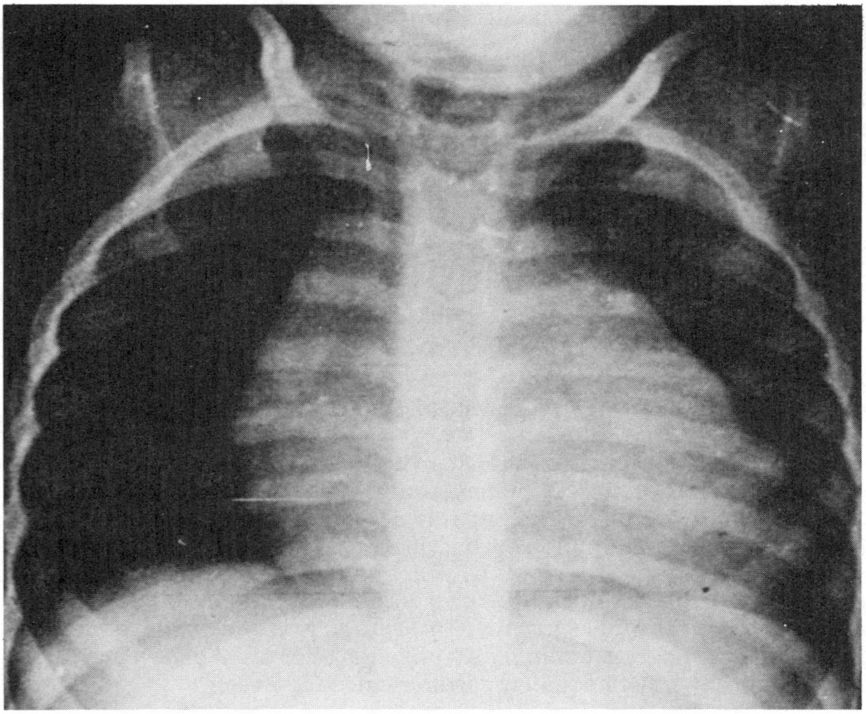

Figure 20-3 Chest roentgenogram of patient with Ebstein anomaly of the tricuspid valve. Note generalized cardiomegaly, prominent right atrium, and reduced pulmonary vascularity.

Course and Prognosis

The clinical course and prognosis are relative to the severity of the anomaly. Milder cases may have minimal manifestations of disease with survival into the sixth decade or beyond. More severely affected patients tend to have gross cardiomegaly and greater frequency of congestive heart failure and dysrhythmias, the two most common causes of death, usually in the third or fourth decades. Infants affected early may not thrive well, but improve after 2-3 months of age. The appearance of profound heart failure, cyanosis, and severe cardiomegaly suggests poor prognosis at any age.

Treatment

Both corrective and palliative surgical procedures have been performed in patients with Ebstein malformation. Palliative procedures include the Glenn operation (superior vena cava to right pulmonary artery anastomosis), systemic-artery-to-pulmonary-artery shunts, and plication of the anomalous tricuspid valve. Corrective procedures have consisted of homograft or prosthetic replacement of the tricuspid valve, with correction of associated lesions such as atrial septal defect. Closure of the atrial septal defect alone also has been performed in some patients. Regardless of the surgical approach, results in general have been far from satisfactory, with inordinately high mortality, both from palliative and corrective attempts. Surgical risk is especially high in young patients with marked cardiomegaly. Palliative procedures probably have no place in therapy of this lesion since little or no improvement has been observed, and mortality in prohibitive. Although those surviving successful valve replacement may be otherwise symptomatically improved, the procedure has not been demonstrated to reduce the risk of fatal dysrhythmia, a major cause of mortality. Corrective surgery should be reserved, therefore, for those demonstrating debilitating congestive heart failure or clinical deterioration. Medical management is preferred for the great majority of patients, as death from natural causes appears to be significantly less than that from surgery.

Differential Diagnosis

Differential diagnosis includes pericardial effusion, secundum atrial septal defect, congenital tricuspid insufficiency, and in the symptomatic neonate, other cyanotic malformations presenting at this age. The major aids in diagnosis are the auscultatory triple or quadruple rhythm characteristics of the lesion, and the electrocardiographic pattern of large P waves, bizarre right bundle branch block, small-amplitude QRS complexes in right precordial leads, or type-B ventricular preexcitation. Transient tricuspid regurgitation occurring in the neonate may be difficult to distinguish from Ebstein anomaly at this age. For this, as well as other lesions, definitive diagnosis may depend on cardiac catheterization.

Bibliography

Bialostozky D, Horwitz S, Espino-Vela J: Ebstein's malformation of the tricuspid valve. A review of 65 cases. Am J Cardiol 29:826, 1972.

Kumar AE, Fyler DC, Mittinen OS, Nadas AS: Ebstein's anomaly. Clinical profile and natural history. Am J Cardiol 28:84, 1971.

Watson H: Natural history of Ebstein's anomaly of the tricuspid valve in childhood and adolescence. An international cooperative study of 505 cases. Brit Heart J 36: 417, 1974.

Chapter 21

ANOMALIES OF THE CORONARY ARTERIES

The coronary arteries are the feeding vessels of the heart. They normally arise from orifices located approximately in the middle of the right and left aortic sinuses of Valsalva, and are named according to the sinus of origin. The principal perfusion of the deep layers of the left ventricular myocardium occurs during diastole while the aortic diastolic pressure exceeds ventricular pressure and the wall is relaxed (Fig. 21-1). It continues throughout diastole until left ventricular wall pressure rises during the next isovolumetric contraction. Coronary flow through the right ventricular wall is continuous throughout the entire cardiac cycle.

There are several congenital anomalies of the coronary arteries. The principal ones to be discussed here are aberrant origin of the left coronary artery, coronary arteriovenous fistula, and multiple aneurysms of the coronary arteries.

Aberrant Origin of the Left Coronary Artery from the Pulmonary Artery

Aberrant origin of the left coronary artery from the pulmonary artery is a rare developmental anomaly where the left coronary artery originates from the pulmonary artery rather than the aorta (Fig. 21-2).

Hemodynamics

The cardiac muscle is able to efficiently extract all available oxygen from coronary blood. It, therefore, tolerates low oxygen tension in the blood perfusing the coronaries. The critical problem in this anomaly is not the low oxygen tension, but rather the low perfusing pressure of the left coronary artery.

At birth, pulmonary vascular resistance is elevated and equals systemic resistance. Therefore, both the right and left coronary arteries are being perfused with the same driving pressure. When the left coronary artery arises from the pulmonary artery, the normal postnatal vascular changes are detrimental. As pulmonary vascular resistance and pressure drop, the perfusing pressure of the left coronary and, therefore, of left ventricular myocardium decreases as well, resulting in poor cardiac output, increased left atrial pressure, and reactive pulmonary hypertension. The increased pulmonary artery pressure in turn improves perfusion of the left coronary, allowing time for the development of intercoronary anastomoses. This is the time when symptoms related to myocardial ischemia develop. Survival and symptomatology depend on the presence or future development of collateral coronary vessels.

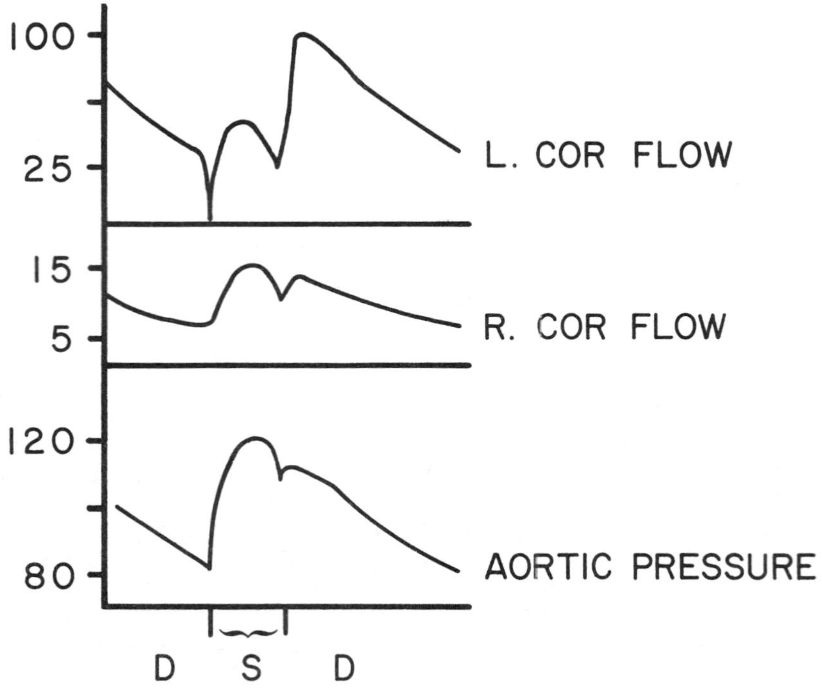

Figure 21–1 Comparison of phasic aortic pressure with left coronary (L. Cor.) and right coronary (R. Cor.) blood flowing during systole (S) and diastole (D).

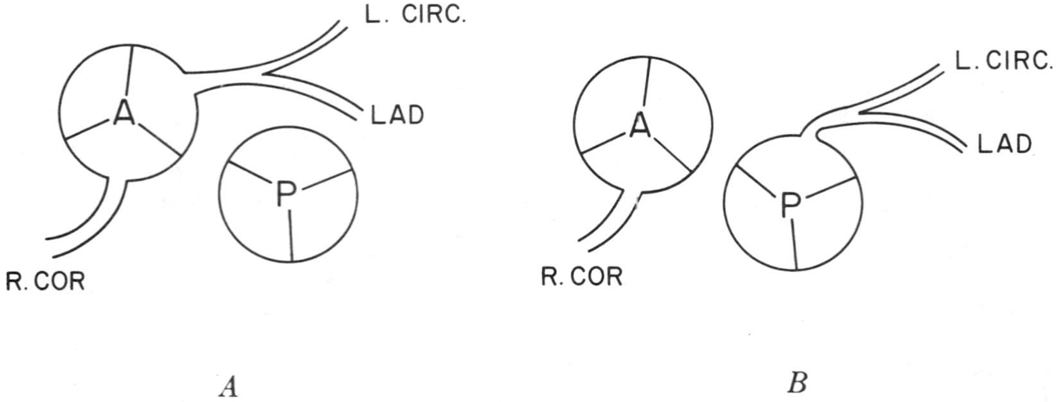

Figure 21–2 (A) Normal anatomy of the coronary arteries with origin of the right coronary artery (R. Cor.) from the right coronary cusp and the left coronary artery from the left coronary cusp. L. Circ. - left circumflex, LAD - left anterior descending. (B) Aberrant origin of the left coronary artery from the pulmonary artery.

If adequate collateral circulation develops between the left and right coronary arteries, the left coronary may be perfused in a retrograde fashion via the right coronary. There is, therefore, a constant pressure and oxygen gradient between the aorta, right coronary, left coronary, and pulmonary artery. At a later stage, these intercoronary vessels may enlarge and no longer act as feeding vessels, but rather as a "steal" with subsequent bypass of that portion of the myocardium.

Usually, patients with adequate intercoronary collaterals are the least symptomatic, whereas the ones with no communication between the left and right coronaries are symptomatic early in the neonatal period. Infarction of the papillary muscles is a leading cause of mitral insufficiency in this anomaly.

Clinical Presentation

The classical picture of an infant who suddenly becomes pale, sweaty, tachycardic, and tachypneic, the so-called infantile angina is not frequently seen. It is more common to see an infant 2-6 months of age presenting with severe congestive heart failure. A murmur of mitral insufficiency is heard in approximately 40% of the cases. Radiographically there is generalized cardiomegaly (Fig. 21-3), with evidence of pulmonary edema. Left lower lobe atelectasis resulting from compression of the bronchus by an enlarged left atrium is commonly seen. The x-ray findings and clinical presentation are indistinguishable from those of patients with endomyocardial disease.

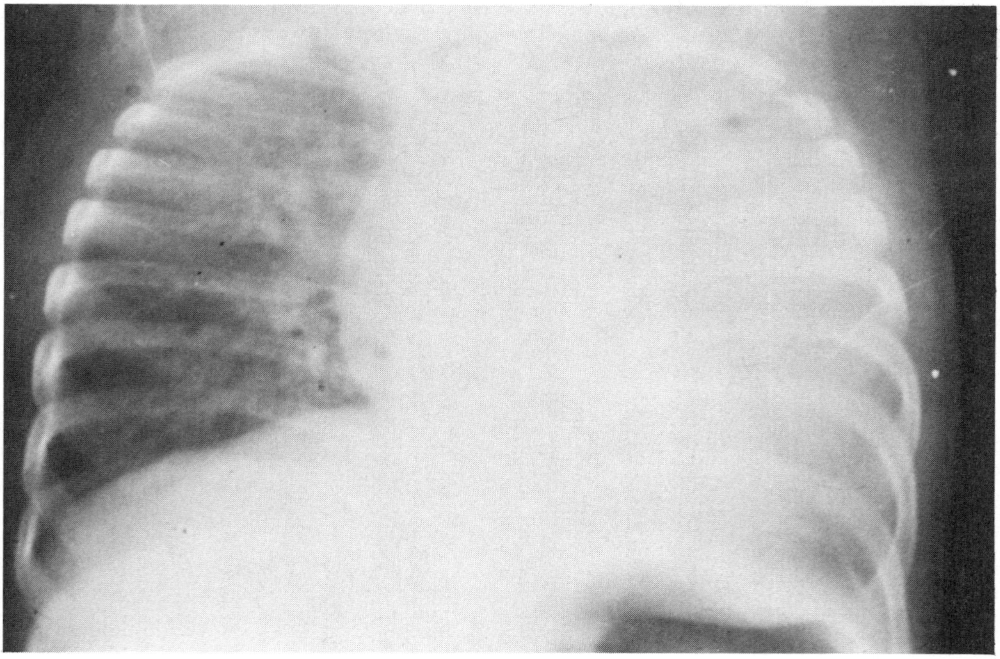

Figure 21-3 Three-month-old with aberrant left coronary artery from the pulmonary artery. There is massive cardiomegaly. The left cardiac border cannot be seen. There is also associated left lower lobe atelectasis. The right lung field appears hazy, indicative of pulmonary edema.

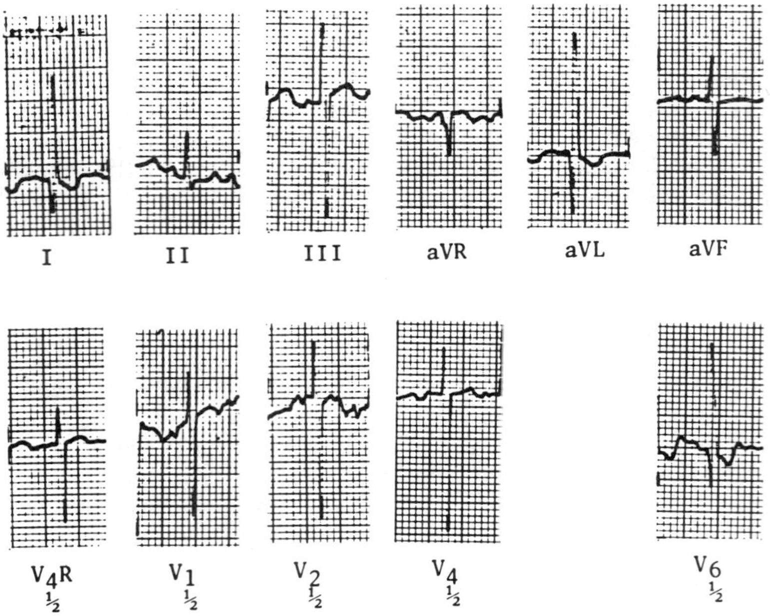

Figure 21-4A Electrocardiogram of the patient discussed in Fig. 21-3. There is left axis deviation and a pattern of atreolateral myocardial infarction manifested by large Q waves in leads I, aVL, and the left precordial leads. There is increased left ventricular voltage and abnormal repolarization. (Also see B.)

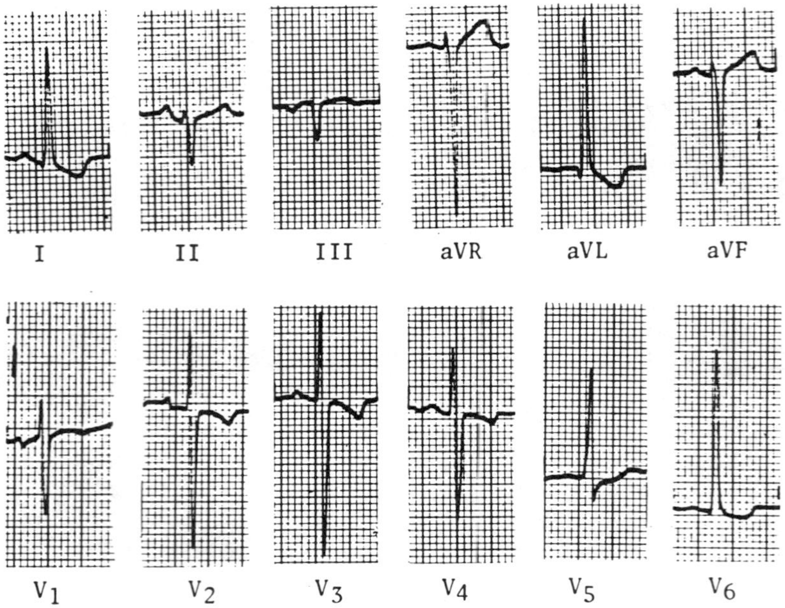

Figure 21-4B The same patient at 3 years of age. There are nonspecific T-wave changes. The Q in I and aVL has decreased in magnitude.

The electrocardiogram often shows left ventricular hypertrophy and a pattern of anterolateral myocardial infarction manifested by deep Q waves in leads I, aVL, and the left precordial leads (Fig. 21-4). This is often associated with inverted T waves in the limb leads and left precordium.

Cardiac Catheterization

The diagnosis is confirmed at catheterization by a left ventricular or aortic root injection. The right coronary artery appears large and tortuous. A small left coronary artery fills in a retrograde fashion from collaterals. When large collaterals are present, the pulmonary artery connection can occasionally be documented.

Course and Prognosis

Review of the literature reveals a total medical and surgical mortality of 89% during the first year of life. Medical mortality alone is close to 95%. If, however, the patients are divided into groups according to the degree of intercoronary anastomosis and proven left-to-right shunt, the results are different. The patients with large intercoronary communication and a shunt at the pulmonary artery level detected by oximetry survived the first year of life, irrespective of the treatment. These patients may first present in adult life with mitral regurgitation related to papillary muscle infarction, or they may experience sudden death, with the anomaly being detected at autopsy. At the other extreme, the patients without any detectable shunt at the pulmonary artery level and no intercoronary connections all died. The intermediate group had a 50% chance of survival, irrespective of the mode of treatment. Those who do survive may develop more collaterals and improve functionally and symptomatically (see Fig. 21-4B).

Accordingly, the following course of treatment is proposed. All patients presenting with this anomaly and evidence of recent myocardial infarction should be treated, as necessary, for cardiac failure or arrhythmias. Cardiac catheterization and angiography should be performed without delay. In infants who demonstrate a sizable left-to-right shunt, conservative treatment is recommended and surgery deferred until stable. In patients where there is no left-to-right shunt, the prognosis is so poor that surgical treatment is advocated without delay.

Ligation of the left coronary artery at the pulmonary artery takeoff is advocated by Nadas et al. for the patients with a sizable left-to-right shunt who are critically ill. This is a palliative procedure, now mostly abandoned, since it does not improve the physiology and does not always improve the outcome. Several surgical procedures such as bypass vein graft from aorta to left coronary artery, as well as subclavian to coronary artery anastomosis, are described. The most promising and physiological procedure, described by Cooley, entails transection of the main pulmonary artery, mobilization of the proximal portion of the left coronary to be attached end-to-side to the aorta. The pulmonary artery is subsequently reanastomosed. This procedure has been performed in several patients with reasonably good results; however, long-term followup is not yet available.

Coronary Arteriovenous Fistula

Coronary arteriovenous fistula is a rare anomaly consisting of a fistulous communication between a coronary artery of normal origin and a cardiac chamber or great vessel. The majority (90%) of coronary artery fistulas involve the right coronary, and empty into the right side, most commonly, into the right ventricle.

Pathophysiology

This anomaly has been attributed to persistence of embryonal vascular sinusoids in the myocardium. Preferential flow of blood occurs through the fistula because it is the pathway of least resistance. This leads to progressive dilatation of the involved coronary and the chamber receiving the shunted blood. The volume of shunted blood may be considerable, imposing a significant volume overload not only on the left heart but on the right side as well. "Coronary steal," causing myocardial ischemia, is not common.

Clinical Presentation

The manifestations depend on the size and location of the fistula and magnitude of the left-to-right shunt. These patients are mostly asymptomatic, the diagnosis being suggested by the presence of a continuous murmur detected on a routine examination. The remainder of the findings depends on the site of drainage of the fistula. The murmur may resemble that of a patent ductus; however, it has a superficial quality to it and is located lower down on the precordium. Since the fistula involves mostly the right-sided chambers, they can present with findings of right-sided volume overload. The abnormal communication can often be visualized at catheterization by left heart angiogram and confirmed by oximetry, demonstrating a left-to-right shunt (Fig. 21-5).

Course and Prognosis

Bacterial endocarditis is a real complication with an incidence of 8%. As previously mentioned, coronary steal is not common. Since there is usually progressive dilatation of the involved coronaries, the current trend is to operate on these patients upon diagnosis, excepting small infants who are asymptomatic. The procedure of choice is ligation of the fistula at its distal end.

Aneurysm of the Coronary Arteries

Acquired aneurysms of the coronary arteries (Fig. 21-6) have recently been described as part of the mucocutaneous lymph node syndrome (Kawasaki disease). This is a febrile illness, first described in Japan, but lately recognized also in the United States, probably of viral etiology, effecting infants and young children. The major clinical findings include fever, hyperemia of the ocular conjunctiva, edema of the hands and feet (initial stages), and desquamation of fingertip (convalescent stage). There are redness and fissuring of the lips and enlargement of the cervical lymph nodes. The laboratory findings usually show elevated erythrocyte sedimentation rate and thrombocytosis.

During the first 3 weeks of the illness, there is a high incidence of myocarditis as suggested by clinical echocardiographic and electrocardiographic abnormalities. Myocardial infarction has rarely been observed in this early stage. Large coronary arteritis occurs during the first week of the disease. This may progress into coronary aneurysm over the next 2 weeks (13% of all patients). The occurrence of coronary aneurysm does not correlate with the presence of signs of carditis. Low-amplitude R and T waves and ST segment changes correlated closely with carditis. In contrast, deep Q waves in II, III, and aVF occur later on and correlate with coronary abnormalities.

The diagnosis of coronary artery aneurysm can be simplified by serial two-dimenstional (2-D) echocardiogram visualization of the main coronary arteries.

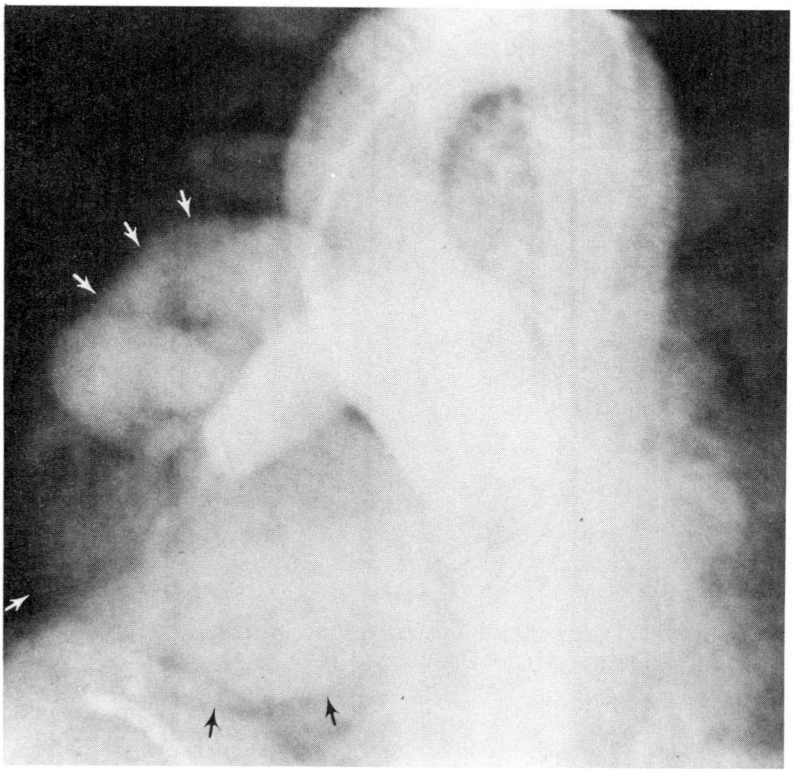

Figure 21-5 Right coronary AV fistula to the right atrium. Aortic root injection demonstrating massive dilatation and tortuosity of the right coronary artery (upper arrows) communicating with the right atrium. Note the dye in the enlarged right atrium (lower arrows).

The appearance of spherical or fusiform shape of the proximal portion of the main coronary artery, especially if progressive, is virtually diagnostic (Fig. 21-7A,B). The major limitation of 2-D echocardiography in the diagnosis of coronary aneurysm is its inability to easily visualize the right coronary artery. It is our practice to perform aortograms in anteroposterior, lateral, and oblique views in patients who exhibit suspicious 2-D echocardiograms. Regression of the aneurysm has been documented in approximately 40% of the patients within the following several months.

The prognosis is usually good, but sudden death occurs in 1-2% of the patients. Postmortem examination reveals coronary arteritis accompanied by multiple aneurysms and thrombosis. It is for this reason that patients with coronary abnormalities are maintained on low-dose aspirin for prolonged periods. In the event of acute occlusion of a major coronary artery, coronary bypass surgery may be lifesaving.

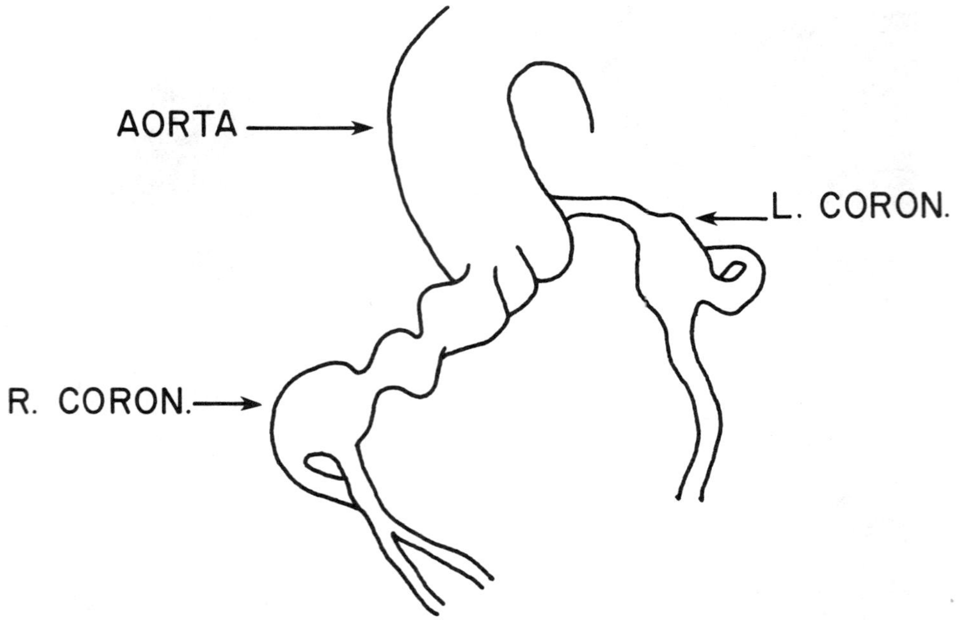

Figure 21–6 Schematic drawing of the aorta and coronary arteries showing multiple sacular aneurysms involving both coronaries.

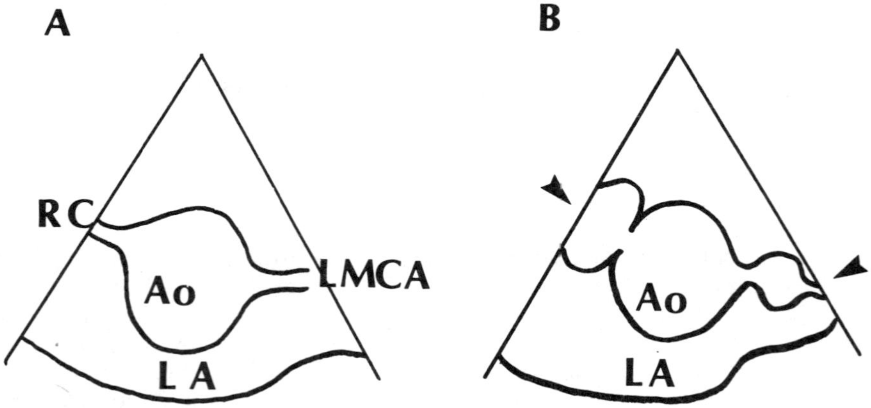

Figure 21–7 (A) Cross-sectional two-dimensional echocardiogram of the normal aorta and coronary ostia. (B) Cross-sectional echocardiogram from a patient with aneurysm of the main left and right coronary arteries (arrow heads). Ao - aorta, LA - left atria, RC - right coronary, LMCA - left coronary.

Bibliography

Askenazi J, Nadas AS: Anomalous left coronary artery originating from the pulmonary artery. Report on 15 cases. Circulation 51:976, 1975.

Edis AJ, Scattenberg TT, Feldt RH, Danielson GK: Congenital coronary artery fistula. Surgical consideration and results of operation. Mayo Clin Proc 47:567, 1972.

Hirashi S, Yshiro K, Oguchi K, Kusano S, Ishi K, Nakazawa K: Clinical course of cardiovascular involvement in the mucocutaneous lymph node syndrome. Am J Cardiol 47:323, 1981.

Kato H, Kojke S, Yamamoto M, Ito Y, Yano E: Coronary aneurysms in infants and young children with acute febrile mucocutaneous lymph node syndrome. J Pediatr 86:892, 1972.

Morens DM, Anderson LJ, Hurwitz ES: National surveillance of Kawasaki disease. Pediatrics 65:21, 1980.

Perry LW, Scott LP: Anomalous left coronary artery from pulmonary artery. Report of 11 cases: Review of indications for and results of surgery. Circulation 41: 1043, 1970.

Pinsky WW, Fagan LR, Mudd JFG, William VL: Subclavian-coronary artery anastomosis in infancy for the Bland-White-Garland syndrome. J Thorac Cardiovasc Surg 72:15, 1976.

Chapter 22

VASCULAR RINGS AND RELATED MALFORMATIONS

Anomalies of the Aortic Arch

The aortic arch and its primary intrathoracic branches as well as the proximal pulmonary arteries and ductus arteriosus arise from six pairs of vascular arches connecting the unpaired ventricle and paired dorsal aortae (Fig. 22-1). Although not seen in normal human development, there is a theoretical potential for bilateral aortic arches, and this hypothetical double arch is illustrated in a simplified diagrammatic form in Fig. 22-2. Alteration in the normal sequence of development may occur at any point in this ring, due to abnormal regression or abnormal persistence at a given location. The normal arch is the result of regression of the eighth segment of the right dorsal aorta. The arch passes to the left of the trachea (left aortic arch), giving rise, in order, to the innominate, left common carotid, and left subclavian arteries. The ductus arteriosus connects the arch just distal to the subclavian artery with the pulmonary artery. In most of the anomalies under consideration here, the abnormal vessels form a ring which more or less completely encircles the mediastinal structures.

When present, symptoms and abnormal physical findings are generally the result of compression of the trachea and/or esophagus. Tracheal obstruction may produce inspiratory stridor, respiratory distress, and frequent lower respiratory infections. Dysphagia may be the result of esophageal narrowing. In our experience, respiratory symptoms generally predominate. Infrequently, growth failure may be seen secondary to chronic poor food intake.

Diagnostic Approach

The diagnosis is primarily made by suspecting its presence when signs of significant and/or prolonged upper respiratory obstruction or swallowing difficulties are present. Physical examination shows no specific features; occasionally, obstruction to one or more of the brachiocephalic vessels may be detected. Congenital heart disease is infrequently associated with the vascular anomaly, and the findings resulting therefrom would be related to the specific type of lesion. The chest x-ray may show the location of the aortic arch; in all discussions relating to position of the arch, the trachea is the point of reference. If the radiographic technique is proper, narrowing of the tracheal or esophageal air column may be seen. A chest x-ray, with barium filling the esophagus, offers significantly more information. In the PA view one may see compression of the esophagus from one or both sides. The aortic arch or, in the case of a double arch, the larger arch produces the larger and

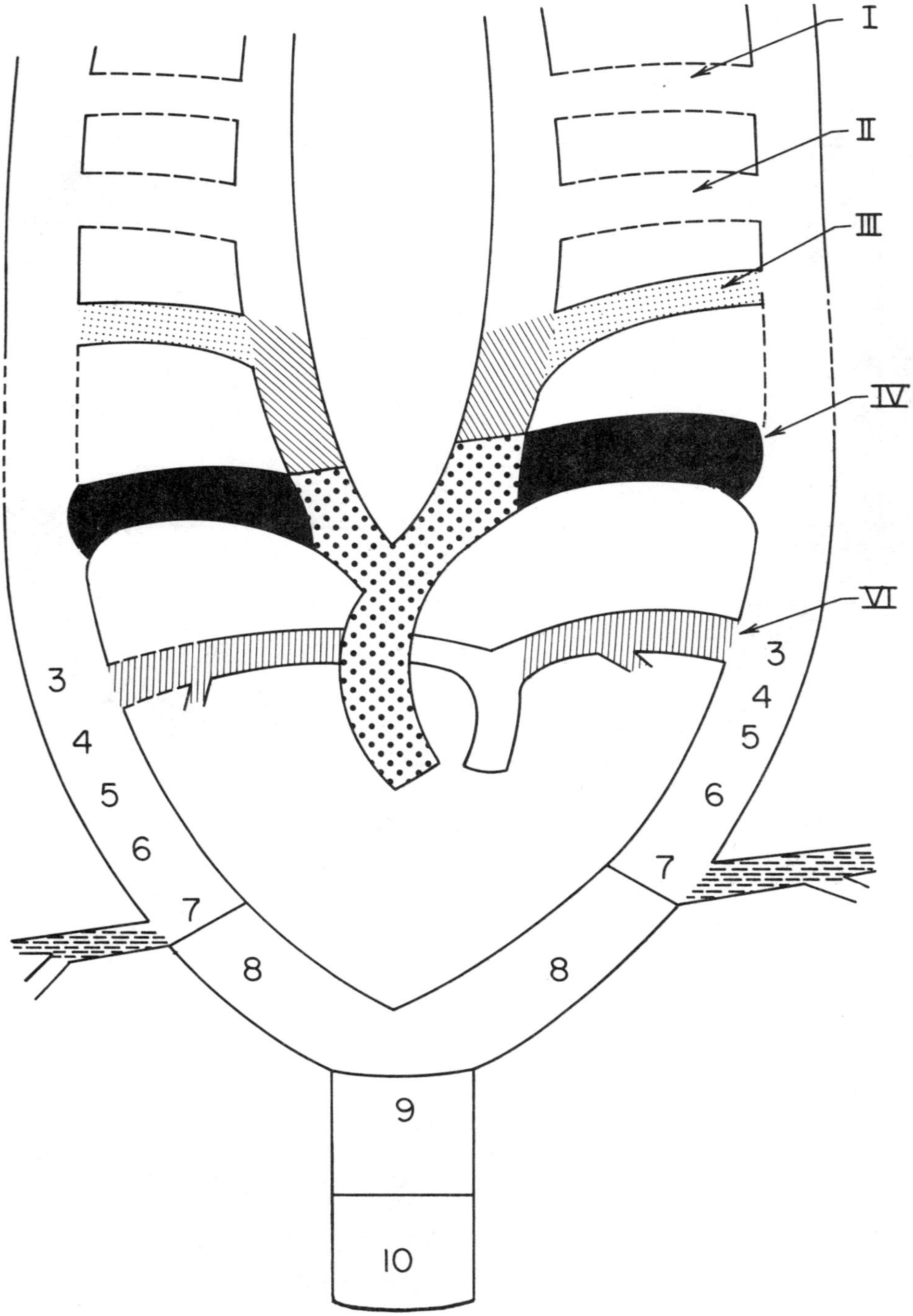

Figure 22-1 Fetal aortic arch system. Roman numerals indicate the paired aortic arches and Arabic numerals the segments of the dorsal aortae. Only the seventh dorsal intersegmental artery is shown. Structures delimited by dashed lines ultimately disappear.

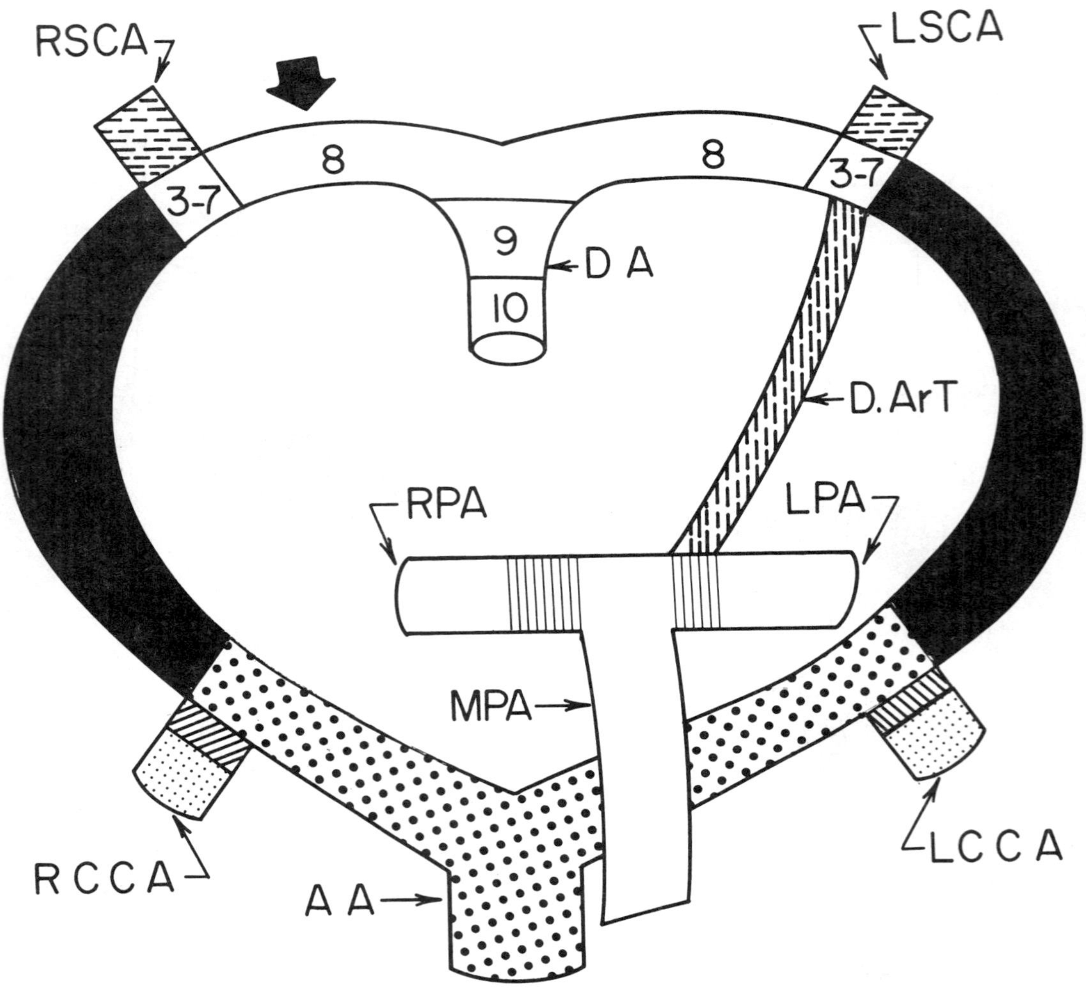

Figure 22-2 Hypothetical double aortic arch system at a stage of further differentiation. Markings identifying the site of embryologic origin are the same as in Fig. 22-1 with the exception of the heavier vertical dashes used to indicate the distal left sixth arch (ductus arteriosus), whereas the lighter vertical lines indicate the proximal sixth arches. Black arrow in this and subsequent figures in this chapter indicates a point of ultimate regression; in normal development this is the eighth segment of the right dorsal aorta. RSCA and LSCA indicate right and left subclavian arteries, respectively. RCCA and LCCA - right and left common carotid arteries, respectively. MPA, RPA, and LPA indicate main, right, and left pulmonary arteries, respectively. AA - ascending aorta, DA - descending aorta. D.ArT refers to ductus arteriosus.

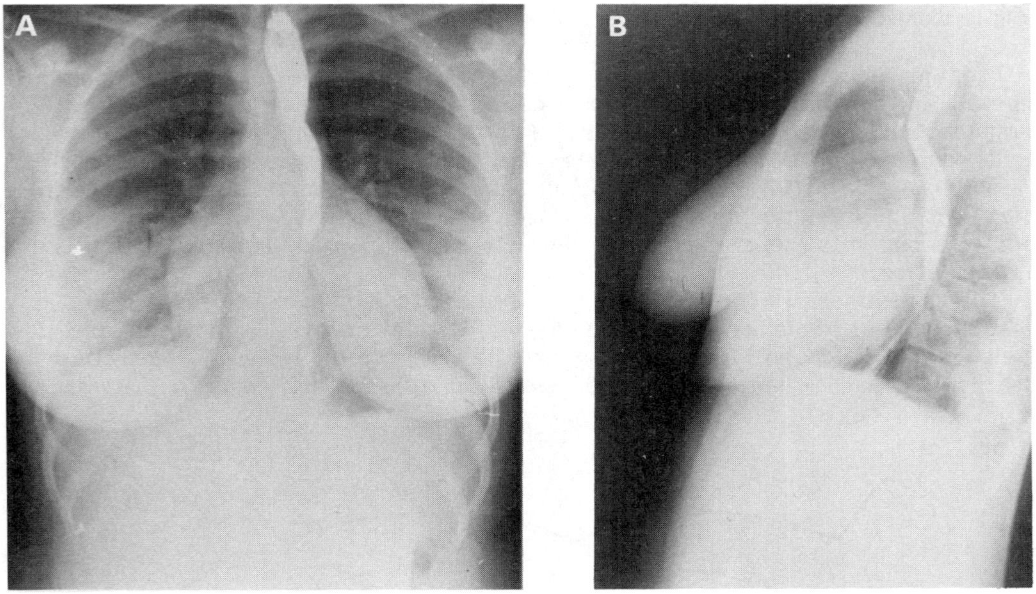

Figure 22-3 (A) Barium esophogram of an adolescent female with a vascular ring (right aortic arch with aberrant left subclavian artery and left ligamentum arteriosum). The density of the right aortic arch is readily identified, together with the more cephalad indentation that it makes on the barium column. A more caudad, somewhat angular indentation on the left side is produced by the ligamentum arteriosum. (B) Lateral view from the same patient. Large posterior esophageal indentation is present due to the dorsal root diverticulum.

more cephalad indentation. An oblique filling defect may be seen due to a portion of the ring which passes posterior to the esophagus (Fig. 22-3). The lateral view will show a larger posterior filling defect and, less frequently, there may be a small, relatively high indentation if the trachea is pulled tightly against the esophagus.

The barium swallow is usually as far as one need go with the diagnostic workup. In this manner the presence of the vascular ring can be identified, as well as the location of the major arch, permitting surgical intervention when indicated. Bronchoscopy and bronchography add little and are potentially hazardous, especially where respiratory compromise exists. If the barium swallow is not conclusive, aortography may be required to delineate anatomy, but this is not often necessary. Numerous other causes of upper airway or esophageal obstruction must be excluded and, here again, the barium swallow will direct the investigator's attention appropriately.

Specific Malformations

Variations in the anatomy of the aortic arch and its brachiocephalic branches are numerous. In this chapter we will consider only those lesions which are more common and are of greater clinical significance.

Double Aortic Arch

From an embryologic standpoint, double aortic arch is the most straightforward anomaly and results from failure of regression of the eighth segment of the right dorsal aorta (Fig. 22-4). The right arch is larger in approximately 75%; uncommonly, one arch or a portion thereof may be atretic. The upper descending aorta is usually on the left of the spinal column, as is the ductus arteriosus (or ligamentum). All the brachiocephalic vessels arise separately, two from each arch. Associated congenital heart disease is seen in less than 1% of individuals with this malformation.

The vast majority of infants with a double aortic arch are symptomatic and most show signs of severe respiratory distress within the first 6 months of life. The barium swallow will generally suggest the presence of two arches and allow identification of the major arch, as previously mentioned. If one arch is atretic,

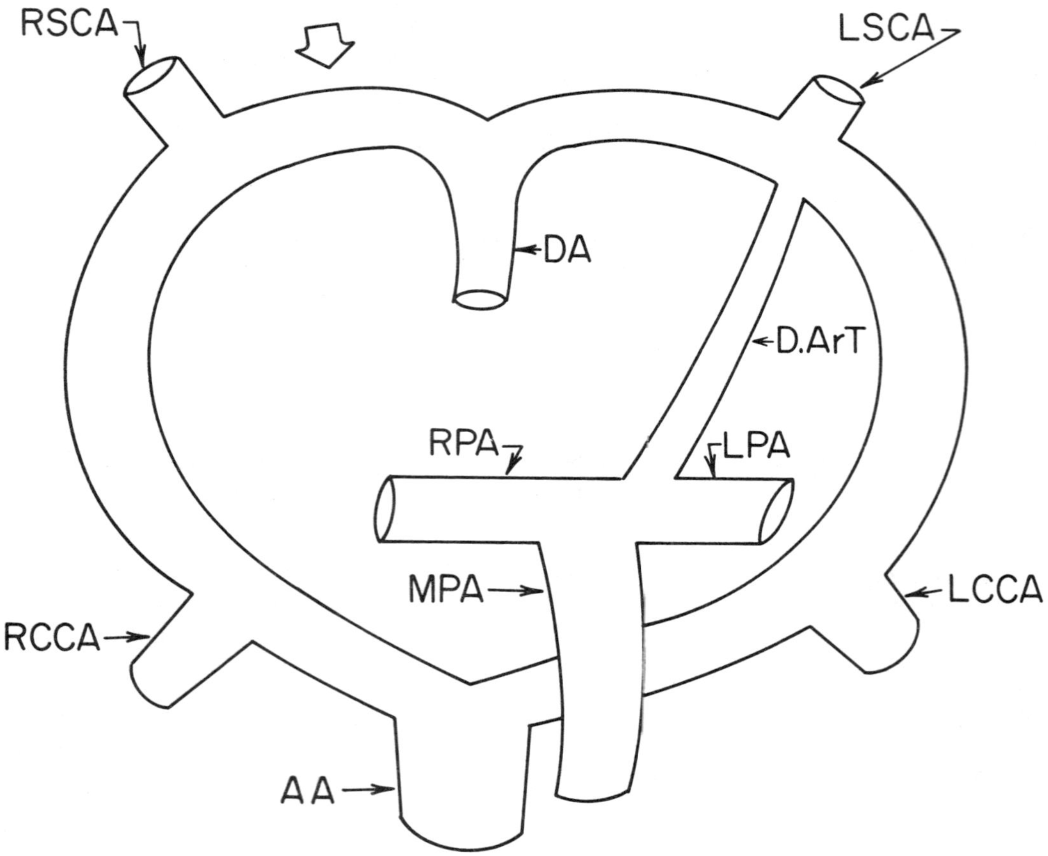

Figure 22-4 Schematic representation of double aortic arch. The open arrow in this and subsequent figures indicates sites of abnormal persistence of a vascular structure, in this case the eighth segment of the right dorsal aorta. RSCA and LSCA indicate right and left subclavian arteries, respectively. RCCA and LCCA - right and left common carotid arteries, respectively. MPA, RPA, and LPA indicate main, right, and left pulmonary arteries, respectively. AA - ascending aorta, DA - descending aorta. D.ArT refers to ductus arteriosus.

this lesion may resemble other vascular rings, but sufficient information will be obtained to permit correction. The distal right arch as it passes behind the esophagus to join the left produces the large posterior indentation.

In the presence of significant symptoms, surgical division of the arch and mobilization of the mediastinal structures are indicated. The smaller arch (usually the left) is divided generally distal to the subclavian artery. Because of softening and deformity of the underlying tracheal cartilages, airway obstruction may require weeks or months to disappear completely, and extremely careful respiratory management in the postoperative period is critical.

Malformations with Right Aortic Arch

The finding of an aortic arch which passes to the right of the trachea almost always means the presence of a vascular ring or congenital heart defect. Right aortic arch anomalies are generally divided into two types.

1. Right arch with mirror image brachiocephalic branching (Fig. 22-5): In this situation there is a right arch with right descending aorta and mirror-image arrangement of the brachiocephalic vessels; this is, the left innominate artery is the first to arise from the arch, followed by right carotid and right subclavian arteries. This lesion results from a regression of the eighth segment of the left dorsal aorta, associated with persistence of the analogous segment on the right. The ductus arteriosus usually connects the innominate artery and left pulmonary artery; therefore, no vascular ring is formed. This type of right aortic arch is associated with cyanotic congenital heart disease in approximately 98% of the cases, usually with tetralogy of Fallot or persistent truncus arteriosus.
2. Right arch with aberrant left subclavian artery: Regression of the left fourth arch and persistence of the eight segment of the right dorsal aorta give rise to a right arch with the left subclavian artery arising as the last brachiocephalic vessel from the arch, and passing posterior to the esophagus, to reach the left arm (Fig. 22-6). The ductus arteriosus usually connects the left subclavian artery and left pulmonary artery, completing the ring. Symptoms are seen less frequently (approximately 20%) and are usually less severe than with double aortic arch, tending to appear between 6 and 24 months of age. Congenital heart disease has been found by some to be associated in approximately 12% of patients.

Findings on barium swallow may be similar to those in double arch, but frequently the left-sided esophageal indentation (due to the ductus arteriosus or ligamentum arteriosum) is smaller. The initial portion of the left subclavian artery, arising embryologically from the eighth segment of the left dorsal aorta, is very dilated and referred to as a dorsal root diverticulum. This produces the large posterior esophageal indentation seen in the lateral view (Fig. 22-3). When symptoms are prominent, surgical division of the ductus or ligamentum with mobilization of the ring is carried out.

Cervical Aortic Arch

This is a rare lesion but one which is important because of the unusual and often confusing physical findings. The aortic arch is elongated, usually extending cephalad into the neck just above the clavicle. The arch is right-sided in almost all the reported cases. Except for the abnormal location of the arch, the anomaly is usually essentially identical to the right arch with aberrant subclavian artery, just described. The left carotid artery arises from the ascending aorta and the right carotid, often from the apex of the arch.

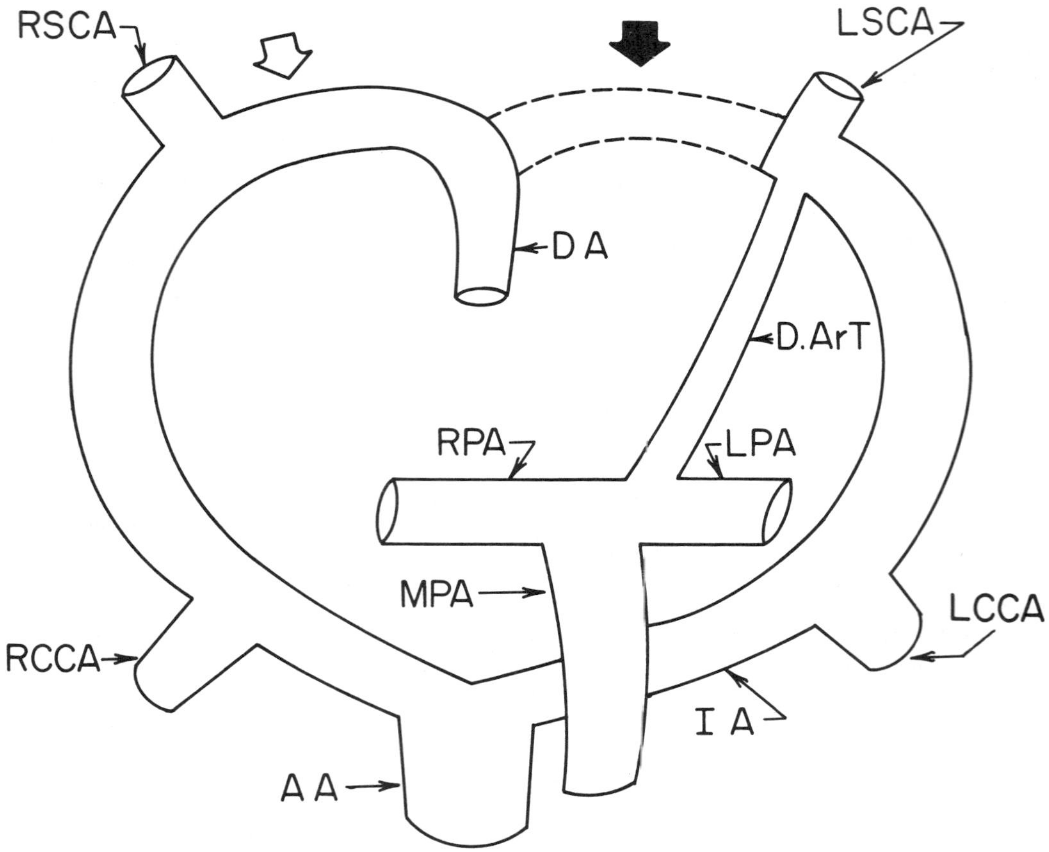

Figure 22–5 Schematic representation of a right aortic arch with mirror-image brachiocephalic branching. Regression of the eighth segment of the left dorsal aorta and persistence of the analogous segment on the right are indicated by the arrows. IA - innominate artery. RSCA and LSCA indicate right and left subclavian arteries, respectively. RCCA and LCCA - right and left common carotid arteries, respectively. MPA, RPA, and LPA indicate main, right, and left pulmonary arteries, respectively. AA - ascending aorta, DA - descending aorta. D.ArT refers to ductus arteriosus.

A left subclavian artery originates from the dorsal root diverticulum and passes behind the esophagus. A ductus or ligamentum on the left completes the ring. The embryology of the anomaly is unclear, but persistence of the third arch as part of the adult structure is thought to be involved by some. All of the right dorsal aorta below the third arch persists, and the left fourth arch regresses, as previously described.

Symptoms and findings may be related to the ring structure, but, not uncommonly, are secondary to the abnormal position of the aortic arch. A pulsatile mass may be present in the supraclavicular fossa, often associated with a thrill. Barium swallow shows findings similar to the lesions previously described except for the more cephalad location of the indentation due to the arch. Since the cervical mass is often the presenting manifestation and may be confused with an aneurysm of a

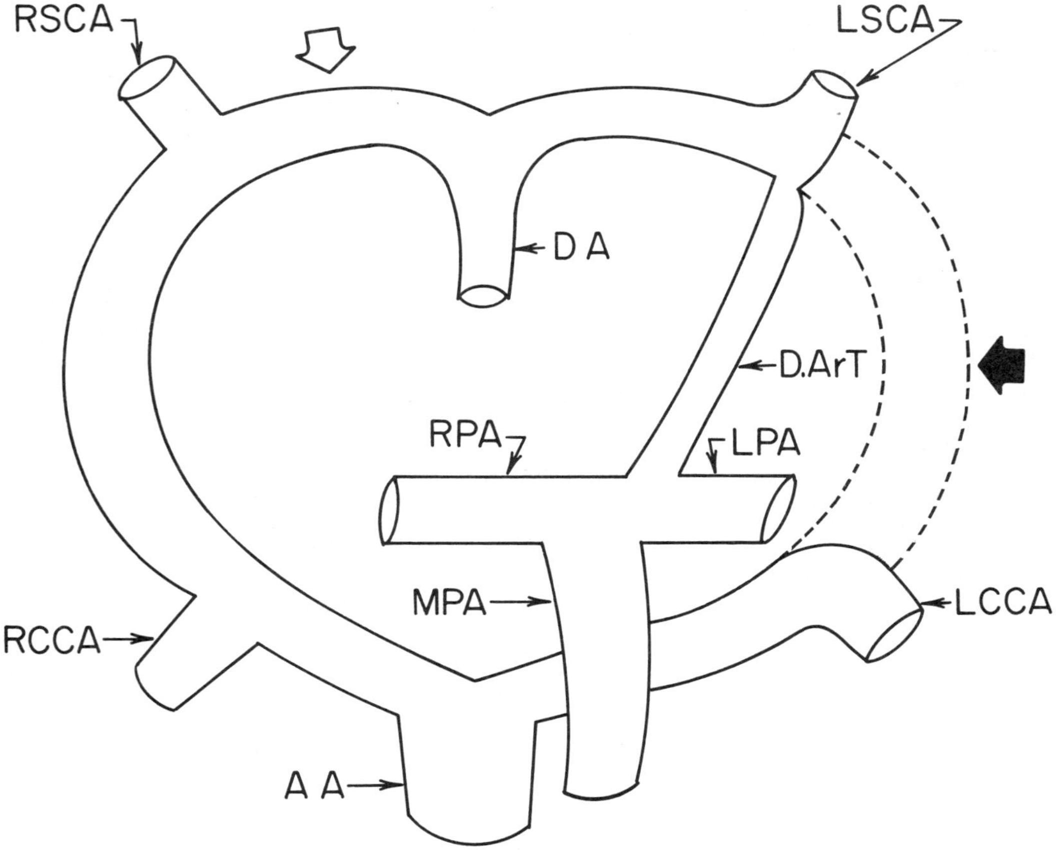

Figure 22-6 Schematic representation of right aortic arch with aberrant left subclavian artery. Arrows indicate abnormal regression of the left fourth aortic arch with persistence of the eighth segment of the right dorsal aorta. RSCA and LSCA indicate right and left subclavian arteries, respectively. RCCA and LCCA - right and left common carotid arteries, respectively. MPA, RPA, and LPA indicate main, right, and left pulmonary arteries, respectively. AA - ascending aorta, DA - descending aorta. D.ArT refers to ductus arteriosus.

brachiocephalic vessel, angiography is frequently employed for more precise clarification.

Malformations with Left Arch

Vascular rings with a left aortic arch are very uncommon. Occasionally, anomalies, which are mirror images of those previously described, are encountered. Far more familiar to most clinicians is the presence of an aberrant right subclavian artery. This results from regression of the right fourth arch and persistence of the right eighth dorsal segment. The ductus is generally in its usual location, and no ring is formed. In the past, much attention was given to this lesion as a cause of dysphagia (dysphagia lusoria), but the frequency with which it is encountered as an incidental finding in totally asymptomatic patients suggests that it causes dysphagia rarely, if at all. The barium swallow shows a narrow oblique posterior indentation extending cephalad and rightwards from the level of T-4 to T-2. For reasons that are unclear, the eighth dorsal segment from which the subclavian artery arises is not dilated if the ductus is on the same side as the arch. If significant dysphagia is truly present, division of the aberrant artery will provide relief.

Anomalous Origin of the Innominate or Left Carotid Artery

Variations in the origin of the brachiocephalic vessels are common and usually produce no problem. Occasionally, the left carotid artery may originate from the innominate artery and follow a course across the anterior aspect of the trachea, such that obstruction results. Alternatively, origin of the innominate artery more distally on the arch may produce the same findings which are those of upper airway obstruction without symptoms of esophageal involvement. Thus, inspiratory stridor is common; several reports allude to apneic episodes which are said to be reflex in origin. Tracheoscopy is usually required to identify the anterior compression; gentle pressure on this area with the bronchoscope will then obliterate the temporal or brachial pulse on the involved side, depending on which anatomic variation is present. Airway obstruction is rarely severe enough to warrant surgery, and spontaneous improvement may occur. If apneic episodes are documented, mobilization and anterior fixation of the obstructing vessel should be carried out.

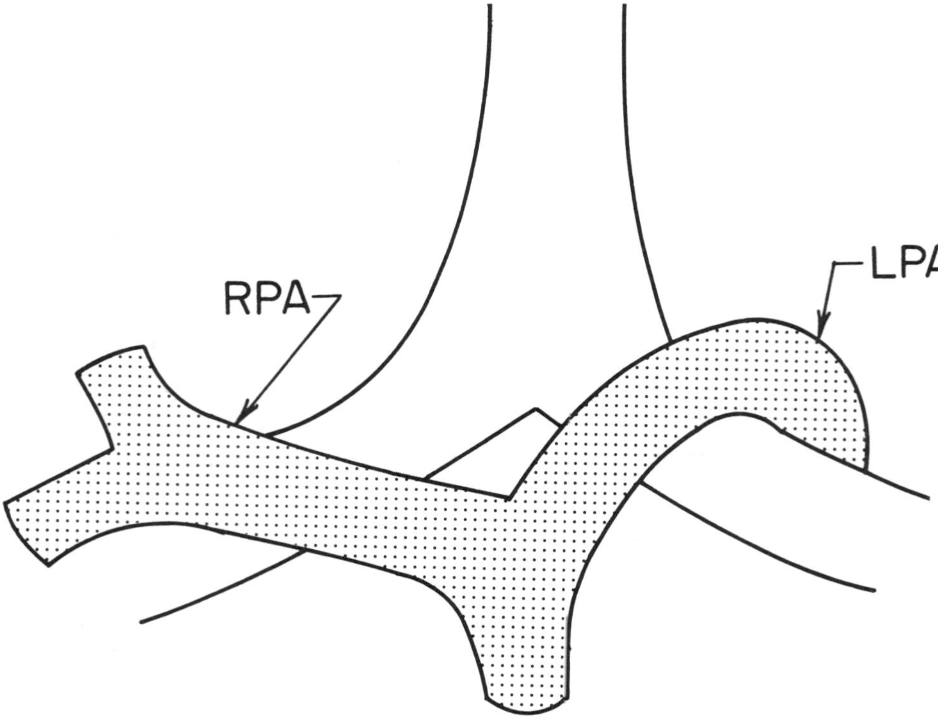

Figure 22–7A Anomalous left pulmonary artery sling. Anterior view of the pulmonary arteries and trachea showing normal relationship between the right (RPA) and left (LPA) pulmonary arteries to their respective bronchi.

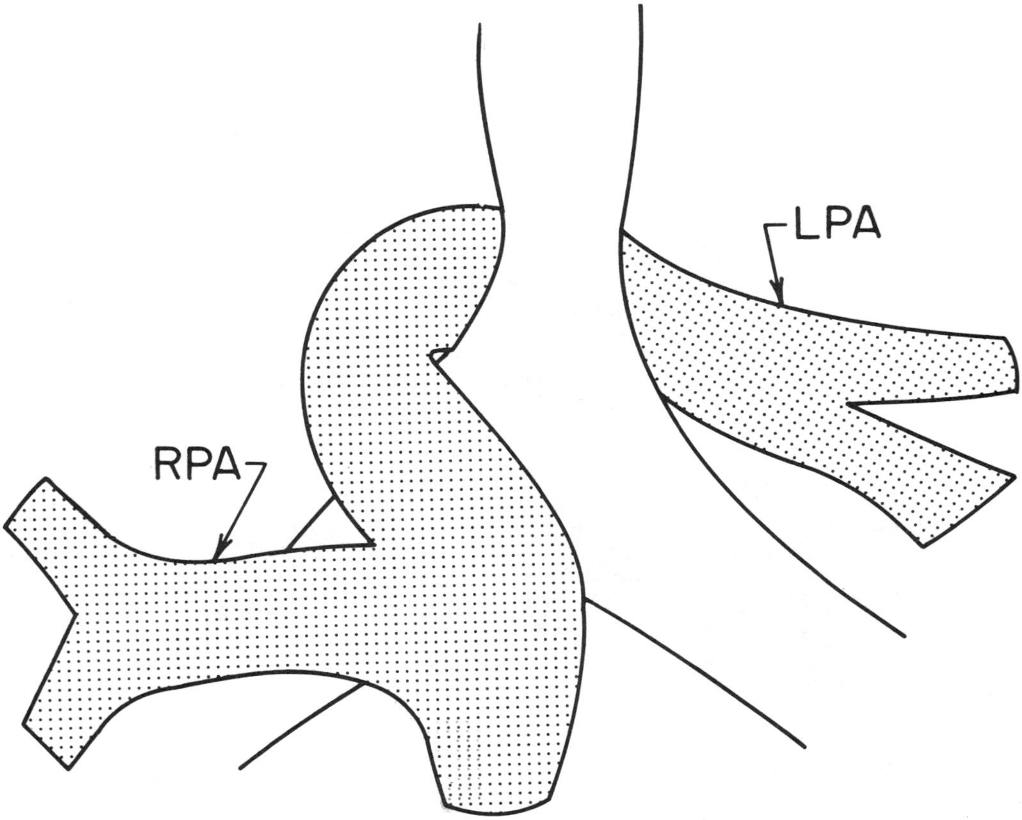

Figure 22-7B Anomalous left pulmonary artery sling. Anterior view showing the abnormally rightward origin of the left pulmonary artery with its subsequent course around the trachea.

Anomalous Origin of the Left Pulmonary Artery (Left Pulmonary Artery Sling)

Anomalous origin of the left pulmonary artery is an uncommon but clinically significant anomaly which usually causes severe airway obstruction. The left pulmonary artery arises from the right pulmonary artery or elongated main pulmonary artery and courses to the right, crossing the superior aspect of the right main stem bronchus at the carina before turning to the left and passing between the trachea and esophagus, to reach the hilum of the left lung (Fig. 22-7). It is thought to have its origin in the failure of the proximal left sixth aortic arch (future left pulmonary artery) to connect with the plexus of vessels developing in the primitive lung bud. While the lung is still in the unpaired state, vascular connections may develop between its right and left halves which then communicate with the right pulmonary artery.

Seen more commonly in males, anomalous left pulmonary artery produces severe lower airway obstruction, usually beginning in the first week of life. Expiratory wheezing and hyperexpansion of the right lung are noted; the degree of

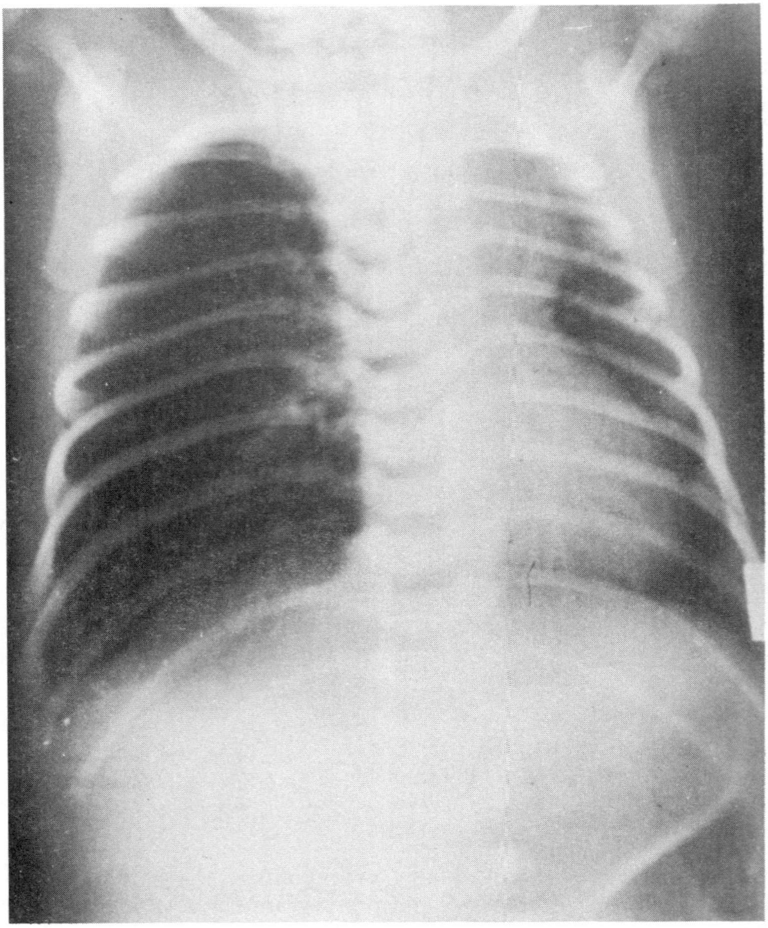

Figure 22-8 Chest x-ray of a 6-week-old infant with LPA sling. Note the prominent hyperinflation of the right lung with displacement of the mediastinum toward the left.

obstruction is progressive, often resulting in death in the first 6 months. Secondary infection of the involved lung is frequent. Chest x-ray shows hyperinflation of the right lung and left shift of the mediastinum (Fig. 22-8). Barium swallow may show anterior indentation on the esophagus, at the level of the carina, which is nearly pathognomonic. Pulmonary angiography is advisable for clarification of vessel anatomy prior to surgical intervention (Fig. 22-9). Division of the left pulmonary artery with reanastomosis to the main pulmonary artery is a difficult procedure in a critically ill infant, but should be carried out because of the poor prognosis with conservative management. It has been performed successfully in a number of patients with good results.

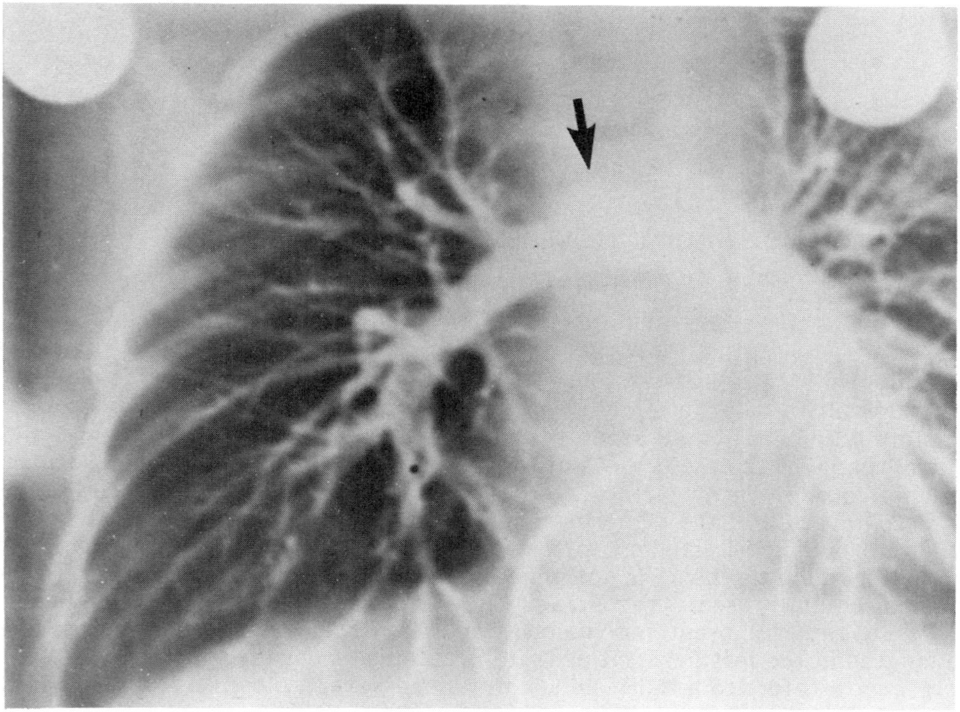

Figure 22–9 Pulmonary arteriogram of the patient shown in Fig. 22–8. The arrow points to the typical density due to the origin of the left pulmonary artery.

Bibliography

Sissman NJ: Anomalies of the Aortic Arch Complex, Heart Disease in Infants, Children and Adolescents, 2nd ed, Moss AJ, Adams FH, Emmanouilides GC, Williams and Wilkins Co., Baltimore, 1977, p. 210.

Stewart JR, Kincaid OW, Edwards JE: An Atlas of Vascular Rings and Related Malformations of the Aortic Arch System, Charles C Thomas, Springfield, Ill., 1964.

Chapter 23

EVALUATION OF CARDIAC MALPOSITIONS

Achieving a clear understanding of the malpositioned heart may be among the most difficult tasks in the field of pediatric cardiology. Embryologists are not in complete agreement on all aspects of the problem, although many of the basic principles appear to be clear. Confusion is compounded by the frequent occurrence of complicated intracardiac defects. The discussion in this chapter will not attempt to cover all of the numerous embryologic variations, rather it will be devoted to providing the student with a basic approach to the analysis of malposition. Defects in which the heart is not in an intrathoracic location will not be covered.

The problem is usually recognized when an abnormal cardiac position is noted on chest x-ray. In normal individuals, the bulk of the cardiac mass and the apex are located in the left chest; this state is referred to as levocardia. The term dextrocardia refers to a right-sided cardiac mass, regardless of how it got in that position. The older terms, dextroversion and dextroposition, are best avoided, as there is much confusion regarding their use in the literature. Dextrocardia may be the result of an embryologic error, or it may be due to a congenital or acquired shift of the mediastinal contents, as with agenesis of the lung, pneumothorax, lobar emphysema, and so forth. A heart which is centrally located is referred to as mesocardia.

Understanding of the very complicated malpositions of embryologic origin is facilitated by systemically analyzing the heart in a segmental manner, as described by Van Praagh.

1. *Determination of visceral situs:* The conventional normal arrangement of the viscera is referred to as situs solitus. When the visceral position is a mirror image of normal (liver on the left, stomach and spleen on the right, trilobed lung with eparterial bronchus on the left, etc.), situs inversus is present. Heterotaxia refers to any other visceral arrangement. This is uniformly present in congenital asplenia or polysplenia where situs of unpaired organs may be difficult to establish. Such an arrangement is referred to as situs ambiguous by some.

Although one is able to gain some impression regarding visceral and cardiac situs from physical examination, a more precise evaluation is obtained from a PA x-ray of the chest and abdomen. The position of the liver and stomach can be identified as well as, frequently, the branching pattern of the bronchi. Concordance of viscera and heart (levocardia in situs solitus and dextrocardia in situs inversus) is associated with a lower incidence of congenital heart defects than is seen when the heart and viscera are discordant (levocardia in situs inversus, dextrocardia in situs solitus). In the latter situation, complex anomalies are the rule as they are in the heterotaxic syndromes of asplenia and polysplenia.

2. *Determination of atrial localization:* The position of the atria is usually determined by the position of the viscera. In situs solitus the morphologic right atrium lies on the right and in situs inversus on the left (Fig. 23-1). This is referred to as visceroatrial concordance and is more reliable in the determination of atrial situs than is the configuration of the P wave on EKG, which can be altered by other factors. In asplenia-polysplenia, morphologic characteristics are difficult to ascertain, but there is a tendency for bilateral right atria in asplenia and bilateral left atria in polysplenia. Rarely, heterotaxia of abdominal viscera only may cause confusion. We have seen cases of apparent situs inversus of the abdominal viscera with normal intrathoracic anatomy and a structurally normal heart. In these atypical cases, the location of the inferior vena cava, as determined by passage of a cardiac catheter or injection of contrast media, defines the location of the morphologically right atrium (venoatrial concordance).

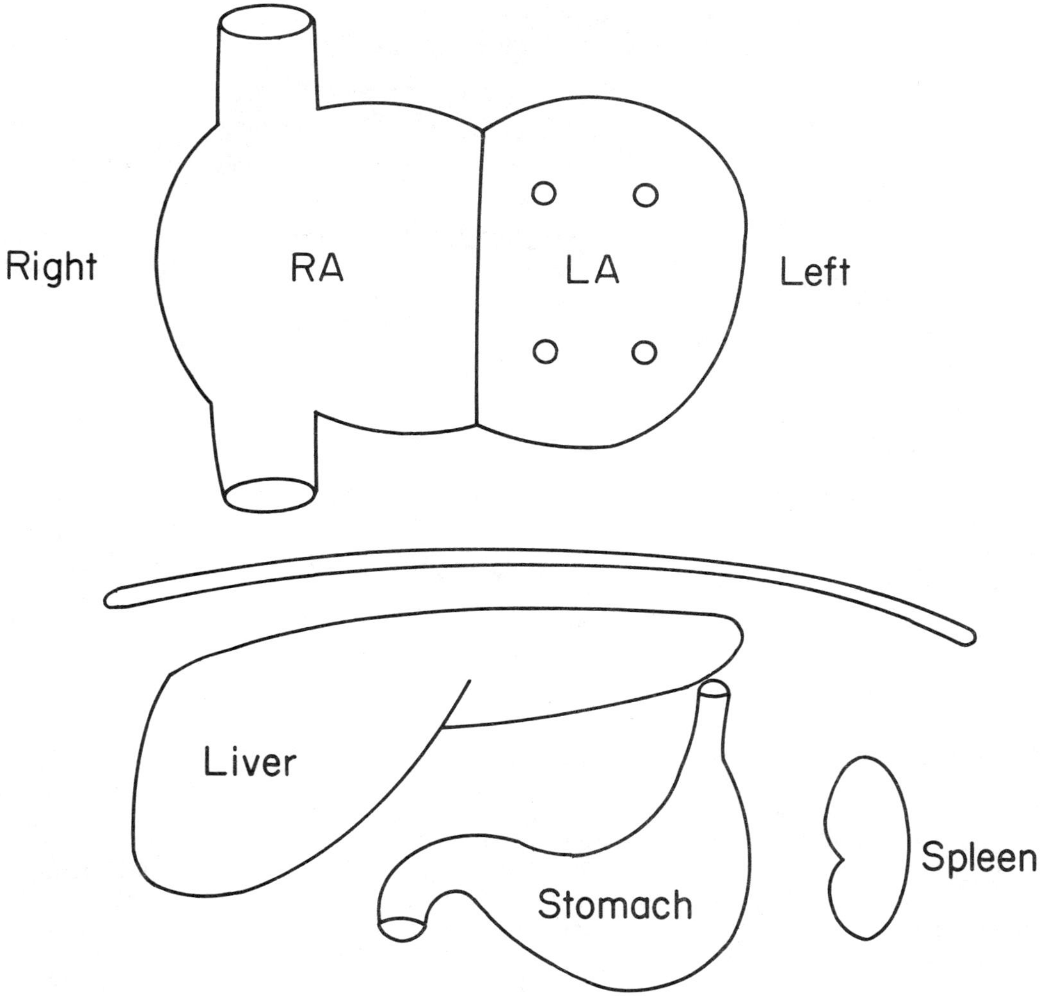

Figure 23-1A Visceroatrial arrangement in situs solitus. RA and LA indicate right and left atria, respectively, with their usual venous connections. (See also B, C, and D.)

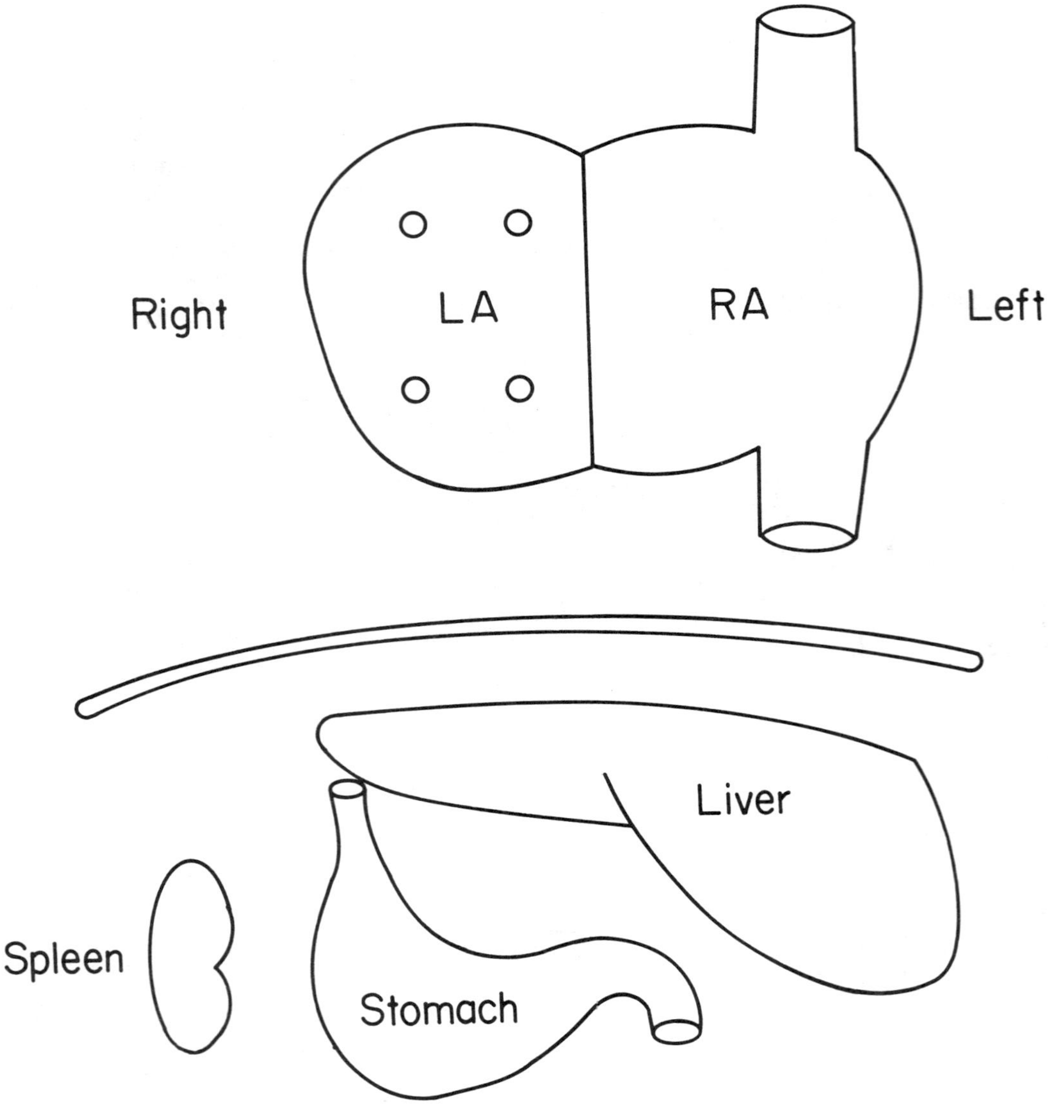

Figure 23-1B Visceroatrial arrangement in situs inversus.

3. *Determination of ventricular position:* As the primitive cardiac tube elongates, it normally forms a loop to the right (Fig. 23-2), referred to as a D-loop. This carries the bulbus cordis (primitive right ventricle) to the right of the ventricular portion (primitive left ventricle). This relationship is maintained as the loop subsequently pivots to lie in the left chest, and the adult right ventricle is to the right of the left ventricle. In situs inversus the cardiac tube loops to the left (L-loop), and the morphologic left ventricle lies to the right of the right ventricle. However, bulboventricular looping may be discordant with visceroatrial situs, and situs solitus with an L-loop, or situs inversus with a D-loop may be encountered. Position of the heart within the chest may vary independently of

bulboventricular looping, and is determined by the degree by which the loop pivots out of its initial location in the right or left chest. Thus, with either a D- or L-loop one may encounter levocardia, dextrocardia, or mesocardia. The morphology of the atrioventricular valves usually goes with the ventricle (e.g., tricuspid valve with right ventricle).

Ventricular position is best determined angiocardiographically. The direction of the Q wave on electrocardiographic chest leads may be helpful, as septal

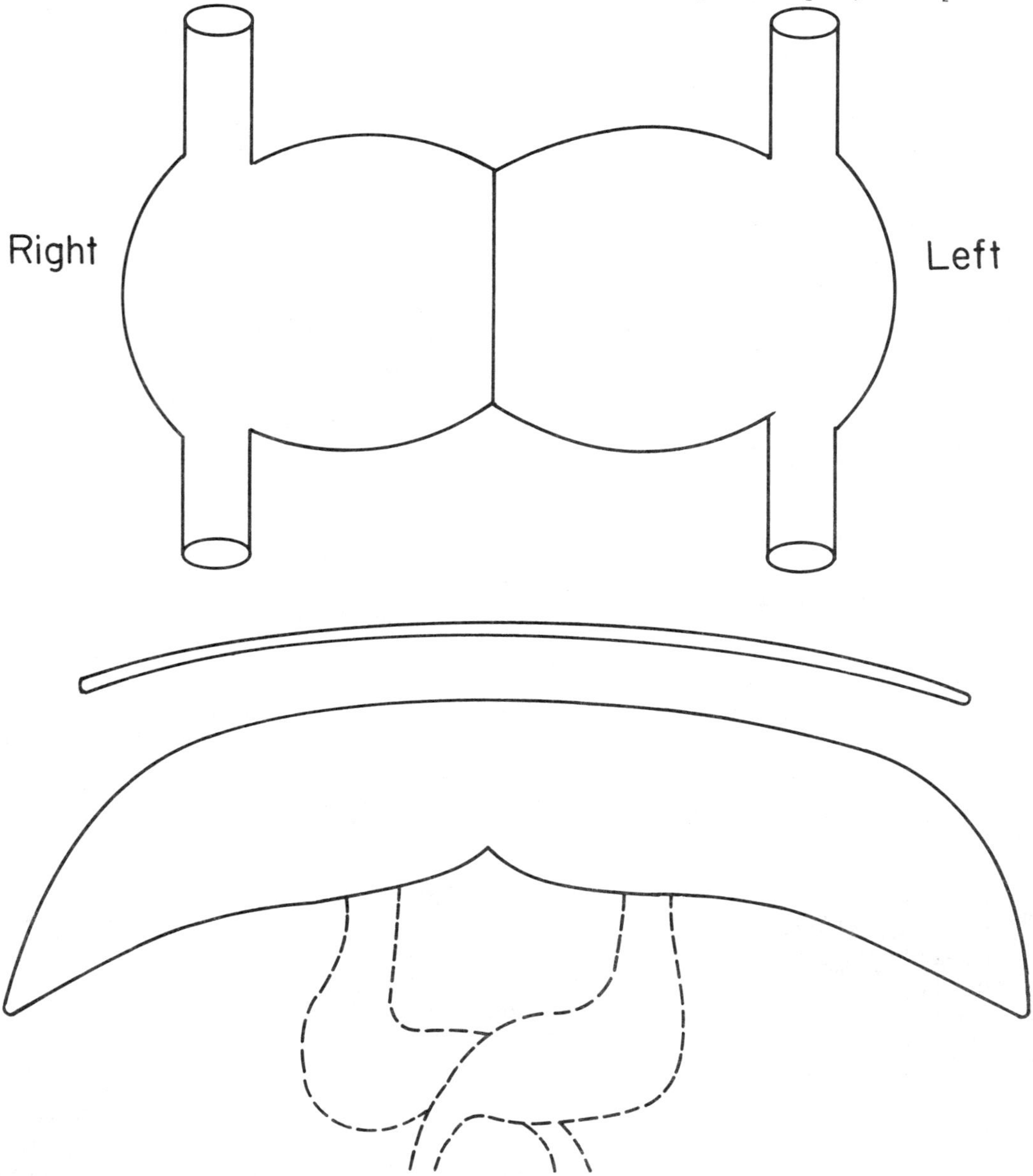

Figure 23–1C Visceroatrial orientation in the asplenia syndrome illustrating the tendency toward bilateral right atria, horizontal and usually symmetrical orientation of the liver, and variability in the stomach position.

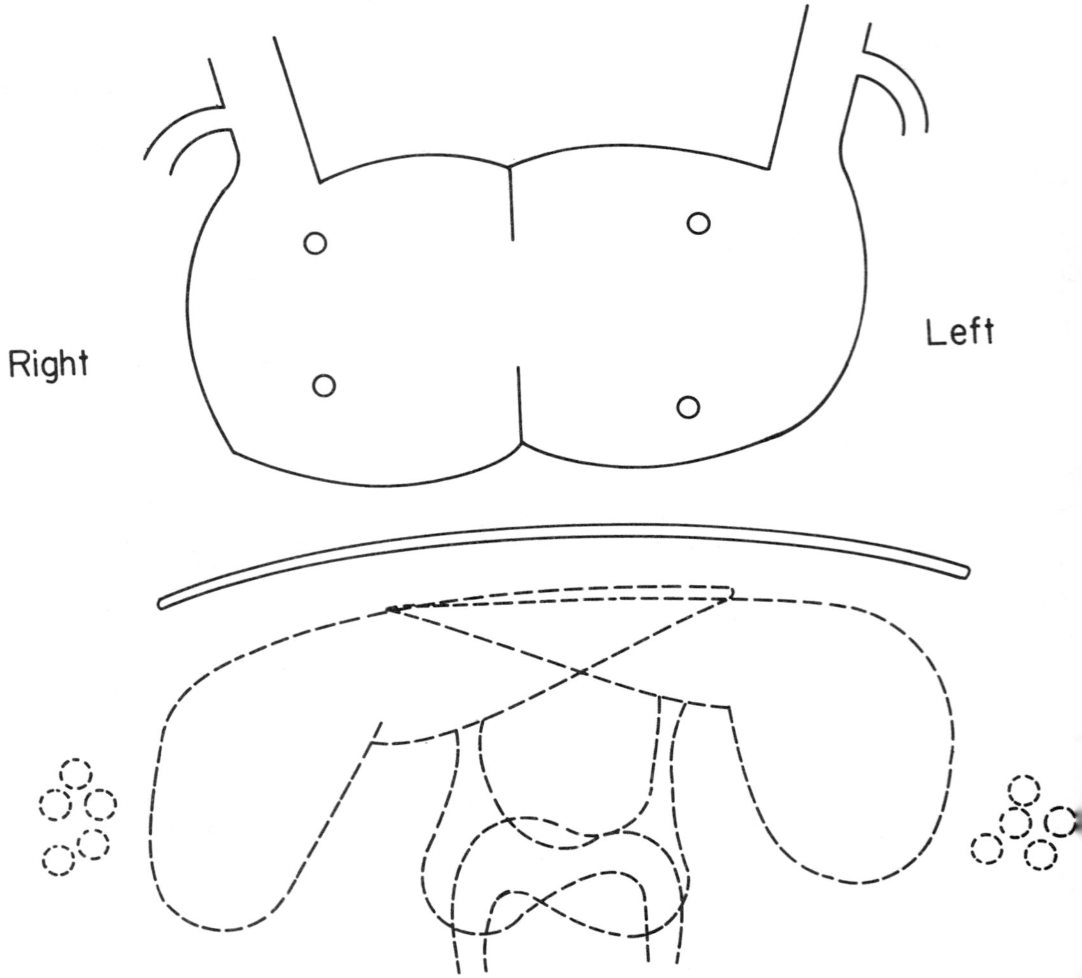

Figure 23-1D Visceroatrial arrangement in the polysplenia syndrome. Abdominal viscera are frequently more asymmetrical than in asplenia.

depolarization progresses from left to right in a normal heart, giving a Q wave in the left chest leads and not in the right. The direction of this vector is altered if the ventricular relationships are abnormal, but may be affected by other factors such as conduction defects (see Chap. 2). On angiocardiography, the right ventricle appears somewhat triangular in shape and shows coarse trabeculations, whereas the left ventricle is more ovoid and smooth walled (Fig. 23-3). At times, this may be difficult to ascertain.

Van Praagh has shown that a D-relationship between great arteries (aortic valve to the right of the pulmonic) almost always means the presence of a D-bulboventricular loop and L-arteries mean an L-loop. This is referred to as the loop rule.

4. *Evaluation of the conotruncus:* Normally, the conus arteriosus expands beneath that portion of the truncus which will form the pulmonary artery, and this conal expansion is felt by some to carry the pulmonary valve to its anterior location over the right ventricle. Because of the presence of the subpulmonic conus,

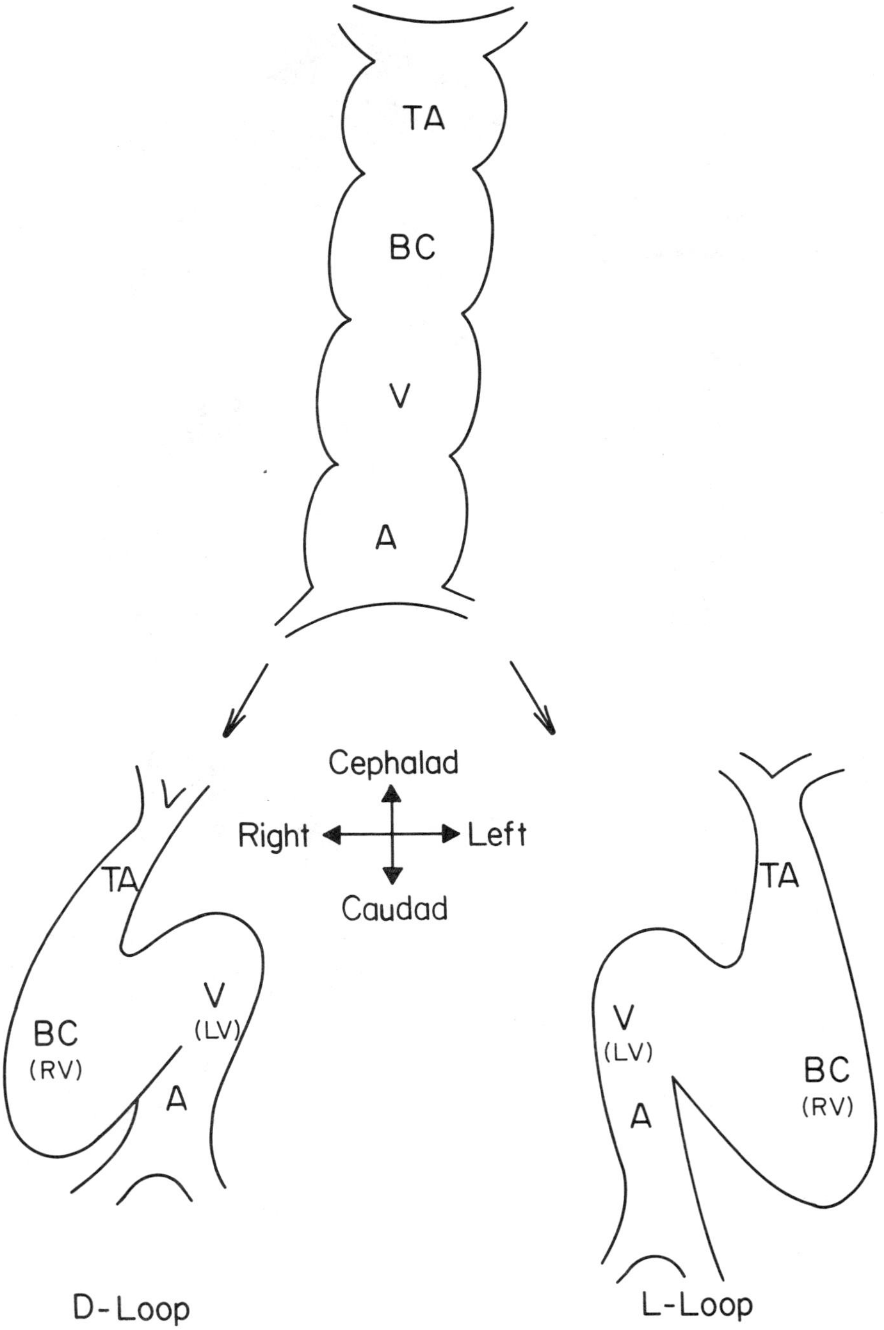

Figure 23–2 The primitive cardiac tube with its segments is shown at the top of the figure and the ventricular orientation produced by D and L looping at the bottom. A - atrial segment, V - ventricular segment (primitive left ventricle), BC - bulbus cordis (primitive right ventricle), and TA - truncus arteriosus. In normal D-looping, the morphologic right ventricle is oriented to the right of the left ventricle. The reverse is true if an L-loop is formed.

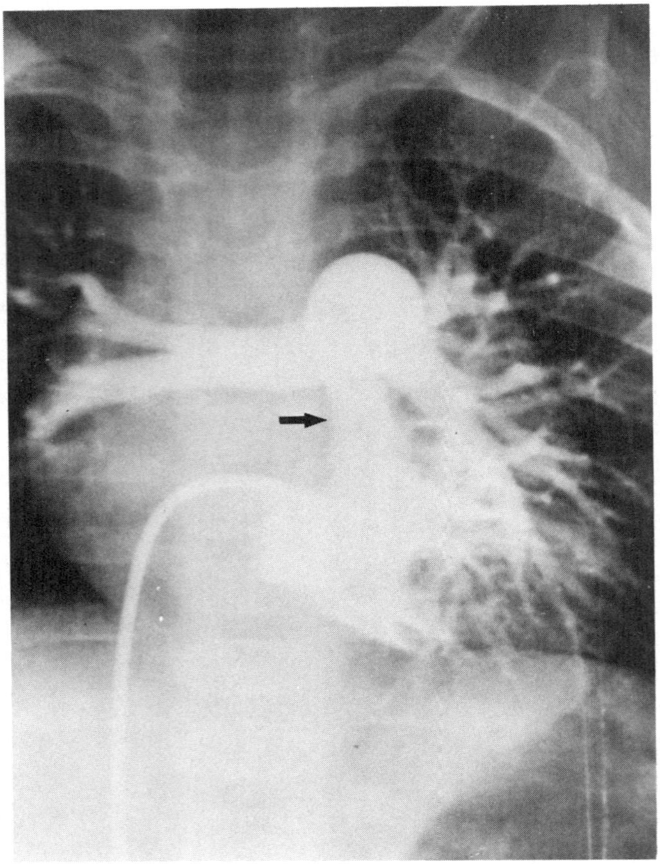

Figure 23–3A Right ventricular angiocardiogram showing typical morphology of that chamber with its somewhat triangular shape and irregular margin due to the coarser trabeculations. The RV infundibulum (subpulmonic conus) is seen as the vertical band of contrast medium (arrow) immediately beneath the circular density of the main pulmonary artery. (See also B.)

the pulmonary valve is anterior to the anterior valve and more cephalad, with no direct continuity between pulmonary and tricuspid valve annuli. The aortic valve with no underlying conus is inferior (caudad) and posterior, and its annulus is in fibrous continuity with the mitral annulus. The side-to-side relationship of the great arteries is determined by bulboventricular looping as previously described. The conal position may assist in the understanding of some of the complex abnormalities of great artery position and can usually be determined from selective ventricular angiocardiography. The position of the conus can be inferred by noting which valve is more cephalad and anterior.

The term transposition of the great arteries refers to their origin from the anatomically inappropriate ventricle, that is, the aorta from the right ventricle and pulmonary artery from the left ventricle. In this situation there is usually a subaortic conus, and the aortic valve is anterior and cephalad to the pulmonic valve. The presence of a conus beneath both valves is characteristic of double-outlet right ventricle. Other abnormal arrangements of the great arteries are

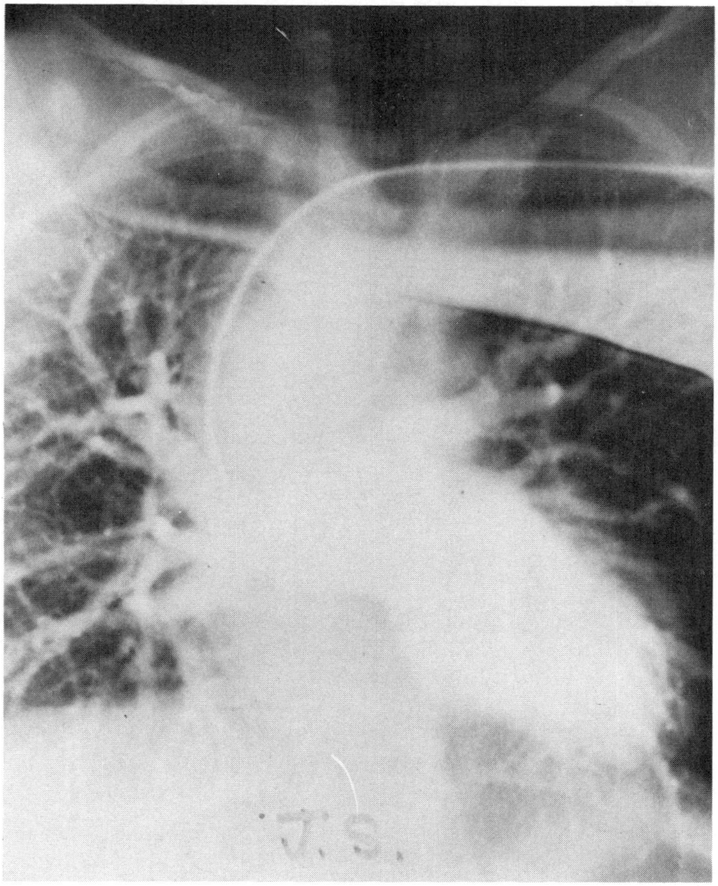

Figure 23-3B Levophase of an angiocardiogram showing filling of the pulmonary veins, left atrium, and left ventricle. Note the ovoid and smooth-walled contour of the latter chamber which is the typical anatomy. The triangular white area near the top of the figure is an artifact.

referred to as malposition. When a D-bulboventricular loop is present, the great arteries are almost always in a D-relationship, as described by the loop rule of Van Praagh. This may be a normal relationship in situs solitus or a D-transposition (Fig. 23-4). Conversely, in the presence of an L-loop, the arteries may be L-normal (situs inversus) or L-transposition.

Convention of Abbreviated Notations

In order to facilitate the description of complicated lesions, at least two conventions of abbreviation have been described. Both sequentially indicate the visceroatrial situs, bulboventricular loop, and arterial arrangement.

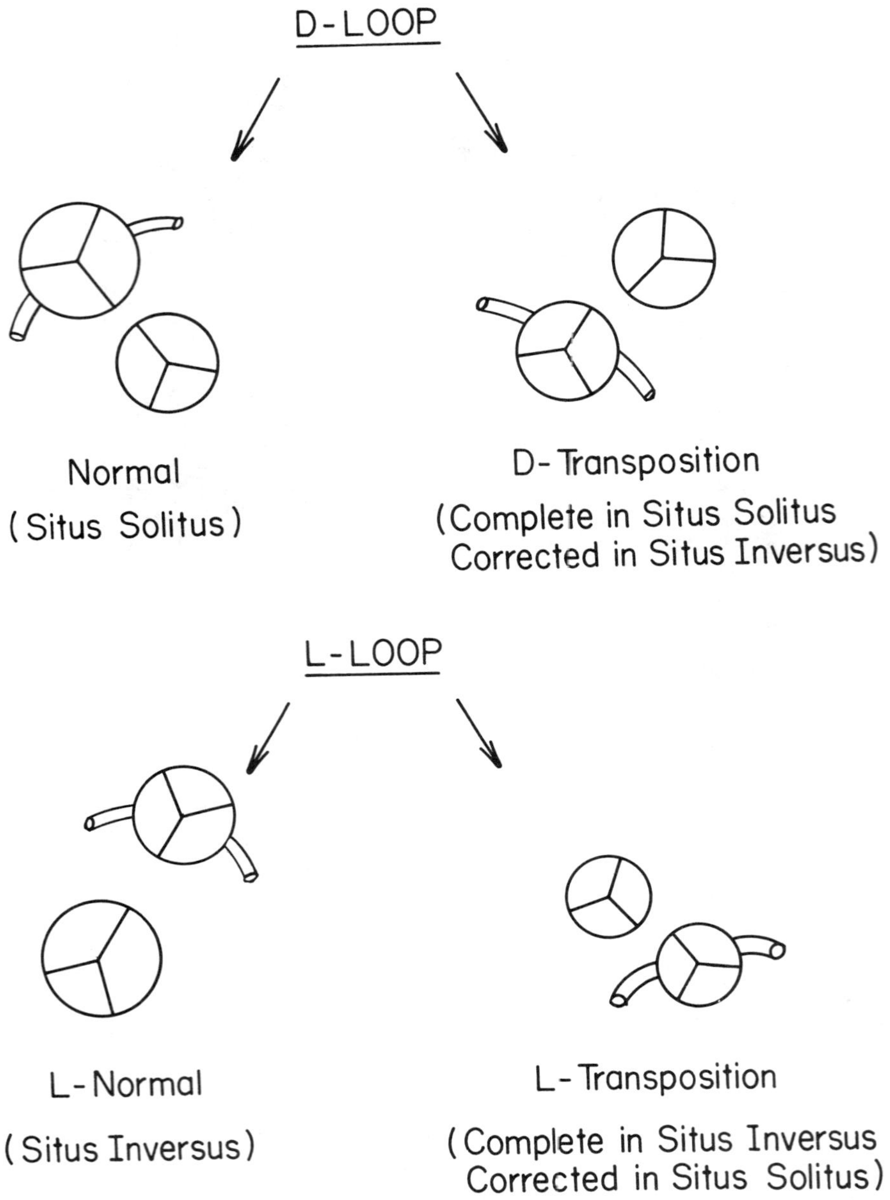

Figure 23–4 Great vessel arrangement as determined by the loop rule. D-looping almost always results in the aortic valve being to the right of the pulmonic ring. If the aorta is both to the right and posterior, the great vessel arrangement is normal. If anterior and rightward to the pulmonary artery, a D-transposition is present which may be complete or physiologically corrected depending upon the body situs. L-looping results in the aortic valve being to the left of the pulmonic. This is the normal arrangement in situs inversus with the aortic valve also posteriorly placed. In L-transposition the aorta is anterior and left of the pulmonary artery and may be complete or physiologically corrected depending again upon visceroatrial situs.

1. Visceroatrial situs
   S: Situs solitus
   I: Situs inversus
   A: Situs ambiguous

2. Bulboventricular loop
   D: D-loop
   L: L-loop
   X: Unknown

3. Arterial (conotruncal) arrangement
   S: Solitus, normally related (D) arteries
   I: Inversus, normally related (L) arteries
   D: D-transposition or malposition
   L: L-transposition or malposition
   A: Anteroposterior transposition or malposition (aorta directly anterior to PA)

Thus, with minimal abbreviation, a normal heart might be described as solitus/D-loop/D-normal or fully abbreviated as [S,D,S]. Other examples are:

Normal heart with sinus inversus: Inversus/L-loop/L-normal or [I,L,I]
Complete transposition in situs solitus: Solitus/D-loop/D-transposition or TGA [S,D,D]
Corrected transposition in situs solitus: Solitus/L-loop/L-transposition or TGA [S,L,L]
Corrected transposition in situs inversus: Inversus/D-loop/D-transposition or TGA [I,D,D]

Bibliography

Stanger P, Rudolph AM, Edwards JE: Cardiac malformations: An overview based on study of fifty-five necropsy specimens. Circulation 56:159, 1977.

Van Praagh R: Terminology of congenital heart disease. Circulation 56:139, 1977.

Van Praagh RV, Weinberg PM, Van Praagh S: Malposition of the Heart, Heart Disease in Infants, Children and Adolescents, 2nd ed., Moss AJ, Adams FH, Emmanouilides GC, Williams and Wilkins Co., Baltimore, 1977, p. 394.

Part IV

ACQUIRED CARDIOVASCULAR PROBLEMS

Chapter 24

PRIMARY ENDOMYOCARDIAL DISEASE

The entities included in this section involve primarily the heart and are therefore designated as primary endomyocardial disease.

Classification

Traditionally, primary endomyocardial diseases are divided into three subgroups: myocarditis, endocardial fibroelastosis (EFE), and hypertrophic cardiomyopathy. The clinical similarities between these entities are striking and often difficult to differentiate on clinical grounds or even on autopsy. The following is a classification of both the primary and secondary endomyocardial diseases; the secondary forms are mentioned for the purpose of differential diagnosis.

1. *Primary endomyocardial disease*
   - A. Myocarditis
   - B. Endocardial fibroelastosis (EFE)
     - 1) Left ventricle
     - 2) Right ventricle
   - C. Hypertrophic cardiomyopathy (HCM) or asymmetric septal hypertrophy (ASH)
     - 1) Obstructive
     - 2) Nonobstructive
2. *Secondary endomyocardial disease*
   - A. Generalized diseases
     - 1) Collagen disease (periarteritis nodosa, dermatomyositis)
     - 2) Systemic hypertension
     - 3) Neuromuscular (Friedreich ataxia, muscular dystrophy)
     - 4) Glycogen storage disease (types II, III, IV)
     - 5) Other (Hurler, Hunter, thalassemia, sickle cell)
   - B. Congenital cardiac anomalies
     - 1) EFE associated with obstructive disease (coarctation, aortic stenosis)

2) Anomalies of the coronary arteries
3) Medial necrosis of the coronaries
4) Neoplasm (rhabdomyoma)

C. Infections

1) Bacteria (diphtheria)
2) Viral (Coxsackie, mononucleosis, rubella, measles)
3) Rickettsial (typhus)

D. Toxic

1) Radiation
2) Anthracycline antibiotics
3) Venoms
4) Iron deposits

Myocarditis

Etiology

Several viruses that are known to produce disease in man can affect the myocardium including varicella, rubella, influenza, mumps, and herpes; however, the viruses most commonly involved in myocarditis are the Coxsackie B subgroups. Other organisms such as toxoplasma, visceral larval migrans, and trichinosis have also been implicated.

It seems that viruses may result in myocardial disease in two ways: (1) direct (active infective) and (2) indirect (autoimmune). The initial stage of the disease is due to direct effect of the viruses on the heart. In chronic cases, however, viruses cannot be isolated, yet the inflammatory process is continuously causing extensive damage. The mechanism for this continued inflammation is not clear but is thought to be autoimmune. The antigenmay be persistent viral particles or a newly formed antigen from necrotic myocardium.

Incidence

The incidence of acute myocarditis in infancy and childhood is difficult to determine because of the impossible task of differentiating it from other inflammatory myocardial diseases. There are two periods of peak incidence, one occurring in the newborn period, the second extending from 1 year of age and over.

Pathological Anatomy

The heart appears dilated, pale, and flabby. Microscopically there are areas of muscle fiber necrosis and interstitial accumulation of mononuclear cells. Viral antigen can be detected in the myocardium of some patients by means of fluorescent antibody technique. Viral particles are also detected in the myocardium and valvular tissue of patients with a picture of cardiomyopathy, supporting the hypothesis of chronic viral myocarditis. The patients who exhibit the autoimmune variety of chronic myocarditis usually show more interstitial changes and less muscle necrosis.

Manifestations

The newborn with myocarditis usually presents within the first few days of life with lethargy, anorexia, and vomiting. Abnormal temperature elevation, respiratory distress, and hepatomegaly are common. Occasionally, the patient presents with a sudden cardiovascular collapse. Examination of the cardiovascular system invariably reveals evidence of enlarged heart, tachypnea, tachycardia, and a gallop rhythm. Significant murmurs are not present. The history often reveals maternal or epidermiologic evidence of nursery infection.

Following the newborn period, the disease is rare within the first 6 months of life and peaks again at 1 year of age. There is often history of preceding acute respiratory illness. The clinical spectrum of the disease varies from the mild form presenting with low-grade fever, slow onset of congestive heart failure, and occasionally ventricular extrasystoles to the sudden onset of severe congestive heart failure. The physical examination is similar to that of the newborn with myocarditis.

Laboratory Data

The sedimentation rate is often elevated, but this is a nonspecific finding indicative of an acute inflammatory process. Viral cultures and rise in specific serum antibody titers are helpful in making the diagnosis.

Electrocardiographic Data

Electrocardiographic findings are nonspecific and manifest an abnormal repolarization. The T waves are low voltage or inverted. There is usually no evidence of hypertrophy. Occasionally, ventricular extrasystoles are present.

Radiologic Features

The radiographic manifestations depend upon the severity of the disease. The findings may range from a normal heart size to marked cardiomegaly. Pulmonary venous congestion, if present, manifests with Kerley B lines and haziness of both lung fields. Left lower lobe atelectasis, related to a compression of the bronchus by a large left atrium, is not uncommon.

Echocardiographic Features

Both M-mode and two-dimensional (2-D) echocardiography are now an essential part of the workup of these patients. The left ventricle appears markedly dilated with decreased contractility and ejection fraction. The ventricular walls and septum are usually of normal thickness. The left atrium may be dilated, and the aortic root motion is decreased, indicating poor cardiac output (Fig. 24-1). The echocardiogram easily excludes pericardial effusion and the cardiomegaly of infants of diabetic mothers who have a thick myocardium with normal contractility.

Differential Diagnosis

The entities to be considered are endocardial fibroelastosis, anomalous origin of the left coronary artery, and pericarditis. The secondary endomyocardial diseases should also be excluded.

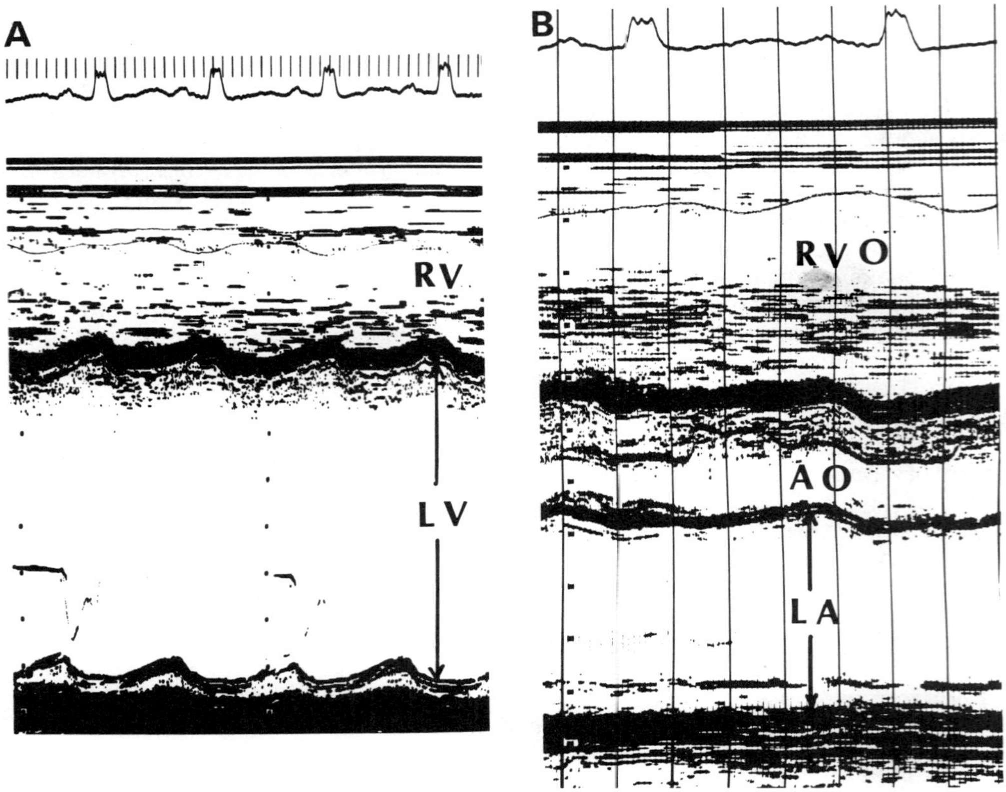

Figure 24-1 M-mode echocardiogram of a patient with dilated cardiomyopathy. (A) The left ventricle is markedly dilated. The septal and posterior wall are thin and exhibit poor contractility. (B) The left atrium is enlarged. The aorta is of normal size but lacks the usual systole motion which indicates poor cardiac contractility and output. The right ventricular outflow tract is dilated. RV - right ventricle, RVO - right ventricle outflow tract, LV - left ventricle, LA - left atrium, Ao - aorta.

1. *Endocardial fibroelastosis:* The clinical presentation and physical examination may be identical in both EFE and myocarditis; however, onset at the newborn period, and after 1 year of age, favors myocarditis. Electrocardiographic manifestation of severe left ventricular hypertrophy favors endocardial fibroelastosis. Occasionally, however, without myocardial biopsy it is impossible to differentiate one from the other. There is now evidence that both entities are related and that endocardial fibroelastosis is a severe manifestation of intrauterine endomyocarditis.

2. *Pericarditis:* Differentiation of myocarditis from acute benign pericarditis is not difficult. The latter patients usually present with chest pain, enlarged cardiac silhouette, but no evidence of failure. In the presence of large pericardial effusion, a friction rub might not be present.

Echocardiogram and cardiac scan are noninvasive techniques available for the identification of significant amount of pericardial fluid. The electrocardiogram may show decreased voltages and ST-segment changes.

3. *Anomalous left coronary artery:* This entity is to be considered in the differential diagnosis of neonatal myocarditis. The physical findings may be indistinguishable. The EKG, however, shows evidence of anterolateral myocardial infarction.

4. *Infant of a diabetic mother:* Occasionally, an infant of a diabetic mother presents in the newborn period with massive cardiomegaly. The differential diagnosis from myocarditis is not difficult since these infants are usually asymptomatic and have no evidence of congestive heart failure. The infants who also have respiratory distress syndrome may present a problem. The cardiomegaly is thought to be part of the generalized macrosomia associated with diabetes. These findings usually regress within 4-6 weeks with no residual abnormalities (Fig. 24-2).

Treatment

Every effort should be made to identify a causative agent. Acute and convalescent titers for viral antibody determination should be drawn. Rising titer for a specific virus establishes the diagnosis. The treatment is mainly supportive and symptomatic. Infants and children who develop congestive heart failure require prolonged periods of bed rest, fluid restriction, and therapy with diuretics and digitalis. Corticosteroids are known to depress interferon production and, therefore, are not used as a primary mode of therapy, since most patients improve on standard therapy alone. There are, however, patients that manifest protracted

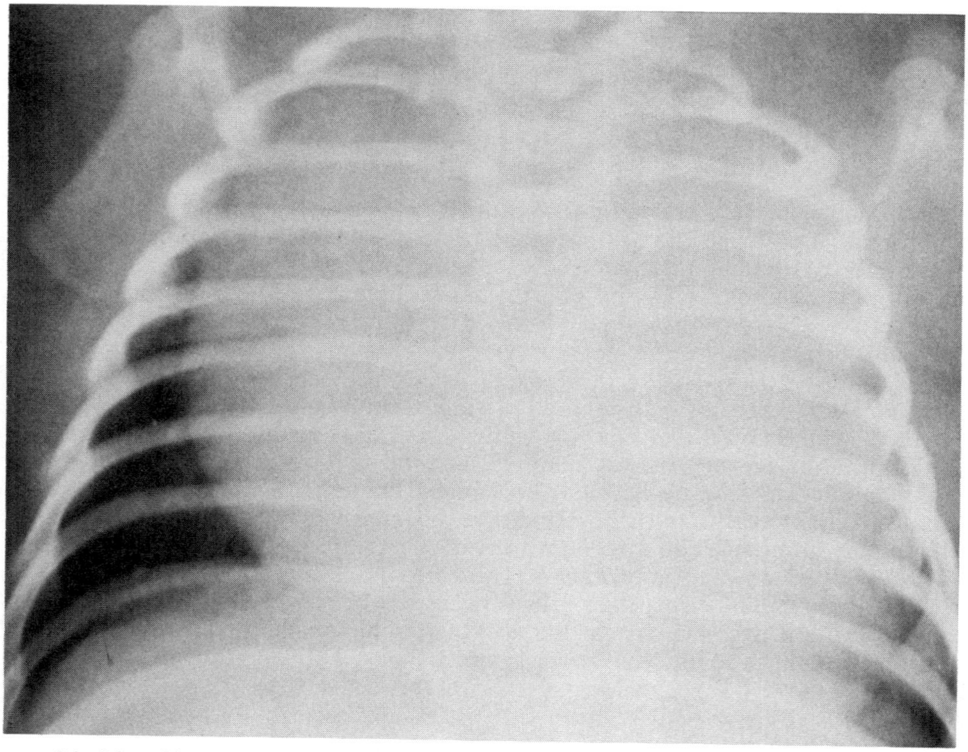

Figure 24-2A Chest radiograph of an infant of a diabetic mother. Radiograph taken at 12 hr of age showing marked cardiomegaly as well as large thymic shadow. There is no evidence of pulmonary edema. (See also B).

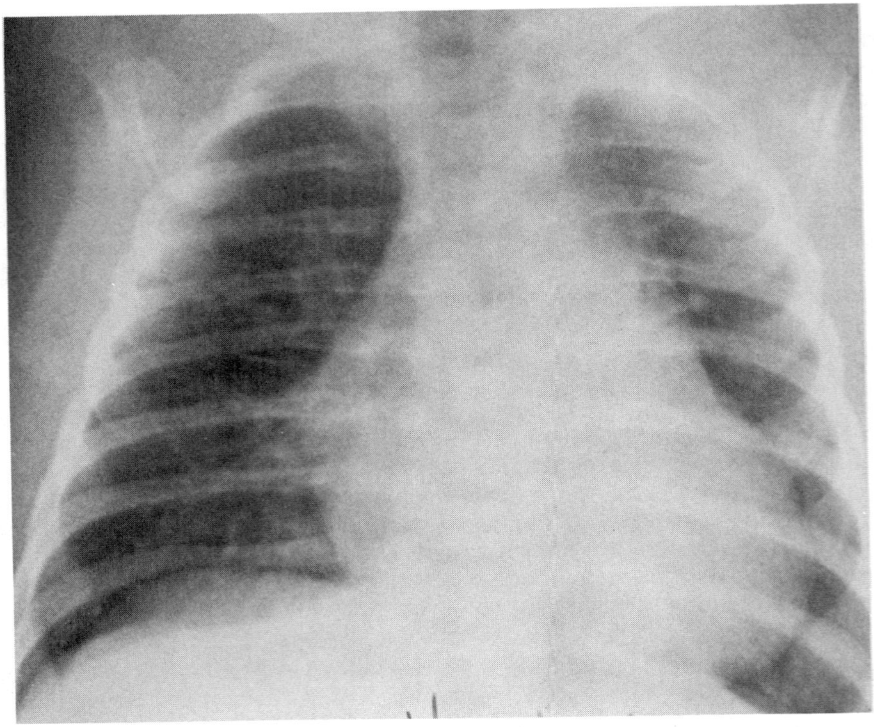

Figure 24-2B The same patient at 30 days of age. Note the decrease in heart size.

course and chronic congestive heart failure that is uncontrollable with standard medications. These are the patients who probably develop autoimmune phenomena and do benefit from the introduction of antiinflammatory agents such as steroids. They often exhibit marked symptomatic improvement and decrease in cardiac size.

Course and Prognosis

The mortality rate of recognized Coxsackie B myocarditis in the newborn period is 50-70%. The true mortality is probably somewhat lower since the milder cases go undetected or are incorrectly diagnosed. Infants and children with the milder form of the disease who do not develop congestive heart failure invariably recover within 6-10 months. More than half of the patients who develop congestive heart failure beyond 6 months of age seem to recover completely, without sequelae.

A few, however, require prolonged treatment. These are the patients who present with an insidious onset, indicating chronicity of the disease. A few of these patients manifest progressive cardiac dilatation, endocardial fibroelastosis, and subsequent death, probably due to arrhythmia.

Endocardial Fibroelastosis

Incidence

Endocardial fibroelastosis is found in 4-8% of all autopsied cases of congenital heart disease. There are no accurate data available regarding the true incidence of clinically detected cases.

Classification

1. Left ventricular
   - A. Isolated
   - B. Complicated
     1) With aortic valve involvement (aortic stenosis, coarctation)
     2) With mitral valve involvement (atresia, stenosis)
     3) With conduction system abnormality (Wolff-Parkinson-White syndrome, complete heart block)
2. Right ventricular
   - A. Isolated
   - B. Complicated
     1) With pulmonic valve involvement (pulmonary atresia)
     2) With tricuspid valve involvement

This section deals with the isolated form and excludes from the discussion the cases associated with other congenital heart lesions. The left ventricle is the most frequently involved chamber in isolated endocardial fibroelastosis. Reports of well-documented isolated right ventricular involvement are scarce.

Pathological Anatomy

At postmortem the heart is markedly enlarged. The left ventricle is dilated and thickened. The left atrium is dilated as well. Macroscopically, there is white opaque glistening, thickened endocardium. The thickening is diffuse, involving the entire endocardial surface, resulting in flattening of the trabeculae carnae. This appearance has been termed sugarcoating or China porcelain and is related to increase in the fibroelastic tissue in and beneath the endocardium, with extension of fibrous bands into the myocardium. The papillary muscles become partially embedded in the fibroelastic process, resulting in shortening of the papillary muscles and chordae tendienae cordis. This distorted valvular architecture may lead to mitral regurgitation.

Microscopically, there is frequent evidence of myocarditis manifested by perivascular cellular infiltration. There is also proliferation of the capillaries, precapillaries, and areas of diffuse fibrosis, necrosis, and dilated lymphatics.

Etiology

Several etiologic theories have been proposed through the years. The theory of fetal endocarditis proposed in 1818 is probably the most plausible one and has recently gained additional support. Fruhling, in France, has presented strong evidence suggesting that endocardial fibroelastosis is a pancarditis probably due to intrauterine or extrauterine Coxsackie B virus infection. He was able to culture Coxsackie B3 from postmortem myocardial specimens obtained from patients with this disease. In some, the virus was also isolated from other organs. Search for other viruses and bacteria was virtually negative. These authors also presented clinical and experimental evidence of transplacental transmission of the virus.

The histologic evidence of inflammatory changes in the myocardium is also in favor of the infectious theory. The process may be infiltrative or degenerative, depending on the intensity of the infection. Persistence of the virus in the heart appears to determine the inflammatory changes and their sequelae. Vascular stasis and blockage of the lymphatics are felt to be the most important factors triggering the excessive fibroelastic process. Analyzing the pathologic manifestation stresses the difficulty in differentiating myocarditis from endocardial fibroelastosis. The acceptance of a common viral etiology for both seems warranted. Accordingly, there are probably various stages of the disease, depending upon the severity of involvement.

Pathophysiology

The abnormal circulatory function in endocardial fibroelastosis appears to result from diffuse left ventricular myocardial disease (Fig. 24-3), leading to decreased contractility. Left ventricular dilatation and subsequent hypertrophy occur. These are both compensatory mechanisms designed to improve cardiac output. With the progression of the disease, left ventricular failure ensues, manifested by the low-cardiac output and pulmonary venous congestion.

Manifestations

There is no apparent sex or race predilection. In the vast majority of patients, the age of onset is between 1 and 6 months of age. In only 18% of the patients the symptoms started after the first year of life. There is usually some evidence of growth retardation expressed as abnormal weight rather than height. The disease is manifested by a fairly rapid onset of congestive heart failure which may be precipitated by an upper respiratory infection. Classic findings of left-sided failure such as dyspnea, tachypnea, grunting, and wheezing are common. Twenty percent of patients have a history of frequent respiratory tract infection, and some have been previously hospitalized for pneumonia. A common respiratory complication present in at least 25% of patients is lower lobe atelectasis, resulting from compression of the bronchus by an enlarged left atrium (Fig. 24-4). The patients may be febrile at the time of admission.

A precordial bulge is usually apparent. The point of maximal impulse is displaced, often to the sixth intercostal space outside the midclavicular line. The first heart sound is normal; the second heart sound may be increased in intensity. A third heart sound is almost always present, but significant murmurs are rare. In chronic cases, a murmur of mitral regurgitation can be heard. Hepatomegaly is invariably present.

The electrocardiogram shows left ventricular overload and T-wave changes. Left atrial enlargement may be seen, but right ventricular hypertrophy is rarely present (Fig. 24-5).

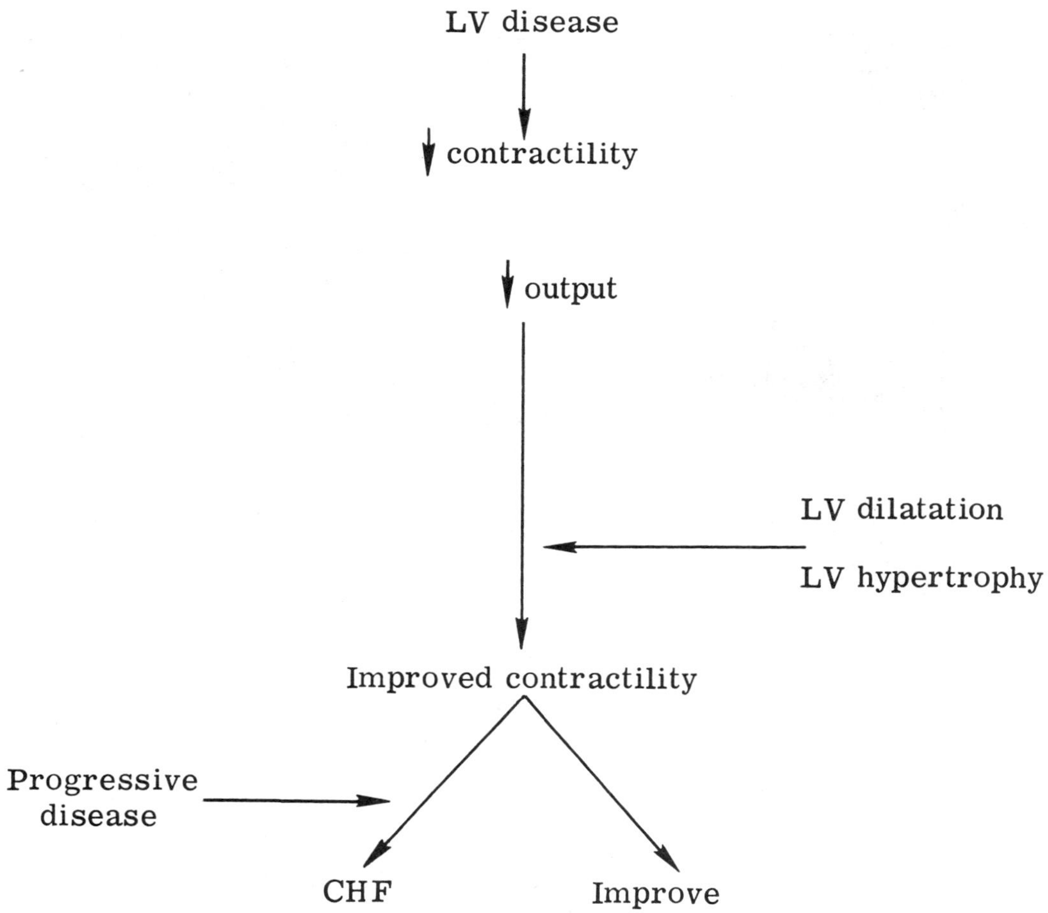

Figure 24-3 Schematic representation of the pathophysiology of primary endomyocardial disease. LV - left ventricle, CHF - congestive heart failure.

The chest radiograph shows massive enlargement of the cardiac silhouette, mainly attributed to left atrium and left ventricle dilatation (see Fig. 24-4). Evidence of left heart failure, such as wet fissures and interstitial edema, is usually present. The echocardiogram is similar to that seen in dilated cardiomyopathy exhibiting a dilated left ventricle with decreased contractility. The left ventricular myocardium is usually thickened. The left atrium is large, and there is an anterior mitral valve-septal separation.

Differential Diagnosis

The entities to be considered are mainly myocarditis, pericardial effusion, aberrant left coronary artery, glycogenosis, and periarteritis nodosa. Myocarditis and pericarditis are discussed under the differential diagnosis for myocarditis. Cardiac involvement in glycogen storage disease may be similar to EFE; however, large liver and tongue, muscle hypotonia, and hypoglycemia suggest the diagnosis. Periarteritis nodosa is a rare multisystem disease usually associated with renal involvement and hypertension.

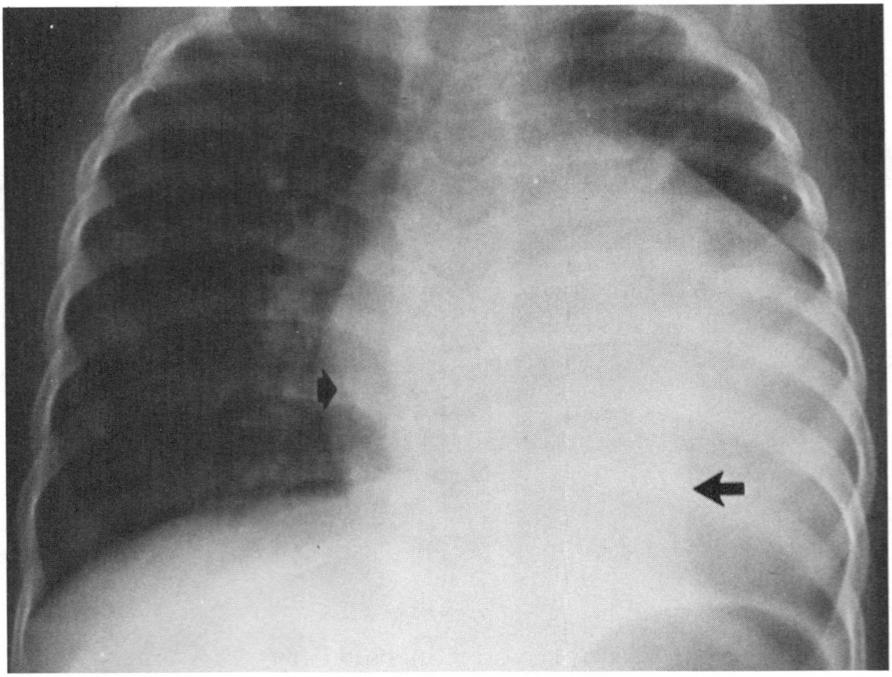

Figure 24–4A A patient with endocardial fibroelastosis. A 3-month-old in congestive heart failure. Note the marked cardiomegaly with left ventricular and left atrial (short arrow) dilatation. The long arrow points to the left lower lobe atelectasis. (See also B.)

Cardiac Catheterization

Right-sided pressures are normal; however, pulmonary wedge pressure and left atrial and left ventricular end-diastolic pressures are elevated. The cardiac output is low. Left ventricular angiogram reveals a markedly dilated, thick-walled left ventricle which contracts poorly. Occasionally, there is evidence of mitral regurgitation. Visualization of both coronaries excludes the possibility of anomalous origin of the left coronary artery from the pulmonary artery.

Treatment

The overall mortality from this disease has been 60%; however, following the introduction of digoxin, the mortality is reduced to approximately 25%. Early institution of treatment cannot be overemphasized. There is now existing evidence that when therapy is delayed for more than 1 month after the onset of symptoms, recovery is never complete. The patients are treated with the usual recommended doses, guided by determination of blood digoxin level. Employing the recommended digitalizing and maintenance doses, we have not encountered any evidence of excessive sensitivity to the drug. As a matter of fact, several of our patients required the higher recommended dose in order to achieve a response or adequate blood level.

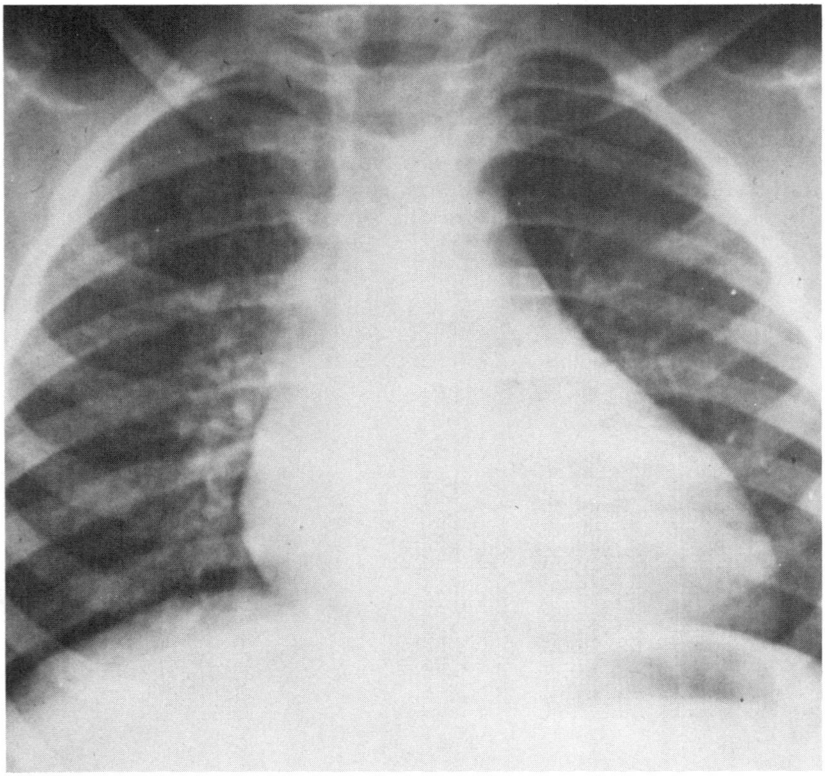

Figure 24-4B The same patient at 3 years of age, now asymptomatic. Note the marked decrease in cardiac size. The left ventricle and atrium are still prominent.

Digitalis therapy should be continued for a minimum of 1 year, or until all evidence of cardiac enlargement and left ventricular overwork have regressed. Termination of therapy prematurely may precipitate congestive heart failure and lessen the chance of complete recovery. The left lower lobe atelectasis, when present, deserves attention; postural drainage and antibiotic treatment, when needed, may be of help.

Complications

Cardiac failure and respiratory tract infection have already been mentioned as complications. Thromboembolic manifestations may occur in 10% of the patients. These originate from the left ventricle and may involve cerebral, renal, and coronary vessels. Myocardial necrosis and fibrosis may be present. Arrhythmias and conduction disturbances are relatively uncommon, but may occur terminally. Iatrogenic complications such as fluid overload are relatively common.

Prognosis

There are several factors that influence mortality. Infants who present between 3-6 months of age have a worse prognosis than those presenting over 1 year. Early medical care is a favorable prognostic sign. The shorter the prodrome, the better the prognosis, since a long prodrome probably indicates chronicity. Patients who show good initial response to digitalis do better. Also, continued treatment for prolonged periods of time has direct bearing on the prognosis. The number of recurrences influences the prognosis adversely.

In most patients who recover completely, the radiologic evidence of an enlarged heart lasts less than 2 years and EKG abnormalities less than 1 year (see Figs. 24-4B, 24-5B). The long-term outlook for the surviving patients is not yet known.

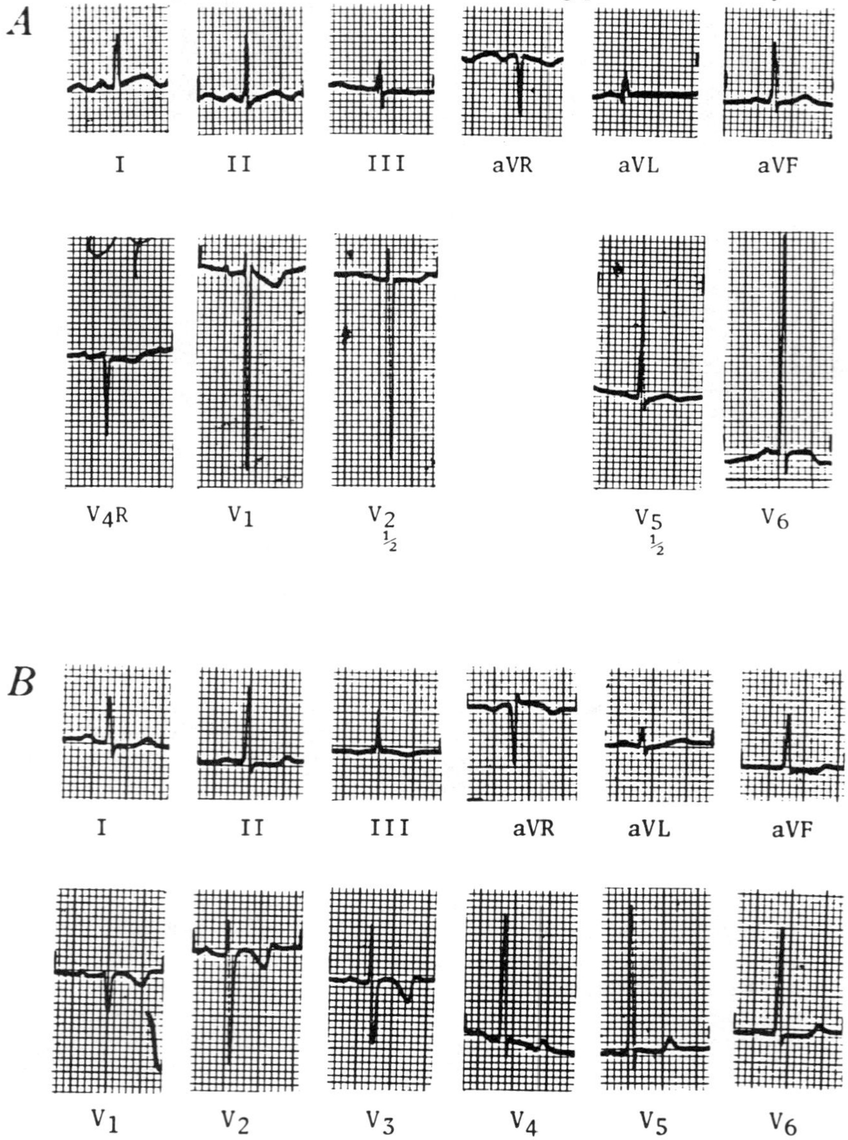

Figure 24-5 Electrocardiogram of a patient with endocardial fibroelastosis. (A) EKG at 3 months of age shows an axis of 45° and left ventricular hypertrophy. (B) EKG of the same patient at the age of 3 years. There are nonspecific ST segment changes and no evidence of hypertrophy.

Asymmetric Septal Hypertrophy (ASH)

Asymmetric septal hypertrophy is a genetically transmitted disease of the heart muscle characterized by disproportionate thickening of the septum, as compared to the left ventricular free wall. The clinical manifestations are variable and are related to the presence or absence of left ventricular outflow obstruction.

Incidence

The incidence of ASH in childhood is not yet known, but several cases have been described from infancy on. This entity usually manifests itself in the second and third decades and is a frequent cause of morbidity and mortality in the adult. This condition is familial and can be seen in 50% of first-degree relatives; however, it can only be detected by echocardiogram in 30% of children of index cases. This supports the fact that the disease does not become manifest until later in life.

Anatomy

The left ventricular cavity may be almost completely obliterated by the greatly hypertrophied muscle involving particularly the interventricular septum (Fig. 24-6). The papillary muscles and trabeculae are also hypertrophied. The mitral valve is usually encroached upon, but the aortic valve is normal.

Microscopically, there are bizarrely shaped and disorganized cells limited to the ventricular septum. The cardiac cells in the remaining left ventricular free wall are hypertrophied but normally arranged. This arrangement is limited mainly to the patients with left ventricular outflow obstruction. In patients with unobstructive ASH, disorganized cardiac muscle cells were found in both septum and left ventricular free wall.

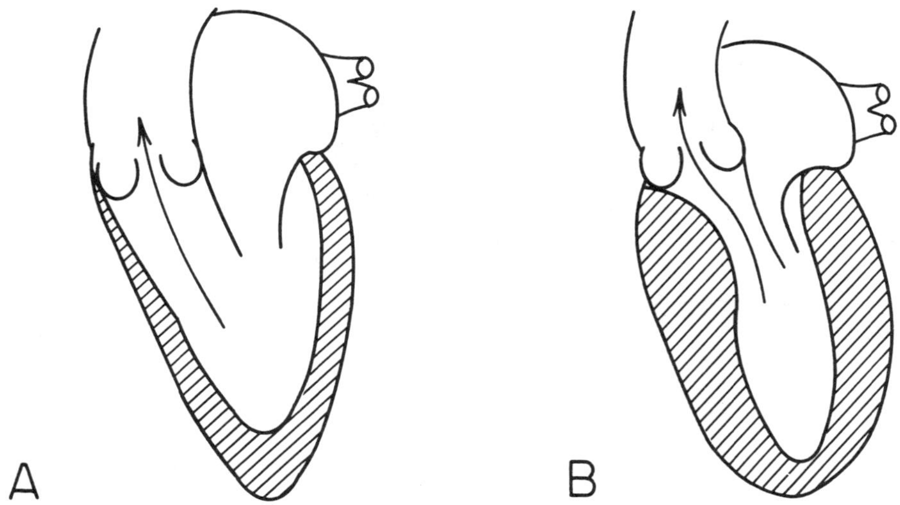

Figure 24-6 Schematic drawing of the left atrium, left ventricle, and aorta. (A) A normal heart with wide-open left ventricular outflow tract. (B) A heart with obstructive asymmetric septal hypertrophy. Note the narrowed left ventricular outflow tract caused by hypertrophied septum.

Hemodynamics

The basic hemodynamic disturbance in patients with hypertrophic cardiomyopathy is decrease in ventricular diastolic compliance. This abnormality is probably the result of severe ventricular hypertrophy. The rapid ventricular diastolic filling phase is thus significantly reduced, and isovolumetric relaxation time is prolonged.

Exercise produces tachycardia with a further reduction in rapid filling phase and an increase in left atrial and pulmonary capillary pressure resulting in dyspnea, pulmonary edema, and congestion. Reduced diastolic complaince also interferes with coronary blood flow, and this leads to the production of angina.

The subvalvular aortic obstruction is functional and may not exist throughout the entire phase of systole (Fig. 24-7). A rapid ejection of blood occurs at the beginning of systole before the muscle clamps down on the outflow tract. Subsequently, the left ventricular pressure increases to above systemic levels, but only a small amount of blood is being ejected. Agents decreasing the left ventricular systolic size or having positive inotropic effect on the left ventricle, such as isoproterenol and digitalis, increase the gradient (see Fig. 24-7B), whereas the beta-adrenergic blocking agents which decrease myocardial contractility (propranolol) decrease the obstruction. These considerations have therapeutic and diagnostic implications.

The hemodynamic spectrum is quite variable. It ranges from those having unobstructive hypertrophic cardiomyopathy, to patients in whom there is no gradient at rest but can be provoked with medications (isoproterenol), to those having a constant outflow obstruction. These patients may be asymptomatic; however, symptoms may also progress, leading to congestive heart failure or syncope and eventual death.

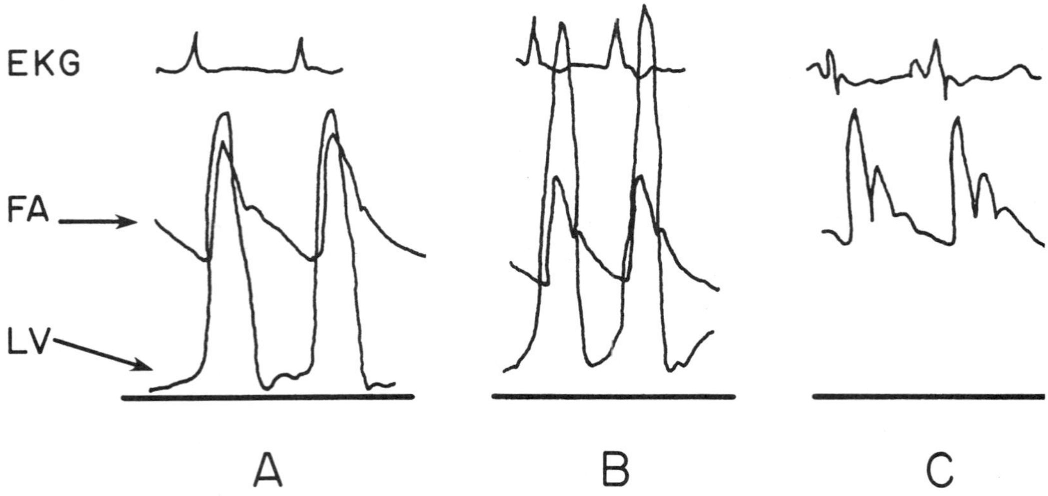

Figure 24-7 Pressure recordings in asymmetric septal hypertrophy. (A) Simultaneous pressure recordings from the left ventricle and femoral artery showing minimal pressure gradient. (B) Effect of isoproterenol. There is striking increase in the left ventricular pressure and decreased aortic pressure confirming the presence of severe provoked left ventricular outflow obstruction. (C) Typical arterial pressure tracing in obstructive asymmetric septal hypertrophy. Note the rapid upstroke, early systolic dip, and second peak in late systole.

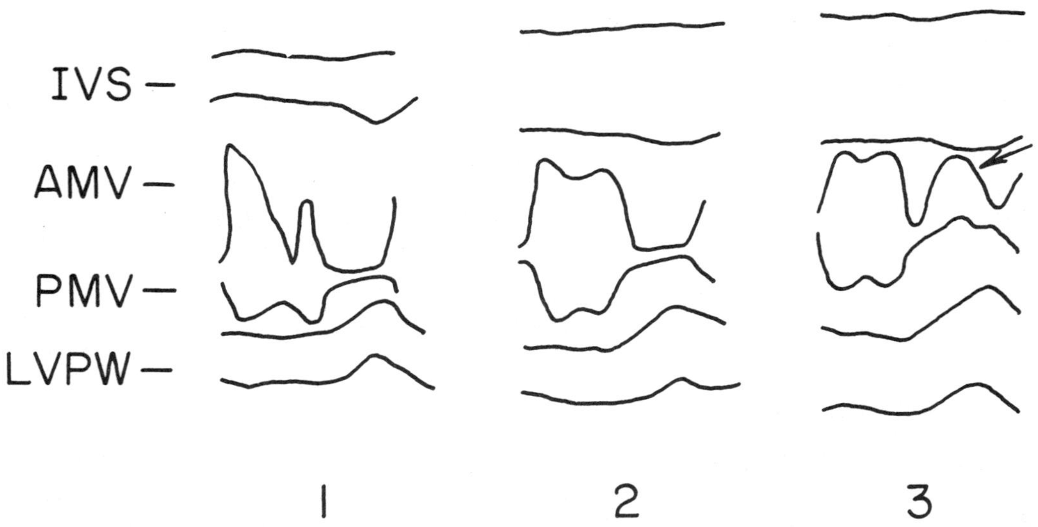

Figure 24-8 Echocardiogram showing septum, mitral valve, and left ventricular cavity. (1) Normal septum and mitral valve echocardiogram. (2) Asymmetric septal hypertrophy without obstruction. Hypertrophied septum and posterior left ventricular wall. Normal mitral valve motion. (3) Obstructive asymmetric septal hypertrophy, markedly hypertrophied septum, and posterior wall. There is abnormal mitral systolic anterior motion encroaching on the septum causing left ventricular outflow obstruction (arrow). IVS - interventricular septum, AMV - anterior mitral valve, PMV - posterior mitral valve, LVPW - left ventricular posterior wall.

Clinical Picture

As previously mentioned, there is a strong familial tendency. Mostly, the patients are asymptomatic and come to the cardiologist's attention because of a murmur discovered in childhood. Symptoms such as fatigue, dizziness, syncope, and angina are present in the more severe cases. On palpatation, a double apical impulse is present which corresponds to the phases of ejection of blood. The peripheral pulse has a double-hump configuration as well (see Fig. 24-7C).

On auscultation, there are often third and fourth heart sounds and a systolic murmur at the apex and left lower sternal border associated with a mid-diastolic murmur. The systolic murmur increases with the Valsalva maneuver and with the inhalation of amyl nitrite.

Chest x-ray shows cardiomegaly with normal pulmonary vascular markings. The electrocardiogram shows left ventricular hypertrophy with strain pattern. The Q wave may be large, indicative of septal hypertrophy. Short PR interval and Wolff-Parkinson-White pattern have been described.

The echocardiogram has been useful in diagnosing this entity. Both the anatomy and physiology are delineated (Fig. 24-8). There is asymmetric hypertrophy of the interventricular septum as compared with the left ventricle posterior wall. Also seen is an abnormal anterior systolic movement of the mitral valve encroaching on the septum, contributing to the left ventricular obstruction. It is only with the use of echocardiogram that asymptomatic patients can be detected and correctly diagnosed.

Cardiac Catheterization

Subaortic pressure gradient can usually be documented. Occasionally, however, there is no gradient at rest, but one can be provoked by administering intravenous isoproterenol (see Fig. 24-7). There is also an increase in the left ventricular end-diastolic pressure commonly seen in patients without outflow obstruction. Simultaneous aortic and ventricular pressure recorded during postextrasystolic beats in these patients is characteristic and shows increased ventricular pressure without corresponding increase in the aortic pressure.

There is increased incidence of asymmetric septal hypertrophy in infants of diabetic mothers. Mostly, these infants are asymptomatic and show regression of the hypertrophy over the first few months of life.

Differential Diagnosis

This entity should be differentiated from aortic valvular stenosis, discrete membranous subaortic stenosis, and an innocent murmur. Innocent murmurs usually decrease with the Valsalva maneuver, whereas the murmur of ASH does not. Cardiac catheterization can usually establish the diagnosis, especially when aided with provocative stimulation and left ventricular angiogram.

Course and Prognosis

This is a severe disease; if progressive, it ultimately leads to death. A few patients, however, have been followed for several years with no progression of the symptoms. Some patients, especially of the nonobstructive group, may deteriorate and develop congestive heart failure. Deaths have been described in infancy where the diagnosis was not suspected and established only on postmortem examination. A recent study of 46 children with ASH showed that 60% of the initial group had progression of symptoms or death. Thirty-one percent of patients in the obstructed group died suddenly. Sudden death was not related to symptoms, EKG, or hemodynamic abnormalities, or to the mode of treatment. Death is thought to be due to ventricular arrhythmia.

Treatment

Administration of a beta-adrenergic blocking agent such as propranolol reduces or abolishes the outflow obstruction by reducing the intensity of muscular contraction. This can usually be documented at cardiac catheterization. On the other hand, digitalis, nitroglycerin, and isoproterenol are contraindicated since they aggravate the obstruction. Recently, calcium antagonist agents such as verapamil and nifedipine have been reported to be useful in the treatment of patients with hypertrophic cardiomyopathy.

Patients with incapacitating symptoms unresponsive to medical management may be considered for surgery. Relief of the obstruction and significant clinical improvement may be achieved by an incision or resection of a portion of the obstructing hypertrophied left ventricular septum. It is important to realize, however, that the basic pathologic process involving the muscle is not halted by surgery.

Unfortunately, neither propranolol nor myotomy-myectomy with complete relief of the obstruction protect against sudden death. Thus, the role of prophylactic medical and surgical therapy in children with obstructive disease remains to be determined.

Bibliography

Greenwood RD, Nadas AS, Fyler DC: The clinical course of primary myocardial disease in infants and children. Am Heart J 92:549, 1976.

Hastreiter AR, Miller RA: Management of primary endomyocardial disease: the myocarditis-endocardial fibroelastosis syndrome. Pediatr Clin North Am 11:401, 1964.

Hirschman SZ, Hammer GS: Coxsackie virus myopericarditis. A microbiological and clinical review. Am J Cardiol 34:224, 1974.

Maron BJ, Edwards JE, Henry WL, Clark CE, Bingle GJ, Epstein SE: Asymmetric septal hypertrophy (ASH) in infancy. Circulation 50:809, 1974.

Maron BJ, Henry WL, Clark CE, Redwood DR, Roberts WC, Epstein SE: Asymmetric septal hypertrophy in childhood. Circulation 53:9, 1975.

Maron BJ, Tajik AJ, Ruttenberg HD, Graham TP, Atwood GF, Victorica BE, Lie, JT, Roberts WC: Hypertrophic cardiopathy in infants: clinical features and natural history. Circulation 65:7, 1982.

Schryer MJP, Kranauchow PN: Endocardial fibroelastosis etiologic and pathogenetic consideration in children. Am Heart J 88:557, 1974.

Chapter 25

ACUTE RHEUMATIC FEVER

Although once the leading cause of heart disease in children, rheumatic fever and rheumatic heart disease now rank second to congenital heart disease in the United States. Nevertheless, the disease remains a serious and major health problem in many countries. In general, both the severity and frequency of the disease appear to have declined in recent decades. Important factors contributing to this are improved socioeconomic conditions and the advent of antimicrobial therapy, effective in the treatment and prophylaxis of group-A streptococcal infections.

Etiology and Incidence

The precise pathogenesis of acute rheumatic fever remains incompletely defined, but the role of infection with certain strains of group-A beta-hemolytic streptococcus is generally accepted. While infection with this organism does not directly produce acute rheumatic fever, it does appear to initiate the disease in a susceptible host. During epidemic streptococcal infection, the incidence of rheumatic fever is approximately 3%. Following endemic infections, the incidence approximates 0.1-0.3%.

Many factors have been considered in the development and prevalence of rheumatic fever. Individual host reaction to streptococcal infection clearly is a factor of major importance. Age also is a factor, since rheumatic fever is rare under 2 years of age and uncommon under 5 years. Most cases occur between 6 and 15 years, with a peak incidence around 8 years of age. First attacks are uncommon after 25 years of age. The age of peak incidence coincides with the period when streptococcal infection also tends to occur with greatest frequency. Many other factors, including socioeconomic deprivation, geography, and seasonal incidence, appear to be of significance primarily in their influence on the frequency of streptococcal disease.

The Streptococcus

Group-A streptococcus may vary greatly in virulence. The most important factors affecting its virulence are the M-protein surface antigen and the hyaluronic acid capsule. The M protein which forms the basis for classification of the streptococcus to the various serotype groups is found on the fimbriae of the cell wall. They also interfere with phagocytosis, rendering the streptococcus more or less virulent.

Rheumatic fever is more common after pharyngeal streptococcal infection than after pyoderma. It appears that the skin strains possess little or no rheumatogenic potential, and the antistreptolysin O responses to skin infection are lower. It is not yet clear whether this is related primarily to the site of infection or to the properties of pyoderma strains.

Pathology

While acute rheumatic fever is a systemic inflammatory disease, only the heart is subject to permanent residual effects. All segments of the heart are involved, but the most serious sequelae result from involvement of the myocardium and endocardium, including the valves. Although all valves may be involved, the disease process has a predilection for the mitral and aortic valves, in that order. Tricuspid involvement is infrequent, and the pulmonic valve is rarely, if ever, affected. The valve leaflets and chordae tendineae cordis are swollen and edematous. Verrucose lesions forming on the lines of valve closure and chordae contribute to valvular insufficiency. These early exudative changes later are replaced by a chronic proliferative process which eventually may lead to valvular stenosis.

Myocarditis is invariably present and, although inflammatory response may be sparse, severe involvement may produce impairment of myocardial function. The characteristic myocardial lesion pathologically is the Aschoff body which can appear in all portions of the myocardium. This lesion, a granuloma, heals by scar formation which may lead to extensive myocardial fibrosis. Scar formation may seriously affect myocardial performance, even though valve function is not severely altered, and may involve, and permanently damage, the conduction system.

Serofibrinous pericarditis commonly occurs but seldom leads to significant pericardial effusion. Pericarditis is a feature of severe rheumatic pancarditis, but usually resolves without complications.

Noncardiac involvement is very common, and inflammatory arthritis is one of the major features of the disease. Pathologic changes are also frequently present in blood vessels, central nervous system, and lungs.

Manifestations

A history of recent upper respiratory infection is obtained in about one-half of cases. This event usually has occurred within the preceding 2 weeks, often is not of sufficient severity to prompt medical attention, and usually is of short duration, even if untreated. Following a latent period of apparent well-being, manifestations of a systemic inflammatory process appear. Some of these are nonspecific, while others are characteristic of the acute rheumatic process. Over 30 years ago, the common clinical and laboratory features of acute rheumatic fever were categorized into major and minor manifestations according to their diagnostic usefulness. These clinical guidelines, commonly referred to as the Jones criteria, subsequently have been modified and revised (Table 25-1). Although the criteria offer a high degree of reliability, they are by no means absolute and require perceptive clinical judgment in their application. As presently constituted, the major manifestations of acute rheumatic fever include: carditis, polyarthritis, chorea, subcutaneous nodules, and erythema marginatum. Minor manifestations consist of nonspecific clinical and laboratory features which include: history of prior rheumatic fever or preexistent rheumatic heart disease, arthralgia, fever, leukocytosis, elevated acute-phase reactants, and prolonged PR interval on electrocardiogram.

Table 25-1 The Revised Jones Criteria for the Guidance of the Diagnosis of Rheumatic Fever *

Major Manifestations	Minor Manifestations
Carditis Polyarthritis Chorea Erythema marginatum Subcutaneous nodules	Clinical Fever Arthralgia Previous rheumatic fever or rheumatic heart disease Laboratory Erythrocyte sedimentation rate, C-reactive protein, leukocytosis, prolonged PR interval
Plus	
Supporting evidence of preceding streptococcal infection (increased ASO or other streptococcal antibodies; positive throat culture for group A streptococcus; recent scarlet fever).	

* Adapted from the American Heart Association

In 1965 the Jones criteria were revised to include a confirmatory role for the preceding streptococcal infection except in patients presenting with chorea or smoldering carditis in which remoteness of the infection is recognized. In an appropriate clinical setting, the presence of two major or one major and two minor manifestations strongly favors the diagnosis of acute rheumatic fever, provided evidence of recent streptococcal infection can be demonstrated.

Major Manifestations

Carditis

The most important and only major manifestation resulting in sequelae is carditis (Fig. 25-1). Although the severity varies considerably, carditis occurs in about 50% of cases in this country and in 80% of cases in the developing countries. It may present acutely or insidiously. The four major signs of carditis are:

1. The appearance of a significant murmur not previously present
2. Cardiac enlargement
3. Congestive heart failure
4. A pericardial friction rub or effusion

Rheumatic carditis almost invariably results in a significant murmur. Three types of murmurs may be present, usually appearing within the first 2 weeks of illness. Most common is the apical holosystolic blowing murmur of mitral regurgitation. Not infrequently, this murmur is associated with a mid-diastolic apical

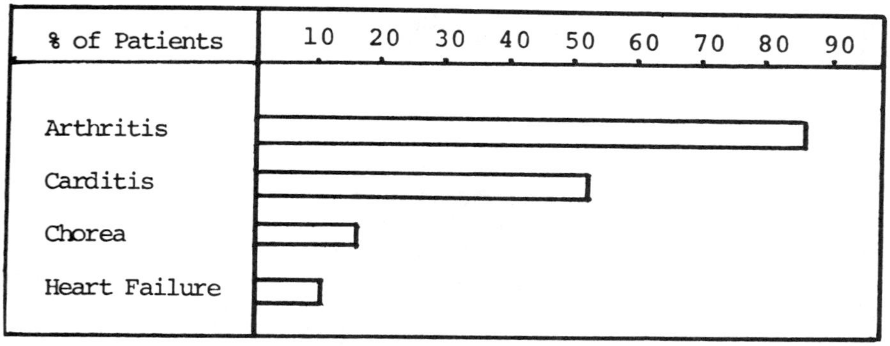

Figure 25-1 The clinical profile of the first attack of rheumatic fever in the United States (adapted from Markowitz and Gordis.)

rumble (Carey-Coombs murmur) of relative mitral stenosis which signifies the presence of definite mitral valvulitis. The third murmur is the basal diastolic murmur of aortic regurgitation. Although less common, this murmur always implies significant carditis and may occur alone or with mitral involvement. True stenosis of valves may evolve over a period of years, but is never seen in the initial acute stages of the disease.

Cardiac dilatation is a common feature of active carditis, implying significant myocardial inflammatory involvement. The degree of cardiac enlargement can be correlated with the severity of carditis.

Congestive heart failure occurs in 5-10% of initial attacks of acute rheumatic fever and, even more frequently, in recurrent rheumatic episodes. Heart failure is more likely in children under 6 years of age and is manifested by the usual features: cough, diaphoresis, fatigue, dyspnea, hepatomegaly, tachycardia, and gallop rhythm. In some cases, only minimal signs and symptoms are present. In a child with a recent attack of rheumatic fever, the presence of heart failure invariably implies active carditis. However, congestive failure also may result from severe valve disease in patients with chronic rheumatic heart disease.

Pericarditis is a less common manifestation, but frequently is associated with severe pancarditis. Rarely is it an isolated feature. Its presence is suggested by chest pain, often relieved by sitting up, and confirmed by auscultatory detection of the typical pericardial friction rub. Pericarditis always implies active disease, and murmurs or other signs of carditis are usually present. Some degree of pericardial effusion is commonly present but rarely leads to complications.

Arthritis

Arthritis, a major manifestation implying true inflammatory joint involvement, must be differentiated from arthralgia, a minor manifestation. Joint symptoms are the most frequent presenting manifestation of rheumatic fever in children over 6 years of age. Characteristically, the arthritis is migratory, affects the large joints, and the pain is disproportionate to objective joint findings. The hips and small joints of the hands and feet are uncommonly involved, and the spine is almost never affected. Severity of involvement varies, but the usual signs of inflammation — heat, redness, tenderness, and pain — are present.

An affected joint frequently resolves within 5 days and, within 2 weeks, all joint symptoms usually subside completely. It is a clinical observation that the severity of arthritis is related inversely to the severity of carditis, for reasons unknown.

Chorea

One of the less common major manifestations, chorea is a disorder of the central nervous system characterized by purposeless involuntary movements, emotional lability, and muscular weakness. This manifestation, more common in girls, occurs most often between ages 7 and 14 years and is rare after 20 years of age. Since a latent period of 1-6 months exists between the streptococcal infection and the appearance of chorea, acute-phase reactants and streptococcal antibody titers are usually normal. Chorea may be the sole manifestation, or occur with other features of rheumatic fever, including carditis.

Characteristically, the onset of chorea is gradual, with irritability and apparent clumsiness. Grimacing, slurred speech, purposeless movements, and muscular weakness soon appear. Often, the first indication is deterioration of handwriting and other school performance. Speech dysfunction, weak spasmodic hand grasp, and hung-up tendon reflexes are typical. Characteristically, on raising the arms above the head, the patient turns the arms so as to oppose the backs of the hands. The condition is usually self-limited with complete recovery within 3 months, although relapses may occur.

Subcutaneous Nodules

Subcutaneous nodules are painless, firm, movable masses of variable size usually found over extensor surfaces of the joints, scalp, or spine. They usually appear only after several weeks of active rheumatic disease, and most often occur in patients with active rheumatic carditis.

Erythema Marginatum

Erythema marginatum, while most commonly seen in acute rheumatic fever, is not limited to this disease. Often delayed in appearance, it is characterized by pink, slightly raised, small macules with sharply demarcated borders and irregular design. The lesions are nonpruritic and most commonly occur over the trunk and inner aspect of upper arms and thighs. Erythema marginatum does not correlate with other evidence of rheumatic activity, is unaffected by suppressive antirheumatic drugs, and may persist intermittently for several months.

Minor Manifestations

Minor clinical manifestations are nonspecific and, therefore, are of secondary diagnostic importance. Arthralgia, a common minor manifestation, is characterized by vague pain in the joint but lacks the objective findings of true arthritis. Fever in excess of 100.4°F (38°C) rectally is almost always present in the acute stage of untreated illness. Rarely does it exceed 104°F, and rarely is rheumatic fever a cause for unexplained fever in a child without other evidence of rheumatic involvement.

Laboratory evidence of an inflammatory process is found in elevation of the erythrocyte sedimentation rate (ESR) and a positive C-reactive protein test (CRP). Although nonspecific, the presence of normal results strongly mitigates against the diagnosis of acute rheumatic fever. The CRP test has the advantages of greater specificity and sensitivity for inflammation. It becomes normal more rapidly than the ESR after antiinflammatory therapy and usually remains positive in the presence of congestive heart failure when the ESR is often normal. Other nonspecific laboratory abnormalities such as anemia and leukocytosis are commonly present.

Supporting Evidence of Streptococcal Infection

With two exceptions, current criteria require evidence of infection with group-A beta-hemolytic streptococcus in support of the diagnosis of acute rheumatic fever. Exceptions are patients whose only rheumatic manifestations are chorea or carditis in which rheumatic activity may have progressed for several months before being recognized.

Evidence of streptococcal infection may be based on clinical or laboratory features. The only acceptable clinical evidence of recent streptococcal infection is a history of the recent occurrence of scarlet fever.

The best evidence of prior streptococcal infection is serological demonstration of abnormal or rising antibody titers against any of several streptococcal antigens. The antistreptolysin O (ASO) antibody test is the one most readily available and most familiar. Among other antibody tests are antistreptokinase (ASK), antihyaluronidase (ASH), and antideoxyribonuclease B (antiDNase B). In children over 5 years of age, single ASO titers of at least 333 Todd units are considered to be elevated, while titers of at least 250 units are considered to be increased in adults. Demonstration of a two-dilution tube change in titer is preferred over single determinations.

Since approximately 20% of patients with acute rheumatic fever may have low or borderline values for the ASO titer, determination of other streptococcal antibody tests is desirable. When two or more such tests are performed, almost all cases of acute rheumatic fever will show an abnormal titer within 2 months of onset of illness. The availability of a commercial slide test for detection of multiple streptococcal exoenzyme antibodies (streptozyme test) has proven useful in this respect.

In general, antibody titers rise within 1-2 weeks following the infection, peak at 3-5 weeks, remain elevated for a variable period of time, and regress gradually over a period of months. Titers tend to rise higher and remain elevated for longer duration in rheumatic patients than in those with uncomplicated streptococcal infection.

Throat cultures provide less reliable evidence than do serological tests for recent streptococcal infection. Negative cultures may be due to spontaneous disappearance of organisms during the interval between acute infection and the onset of rheumatic symptoms, or growth may be suppressed by prior antibiotic therapy. Furthermore, a positive culture may only reflect the carrier state, rather than recent active infection.

Electrocardiogram

Electrocardiographic features of acute rheumatic fever are nondiagnostic and characterized by conduction abnormalities or changes related to myocarditis or pericarditis. Prolongation of the PR interval is the most common conduction abnormality, occurring in 25-40% of cases during the acute stage. However, this is not specifically related to myocardial inflammation and has no prognostic implications. Apparently a result of increased vagal tone, PR prolongation may revert to normal, following atropine administration. Occasionally, second- or third-degree atrioventricular block may be observed.

Myocarditis may exist without specific electrocardiographic abnormality, but is suggested by the presence of flat or inverted T waves, relatively low QRS voltage and, perhaps, QT prolongation. More characteristic changes may occur with pericarditis, notably ST-segment elevation and changes of T-wave morphology (Fig. 25-2).

Radiologic Features

Definite cardiomegaly or a clear increase in heart size during the course of rheumatic fever is considered evidence of carditis. The cardiac contour, in the absence of preexisting valvular lesions, is nonspecific. Differentiation between cardiac dilatation and pericardial effusion may be difficult at times. The degree of cardiac dilatation is an indication of the severity of carditis, and improvement is usually indicated by diminishing heart size. Persistent cardiomegaly suggests significant residual cardiac disease. In the presence of congestive heart failure, the usual signs of pulmonary venous and lymphatic distension are observed (Fig. 25-3).

Differential Diagnosis

Some of the difficulties in diagnosis are related to the limitation of the Jones criteria and tremendous variability of the disease. There are other diseases, however, that may fulfill the Jones criteria and should always be considered in the differential diagnosis.

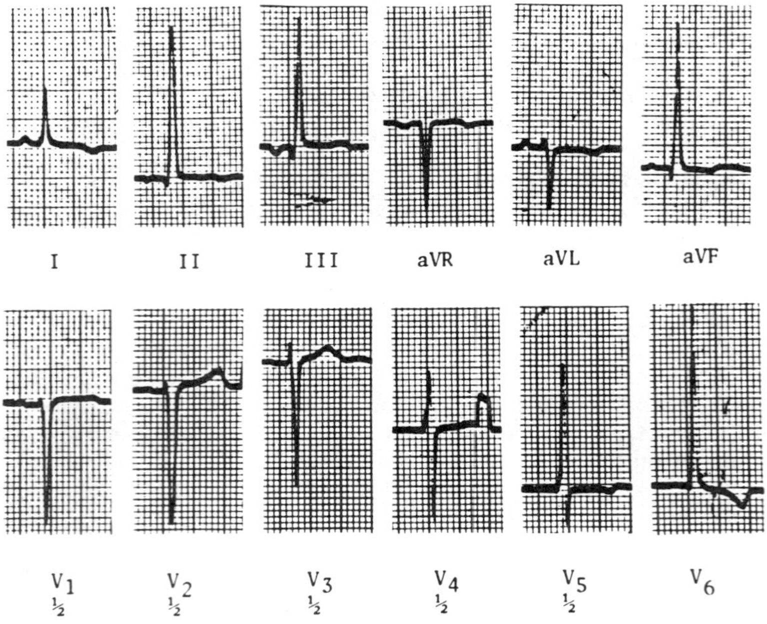

Figure 25-2 Electrocardiogram of a young boy with recurrent acute rheumatic fever with isolated aortic regurgitation. Severe left ventricular hypertrophy is present (note one-half standard precordial leads) with T-wave inversion in left precordial leads.

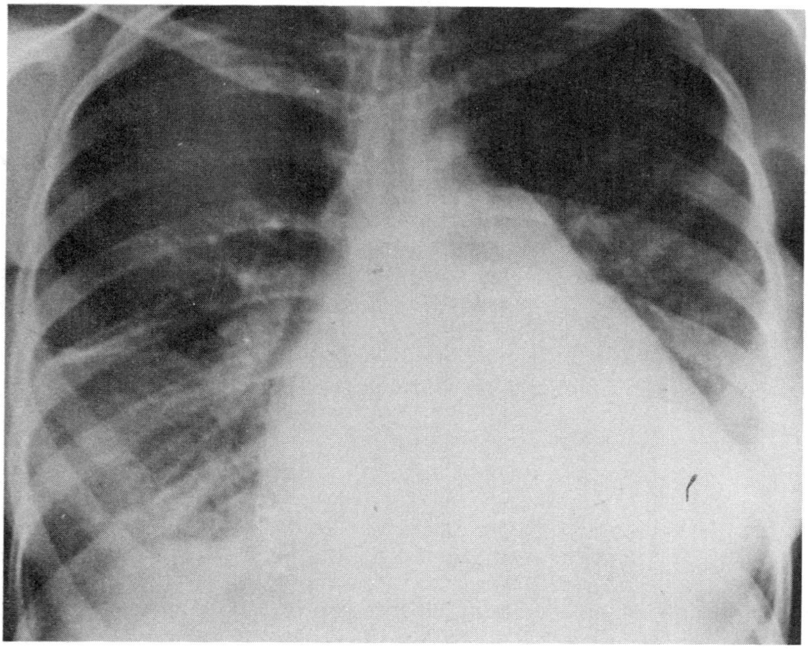

Figure 25–3A Chest roentgenogram of patient with acute rheumatic myocarditis and mitral regurgitation. Film taken on admission showing severe cardiomegaly and pulmonary edema. (See also B.)

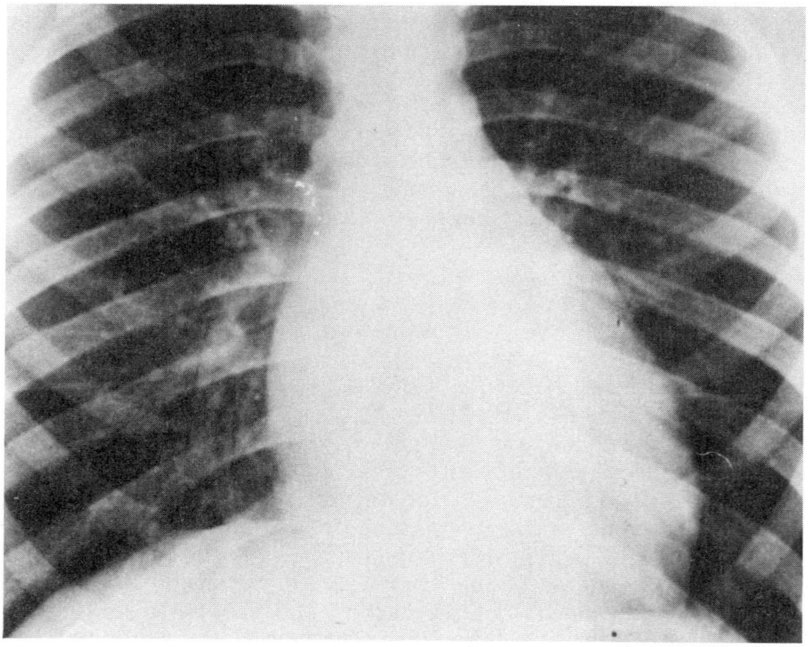

Figure 25–3B Followup film after therapy with anticongestive measures and steroids. The heart is near-normal size and lungs are clear. Note bulge of mid-left cardiac border caused by residual enlargement of left atrial appendage.

Rheumatoid arthritis may mimic rheumatic fever. The presence of pericarditis may further confuse the issue. The chronic nature of the arthritis and the subsequent appearance of splenomegaly and lymphadenopathy help establish the diagnosis of rheumatoid arthritis. Polyarthritis may occur early in the course of periarthritis nodosa, lupus erythematosus, and dermatomyositis; the arthritic symptoms are usually mild in these diseases. In the differential diagnosis of polyarthritis, the exclusion of hypersensitivity reaction (serum sickness) is important.

There are cardiac conditions that simulate rheumatic heart disease. Innocent murmurs should never be confused with actual carditis. Myocarditis, pericarditis, and congenital heart disease (aortic and mitral regurgitation) are usually not difficult to exclude. Cardiac enlargement, loud murmur, and joint involvement are common in patients with sickle-cell disease.

Chorea is usually a straightforward diagnosis; however, choreiform movement may be caused by organic central nervous system involvement.

Course and Prognosis

The course of rheumatic fever is quite variable. Untreated, the average duration of the attack is 3 months, but may be as long as 6 months or more if severe carditis is present. Joint symptoms usually abate within 2-4 weeks even if untreated. Signs of minimal carditis usually subside rapidly.

In any case, the disease appears to run its course, regardless of therapy employed. Antiinflammatory agents are effective only in suppressing manifestations of the disease to a subclinical level, but do not shorten the duration of the inflammatory process. If therapy is discontinued before the disease has subsided, rebound manifestations commonly occur.

The only sequela of rheumatic fever is residual heart disease. The incidence of residual cardiac involvement following an attack of acute rheumatic fever is related to the severity of myocarditis. Gross cardiomegaly and congestive heart failure have the worst prognostic implications.

However, following the initial attack, approximately two-thirds of patients with residual isolated mitral regurgitation who are maintained on uninterrupted prophylaxis will demonstrate disappearance of the murmurs within 5-10 years. The murmur of aortic regurgitation is less likely to disappear (approximately 25%) but frequently becomes less intense.

Treatment

Suppressive Therapy

Although no specific therapy is available for acute rheumatic fever, the manifestations can be suppressed by antiinflammatory agents. Drugs commonly employed are salicylates and adrenal corticosteroids. Numerous studies to evaluate the efficacy of these compounds, given alone or in combination and in variable dosage schedules, suggest that neither appears to prevent or minimize cardiac damage nor shorten the course of the illness. Steroid therapy, however, does appear to benefit the acute cardiac complications and may be lifesaving at times.

In the face of mild arthritis or resolving arthritis alone, we do not treat with aspirin. This is particularly contraindicated if the diagnosis is not definite. Arthritis with minimal or no carditis (no cardiomegaly) may be effectively relieved by aspirin in a dosage of 100 mg/kg/day for the first 48 hr, followed by 60-75 mg/kg/day thereafter in four divided doses. A blood salicylate level of 25-30 mg% should be achieved and maintained until all signs of rheumatic activity have subsided, as indicated by clinical findings and normalization of acute-phase reactants. Usually, this varies from 2-4 weeks.

Patients with moderate-to-severe carditis should receive prednisone (or similar steroid) in a dosage of 2 mg/kg/day in four divided doses until cardiac findings are stable and the general condition improved. Satisfactory response is usually attained in 7-10 days, after which time the dosage is tapered. Rebound phenomena can be minimized by the addition of aspirin therapy to overlap the last week of steroid treatment. Depending on initial severity and individual response, the total duration of therapy may extend up to 4 months or longer. The response to suppressive therapy is often dramatic, with prompt lysis of fever and relief of joint symptoms, although carditis responds more slowly.

Supportive Measures

Other measures, though less dramatic, are clearly important. Strict bed rest is indicated during the acute illness, and ambulation should be gradual thereafter. Congestive heart failure should be treated with the usual anticongestive measures.

All patients, regardless of presenting manifestations, should receive antibiotic therapy to eradicate any potential streptococcal foci. Penicillin is the drug of choice and is most efficacious when given as a single intramuscular injection of respository benzathine penicillin G in a dose of 600,000 U for patients weighing less than 60 lb and 1.2 million U for those over 60 lb. Oral penicillin is effective if given in appropriate dosage for 10 full days. Penicillin G in a dose of 200,000-250,000 U three or four times daily is adequate for both children and adults. Erythromycin 20 mg/lb/day in divided doses (not to exceed 1.0 g/day) may be substituted in patients allergic to penicillin.

Prevention of Recurrences

Of major importance in the management of the rheumatic patient is prevention of recurrent attacks. Prevention of recurrences depends on prevention of group-A beta-hemolytic streptococcal infections. Rheumatic subjects are generally at high risk to develop recurrent rheumatic fever following subsequent streptococcal infection. Factors related to recurrences include the time elapsed since the previous attack, age of the patient, severity of carditis, and the number of previous episodes. The risk of recurrence is highest in younger individuals with recent attack and severe cardiac involvement. Each recurrence carries the risk of carditis with its potentially damaging effects. Therefore, all patients with a well-documented history of rheumatic fever or Sydenham's chorea or those with definite evidence of rheumatic heart disease should be placed promptly on continuous antibiotic prophylaxis to prevent infection with the group-A beta-hemolytic streptococcus.

This is most effectively accomplished by injection of 1.2 million U benzathine penicillin G every 28 days for children weighing over 60 lb and 0.6 million U for those under 60 lb. This approach is especially recommended for those with significant rheumatic heart disease. Oral prophylaxis is less satisfactory since the variable of patient compliance is present. Even in compliant patients oral prophylaxis is somewhat less effective than intramuscular benzathine penicillin G. Recommended oral dosage is 200,000-250,000 U twice a day.

Oral sulfadiazine is similarly effective prophylaxis in a dose of 1.0 g daily for patients over 60 lb and 0.5 g daily for those under 60 lb.

All patients with evidence of rheumatic valvular heart disease should receive additional short-term antibiotic prophylaxis to prevent possible infective endocarditis. This should be administered in accordance with current recommendations (Chap. 26).

Bibliography

Committee on Rheumatic Fever and Bacterial Endocarditis, American Heart Association: Prevention of rheumatic fever. Circulation 55:1, 1977.

Committee to Revise the Jones Criteria. Jones Criteria (revised) for guidance in the diagnosis of rheumatic fever. Circulation 32:664, 1965.

DiSciascio G, Taranta A: Rheumatic fever in children. Am Heart J 99:635, 1980.

Gordis L: Effectiveness of comprehensive care programs in preventing rheumatic fever. N Engl J Med 289:331, 1973.

Markowitz M, Gordis L: Rheumatic Fever. W. B. Saunders Co., Philadelphia, 1972.

Stollerman GH: Rheumatic Fever and Streptococcal Infections. Grune and Stratton, New York, 1975.

Tompkins DG, Boxerbaum B, Liebman J: Long-term prognosis of rheumatic fever patients receiving regular intramuscular benzathine penicillin. Circulation 45:543, 1972.

Chapter 26

INFECTIVE ENDOCARDITIS

The changing nature of endocarditis became apparent in recent years with increased involvement of fungi, rickettsiae, and viruses. The preferred terminology is, therefore, infective endocarditis rather than bacterial endocarditis.

Incidence

Since the introduction of penicillin and sulfonamides, the mortality of patients with endocarditis has declined markedly. It is, however, by no means a rare complication of congenital heart disease, and patients of all ages are affected. The true incidence is difficult to ascertain, but hospitalized patients with this disease account for approximately 0.55/1000 pediatric admissions, as compared to 0.2/1000 admission during 1943-1952. This increase in incidence is probably related to increased survival of patients with congenital heart disease beyond infancy and early childhood.

Pathogenesis

Transient invasion of the bloodstream by microorganisms occurs frequently in normal subjects. These microorganisms can become implanted in endocardial surfaces that have been previously damaged, congenital malformed valves, and areas of jet lesions (Fig. 26-1). Vegetations form as small granular masses which can become quite large and friable and may account for continuous seeding of the bloodstream.

The healing process starts with deposition of fibrous tissue which ultimately covers the injured surface and seals off the vegetation, resulting in sterilization of the bloodstream. Organisms may remain viable within these vegetations and account for exacerbation of the disease. Portions of these vegetations may embolize to distant parts of the body. If they contain viable organisms, an abscess may result.

Portal of Entry

Oral surgical procedures are the most common and easily preventable sources of bloodstream invasion. Vigorous brushing or orthodontal manipulations, especially of diseased gums, will produce bacteremia. This is also true after extraction of

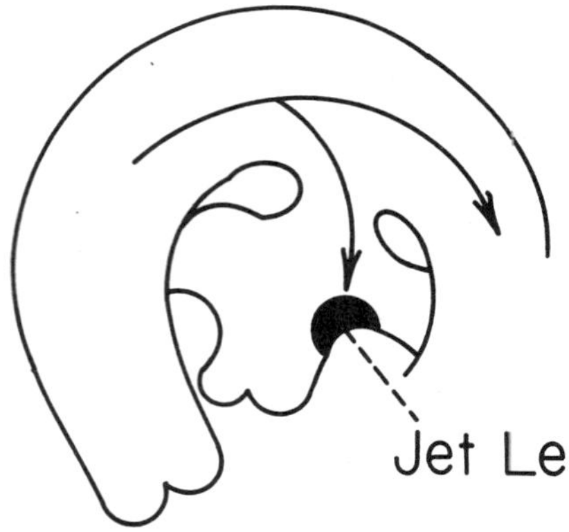

Figure 26-1 Patent ductus arteriosus, high-velocity stream producing the jet lesion on the left pulmonary artery opposite the defect.

diseased teeth. Other described causes are tonsillectomy, reduction of open fractures, and extensive burns. Cardiac surgery has become an increasingly important portal of entry, especially when prosthetic material is used. Endocarditis following cardiac catheterization is extremely rare and is usually associated with suppurative arteritis. It has also been shown that cystoscopy in the pediatric population is not associated with demonstrable bacteremia.

Sites of Vegetations

Vegetations usually occur at the location of a jet lesion. The jet effect is produced by blood flowing from a zone of higher pressure to one of relatively low pressure, as in mitral insufficiency, ventricular septal defect, and patent ductus arteriosus. In a ventricular septal defect the vegetations are located on the right-sided rim of the defect or right ventricular outflow tract. In patent ductus arteriosus this occurs in the left pulmonary artery just opposite the defect (see Fig. 26-1).

In a recent series from Boston Children's Hospital, tetralogy of Fallot was the single most common underlying lesion, accounting for 38% of all patients (Table 26-1). Aortic stenosis ranked second, followed by ventricular septal defect. A review of bacterial endocarditis from the Mayo Clinic cites ventricular septal defect as the most common underlying lesion (35%), followed by aortic stenosis (19%) and tetralogy of Fallot (16%). Patent ductus arteriosus was a common underlying lesion for bacterial endocarditis in the preantibiotic era. In recent years, patent ductus arteriosus and pulmonic stenosis were rarely the cause of endocarditis, and in no case was an atrial septal defect involved.

Bacteriology

The most common causative microorganism is *Streptococcus viridans*, accounting for approximately 50% of the cases. The enterococcus group of streptococci accounts for 20% of the cases in adults; rarely is it a causative agent in pediatrics. *Staphylococcus aureus* coagulase positive is increasingly being isolated and accounts for approximately 40% in most series. The Mayo Clinic cites an incidence of 50%. These organisms are almost always resistant to penicillin.

Staphylococcus albus, pneumococcus, and gram-negative bacteria have been described. Viruses, mainly the Coxsackie B group, have also been implicated as

Table 26-1 Underlying Cardiac Abnormality in 68 Cases with Bacterial Endocarditis (1963-1972) (%) *

Tetralogy of Fallot	38
Aortic stenosis	16
Ventricular septal defect	13
D-transposition of the great vessels	5.8
Postsurgery	4.4
Patent ductus arteriosus	0

* Adapted from Johnson DH, et al.: Circulation 51:581, 1975.

a cause of endocarditis. Fungal endocarditis, mainly with *Candida albicans,* has been reported postcardiac surgery in patients who are debilitated and have received prolonged courses of antibiotics.

Manifestations

The typical history is that of a known heart patient who was well and gradually develops fever, chills, malaise, fatigue, and night sweats. The most common findings are fever, anemia, splenomegaly, and embolic phenomena with petechiae (Fig. 26-2).

Hepatomegaly, hematuria, and joint pain are less frequent manifestations. The petechiae are usually scattered and may persist even after bacteriologic cure. Embolic phenomena are relatively common and occur mostly to the lungs, spleen, brain, and kidney. Congestive heart failure may be present, especially in the presence of significant damage to the valve cusps and chordae tendineae cordis. Rarely is the failure due to myocardial abscesses.

Echocardiographic Findings

Recently M-mode and two-dimensional echocardiography has become a useful adjunct to the evaluation of patients with infective endocarditis. Two-dimensional echocardiography seems to be superior in identifying the presence of an infective mass (vegetation) within the heart. It may also identify patients with more severe disease such as "flail" aortic leaflet and flail mitral leaflet who may require early surgery.

Laboratory Findings

Anemia is almost invariably present, as well as leukocytosis. The erythrocyte sedimentation rate is elevated, but this is a nonspecific finding. A blood sample obtained from the ear lobe frequently shows a large number of histiocytes or macrophages. Microscopic hematuria is found in roughly 25% of the patients. Evidence of renal failure may be present. Positive blood cultures can be obtained in 80-87% of the cases. Several studies report that 77% of positive blood cultures are obtained at first culture and that bacteremia is constant and, therefore, obtaining the culture at a time of a temperature spike is unnecessary.

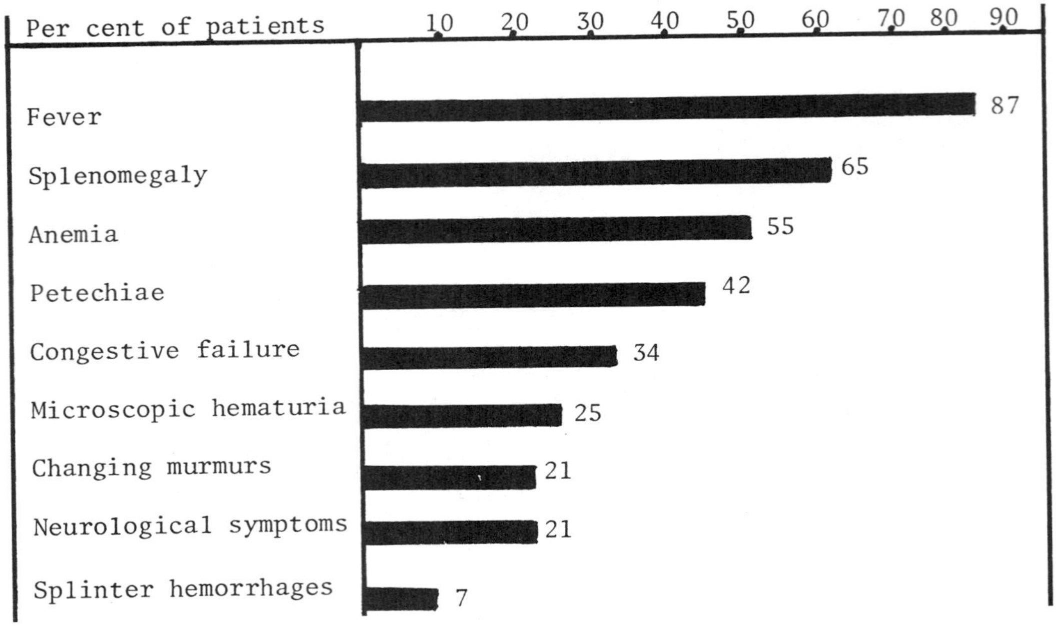

Figure 26-2 Admission findings in 149 episodes of infective endocarditis. (Adapted from Johnson DH, et al.: Circulation 51:581, 1975.)

Differential Diagnosis

Rheumatic fever should always be considered and excluded. Among the major manifestations of rheumatic fever, only carditis could be mistaken for infective endocarditis. Positive blood culture indicates endocarditis, whereas high antistreptococcal antibody titers point toward rheumatic fever. Other systemic diseases occuring in patients with known congenital heart disease such as nephritis, pneumonia, and brain abscess should be considered. Premature treatment of a febrile illness without the proper diagnosis can sometimes mask acute bacterial endocarditis.

Treatment

When the diagnosis is suspected, at least six blood cultures are obtained within the first 48 hr. All other possibilities are simultaneously explored and excluded. In the presence of a known congenital heart disease, unexplained fever, changing murmurs, and enlarging heart, treatment is begun at the end of 2-5 days even if the cultures are negative. Since *S. viridans* and *S. aureus* are the most common causative organisms, a semisynthetic penicillin (oxacillin or nafcillin) is given (Table 26-2). Upon identification of the organism, therapy could be more specific. Penicillin G is the drug of choice for *S. viridans*. For patients allergic to penicillin, vancomycin 10 mg/kg IV can be given every 6 hr. If enterococcus is identified, streptomycin is added. This usually is given for 2 weeks only and is stopped if signs of renal insufficiency develop. Staphylococcus is best treated by one of the synthetic penicillins alone.

Table 26–2 Antibiotic Treatment in Endocarditis

Organism	Antibiotic	Dose (kg/day)	Doses per day	Duration (weeks)
Streptococcus viridans	Penicillin	250,000 U IV	4-6	4
Staphylococcus aureus	A. methicillin	300 mg IV	4-6	6 [a]
	or			
	B. nafcillin	200-300 mg IV	4-6	6 [a]
	or			
	C. oxacillin	200-300 mg IV	4-6	6 [a]
	or			
	D. vancomycin [b]	30-40 mg IV	3	6 [a]
Enterococcus	A. Penicillin G,	250,000 U IV	4-6	4-6 [a]
	streptomycin	20 mg IM (Max. 500 Mg)	2	2
	or			
	B. Ampicillin,	300 mg IV	6	4-6 [a]
	gentamycin [c]	4.5-7.5 mg IV	3	4-6 [c]

[a] Intravenous therapy for 4 weeks; the latter 2 weeks could be given IM or orally.
[b] For patients allergic to penicillin.
[c] Gentamycin dose is modified according to the patient's age and renal function.

Occasionally, persistent low-grade fever may be due to local irritation at the injection site or to phlebitis. Each patient should be evaluated individually and a decision made regarding the antibiotic therapy.

Course and Prognosis

Since the introduction of antibiotics, the recovery rate from bacterial endocarditis is approximately 70–80%. The success of the treatment depends on the phase of recognition of the disease and institution of treatment. Any delay in therapy worsens the prognosis: patients with negative blood cultures, embolic phenomena, and congestive heart failure have the poorest prognosis. Also staphylococcal, *Escherichia coli,* or pseudomonas endocarditis is more difficult to treat.

Postopen heart surgery endocarditis, especially after insertion of prosthetic material such as valves, conduits, or patches, is a serious disease. It may be resistant to antimicrobial agents. It is now recommended that patients with congenital heart disease or acquired valvular disease should receive antibiotic prophylaxis for dental manipulation or during oral surgery (tonsillectomy and adenoidectomy).

Table 26–3 Prophylaxis of Infective Endocarditis

Regimen A: For dental procedures and oropharyngeal surgery in patients with congenital heart disease, rheumatic-fever-acquired valvular disease, and mitral valve prolapse syndrome with mitral insufficiency.

Penicillin: Parenteral-oral combined: 600,000 U of procaine penicillin G mixed with 30,000 U/kg of crystalline penicillin G not to exceed 1,000,000 U, intramuscularly, 1 hr prior to procedure, followed by penicillin V, 250 mg orally every 6 hr for eight doses. For children over 60 lb, penicillin V, 500 mg is substituted

Oral: 1.0 g of penicillin V 1 hr prior to procedure and then 250 mg every 6 hr for eight doses. For children above 60 lb, penicillin 2.0 g, 1 hr before the procedure, then 500 mg orally every 6 hr for eight doses.

For patients suspected to be allergic to penicillin or for those on continual oral penicillin for rheumatic fever prophylaxis who may harbor penicillin-resistant streptococci:

Erythromycin: Oral: The dose for small children is 20 mg/kg orally 1.5 hr prior to the procedure and then 10 mg/kg every 6 hr for eight doses.

Regimen B: For patients with prosthetic heart valves or for gastrointestinal and genitourinary tract manipulation:

Penicillin: Follow recommendations in Regimen A.

or

Erythromycin: Follow recommendation in Regimen A.

plus

Streptomycin: 20 mg/kg intramuscularly (not to exceed 1 g) 1 hr before the procedure, then every 12 hr for two doses.

or

Gentamycin: 2 mg/kg intramuscularly 1 hr before the procedure then every 8 hr for two additional doses.

The routine use of antibiotics for simple urinary tract manipulation is not necessary. Genitourinary tract surgery in the presence of bacterial infection and gastrointestinal tract surgery also require prophylaxis. These regimens are outlined in Table 26-3 A and B.

The indiscriminate use of antibiotics during febrile episodes in children who have congenital heart disease is unwarranted.

Bibliography

AHA Committee Report: Prevention of bacterial endocarditis. Circulation 56: 139A-143A, July 1977.

AHA Committee Report: Treatment of infective endocarditis due to viridans streptococci. Circulation 63:730A, 1981.

Johnson CM, Hable Rhodes K: Pediatric endocarditis. Mayo Clin Proc 57:86-94, 1982.

Johnson DH, Rosenthal A, Nadas AS: A forty-year review of bacterial endocarditis in infancy and childhood. Circulation 51:581, 1975.

Lerner IL, Weinstein L: Infective endocarditis in the antibiotic era. N Engl J Med 274:199-206, 388-398, 1976.

Speck WT, Dresdale SS, Krongrad E, Gersony WM: Absence of bacteremia after instrumentation of the genitourinary tract in children. J Pediatr 85:224, 1974.

Speck WT, Spear SS, Kongrad E, Mandel L, Gersony WM: Transient bacteremia in pediatric patients after dental extraction. Am J Dis Child 130:406, 1976.

Weinstein L, Schlesinger JJ: Pathoanatomic, pathophysiologic and clinical correlation in endocarditis. N Engl J Med 291:832, 1974.

Chapter 27

DISEASES OF THE PERICARDIUM

Numerous inflammatory diseases, both infectious and noninfectious, can involve the pericardial space and its contiguous structures. The potential for disaster requires the physician to be familiar with the manifestations, complications, and treatment. The common and less common causes of pericarditis are in the following list. This section will deal mainly with pyogenic pericarditis and "acute benign" or viral pericarditis.

Common causes of pericarditis are:
Rheumatic fever
Purulent pericarditis
Acute viral pericarditis
Rheumatoid arthritis
Uremia
Neoplastic diseases
Postpericardiotomy syndrome

Less common causes of pericarditis are:
Tuberculosis
Systemic lupus erythematosus
Chronic constrictive pericarditis
Congenital hypoplastic anemia
Radiation pericarditis

Pathophysiology

The pericardium is a thin sac which normally envelops the heart and the proximal portion of the great vessels. It consists of parietal and visceral layers, with a potential cavity between them, the pericardial sac. The intimate relationship of the pericardium with its contiguous structures (pleura, lung, mediastinum) is of importance when considering the etiology of the disease. The most dramatic and life-threatening form of pericardial disease is cardiac tamponade. It is a clinical syndrome caused by the accumulation of fluid in the pericardial sac. The more rapidly the fluid accumulates, the larger the amount, and the more rigid the pericardium, the more serious the consequences. When fluid accumulates slowly, it is well tolerated; however, when there is a sudden accumulation, it interferes with the diastolic filling of the heart. To counteract this, there are several compensatory mechanisms that come into play (Table 27-1).

Table 27-1 Pericardial Tamponade: Compensatory Mechanisms

1. Reflex vasoconstriction
2. Increased venous pressure
3. Tachycardia

The right and left atrial and systemic and pulmonic venous pressures increase in an attempt to increase cardiac filling. There is also an attempt to increase cardiac output by increasing the heart rate. To prevent fall in systemic pressure, there is a reflex vasoconstriction which results in adequate systemic mean pressure with narrow pulse pressure. If the intrapericardial pressure rises further, the patient may succumb.

Pulsus paradoxus is often present in patients with tamponade. Normally, during inspiration, increase in the negative intrathoracic pressure causes augmentation in venous return into the right heart, increasing the right ventricular output. Concomitantly, there is a decrease in pulmonary venous return into the left heart, therefore decreasing left ventricular output (Fig. 27-1). In the normal subject, the fall of systemic pressure during inspiration is 8-10 mmHg. In the presence of tamponade, this fall is exaggerated above 10 mmHg. The mechanisms responsible for this phenomenon are not completely understood; however, it seems that in tamponade, inspiration appears to augment right ventricular filling more than normal. Because of the limiting rigid pericardial envelope, the right ventricular dilatation appears to interfere with left ventricular filling and, therefore, with cardiac output. Echocardiographic studies have shown that there is an inspiratory shift of the interventricular septum towards the left ventricle that results in increase in the right ventricular volume at the expense of the left ventricle (Fig. 27-2). Accordingly, left ventricular output decreases in inspiration, and consequently systemic blood pressure falls.

It is important to remember that increased heart rate, narrow pulse pressure, and increased venous pressure all represent compensatory mechanisms and should not be interfered with, or it may prove fatal.

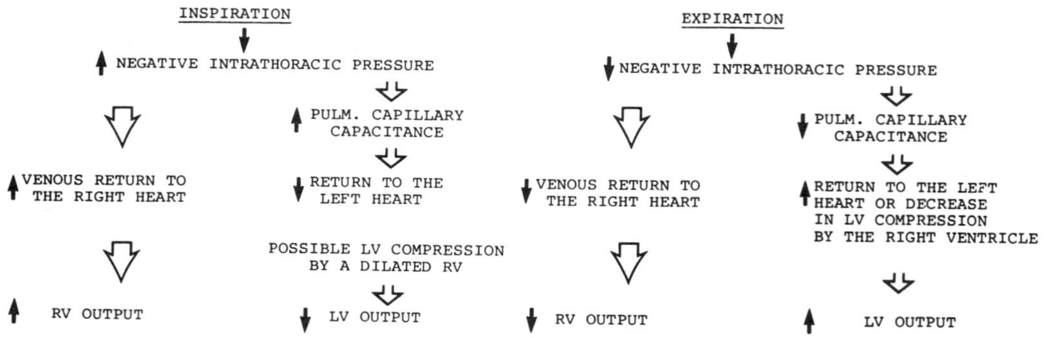

Figure 27-1 Suggested mechanism of pulsus paradoxus.

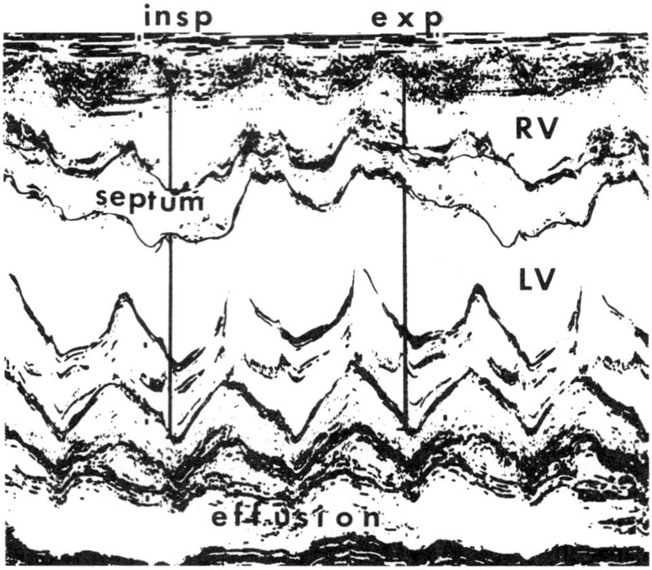

Figure 27-2 Echocardiogram of a 3-year-old with pericardial tamponade. Pericardial effusion and pronounced respiratory changes in right ventricular internal diameter and left ventricular internal diameter are present. RV - right ventricle, LV - left ventricle, Insp. - inspiration, Exp. - expiration.

Pyogenic Pericarditis

Pyogenic pericarditis is a rare, but therapeutically important disease. It is commonly associated with another site of infection which varies, depending on the etiology.

Causative Organism

The most common bacteria involved are *Staphylococcus aureus* (44%), *Haemophilus influenzae* (22%), neisseria meningitides (9%), and streptococcus pneumoniae (6%). *S. aureus* is usually associated with respiratory tract infection; however, distant infections, such as osteomylitis, have also been described. *H. influenzae* pericarditis is usually a disease of infants and children and is commonly associated with respiratory tract infection, either croup or bronchitis. Neisseria meningitis pericarditis is often associated with meningitis. Many other bacteria such as *Salmonella, Escherichia coli, Klebsiella,* and so forth, have been described, but are uncommon.

Clinical Features

The presenting signs and symptoms may vary according to the organism, the site of the associated infection, and the age of the patient. Fever, tachypnea, tachycardia, and chest pain are almost always present. The pain usually improves upon sitting up and leaning forward. The presence of neck vein distention, weak pulses, pulsus paradoxus, and enlarged liver is related to the amount of pericardial fluid and the presence of tamponade (Table 27-2). Search for associated infection is imperative in order for the therapy to be effective.

Table 27-2 Clinical and Laboratory Manifestations of Pericardial Tamponade

Tachycardia	
Tachypnea	
Peripheral vasoconstriction	
Elevated venous pressure:	distended neck veins, enlarged liver, hepatojugular reflux
Pulsus paradoxus	
EKG: low voltages, ST-T changes	
X-ray: large cardiac silhouette	
Echo: pericardial effusion	

Electrocardiographic Features

Of the patients, 40-80% exhibit an abnormal electrocardiogram. Low voltages are always looked for, but are not frequently seen (Fig. 27-3). The most constant findings are ST-segment elevation or depression and T-wave changes (usually inverted). According to a recent review, the ST-segment abnormalities reverted to normal 2-3 days after therapy was begun. In our experience, however, T-wave abnormalities may linger for weeks.

Radiographic Features

The cardiac silhouette may be normal in the absence of significant effusion. Evidence of pneumonia, empyema, and so forth, should always be sought for. In the presence of a large pericardial effusion, there are various degrees of cardiomegaly. The heart appears globular and assumes the shape of a water bottle (Fig. 27-4A,B). The lungs are usually clear, except in the presence of cardiac failure and/or cardiac tamponade.

Echocardiographic Features

Echocardiography is the most useful tool in diagnosing pericardial fluid. Relatively small amounts of fluid can be detected with ease either with the M-mode or two-dimensional methods. In the normal echocardiogram, the pericardium is closely related to the epicardium, and the two layers usually appear as one. In patients with pericardial effusion, the two layers are separated by fluid which appears as echo-free space (Fig. 27-5). It may be seen anterior or posterior to the heart or in both locations. An important feature is that pericardial effusion cannot accumulate behind the left atrium because the pulmonary veins bind the pericardium to the left atrial wall. If fluid is seen behind the left atrium, one may presume it is pleural rather than pericardial. In the presence of tamponade, there is excessive right ventricular dilatation and left ventricular compression with every inspiration (Fig. 27-2). This may be the counterpart of the clinical pulsus paradoxus.

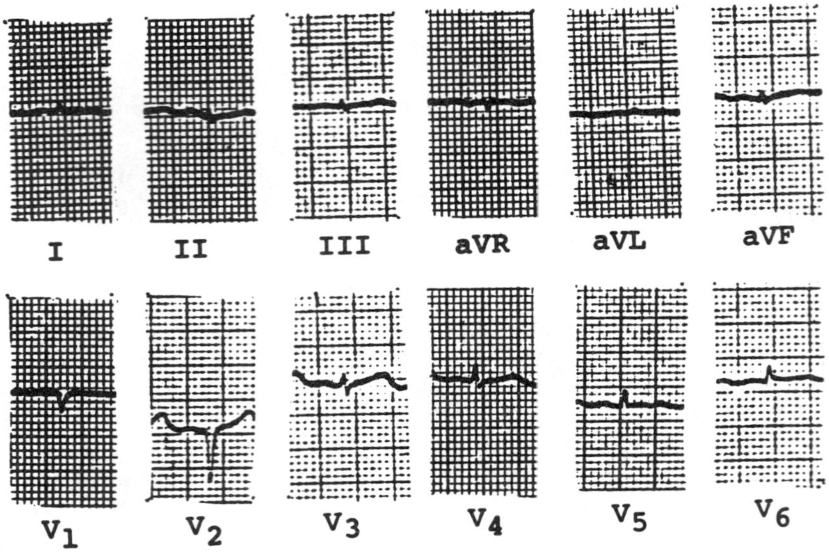

Figure 27–3 Electrocardiogram of a 12-year-old girl with lupus and pericardial effusion. Note the complexes are very small and the T waves are flat.

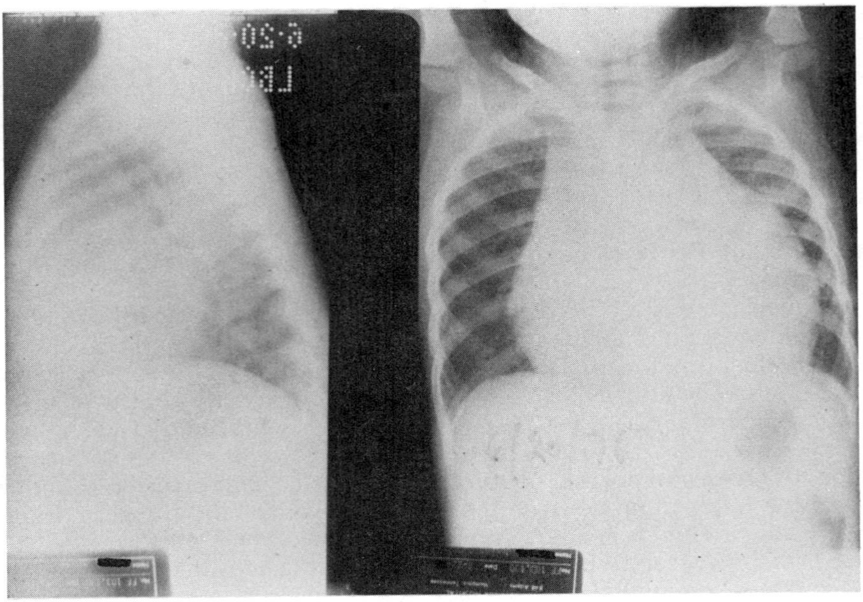

Figure 27–4A Chest x-ray of a child with purulent pericarditis without tamponade. The cardiac silhouette is enlarged resembling a water bottle configuration.

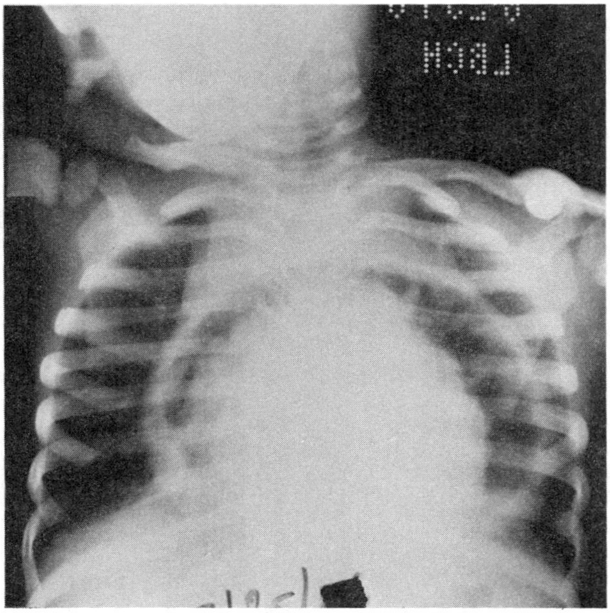

Figure 27-4B Chest x-ray of the same child following pericardiocentesis. There is air in the pericardial sac (introduced following the procedure). The cardiac silhouette is not enlarged. The pericardium appears thickened.

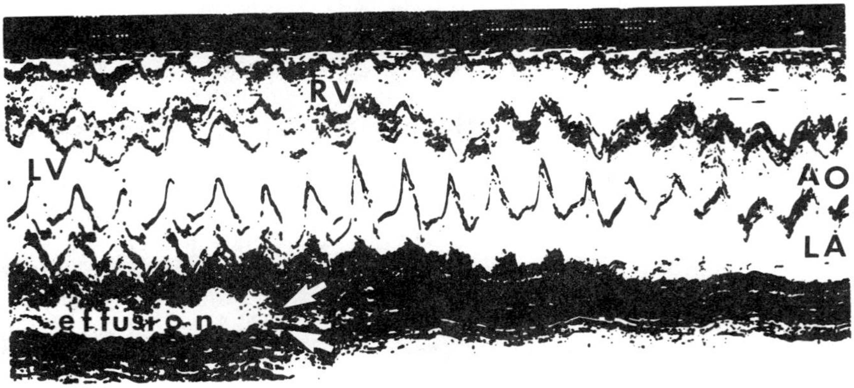

Figure 27-5 M-mode echocardiographic sweep from the LV to the aorta. There is posterior pericardial effusion seen at the level of the left ventricle. The effusion stops behind the left atrium (white arrows). LV - left ventricle, RV - right ventricle, Ao - aorta, LA - left atrium.

Laboratory Findings

The white blood cell count is usually elevated with immature forms. The urinalysis is usually normal, but hematuria may be present with generalized septicemia. The only way of establishing the diagnosis is by direct examination and culture of the pericardial fluid, obtained by pericardiocentesis. This has both diagnostic and therapeutic implications. In the event that an organism cannot be grown, countercurrent immunoelectrophoresis (CIE) can be performed on the fluid, and with certain bacteria, it may also be found in the urine.

In the presence of bacterial infection, the pericardial fluid may be grossly purulent and thick. It exhibits marked leukocytosis, the protein may be variable, but the glucose is almost always low.

Treatment and Prognosis

Survival from purulent pericarditis appears to depend upon the mode of therapy. There are no survivors in untreated patients. Survival certainly improved with the introduction of antibiotics; however, the best survival (80%) was obtained with a combination of pericardial drainage and antibiotics.

The frequent occurrence of loculation in purulent pericarditis made the practice of percutaneous insertion of a small polyethylene tube into the pericardial space unrewarding. Surgical creation of pericardial window with placement of a large tube into the pericardium may be necessary. It is important to keep in mind that purulent pericarditis is a fatal disease. Early aggressive diagnosis and treatment improve survival markedly. Careful identification of the organism is most important, and early specific antibiotic therapy is mandatory. Therapy should be continued for 4-6 weeks, depending on the clinical response. Although pericardial constriction infrequently occurs, all patients should be followed carefully for this complication. When present, pericardiectomy is indicated and may be lifesaving.

Viral Pericarditis

Patients with acute benign pericarditis characteristically present with signs and symptoms of pericarditis, yet no etiology could be established. Viral infections of the pericardium have been documented to occur with Coxsackie, ECHO, adenovirus, and influenza virus. In two recent reports, however, viral etiology was documented in 20% of the cases only.

The disease usually follows upper respiratory infection. The first symptoms are fever with pericardial pain and dyspnea. The patients may appear sick, anxious, sitting up in bed, leaning forward. On auscultation, a pericardial friction rub is heard without a murmur. The electrocardiogram often shows ST-T wave changes (Fig. 27-3). These changes are similar to those seen with purulent pericarditis. Cardiomegaly may or may not be present (Fig. 27-4). Echocardiogram is helpful to determine whether or not pericardial effusion is present or not (Fig. 27-5).

When the diagnosis is in doubt or in toxic patients with evidence of pericardial effusion, pericardiocentesis is indicated. The fluid is serous or serosanguineous, and may show polymorphonuclear or mononuclear cells. Gram-stain, bacterial, and viral cultures should be done, and cytology in order to rule out malignancy.

The treatment is symptomatic and includes bed rest and salicylates for fever and pain. The use of steroids is controversial. Some reports suggest that there is hastened resolution of the pain and pericardial fluid. However, the incidence of rebound phenomenon is increased. There is also no convincing evidence that the use of steroids reduces the incidence of myocardial scarring or pericardial constriction. Surgical intervention is usually not indicated and is reserved for the patients with tamponade. Recurrent attacks have been reported in 15% of the patients. The differential diagnosis should be directed principally toward excluding rheumatic fever, rheumatoid arthritis, and lupus.

Tuberculous Pericarditis

Tuberculous pericarditis is not common in the pediatric age group. It usually occurs as a direct spread of the infection from adjoining lung fields or adjacent lymph nodes. The diagnosis is established by examination of the pericardial fluid for acid-fast bacilli. The prognosis of untreated patients is poor. Tamponade occurs relatively frequently, and longstanding disease often results in extensive scarring and pericardial constriction. In patients who develop this complication, pericardiectomy is necessary. Chemotherapy, guided by the sensitivity of the organism, has improved the prognosis significantly.

Constrictive Pericarditis

Constrictive pericarditis is a relatively rare disease of childhood. It may present with a chronic course consisting of ascites, dyspnea, and failure to thrive. These symptoms may be present for months or years before the correct diagnosis may be made. On the other hand, the symptoms may manifest following an acute pyogenic or viral pericarditis. It is more common following tuberculous pericarditis than other bacterial infection. In over 50% of the patients, the etiology could not be determined.

The chest x-ray often reveals a small heart; however, pulmonary venous congestion may be present. The electrocardiogram invariably shows ST-T changes and low voltages. The echocardiogram fails to reveal fluid, and the cardiac contractility is usually normal.

The hemodynamic findings are a result of impaired ventricular filling and reduced stroke volume. Central venous pressure tracing demonstrates deep, steep X and Y descents corrresponding to early ventricular ejection and filling. Ventricular pressure tracing demonstrates an early diastolic dip and a late diastolic plateau (square root sign), with equal end-diastolic pressure in both ventricles. In contrast to cardiac tamponade, pulsus paradoxus is often absent.

The treatment of choice is extensive pericardiectomy. Of the patients, 50% are thus cured, and 20% are improved. Occasionally, extensive fibrosis may render this procedure extremely hazardous.

Other Causes of Pericarditis

Several other causes of pericarditis should be kept in mind including collagen disease such as systemic lupus erythematosus, rheumatoid arthritis, and so forth. It is often associated with rheumatic fever and malignancy. Pericarditis is diagnosed with increased frequency in patients with chronic renal disease and uremia.

Postpericardiotomy syndrome is seen frequently in the pediatric age group. The patients usually present 1-2 weeks following open heart surgery, with fever, leukocytosis, and pericardial effusion. Occasionally this may progress to develop tamponade. Symptomatic treatment with bed rest and aspirin is usually sufficient. The disease is self-limited, but recurrences are not unusual. Recently, viral etiology has been implicated. No specific virus has been isolated, rather it is a virus that is responsible for community outbreak at the time.

Bibliography

Carmichael DB, Sprague H, Wyman D, Bland EF: Acute non-specific pericarditis clinical laboratory and follow-up considerations. Circulation 3:321, 1951.

Feldman WE: Bacterial etiology and mortality of purulent pericarditis in pediatric patients. Am J Dis Child 133:641, 1979.

Fowler NO: Autoimmune heart disease. Circulation 44:159, 1971.

Fowler N, Manitsas G: Infectious pericarditis. Prog Cardiovasc Dis 16:323, 1973.

Okoroma EO, Perry LW, Scott LP: Acute bacterial pericarditis in children: report of 25 cases. Am Heart J 90:709, 1975.

Reddy PS, Curtis EI, O'Toole JD, Shaver JA: Cardiac Tamponade: Hemodynamic observation in men. Circulation 58:265, 1978.

Spodick DH: Acute Pericarditis. Grune & Stratton Co., New York, 1959.

Strauss AW, Santamaria M, Goldring D: Constrictive pericarditis in children. Am J Dis Child 129:822, 1975.

Van Reken D, Strauss A, Hernandez A, Feigin RD: Infectious pericarditis in children. J Pediatr 85:165, 1974.

Yamcey CL, Doughty RA, Cohlan BA, Athreya BH: Pericarditis and cardiac tamponade in juvenile rheumatoid arthritis. Pediatrics 68:369, 1981.

Chapter 28

RHYTHM AND CONDUCTION DISORDERS

The normal electrical rhythm of the heart depends upon the spontaneous, repetitive initiation of a wave of depolarization in the sinoatrial node with sequential spread to the atria, atrioventricular node, and remainder of the conduction system, as discussed in Chap. 2, Fig. 2-13. Disorders of rhythm can basically be divided into abnormalities of generation of the excitation impulse and abnormalities of spread through the conduction system. In general, arrhythmias are neither as common in children nor as varied as those seen in adults; but neither are they rare, and a basic understanding of the more common types is essential. The present discussion will be directed primarily toward the basic of electrocardiographic interpretation of arrhythmias and associated clinical problems and treatment. Detailed analysis of the electrophysiologic mechanisms involved is avoided but is available in the Bibliography at the end of the chapter.

Although many of the simpler rhythm disturbances will be readily recognized, the more complicated ones will remain confusing unless an orderly approach to the electrocardiogram is adopted. The following approach is suggested.

1. *What is the broad general category of disturbance?*
   The majority of rhythm disturbances come to attention because the rate is abnormal (too fast or too slow) or because the rhythm is irregular. This broad generalization allows one to focus his attention more productively. If the rhythm is irregular, it is of extreme value to look at the rhythm strip as a whole to decide if there is definable pattern to the irregularity. Often a recurrent pattern of irregularity (so-called regular irregularity or group beating) can be identified.
2. *What is the relationship between P waves and QRS complexes?*
   If a period of normal sinus rhythm with 1:1 atrioventricular conduction is present, this provides a useful reference for analysis of the rhythm disorder. Frequently, the relationship between atrial and ventricular complexes is readily recognized, but in more complicated disturbances, careful measurement of sequential PP intervals throughout the tracing is essential and best done with calipers. Having defined the atrial mechanism, it is a relatively simple task to ascertain whether the QRS complexes are occurring in regular relationship to the P waves or independently. Sequential RR intervals should be measured as this may at times provide the only clue to the presence of an independent pacemaker activating the ventricles. An analysis of the configuration of the atrial complexes and relative frequency of P waves and QRS complexes is important also. The PR interval should be serially measured, and P waves hidden by QRS-T complexes looked for.

3. *Is the QRS complex normal?*
   Regardless of the nature of the rhythm disorder, the presence of a QRS complex which is normal in duration indicates that activation of the ventricles is occurring from a depolarization wave which has originated above the bifurcation of the bundle of His. If the QRS complex is prolonged, it may be caused by disease of the bundle branch system or by a subsidiary pacemaker below the bifurcation of the His bundle.

Such an approach is an oversimplification, but provides some general orientation toward analysis. To spell out in a stepwise manner the approach to analyzing all possible rhythm disorders is not a practical undertaking. This approach and some familiarity with the EKG characteristics of the common arrhythmias will allow most of these to be recognized.

Disorders of Impulse Generation

Sinus Arrhythmia

Sinus arrhythmia is typical of children and is not an abnormal mechanism but rather an expression of intact neuroregulatory controls. The cardiac impulse originates in the sinoatrial node and spreads normally through the conduction system. The EKG shows variable intervals between P waves (PP interval), as shown in Fig. 28-1. The P wave is of normal configuration and directed leftward and inferiorly, reflecting its sinus node origin. There is no change in P-wave configuration or PR interval. Careful correlation of the cardiac rhythm and physical examination reveal that the rate varies with respiration, becoming more rapid during inspiration. This inspiratory tachycardia results from a normal decrease in vagal tone produced by the increased cardiac filling associated with inspiration. Obviously, no symptoms are produced by sinus arrhythmia, and no treatment is necessary.

Bradyarrhythmias

An abnormally slow cardiac rate may result either from failure of the sinoatrial node to discharge appropriately, or from failure of the excitation wave to reach the ventricles. The latter is referred to as an atrioventricular block and is discussed later in this chapter. The degree of slowing which would be considered abnormal will vary with age; rate of less than 100/min would be slow for a newborn,

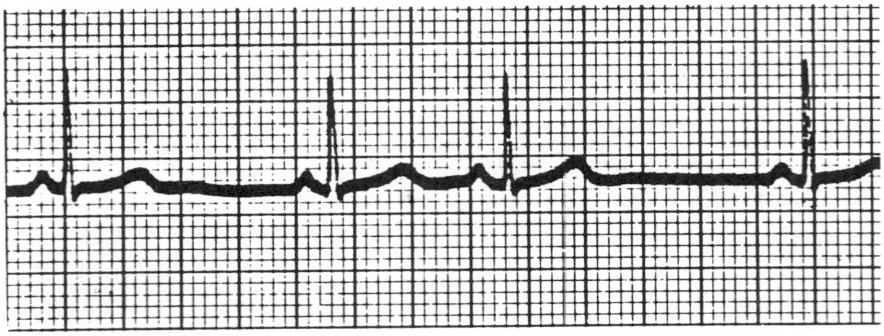

Figure 28-1 Sinus arrhythmia. Each QRS complex is preceded by a P wave of unchanging configuration with constant PR interval indicating that the irregularity in rhythm is not the result of a shifting pacemaker or a change in AV conduction. The arrhythmia results from alteration in the sinoatrial nodal discharge rate.

whereas this limit would be decreased to 60/min in adults. Although cardiac filling and therefore stroke volume are increased at slower rates, excessive slowing will limit the cardiac output which may reduce exercise tolerance and produce easy fatigability. In more severe forms, particularly if the rate slows abruptly, cardiac output may be so reduced as to produce syncope.

Sinus Bradycardia

Sinus bradycardia is defined as sinus rhythm at an abnormally slow rate for age, with normal conduction to the ventricles. Sinus bradycardia is not uncommon, especially in trained athletes. If the patient is asymptomatic with normal exercise tolerance and shows an appropriate increase in sinus discharge rate with exercise, no treatment is indicated.

Sinus Node Dysfunction (Sick Sinus Syndrome)

Several electrophysiologic abnormalities are grouped in this category, having in common an inappropriate slowing of sinus node discharge rate and an inability to accelerate the cardiac rate adequately with exercise. Symptoms of fatigue and syncope are common. Causes are multiple and are usually divided into intrinsic disease of the sinoatrial node including inflammatory and metabolic causes or abnormalities of rate regulation, such as excessive vagal tone or increased sensitivity to vagal impulses. In the pediatric age group the most common cause appears to be intraatrial surgery such as repair of transposition of the great arteries or total anomalous pulmonary venous drainage, with injury to the sinoatrial node. All cells along the conduction system have the intrinsic property of automaticity, that is, the ability to spontaneously depolarize and function as a subsidiary pacemaker. The spontaneous rate decreases progressively from the sinoatrial node inferiorly to the ventricular Purkinje fibers. Thus, the more rapidly discharging sinoatrial node normally functions as the cardiac pacemaker, and spontaneous discharge of cells further along the conduction system is not seen. If the sinus node is discharging at a rate slower than the spontaneous rate of a lower center, the latter will "escape" sinoatrial node control and serve as the pacemaker for the ventricles. Such an escape rhythm is protective and will often prevent dangerous slowing of the ventricular rate.

The syndrome of symptomatic sinus node dysfunction results from an abnormal slowing of sinus rate together with failure of an adequate escape mechanism. Fig. 28-2 is a tracing from a 10-year-old boy with marked exercise intolerance. P waves are seen only infrequently. The majority of QRS complexes show no preceding P waves and originate from a lower pacemaker. The normal duration and configuration of these complexes indicate that the pacemaker is located above the bifurcation of the His bundle (i.e., in the atrioventricular junction). The escape interval is extremely prolonged, at times exceeding 1800 msec (effective rate less than 33/min). When a normal sinus discharge occurs and captures the atria (last beat in leads V_2 and V_3), it is conducted normally to the ventricles.

The rate may change abruptly in some of these patients for reasons that are not clear. Occasionally, periods of marked bradycardia alternate with runs of pathologic tachycardia, usually atrial flutter or fibrillation. If the basic problem is one of excessive vagal control, treatment with atropine or other anticholinergic agents may be effective in increasing the cardiac rate. This can be assessed by evaluating the response to an intravenous dose of atropine. Failure of cardioacceleration following atropine indicates that implantation of artificial pacemaker will probably be

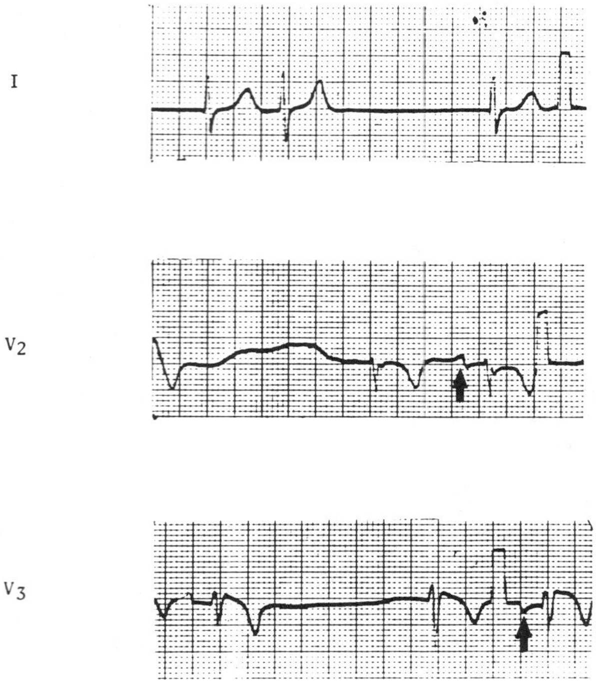

Figure 28–2 Selected leads from tracing of a 10-year-old boy with sinus node dysfunction. See text for discussion. Arrows indicate conducted P waves.

necessary. Pacemaker implantation is generally necessary prior to medical therapy of atrial flutter or fibrillation, as the ventricular rate may be slowed even more severely by antiarrhythmic medications.

Atrioventricular Dissociation

Atrioventricular (AV) dissociation refers to the presence of two independent pacemakers, one driving the atria and the other the ventricles. There is no abnormality of atrioventricular conduction. Again, several electrophysiologic mechanisms may be responsible, but as most commonly seen in children there is marked sinus node slowing with the escape of a lower subsidiary pacemaker, usually in the AV junction. Thus, sick sinus syndrome may be a type of AV dissociation. The first four beats of Fig. 28-3 show normal sinus rhythm. The sinus rate then slows, and beats 5-7 show the escape of a junctional pacemaker (QRS configuration slightly different but the duration remains normal). The P waves, partially hidden at the start of these complexes, are not conducted into the ventricles. The ventricular rate during the period of dissociation is approximately 58/min as contrasted with 75/min during normal sinus rhythm. The sinus rate then increases, and the last beat shows normal-conducted sinus rhythm (sinus node is said to "capture" the ventricles).

This type of dysrhythmia may result from a variety of diverse causes. Altered vagal tone, with sinus node slowing, may result from nonspecific causes such as pneumonia or sepsis or may be an idiopathic phenomenon seen at rest but disappearing with exercise. It may also occur following open heart surgery. Probably

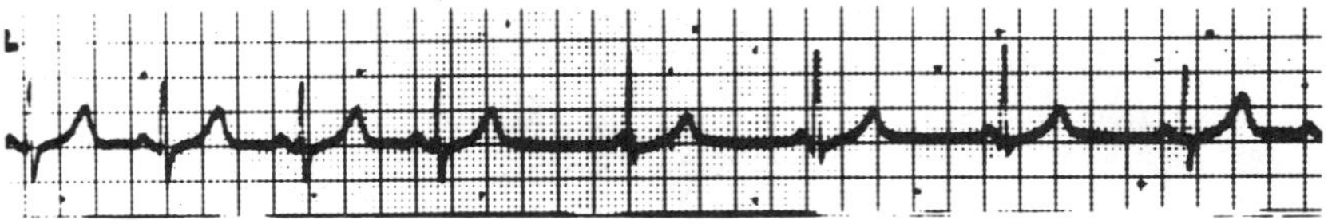

Figure 28-3 Atrioventricular dissociation. Counting from the left, beats 1-4 show normal sinus rhythm. Beats 5-7 demonstrate AV dissociation as discussed in the text. The last P wave is again conducted normally.

the most important etiology of AV dissociation is digitalis toxicity, and the presence of this dysrhythmia in a child on digitalis should be regarded as presumptive evidence of toxicity until proven otherwise. Treatment is primarily directed toward the underlying problem. A healthy child with no definable underlying etiology and showing an appropriate increase in cardiac rate with exercise may require no treatment. Atropine may accelerate the cardiac rate and abolish the arrhythmia; this is particularly useful in cases of digitalis toxicity. As previously mentioned, excessive sinoatrial (SA) node slowing, with an ineffective escape mechanism, may require implantation of a pacemaker.

Premature beats

A beat occurring earlier than expected in relation to the preceding one may be described as premature. The EKG pattern varies according to whether the beat arises in the atria or AV junction (supraventricular) or in the ventricular Purkinje network. Although the premature beat may result from the spontaneous discharge of an ectopic focus competing with the sinoatrial node, the majority appear to be on the basis of a phenomenon known as reentry. This involves conduction over pathways with different refractory periods as schematically depicted for the distal Purkinje network in Fig. 28-4. Reentry circuits may also occur in the atrial myocardium, AV node, or SA node. Anatomically, larger circuits may include the bundle branches or bypass tract (q.v.).

Supraventricular premature beats generally show no change in configuration or duration of the QRS complex, as compared to the basic sinus rhythm. P waves may be seen preceding or following the QRS complex but may also occur simultaneously with the QRS and, therefore, be difficult to detect. If the reentry focus is in the region of the AV junction, the premature excitation wave excites ventricles over the normal pathway, but spreads to the atria in a retrograde manner (i.e., from inferior to superior) and inverted P waves are seen in leads II, III, and aVF. This atrial activation generally depolarizes the sinoatrial node as well, prior to the next spontaneous discharge. The SA node is then reset and starts a new sequence. The pause following the premature beat is not fully compensatory (v.i.). At times, the premature beat may reach the lower conduction system when a portion of it (usually the right bundle branch) has not completely recovered and is still partially refractory to the passage of the depolarization wave. Thus, conduction of the premature beat through this area may be somewhat delayed, producing a wide QRS complex resembling a bundle branch block, and often difficult to differentiate from a beat of ventricular origin. This phenominon is known as aberrant conduction.

A prolonged QRS complex, which is usually different in configuration from the basic pattern, characterizes ventricular premature beats (PVC) (Fig. 28-5). The T wave is usually directed opposite to the QRS complex, and P waves, if seen, have

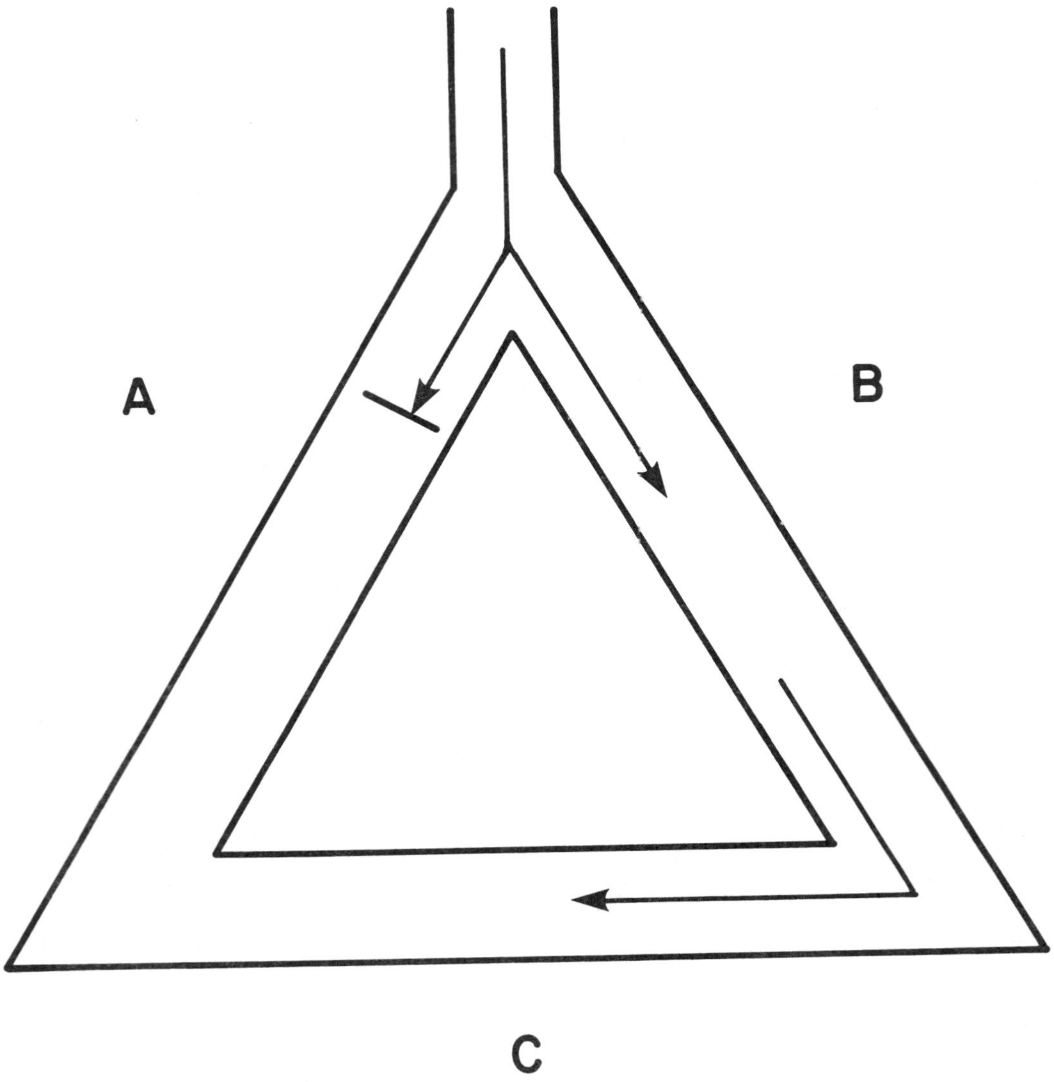

Figure 28–4A Schematic representation of the reentry mechanism. A and B refer to distal fibers of the Purkinje network supplying an area of myocardium, C. If an impulse reaching the upper ends of A and B simultaneously is blocked in its passage down one fiber, conduction will proceed down the other fiber activating the myocardium as shown. (Also see B.)

no relation to the premature QRS. The SA node is usually not discharged by the premature ventricular beat; thus, the PP interval between the sinus beat preceding and that following the PVC is twice the basic PP (or RR) interval, and the pause following the PVC is said to be fully compensatory.

Both supraventricular and ventricular beats may occur commonly in the absence of any cardiac disease, although they are noted in the presence of myocardial inflammation, cardiomyopathies, and drugs such as caffeine, phenylephrine, and so forth. As an indication of digitalis toxicity, PVC are common in adults but unusual

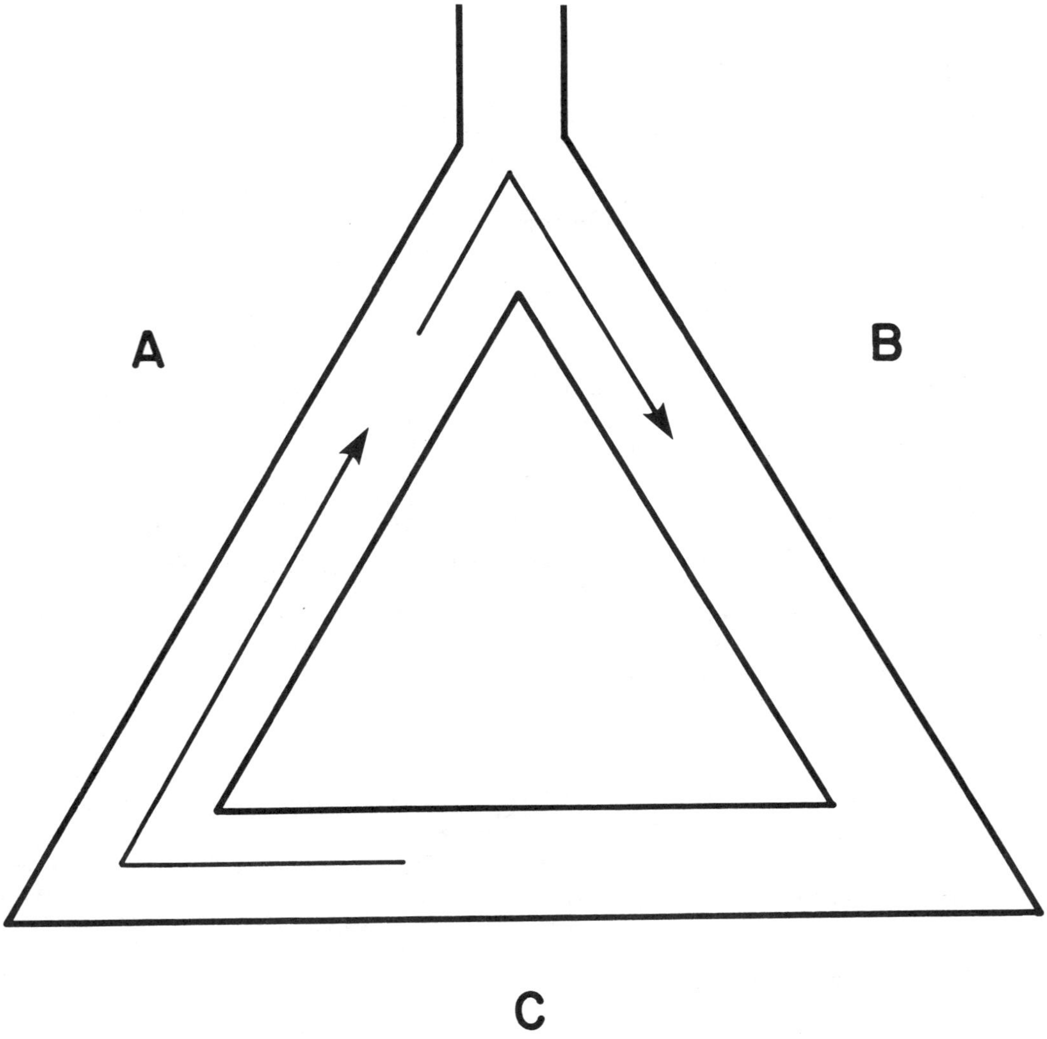

Figure 28-4B If the same impulse then reaches the distal end of fiber A following its recovery from refractories, retrograde conduction may be possible, subsequently reexciting fiber B. Activation of myocardium at C may occur by this mechanism, independent of any normally transmitted impulse.

in children. Any child with frequent premature beats should have a 24-hr ambulatory EKG monitoring (Holter monitor) as it has been clearly shown that the resting EKG frequently will miss more serious dysrhythmias such as runs of pathologic tachycardia. Another useful technique is the obtaining of an EKG during and immediately following exercise as, occasionally, a potentially serious arrhythmia may be provoked in such a manner (see Fig. 28-6). Echocardiography is helpful in excluding underlying heart disease such as an occult cardiomyopathy. Benign premature beats with no underlying cardiac disease produce no symptoms and usually disappear with exercise; no therapy is required. Ventricular premature beats

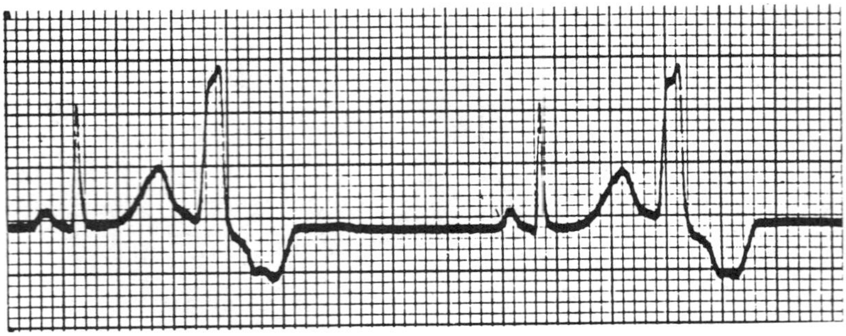

Figure 28–5 Premature ventricular beats. The notches seen on the downslope on the premature-beat T waves are P waves, probably originating from the SA node but not conducted into the ventricles.

which originate from more than one focus (multifocal, characterized by varying QRS morphology) or occur early, coinciding with the preceding T wave, are more likely to precipitate serious tachyarrhythmias at least in adults. Such a patient should be evaluated very carefully and serious consideration given to treatment. If prophylactic therapy to suppress premature beats is indicated, the drugs of choice are as subsequently described under tachyarrhythmias.

Tachyarrhythmias

When an ectopic focus generates an impulse faster than the sinus discharge rate, it assumes control of the heart and ectopic tachycardia results. The most common type of tachycardia has its origin in the sinoatrial node and is a physiologic response to stress. From an electrophysiologic standpoint there is evidence for both reentry and automatic ectopic focus mechanisms to account for the pathologic tachycardias. It is traditional to divide the tachyarrhythmias according to whether the pacemaker (reentrant or automatic ectopic) is above or below the His bundle bifurcation (supraventricular or ventricular). Such a categorization is useful because of etiologic and therapeutic differences.

Supraventricular Tachycardia

Paroxysmal supraventricular tachycardia (PSVT) is the most common pathologic tachyarrhythmia in childhood. Although seen at any age, the period from 1–4 months is that of greatest risk, and in this group the incidence in males is greater than in females. The occurrence of PSVT is often overlooked for up to several hours, as rates of 300/min may be tolerated for a surprising period of time in the young infant. Eventually, the child becomes fussy, tachypneic, and feeds poorly. Pallor may be present. Congestive heart failure eventually develops and is seen within 48 hr in approximately 50%. The child's condition may deteriorate rapidly from that point.

In up to half of the reported cases, no specific etiology has been defined. Preexcitation of the Wolff-Parkinson-White (WPW) type is said to be present in approximately 10% of children with PSVT, although the typical EKG pattern is not seen until reversion to normal sinus rhythm, since anterograde atrioventricular condition usually proceeds via the normal conduction system during the tachycardia.

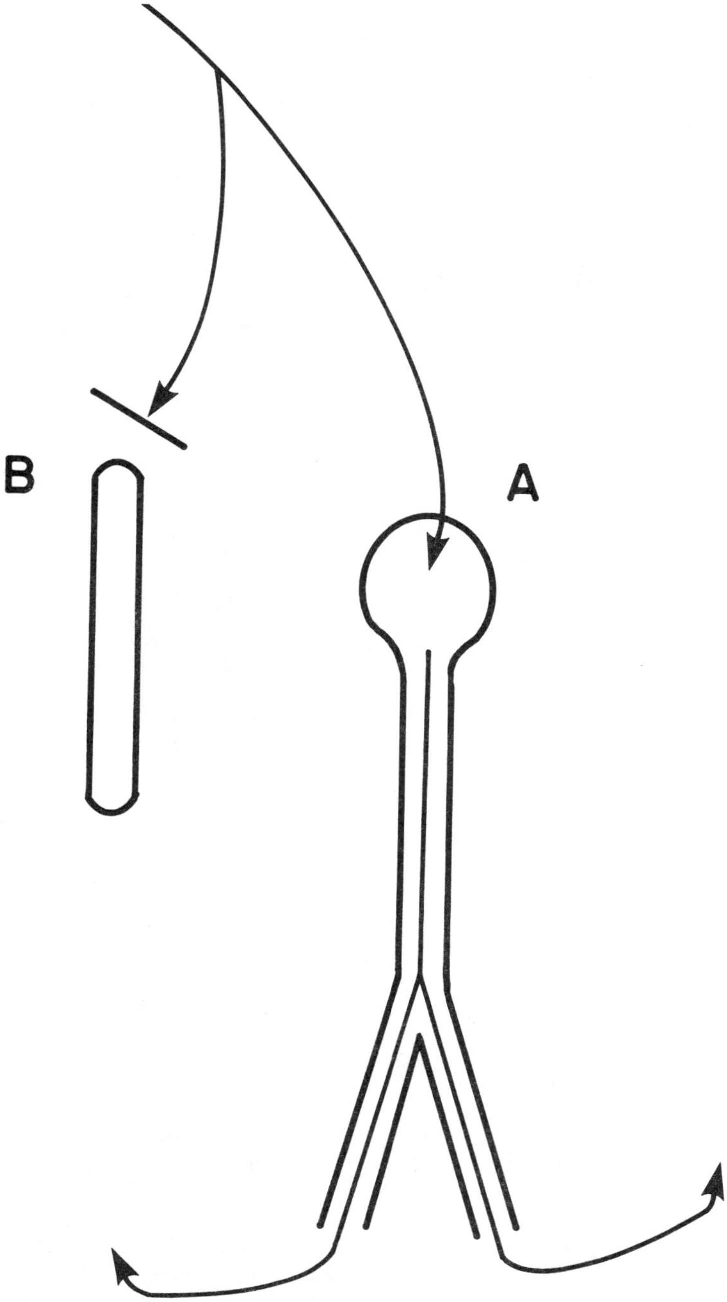

Figure 28–6A Postulated mechanism of tachycardia in the WPW syndrome. A refers to the normal conduction system, whereas the bar labeled B represents the bundle of Kent. A properly timed supraventricular premature beat may arrive simultaneously at points A and B at a time when the normal conduction system has recovered from refractoriness, whereas the bypass tract with its longer refractory period has not. Conduction would thus proceed anterograde down the normal conduction system activating the myocardium in the normal manner. (See also B.)

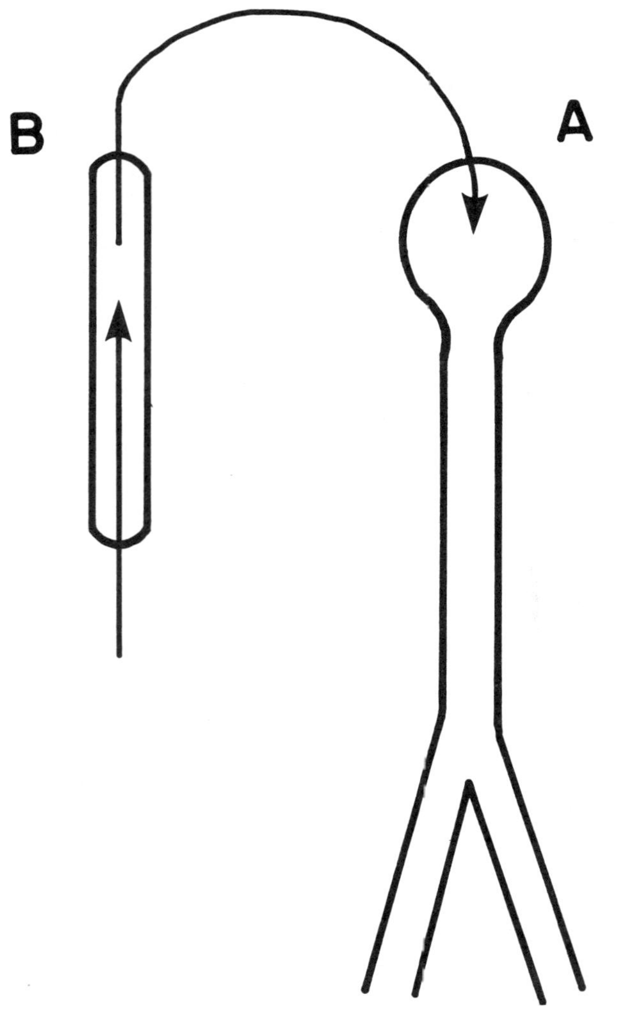

Figure 28-6B If, following activation of ventricular myocardium, the excitation wave reaches the distal end of the bypass tract following its recovery from refractoriness, retrograde conduction may occur with subsequent reactivation of the normal conduction system setting up a reentry circuit.

In our experience, the vast majority of infants whose onset of PSVT is either in utero or within the first 2 weeks of life has had WPW syndrome. Congenital heart disease is said to be present in another 20-30%, although the causal relationship is not clear. PSVT is a common complication of intraatrial surgery for repair of congenital heart defects. The remainder have other definable causes, such as myocarditis, including acute rheumatic fever, cardiac tumors, or drugs. The arrhythmia is seen not infrequently in the cardiac catheterization laboratory following stimulation of the atrial endocardium. The development of techniques for intracardiac electrophysiologic study has vastly increased our understanding of PSVT so studied. In over half of these, the circuit involved a bypass tract, usually of the

Kent type. The mechanism most commonly accepted for these tachyarrhythmias is illustrated in Fig. 28-6 and depends upon the observed fact that the refractory period of the bypass tract is usually greater than that of the conduction system. Thus, a premature supraventricular beat falling at the right time might pass down the normal conduction system but block at the bypass tract. Following completion of ventricular depolarization, recovery of the bypass tract may permit retrograde conduction back to the atria which then returns to the ventricle via the normal conduction pathway, the QRS complex is normal, and the WPW pattern is not seen until sinus rhythm is restored (see Fig. 28-6B). In some cases anterograde conduction to the ventricles during tachycardia may be via the bypass tract, and the electrocardiographic picture of pseudoventricular tachycardia results.

The EKG shows a rapid regular tachyarrhythmia with ventricular rate exceeding 250/min in infants and 160/min in older children (Fig. 28-7). QRS complexes are typically normal, although occasionally a widened QRS may be present, due to aberrant conduction, and may be difficult to differentiate from ventricular tachycardia. P waves are frequently not visible due to simultaneous activation of atria and ventricles or to superimposition on T waves. The former is especially true in PSVT due to AV nodal or bypass tract reentry (low right atrial P waves, upright in lead I and inverted in II, III, and aVF may also be seen). High right atrial P waves (i.e., of normal morphology) may be detected in SA nodal reentry or atrial ectopic tachycardia. Normal P waves occurring randomly, with no relation to the QRS complex, are typical of junctional ectopic tachycardia. Left atrial P waves may be encountered with Kent bundle reentry or atrial ectopic tachycardia. Varying morphology of P waves characterizes atrial muscle reentry. ST-T changes of a nonspecific nature or resembling those seen in ischemia may be present.

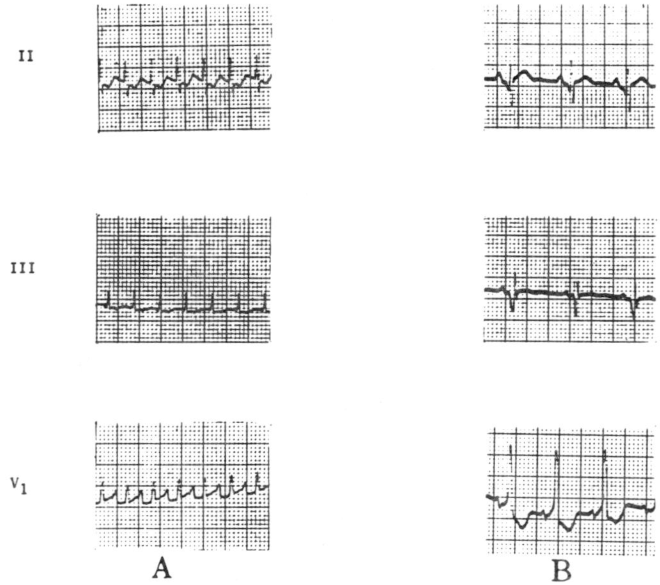

Figure 28-7 Paroxysmal supraventricular tachycardia at a rate of 290/min, is seen in panel A. Characteristic features are the rapid ventricular rate with a narrow and normal-appearing QRS complex. In panel B tracing from the same infant is shown following return to normal sinus rhythm. There is a very short PR interval with a delta wave which is negative in leads II and III and upright in V_1 showing the typical pattern of the WPW type of preexcitation. The preexcitation pattern is characteristically not seen during the tachyarrhythmia as discussed in the text.

Table 28-1 Treatment of Paroxysmal Supraventricular Tachycardia

I. Termination of tachycardia

 A. Digoxin:* Traditional drug of choice if hemodynamically stable.

 B. Verapamil:* May replace digoxin.

 C. Vagal stimulation:

  1. Reflex
   Carotid massage
   Gagging
   Anal dilatation
    Often ineffective. Avoid eyeball pressure.

  2. Pharmacologic reflex
   Phenylephrine*
   Other alpha-adrenergic stimulators
    Significant elevation of blood pressure must be achieved.

  3. Direct
   Edrophonium *

 D. Propranolol *

 E. Quinidine:* Rarely useful. Serious side-effects if given IV.

 F. Atrial pacing

II. Prevention of recurrent attack

 A. Digoxin*

 B. Propranolol*

 C. Quinidine*

* See Table 29-1 on p. 454 for dosage.

PSVT constitutes an emergency requiring prompt medical treatment, for once congestive heart failure occurs, deterioration can be precipitous. Principles of treatment are outlined in Table 28-1. Vagal stimulatory maneuvers, in our experience, have rarely been successful. Ocular pressure should be avoided because of the risk of a detached retina. Digoxin is the mainstay in our treatment regimen, as in most other centers. This is given orally or intravenously over a 16-24-hr period with a vast majority of children responding with return of sinus rhythm. Vagal maneuvers may occasionally be successful after digitalis has been administered. If PSVT persists after full digitalization, intravenous phenylephrine or propranolol may be added. Intravenous edrophonium has been useful, particularly in the catheterization laboratory, and has now become our drug of choice for treatment of PSVT in this setting. If congestive heart failure is present when the child is first seen, conversion to normal sinus rhythm should be achieved as rapidly as possible, therefore, DC cardioversion should be carried out as the first step. This should be done only by an experienced operator using a synchronized cardioverter. The initial dose is usually 2 watt sec/kg and may be increased stepwise if unsuccessful. DC cardioversion carries a risk of producing serious arrhythmias in a patient receiving digitalis and, for this reason, should be the initial treatment if the patient is significantly compromised by the arrhythmia.

These recommendations will be effective only in the case of reentry tachycardias and, in the case of digoxin, propranolol, or vagal maneuvers, only if this circuit includes the AV node as with AV nodal reentry or reentry involving the Kent type of bypass tract (manifest or concealed WPW). In the latter case, treatment is directed toward altering the critical relationship between the refractory periods in the normal conduction system and in the bypass tract. Digoxin, propranolol, and the vagal maneuvers, of course, increase refractoriness in the AV node (Table 28-2); the effect of digoxin on the bypass tract is unpredictable but, in some patients, the refractory period is decreased. Rarely, when the tachycardia is the result of atrial flutter or fibrillation, rather than reentry, the use of digoxin may facilitate anterograde conduction over the bypass tract at a very rapid rate, possibly resulting in ventricular tachycardia or fibrillation. For this reason, some workers prefer to use the type-I antiarrhythmic agents, quinidine, procainamide, or disopyramide which increase refractoriness in the bypass tract.

Verapamil blocks calcium entry into the cell and has its greatest effect on the SA and AV nodes and, therefore, on reentry circuits that include them. The response in terminating reentrant tachycardia has been excellent, and verapamil will probably replace digoxin as the drug of choice because of its rapid effect. The cases which fail to respond can be managed with DC cardioversion in contrast to

Table 28-2 Effect of Drugs on Impulse Conduction*

	AV Node		His-Purkinje		Bypass Tract	
	ERP	CV	ERP	CV	ERP	CV
Digitalis	+	–	?	?	–	?
Propranolol	+	–	?	0	0	?
Verapamil	+	–	0	0	0	0
Quinidine	±	±	+	–	+	?
Procainamide	0	±	+	–	+	?
Disopyramide	0	±	+	–	+	?
Lidocaine	0	±	?	?	+	?
Diphenylhydantoin	–	+	–	0	–	?

* + - increased, - - decreased, ± - inconsistent, ? - unknown, 0 - no effect, ERP - effective refractory period, CV - conduction velocity.

the situation with digoxin. A major side-effect of verapamil is depression of myocardial function, a characteristic which may be made use of in management of hypertrophic obstructive cardiomyopathy. For this reason it should not be used in the presence of congestive heart failure unless it can be determined with certainty that the failure is the result of rate and not depressed myocardial function. Administration of beta-adrenergic blocking drugs, especially by the IV route, within 48 hr should be considered a contraindication to the use of verapamil.

Automatic ectopic tachycardia resulting from abnormally increased automaticity in the atrial myocardial or junctional cells may be extremely resistent to pharmacologic therapy. Digoxin may be of value in the management of accompanying congestive heart failure, but is usually ineffective in slowing the rate. Propranolol at high doses (up to 16 mg/kg/day) has been reported to be effective in junctional ectopic tachycardia, but its use in such a manner should be under the supervision of a cardiologist. Because of its effect in decreasing automaticity, especially in myocardial cells, quinidine may result in conversion to sinus rhythm.

Two other modalities need to be considered in patients refractory to pharmacologic therapy: pacing and surgery. An electrical stimulus introduced via an electrode catheter positioned in the right atrium or coronary sinus may, if appropriately timed, interrupt the reentry circuit and terminate the tachycardia; there is no effect on automatic ectopic rhythms. As most commonly used, the atrium is paced at a rate in excess of the atrial rate during the tachycardia (overdrive pacing); this requires the use of a specially designed basic generator capable of rates up to 800/min. Capture of the atria is confirmed by EKG monitoring and is often accompanied by a 2:1 or a greater AV block with slowing of the ventricular response. Pacing is continued for 1-2 min and then abruptly terminated; return of normal sinus rhythm frequently results. This technique can be used in digitalized patients as toxic dysrhythmias do not result.

The development of sophisticated techniques for electrophysiologic diagnosis has made a surgical approach to the treatment of refractory tachycardias feasible. Generally used for prevention of recurrence, surgery has also been used to terminate prolonged unresponsive episodes. The most common application has been interruption of a reentry circuit involving a bypass tract. Identification of the mechanisms of the tachycardia and approximate localization of the bypass tract by intracardiac electrophysiologic studies is mandatory; precise localization is achieved on the operating table by epicardial mapping techniques. Surgical excision of automatic foci has also been achieved.

After conversion to normal sinus rhythm, prophylactic treatment in order to prevent a recurrence should be instituted. The young infant with PSVT who responds to digitalis should remain on this agent for approximately 6-12 months. Infants with the WPW syndrome usually show permanent disappearance of the preexcitation pattern by 4-6 months of age. Although normalization of the EKG pattern is no guarantee that the bypass tract has become nonfunctional, experience has shown that the vast majority can be taken off digoxin by a year of age and do well. Persistence of the WPW pattern is an indication for more prolonged treatment; it has been the practice of us and others to maintain the child on digoxin until he is 3 or 4 years of age, and then, if there have been no recurrences of tachycardia, discontinue it. At this age the child can readily inform the parents if recurrences develop. With other etiologies the duration of prophylactic treatment will depend upon the duration of the underlying problem. Failure to prevent recurrences with digoxin will necessitate the addition of a second drug, providing that the serum level digoxin is within the therapeutic range. Propranolol or quinidine are most commonly employed in this situation.

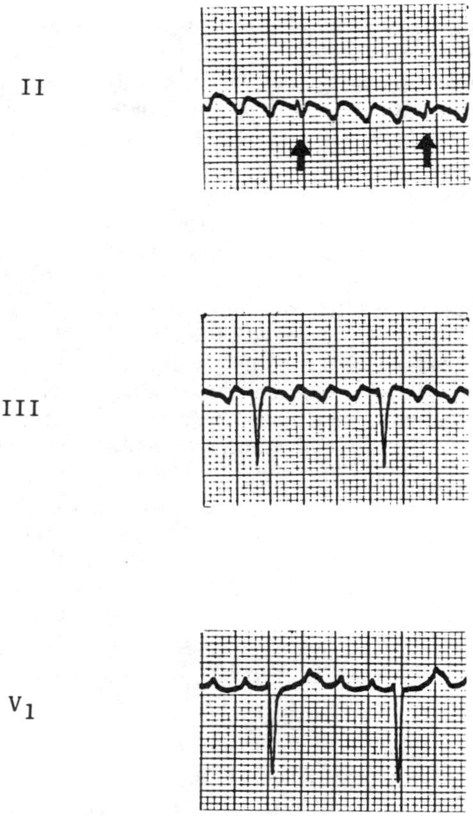

Figure 28-8 Atrial flutter. Note the rapid regular atrial activity at approximately 300/min with typical sawtooth configuration seen in leads II and III. A 4:1 AV block is present. Arrows in lead II indicate a low-voltage QRS complex.

Atrial Flutter

Flutter may be difficult to differentiate from simple PSVT on EKG, but in most cases the frequency of atrial depolarization is so high that some of the atrial excitation waves reach the AV junction while it is still refractory from a preceding depolarization and thus are blocked at that point so that ventricular excitation does not occur. The ventricular rate is usually slower than with simple PSVT. The characteristic feature of the EKG pattern of flutter is regularly occurring oscillations of atrial depolarization called flutter waves. These are best seen in the inferior limb leads (II, III, aVF) and right chest leads. They have a typical triangular or sawtooth waveform (Fig. 28-8) and occur at a rate of 200-400/min. Although occasionally 1:1 AV conduction is present, it is more common to see two, three, or four flutter waves for every QRS complex.

Although seen far less commonly than PSVT, flutter has a more serious implication, as its presence means significant underlying heart disease. We have seen it most commonly in patients whose congenital heart disease results in dilated atria, or following intraatrial surgery (e.g., for ASD or Mustard procedure for transposition of the great arteries), and, less frequently, due to cardiac catheterization, digitalis toxicity, or acute rheumatic fever.

Synchronized DC cardioversion is the most effective way of treating this tachyarrhythmia and should be considered the treatment of choice if the patient is not on digoxin. In the latter circumstance, digoxin may be discontinued for 48 hr (if not required for management of congestive failure) and cardioversion carried out. Since digoxin will slow the ventricular rate in atrial flutter by prolonging refractoriness in the AV node, it may be necessary to control the rate with propranolol or verapamil prior to the cardioversion. Alternatively, rapid atrial pacing may be used for cardioversion without discontinuation of digoxin.

If the arrhythmia is not the result of digitalis toxicity, this drug may occasionally be effective in restoring normal sinus rhythm, often first converting flutter to atrial fibrillation. In some instances, fibrillation may persist, and discontinuation of digoxin may then result in a return of sinus rhythm. Rarely, when flutter is chronically persistent despite all treatment, digitalis is used to increase the degree of AV block and maintain a slower ventricular rate. Quinidine has been used to convert flutter and was successful in 30-50% of adults; but it is a difficult drug to utilize in this way in children. It should never be given without prior digitalization, for the effect of quinidine on increasing AV conduction may result in a 1:1 conduction and a ventricular rate in excess of 300/min. DC cardioversion is preferable, with quinidine utilized together with digitalis to prevent further attacks, if needed. The combination of quinidine and propranolol may also be effective in this regard. The duration of prophylactic treatment again depends upon the underlying etiology; if a specific cause can be identified and alleviated, no further treatment may be necessary. In the presence of chronic cardiac disease or following surgery, long-term prophylactic therapy is frequently necessary.

Atrial Fibrillation

Rapid irregular atrial activity at a rate of 300-700/min with irregular ventricular response characterizes fibrillation (Fig. 28-9). Atrial complexes are of low amplitude and vary erratically in frequency, amplitude, and configuration. Because of the extremely high frequency of impulses bombarding the AV junction, a greater degree of block is seen than with flutter. Impulses are conducted to the ventricles with no predictable pattern. Predisposing factors are the same as described for atrial flutter. Treatment is similar, with attention to the elimination of underlying causes. When fibrillation occurs in the presence of congenital heart disease, DC cardioversion is probably the procedure of choice, with digitalis and quinidine as prophylactic therapy. Restoration of normal sinus rhythm may be impossible until corrective surgery, such as closure of a large ASD or mitral valvulotomy, is carried out. Conversion should be attempted as early as possible since fibrillation of long duration may persist even after underlying factors are eliminated.

Ventricular Tachycardia

Nadas and Fyler estimate that 5% of tachyarrhythmias in children are ventricular in origin; that figure is considerably higher than in our experience, if arrhythmias occurring in the catheterization laboratory are excluded. Runs of ventricular tachycardia like PVC are common during catheterization. Fortunately, they are usually brief and terminate following repositioning of the catheter. Spontaneous paroxysmal ventricular tachycardia usually indicates the presence of a severe myocardial disease such as a cardiomyopathy or major metabolic disturbance. We have seen this arrhythmia in a young infant during episodes of paroxysmal hyperpnea associated with tetralogy of Fallot and also with mitral valve prolapse. It may also

II

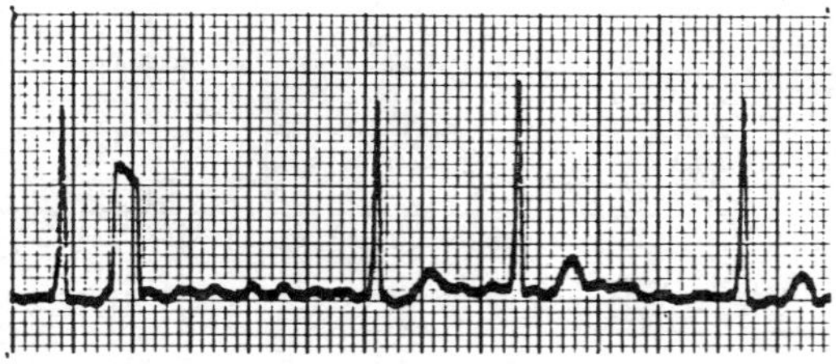

III

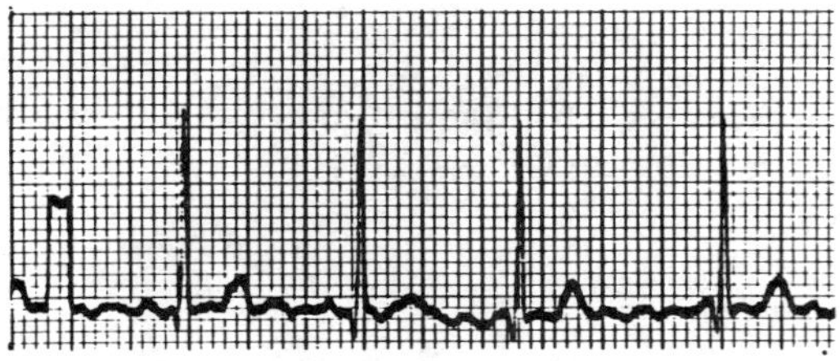

Figure 28-9 Atrial fibrillation. Atrial activity appears as exceedingly rapid, low-amplitude undulations which vary irregularly in both form and frequency. Gross ventricular irregularity characteristic of this arrhythmia is also seen.

occur as a manifestation of digitalis toxicity. An occasional patient will show runs of ventricular tachycardia which are generally of short duration, with no evidence of type of underlying heart disease.

Wide bizzare QRS complexes at a rate of 140-180/min are the electrocardiographic hallmark of ventricular tachycardia (Fig. 28-10). A very slight degree of irregularity in ventricular complexes is common. Differentiation from PSVT with aberrant conduction may be difficult. If P waves can be recognized during ventricular tachycardia, they occur independently of the QRS complexes. Diagnosis of ventricular tachycardia is favored by the presence of fusion beats on EKG after the arrhythmia is terminated and by the lack of slowing or other response to vagal stimulatory maneuvers. The former results from depolarization of a ventricle, partially from a normally conducted impulse, and partially from a PVC. The QRS complex is intermediate in form and duration between the normal lead and the PVC, generally with a preceding P wave (Fig. 28-11).

In general, the cardiac output is more severely compromised with ventricular tachycardia than with PSVT. Conversion to normal sinus rhythm should be carried out promptly. Intravenous lidocaine may be effective in many cases, but the duration of effect is brief and the arrhythmia may recur. If ineffective or if the patient is severely compromised hemodynamically, DC conversion should be carried out promptly if the arrhythmia is not due to digitalis toxicity. If the tachycardia recurs, continuous infusion of lidocaine is indicated. Intravenous procainamide may also be effective. Prophylactic treatment should be given in recurrent attacks if there is significant underlying chronic heart disease; quinidine or procainamide are the drugs of choice. Propranolol has been reported as effective in selected cases.

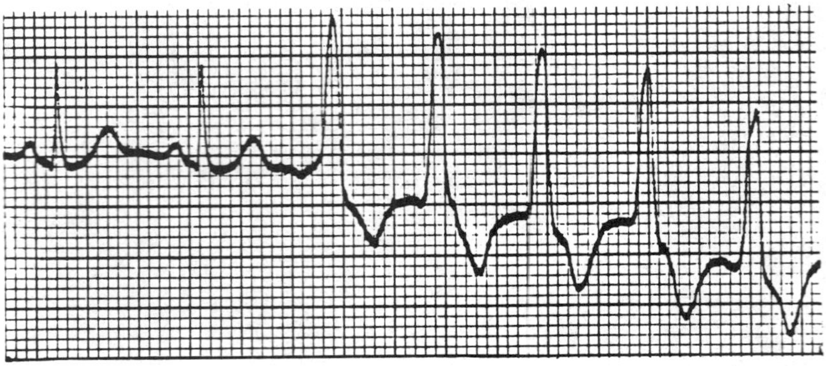

Figure 28–10 Postexercise EKG from the child shown in Fig. 28–5 reveals the abrupt onset of ventricular tachycardia at a rate of 140/min.

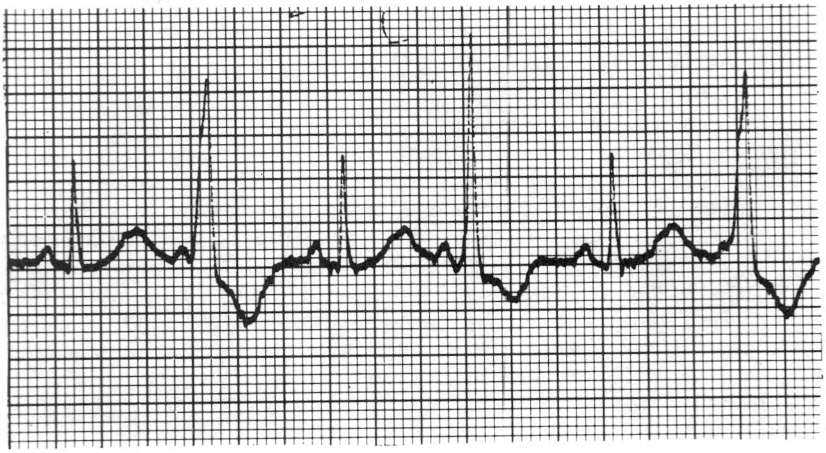

Figure 28–11 Fusion beats. This rhythm strip is from the same child as in Fig. 28–10. From the left, beats 1, 3, and 5 are normally conducted. Beats 2, 4, and 6 are premature and show a conduction abnormality. P waves are seen before each of the premature beats (partially hidden in beat 6). Width of the QRS complex varies inversely with the PR interval; thus, in beat 4 the longer interval between sinoatrial discharge and the ventricular beat allowed the impulse from the former to be partially conducted into the ventricles depolarizing a portion of ventricular myocardium normally. QRS complex is, therefore, less prolonged than in beats 2 and 6 where the majority of ventricular myocardium was depolarized from the ventricular focus.

Disorders of Impulse Conduction

The orderly sequence of progression of the excitation wave from sinoatrial node to ventricular myocardium may be disturbed at several levels: the atrioventricular junction (AV node and His bundle), the bundle branches, or by the presence of an alternative pathway, partially or completely, bypassing the conduction system (pre-excitation, see Chap. 2).

Abnormalities of Conduction Through the Atrioventricular Junction (AV Block)

A wide variety of situations may result in prolongation of the time required by the conduction system to recover or repolarize following a passage of a wave of depolarization. During this prolonged recovery period, a stimulus arising from above may fail to transmit further if it occurs sufficiently early during the so-called absolute refractory period or, alternatively, may transmit down the conduction system at a slower velocity than normal if it falls somewhat later during the relative refractory period. Such AV blocks may be extremely complicated on occasion and the exact mechanism be defined only through detailed intracardiac electrophysiologic studies. In the majority of instances in children the type of block can be readily identified.

First-Degree AV Block

First-degree AV block is defined as a prolongation of conduction time through the atrioventricular junction, manifested as a prolonged PR interval. One-to-one atrioventricular conduction is maintained. This is not necessarily a sign of disease of the conduction system but often is the result of increased vagal tone, for many reasons, including acute rheumatic fever and digitalis. Prolongation of the PR interval due to digitalis is generally not regarded as a sign of toxicity but is an indication for careful evaluation of the patient status including determination of serum digoxin level. It may also be present in certain types of congenital heart disease, most notably, endocardial cushion defects. No impairment of cardiac function is produced, and no treatment is necessary.

Second-Degree (2°) AV Block

If the absolute refractory period of the AV node or His bundle is sufficiently prolonged, some impulses arising in the sinoatrial node may block at the AV junction and not reach the ventricles. A number of different mechanisms have been identified, and these can be among the most difficult of the arrhythmias to analyze. The most common seen in children is known as Wenckebach phenomenon (Mobitz type I, second-degree block) in which there are recurrent groups of complexes, with progressive lengthening of the PR interval until the cycle is terminated by a P wave which is blocked at the AV junction (Fig. 28-12). The ratio of P waves to QRS complexes may vary from 2:1, 3:2, to as high as 8:7, or rarely larger. The number of complexes in each cycle may vary as well. This type of 2° block may be the result of intrinsic disease of the AV node or His bundle, but also may be seen with increased vagal tone. It may also occur in normal hearts at rapid rates. Generally, no symptoms are produced, and no specific treatment is indicated. Any underlying etiology should be treated as necessary.

When P waves are blocked intermittently and conducted cycles show a normal and/or nonvarying PR interval, the pattern is referred to as Mobitz type II, 2°

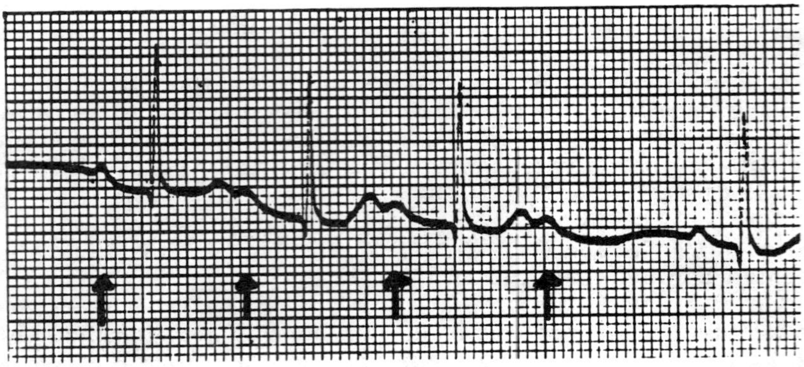

Figure 28–12 Mobitz type I, 2° AV block (Wenckebach). Arrows indicate P waves. Note the progressive prolongation of the PR interval. The fourth P wave is blocked at the AV junction and does not reach the ventricles terminating the cycle.

block (Fig. 28–13). This type of block generally indicates the presence of a significant intrinsic abnormality of the conduction system. Two or more P waves may be seen for each QRS complex, and the pattern may be regular or quite variable. If a 2:1 block is present, the QRS complex is usually normal in configuration, and the block is most often in the AV node or His bundle. When higher grades of block occur (4:1 or greater), the QRS complex is often widened and, under these circumstances, diffuse disease of the distal His bundle and/or bundle branches is generally present. This carries a more ominous prognosis, and symptoms of fatigue and/or syncope may occur, necessitating insertion of an artificial pacemaker.

Third-Degree (3°) AV Block

Third-degree or complete heart block is present when there is failure of the depolarization wave to reach the ventricles at any time. The EKG shows total independence of P waves and QRS complexes with the atrial rate faster than the ventricular, in contrast to AV dissociation (q.v.). If the escape pacemaker driving the ventricles is in the AV junction, the QRS complex is normal; if located distal to the bifurcation of the His bundle, the QRS is generally widened. The RR interval is usually regular, reflecting the lack of ventricular capture by impulses conducted from the atria.

In children 3° block is usually of congenital origin, or occurs following open heart surgery. In the former, the block is generally in the atrioventricular node, and a junctional escape pacemaker is present (Fig. 28–14). The QRS complex is

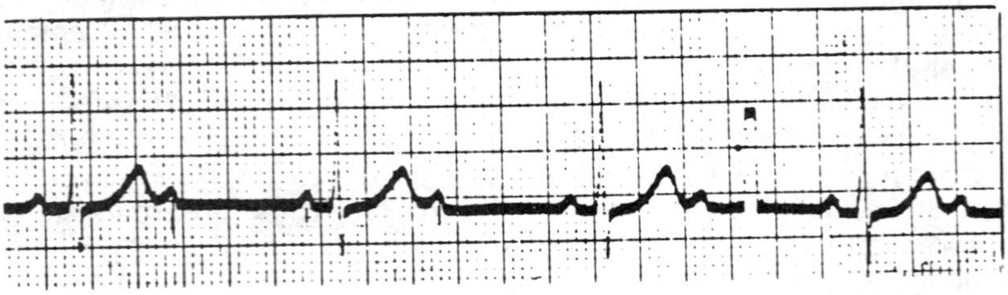

Figure 28–13 Mobitz type II, 2° AV block. Illustrated is a 2:1 block showing the typical regular relationship between P waves and QRS complex. Normal intraventricular conduction present.

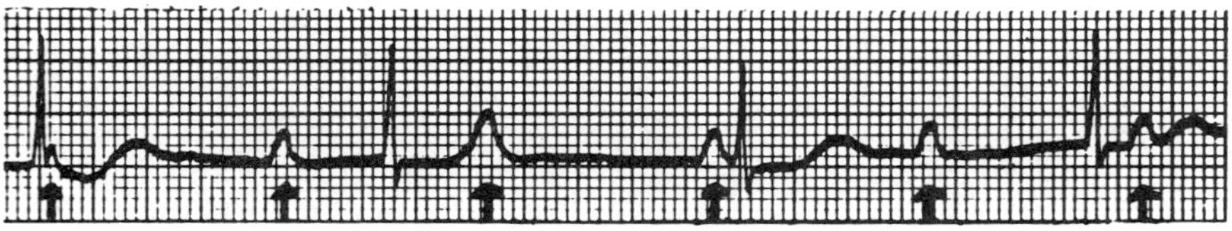

Figure 28-14 Atrioventricular block, 3° (complete). Arrows indicate P waves which bear no constant relationship to the QRS complexes, indicating that none are conducted to the ventricles. QRS complex shows normal duration and configuration consistent with a secondary pacemaker located in the atrioventricular junction.

normal, and the ventricular rate is usually 45-70/min, showing small variations with exercise. Complete heart block has been detected in utero and may occur as an isolated phenomenon or in the presence of congenital heart disease. The ventricular rate in a newborn may be as fast as 60-80/min, especially if the heart is otherwise normal. Although the ventricular rate may slow somewhat with age, prognosis is generally good, and many patients lead relatively normal lives with little or no exercise limitation and require no treatment. An occasional infant with or without congenital heart disease will demonstrate a severely reduced ventricular rate and congestive heart failure. Implantation of a pacemaker is then required, as in older patients who experience extreme fatigue or syncope. When 3° block is the result of open heart surgery, or in the adult with acquired block, there is usually diffuse disease involving the His bundle or bundle branches. The lower pacemaker is usually in the Purkinje network, and ventricular rate is less than 45/min with prolonged QRS complex. Symptoms of fatigue, syncope, or sudden death are common, and pacemaker implantation is often required.

Abnormalities of Conduction in the Bundle Branches

The EKG criteria for the diagnosis of conduction defects involving the bundle branch system have been discussed in detail in Chap. 2. Blocks involving the right bundle branch or the anterior fibers of the left bundle branch may be congenital, either occurring by themselves or related to certain congenital heart defects. They may also be the result of surgical trauma; virtually all cases of block of the entire left bundle (complete left bundle branch block) in children are the result of surgery. Regardless of the etiology, right bundle branch block by itself does not appear to cause any severe impairment of ventricular function. Neither does left bundle branch block, whether complete or fascicular.

In the postsurgical patient there is significantly greater concern when a pattern of combined bundle branch block (e.g., right bundle branch block and left anterior fascicular block) develops. If the right bundle branch block is the result of damage to the proximal right bundle and not due to division of the moderator band or extensive division of Purkinje fibers related to the ventriculotomy, the implication is that of major conduction system damage, with increased likelihood of progression to complete heart block or sudden death. These patients may require a pacemaker. Identification of the site of damage to the right bundle is generally not feasible without intracardiac electrophysiologic studies, although those of greatest risk are the patients who have had a brief period of complete (3°) AV block in the immediate postoperative period with subsequent return to normal sinus rhythm.

Bibliography

Bellet S: Clinical Disorders of the Heart Beat, 3rd ed., Lea and Febiger, Philadelphia, 1971.

Fisch C: Complex Electrocardiography, F. A. Davis Co., Philadelphia, 1973.

Garson A Jr, Gillette PC: Electrophysiologic studies of supraventricular tachycardia in children. I. Clinical-electrophysiologic correlation. Am Heart J 102:233, 1981.

Garson A Jr, Gillette PC: Electrophysiologic studies of supraventricular tachycardia in children. II. Prediction of specific mechanism by noninvasive features. Am Heart J 102:383, 1981.

Nadas AS, Fyler DC: Pediatric Cardiology, W. B. Saunders Co., Philadelphia, 1972, pp. 191-216.

Narula OA: His Bundle Electrocardiography and Clinical Electrophysiology, F. A. Davis Co., Philadelphia, 1975.

Part V

THERAPEUTIC

PRINCIPLES

Chapter 29

MEDICAL TREATMENT

Throughout this text the major therapeutic emphasis has been on surgical palliation or correction of congenital defects. Several problems do exist, however, where nonsurgical therapy is the primary or the sole modality employed. Treatment of arrhythmias and hypoxic spells have been discussed in previous chapters; the doses of antiarrhythmic agents commonly employed in pediatrics is listed in Table 29-1.

Congestive Heart Failure

The most common situation requiring definitive treatment in pediatric cardiac patients is that of congestive heart failure. The clinical manifestations are covered in Chap. 1 and the pathophysiology briefly discussed in Chap. 3. Treatment of failure can be logically based on an understanding of the abnormal mechanisms involved.

General Therapeutic Measures

Respiratory distress is the symptom most distressing to the patient; significant symptomatic relief may be achieved by placing him in the semisitting position. Infants may be placed in any one of a variety of the commercially available seating devices. If there is significant fluid accumulation, restriction of fluid intake is of value, at least during the initial period of treatment. Restriction does not have to be severe and, only rarely, continued for more than a day or two. Oral intake is usually temporarily withheld in infants, as vomiting is commonly present. If arterial hypoxemia is the result of pulmonary edema, administration of oxygen during the initial treatment phase may make the patient more comfortable until other modalities have achieved their desired effect. Marked sodium restriction is rarely needed, either acutely or chronically. Avoidance of added salt and a few selective foods, such as potato chips, is usually all that is necessary. Infants are routinely placed on a formula containing 6-7 mEq/L of sodium rather than the more conventional preparations which contain twice the amount. Utilization of a commercially available formula containing 1 mEq/L of sodium is probably unnecessary. This product is significantly more expensive and less palatable than preparations with a slightly higher salt content.

Table 29-1 Drug Dosages

Drug	Route	Initial	Maintenance	Toxicity	Comments
Digitalis					
Digoxin	p.o.	Premature: 0.03 mg/kg Full-term: 0.04 mg/kg Infants up to 2 years: 0.06-0.08 mg/kg Children over 2 years: 0.04-0.06 mg/kg	25-30% of initial dose daily in two divided doses	Nausea, vomiting, arrhythmias	See text for details regarding administration
	IV	2/3-3/4 of oral	Same as above		
Diuretics					
Furosemide	IV or IM	0.5-2.0 mg/kg		Nausea, vomiting, electrolyte depletion; hearing loss	Agent of choice in pulmonary edema because of rapid action
	p.o.	0.5-1.0 mg/kg/day		-	-
Chlorothiazide	p.o.	20-40 mg/kg/day in two doses	-	Potassium depletion, hyponatremia	Potassium supplementation essential unless spironolactone or triamterene given concurrently
Hydrochlorothiazide	p.o.	2-4 mg/kg/day	-	Same as above	Same as above
Spironolactone	p.o.	1.5-3.0 mg/kg/day in two to three doses	-	Hyperkalemia, hyponatremia	Most effective in combination with chlorthiazide or furosemide, maximal effect may take 3-5 days
Triamterene	p.o.	2-4 mg/kg/day	-	Nausea, vomiting, potassium retention	Same as above

Antiarrhythmics					
Quinidine	p.o.	15-60 mg/kg/day of quinidine base divided into three or four doses	-	Nausea, vomiting, tinnitus, intraventricular conduction defects	Quinidine sulfate is 80% quinidine base by weight; gluconate is 60%; for prevention of recurrent tachyarrhythmias
Procainamide	p.o.	15-50 mg/kg/day		Hypotension, ventricular arrhythmias; Lupuslike syndrome	Same as above
	IV	2-6 mg/kg over 5 min, maximum 500 mg	20-80 µg/kg/min		
Propranolol	IV	0.01-0.05 mg/kg every 10 min	Repeat every 6-8 min if needed	Myocardial depression; heart block	For conversion of tachyarrhythmias in digitalis toxicity and for hypoxic spells in cyanotic CHD; use with extreme caution if congestive failure present
	p.o.	0.5-2.0 mg/kg/day in three to four divided doses	-	Same as above	For prevention of recurrent arrhythmias; in obstructive cardiomyopathy
Lidocaine	IV	0.5-1.0 mg/kg	Repeat every 20-60 min as needed	Myocardial depression, hypotension, heart block, prolonged QT	Effective in converting ventricular tachycardia, less so for supraventricular; EKG monitoring essential; use only cardiac preparation
	IV	20-50 µg/kg/min every 4-6 hr	-	Same as above	As continuous infusion in recurrent life-threatening arrhythmias; use with extreme caution
Verapamil	IV	0-1 year: 0.1-0.2 mg/kg 1-15 year: 0.1-0.3 mg/kg over 2 min	Repeat in 30 min if needed	Myocardial depression, hypotension, and bradycardia	Do not exceed 5 mg; should not use if beta-blocking agents have been given (especially IV) within 12-48 hr
Atropine	IV	0.01-0.03 mg/kg every 4-6 hr	-	Dry mouth, blurred vision, hyperpyrexia, hallucinations	For acceleration of sinus rate; of benefit in digitalis toxicity

Table 29-1 (continued)

Drug	Route	Initial	Maintenance	Toxicity	Comments
Edrophonium	IV	0.1-0.2 mg/kg (max. dose; 10 mg)	-	Nausea, vomiting, perspiration, abdominal cramps	Beneficial in conversion of supraventricular tachycardias
Phenytoin	IV	a. 3-5 mg/kg over 5 min	-	Myocardial depression, hypotension	Primarily useful in digitalis toxicity; ventricular tachycardias
		b. 15 mg/kg over 1 hr			Loading dose for serious ventricular ectopy; start oral at the same time
	p.o.	3-5 mg/kg/day in two to three doses	-	Ataxia, gingival hyperplasia, hematologic effects	Same as above
Inotropic Agents					
Calcium gluconate	IV	30 mg/kg	Repeat every 30-60 min p.r.n.	Bradycardia, cardiac arrest, slough if given subcutaneously	For improvement of myocardial contractility, especially with ineffective output following cardiac arrest
Calcium chloride	IV	Infants: 0.5-1.0 cc of 10% solution Children: 1-4 cc of 10% solution Not over 1-2 cc/min	Same as previously shown	Same as previously shown	Same as previously shown; use with extreme caution
Isoproterenol	IV	1 mg in 250 cc 5% glucose (4.0 μg/cc) start infusion at 0.25 μg/kg/min and increase slowly to desired effect	-	Ventricular excitability	Accelerates rate and improves myocardial contractility; some peripheral vasodilatation; volume must be maintained

Epinephrine	IV	1.25 mg in 250 cc (5.0 µg/cc), 0.25-1.0 µg/kg/min	-	Tachycardia, hypertension	Improve myocardial contractility; rate acceleration
		Arrest: 0.1 cc/kg of 1:10,000 solution slowly		-	May initiate electrical activity in a systole; do not give intracardiac if vein is accessible
Dopamine	IV	Dilute one amp. (5.0 cc) in 500 cc 5% dextrose, final conc. 400 µg/cc.	-	Ectopic beats, nausea, vomiting, tachycardia	Maintain blood volume; peripheral vasoconstriction may occur with larger doses
		Start infusion at 2-5 µg/kg/min, increase stepwise to max. of 20-50 µg/kg/min as necessary	-		
Vasopressors					
Phenylephrine	IV	5-10 µg/kg, continuous infusion: 10 mg in 250 cc-5% glucose (40 µg/cc): may increase to 50 mg/250 cc	-	Hypertension, bradycardia, ventricular arrhythmia	For conversion of supraventricular tachycardia, continuous infusion preferable to produce elevation of BP; also for hypoxic spells
Metaraminol	IV	15-100 mg in 500 cc-5% glucose as continuous infusion	-	Same as above	Same as above
Miscellaneous					
Sodium bicarbonate	IV	1 mEq/kg	-	Hypertonicity CNS bleeding in newborns, alkalosis	Correction of acidosis in cardiac arrest, severe hypoxemia, hypoxic spells

Table 29-1 (continued)

Drug	Route	Initial	Maintenance	Toxicity	Comments
Sodium nitroprusside	IV	0.5-10.0 μg/kg/min continuous infusion	-	Hypotension, metabolic acidosis, cyanide poisoning	For peripheral vasodilatation in hypertensive crises or to reduce left ventricular afterload
Prazosin	p.o.	25 μg/kg every 6 hr	-	Hypotension	Same as above
Hydralazine	p.o.	Start with 2 mg/kg/day; may increase two to five times over 4 weeks	-	Hypotension, tachycardia, lupuslike syndrome	Same as above

Digitalis

When the underlying basis of congestive failure is diminished myocardial contractility, agents exerting a positive inotropic effect are essential to the therapeutic plan. Digitalis is the main stay of this approach and, of the various forms available, digoxin is the one employed in most pediatric centers because of its relatively rapid onset of action, fairly rapid elimination, and the ease of administration.

In treating a pediatric patient with congestive failure, a loading or "total digitalizing" dose is usually employed to elevate body stores of the drug to a desired level within a relatively short period of time (i.e., usually 18-24 hr). This loading can be achieved more rapidly if the severity of the clinical state warrants but there is greater risk of toxicity. Doses employed are listed in Table 29-1. The drug may be administered orally in mild congestive failure, but in more severe decompensation, absorption from the gastrointestinal tract may be delayed or erratic so that the intravenous route is preferred. Intramuscular administration offers no benefit, as blood flow to large muscle groups may be decreased and absorption variable. The drug is also irritating and may produce muscular fibrosis if given for more than a very short period of time by this route. Most frequently in our institution we follow the practice of administering one-half of the calculated total digitalizing dose initially, followed by one-fourth 12 hr later, and a final one-fourth 24 hr after the initial dose. There is no particular benefit to this approach over fractionating the total digitalizing dose into fourths, thirds, and so forth. Our house staff officers are instructed to write each dose in both milligrams and cubic centimeters to minimize the chance of error in administration and to not write orders for more than three-fourths of loading dose, initially. An electrocardiographic rhythm strip is obtained prior to ordering the final quarter and compared to a predigitalization tracing. If there is no marked change in the PR interval and no arrhythmias, the final dose is ordered; otherwise, a more cautious approach is taken. Once total loading is accomplished a smaller maintenance dose is given daily to replace urinary losses and maintain body stores nearly constant. The total daily maintenance dose is usually 20-30% of the loading dose divided in half and given every 12 hr to minimize fluctuations in serum and tissue levels.

Diuretics

In the presence of pulmonary edema or significant systemic venous reservoir overexpansion, diuretics are used to mobilize this fluid and promote renal excretion. Significant symptomatic improvement may occur well in advance of the maximum digitalis effect. Parenteral administration is generally preferred in treatment of acute failure in infants or whenever the decompensation is severe. Furosemide has largely replaced the mercurial diuretics because of its rapid action and effectiveness (see Table 29-1). When chronic failure is not adequately controlled by digoxin alone, oral diuretics are administered concomitantly. We prefer a thiazide diuretic for this purpose or, alternatively, furosemide in more severe cases. Supplemental potassium must be given to prevent hypokalemia; a dose of 1-2 mEq/kg/24 hours usually suffices. If the response is not satisfactory, the addition of spironolactone to the regimen may be effective, although this agent is generally much less efficacious if used alone. If a thiazide diuretic and spironolactone are used in combination, potassium supplementation is not necessary, as spironolactone is a potassium-sparing agent (which may produce hyperkalemia if used by itself). Triamterene is an effective alternative potassium-sparing diuretic.

Other Therapeutic Agents

In selective cases, myocardial decompensation may be so profound as to be unresponsive to the above approaches, and additional positive inotropic agents may be required to maintain cardiac output. In the pediatric patient, this situation occurs most often following open heart surgery. Careful intravenous infusion of isoproterenol or dopamine may be lifesaving under these circumstances but is generally necessary for only a few days. At any given level of myocardial contractility, the effective cardiac output will vary inversely with the ventricular afterload (see Chap. 4). Consequently, recent approaches to this problem have been directed at afterload reduction which may be achieved mechanically or pharmacologically. In postoperative or coronary care situations, balloon counterpulsation has been very effective in improving cardiac output. A catheter with an elongated balloon is inserted into the femoral artery and passed to the descending aorta. Synchronized with the electrocardiographic signal this unit inflates the balloon during each diastolic period, aiding maintenance of peripheral and coronary flow; collapse during systole aids ventricular emptying. Balloon catheters of a proper size for use in children are not currently available. Peripheral vasodilatation, if not excessive, will unload the left ventricle as well. In the in-hospital situation this may be achieved through the use of intravenous nitropusside or isoproterenol; chronic ventricular unloading on an outpatient basis has been of value in some conditions (e.g., mitral regurgitation or cardiomyopathy), using a variety of arterial and/or venodilating agents. Prazosin or Hydralazine (Table 29-1) have had the greatest utilization in children. Whenever feasible, initiation of chronic ventricular unloading therapy should be based on the response to the intravenous administration of drugs in this class as judged by measurement of arterial pressure, ventricular filling pressure and cardiac output.

The effectiveness of any treatment regimen for congestive failure depends on the nature of the underlying cause and the severity of the myocardial insult. Not uncommonly with congenital heart defects, the workload imposed by the structural abnormality is sufficiently excessive that, even with the measures outlined above, adequate myocardial function is not achieved and the patient remains symptomatic. Under these circumstances some type of palliative or corrective surgical intervention is required. It is of extreme importance to be aware that the clinical manifestations of congestive failure may be produced by conditions in which myocardial contractility is not impaired. Examples of this would include any form of severe pulmonary venous obstruction such as may be present in some patients with total anomalous pulmonary venous drainage or mitral stenosis or peripheral edema and hepatomegaly, resulting from interference with right ventricular filling, as with tricuspid stenosis or constrictive pericarditis. In these conditions the problem is one of mechanical obstruction to ventricular filling, and digitalis or other agents designed to improve myocardial contractility are of little benefit. An exception to this last statement exists in those patients whose venous obstruction is complicated by a tachyarrhythmia (e.g., atrial fibrillation). Under these circumstances digitalis is of value in slowing the ventricular rate and allowing more time for filling. The medical therapy of patients with pulmonary or systemic edema secondary to venous obstruction would logically be directed primarily toward the use of diuretics.

Digitalis Toxicity

Although all therapeutic agents employed have toxic side-effects, digitalis toxicity is of particular importance because of its frequency and potentially lethal results. As the more purified form of cardiac glycosides have become available, the incidence of gastrointestinal or visual side-effects commonly seen with the use of digitalis leaf have become much less frequent. Conversely, there is a much narrower margin of safety between therapeutic effectiveness and potentially life-threatening side-effects. This is a not uncommon problem in children, occurring in as many as one-third of patients in some series. Toxic manifestations are most frequently noted during the initial loading phase and are more likely to occur in newborn infants, especially premature. This age predilection may be the result of reduced renal function with consequent higher serum and, therefore, higher tissue levels of the drug. Certain cardiac abnormalities such as myocardial inflammation or ischemia may render the heart more susceptible to the toxic side effects. Hypokalemia and hypercalcemia are other frequent predisposing factors.

The ability to measure serum levels of digoxin has increased immeasurably the understanding of the pharmacokinetics of this drug and factors involved in toxicity. Available in most centers, this assay is easy to obtain and is generally performed by radioimmunoassay technique. Small quantities of serum are required, making it applicable to even the smallest prematures. A blood sample for assay is drawn 5-9 hr following the last oral dose of the drug (plateau phase level) or immediately prior to the next dose (trough level). If repeated levels are obtained on the same patient, they should all be drawn at the same time relative to the preceding dose, otherwise comparison is difficult. Several series have demonstrated higher serum level in infants and small children than are seen in adults, presumably related to the larger doses employed in younger age groups. The reason why higher doses appear to be necessary in infants is not clear, as pharmacokinetic studies of the rate of tissue binding and elimination of the drug show no significant differences when compared to adults.

The toxic manifestations of concern are a variety of arrhythmias and conduction defects. Some of the electrocardiographic manifestations in digitalized patients are seen at normal serum levels, and are more properly classified as digitalis "effect," rather than toxicity. Thus, shortening of the QT interval and sagging of the ST segment are indications of the presence of the drug and are of no real concern. Some prolongation of the PR interval is not uncommon and appears to be secondary to the vagal effect of the drug. Even a first-degree atrioventricular block is not felt by most to be a manifestation of toxicity. Significant lengthening of the interval should, however, serve as a warning to the physician to proceed with some caution. As mentioned in Chap. 28, ventricular ectopic beats or ventricular tachyarrhythmias appear to be significantly less common in children than adults. We have far more frequently noted the occurrence of atrioventricular dissociation in toxic patients. More severe degrees of atrioventricular block, sinus node dysfunction, and supraventricular tachyarrhythmias have been reported.

Any patient receiving digitalis who manifests the appearance of an arrhythmia should be regarded as toxic until proven otherwise. The drug should be withheld and the serum level drawn immediately. Although there is a large range of overlap between the serum levels of toxic and nontoxic patients, levels of greater than 3.5 mg/ml in infants constitute presumptive evidence of toxicity. Toxic arrhythmias may occur at lower levels, however, in the presence of predisposing conditions, as previously discussed. Atropine is an extremely effective agent in counteracting the vagal-related side-effects, such as bradycardia and atrioventricular dissociation. Intravenous potassium is indicated when hypokalemia is present and may be effective in occasional patients with ventricular ectopic rhythms and normal serum potassium levels. It should not be given in the presence of atrioventricular conduction defects, as it may increase the severity of the block. Phenytoin appears to be of particular value in digitalis-induced tachyarrhythmias and exhibits much less depression of myocardial contractility than does propranolol which, although useful in treating the arrhythmias, may also worsen the congestive failure for which the digitalis was given in the first place. Lidocaine also has a place in the treatment of the ventricular tachyarrhythmias. All patients exhibiting manifestations of digitalis toxicity, as well as those who have accidentally ingested a potentially toxic dose, should be observed carefully with appropriate monitoring until the condition has stabilized.

Cyanosis

Until recently there has been no effective nonsurgical attack on hypoxemia. Cyanotic congenital heart defects which are associated with large pulmonary blood flow and good venoarterial mixing generally present with manifestations of congestive failure and relatively mild hypoxemia. More severely cyanotic infants usually have lesions characterized by a marked reduction in pulmonary blood flow, or the inability of pulmonary venous blood to reach the aorta as in transposition of the great arteries. The administration of increased concentrations of inspired oxygen to these patients is of little value when pulmonary flow is inadequate to transport it or when the pulmonary venous blood is primarily returned to pulmonary artery. Thus, treatment directed at the alleviation of hypoxemia has consisted of creation of a surgical shunt to increase pulmonary blood flow or an atrial septal defect to improve venoarterial mixing in transposition of the great arteries. This basic approach has not changed and is still the only way to achieve long-term palliation. Many of these infants are critically hypoxemic at the time of surgery and, as a result, surgical morbidity and mortality has been significant. With an increased understanding of vasoactive substances affecting the ductus arteriosus (see Chap. 4), evidence has accumulated suggesting that the E-series prostaglandins (PGE_1 and PGE_2) play a role in maintaining ductus patency in utero. Subsequent investigations have shown them to be effective in dilating the ductus in newborn infants with severe cyanotic congenital heart defects where the ductus is the primary source of pulmonary blood flow, such as in various lesions with pulmonary atresia. Continuous infusion of PGE_1 at the aortic end of the ductus or intravenously, at a rate of 0.05-0.1 µg/kg/min has uniformly produced rapid and sustained increases in arterial pO_2 (Fig. 29-1). This infusion is continued until the surgical shunt is established. In the absence of an arterial line, intravenous infusion appears to be equally effective. Dilatation of the ductus will often increase pulmonary blood flow and transposition of the great arteries and thereby improve venoarterial mixing. Another situation where dilatation of the ductus may be lifesaving is in the patient with interruption of the aortic arch or severe coarctation of the aorta; here the desired goal is improved perfusion of the lower body (especially the kidneys) rather than relief of hypoxemia.

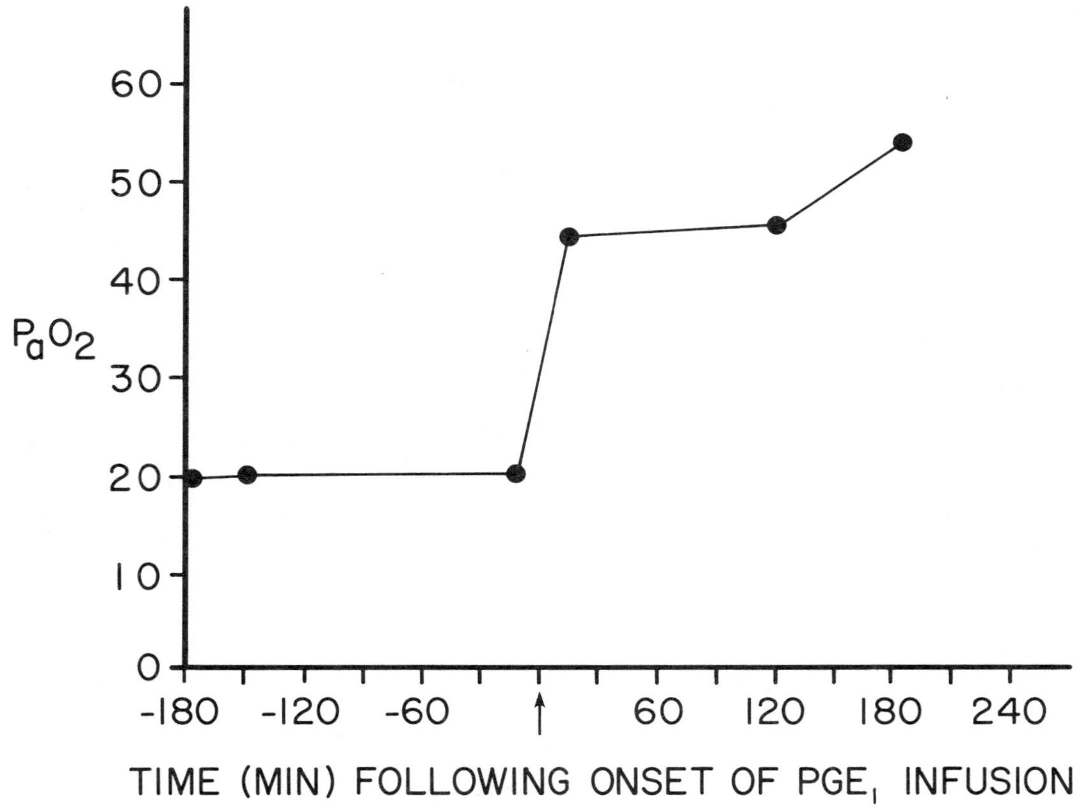

Figure 29–1 Response of arterial pO_2 following initiation of prostaglandin E_1 infusion in a newborn infant with pulmonic atresia. Infusion into the aorta at the upstream end of ductus arteriosus was begun at point marked (arrow) and was followed by a prompt rise in arterial pO_2 which was sustained for the duration of the infusion.

INDEX